Environmental and Occupational Health in Brazil

Environmental and Occupational Health in Brazil

Editors

Rejane C. Marques
José Dórea
Rafael Junqueira Buralli

MDPI • Basel • Beijing • Wuhan • Barcelona • Belgrade • Manchester • Tokyo • Cluj • Tianjin

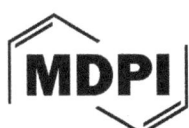

Editors

Rejane C. Marques
Graduate Program in
Environmental Sciences and
Conservation
Federal University of Rio de
Janeiro
Macaé
Brazil

José Dórea
Nutrition Department
University of Brasília
Brasília
Brazil

Rafael Junqueira Buralli
Department of Preventive
Medicine, Faculty of
Medicine
University of São Paulo
São Paulo
Brazil

Editorial Office
MDPI
St. Alban-Anlage 66
4052 Basel, Switzerland

This is a reprint of articles from the Special Issue published online in the open access journal *International Journal of Environmental Research and Public Health* (ISSN 1660-4601) (available at: www.mdpi.com/journal/ijerph/special_issues/environmental_Brazil).

For citation purposes, cite each article independently as indicated on the article page online and as indicated below:

LastName, A.A.; LastName, B.B.; LastName, C.C. Article Title. *Journal Name* **Year**, *Volume Number*, Page Range.

ISBN 978-3-0365-8407-2 (Hbk)
ISBN 978-3-0365-8406-5 (PDF)

Cover image courtesy of Rafael Junqueira Buralli

© 2023 by the authors. Articles in this book are Open Access and distributed under the Creative Commons Attribution (CC BY) license, which allows users to download, copy and build upon published articles, as long as the author and publisher are properly credited, which ensures maximum dissemination and a wider impact of our publications.
The book as a whole is distributed by MDPI under the terms and conditions of the Creative Commons license CC BY-NC-ND.

Contents

About the Editors ix

Thayssa C. S. Bello, Rafael J. Buralli, Mônica P. L. Cunha, José G. Dórea, Fredi A. Diaz-Quijano and Jean R. D. Guimarães et al.
Mercury Exposure in Women of Reproductive Age in Rondonia State, Amazon Region, Brazil
Reprinted from: *Int. J. Environ. Res. Public Health* **2023**, 20, 5225, doi:10.3390/ijerph20065225 . . . 1

Luciana Leirião, Michelle de Oliveira, Tiago Martins and Simone Miraglia
A Multi-Pollutant and Meteorological Analysis of Cardiorespiratory Mortality among the Elderly in São Paulo, Brazil—An Artificial Neural Networks Approach
Reprinted from: *Int. J. Environ. Res. Public Health* **2023**, 20, 5458, doi:10.3390/ijerph20085458 . . . 15

Neice Muller Xavier Faria, Rodrigo Dalke Meucci, Nadia Spada Fiori, Maria Laura Vidal Carret, Carlos Augusto Mello-da-Silva and Anaclaudia Gastal Fassa
Acute Pesticide Poisoning in Tobacco Farming, According to Different Criteria
Reprinted from: *Int. J. Environ. Res. Public Health* **2023**, 20, 2818, doi:10.3390/ijerph20042818 . . . 39

Gilvania Barreto Feitosa Coutinho, Maria de Fátima Ramos Moreira, Frida Marina Fischer, Maria Carolina Reis dos Santos, Lucas Ferreira Feitosa and Sayonara Vieira de Azevedo et al.
Influence of Environmental Exposure to Steel Waste on Endocrine Dysregulation and *PER3* Gene Polymorphisms
Reprinted from: *Int. J. Environ. Res. Public Health* **2023**, 20, 4760, doi:10.3390/ijerph20064760 . . . 57

Homègnon A. Ferréol Bah, Victor O. Martinez, Nathália R. dos Santos, Erival A. Gomes Junior, Daisy O. Costa and Elis Macêdo Pires et al.
Determinants of Exposure to Potentially Toxic Metals in Pregnant Women of the DSAN-12M Cohort in the Recncavo Baiano, Brazil
Reprinted from: *Int. J. Environ. Res. Public Health* **2023**, 20, 2949, doi:10.3390/ijerph20042949 . . . 79

Cristiano Barreto de Miranda, João Silvestre Silva-Junior, Klauss Kleydmann Sabino Garcia, Flávia Nogueira e Ferreira de Sousa and Frida Marina Fischer
Vocational Rehabilitation and Length of Stay at Work after Work-Related Musculoskeletal Disorders: A Longitudinal Study in Brazil
Reprinted from: *Int. J. Environ. Res. Public Health* **2023**, 20, 2334, doi:10.3390/ijerph20032334 . . . 95

Aline Souza Espindola Santos, Josino Costa Moreira, Ana Cristina Simoes Rosa, Volney Magalhães Câmara, Antonio Azeredo and Carmen Ildes Rodrigues Froes Asmus et al.
Persistent Organic Pollutant Levels in Maternal and Cord Blood Plasma and Breast Milk: Results from the Rio Birth Cohort Pilot Study of Environmental Exposure and Childhood Development (PIPA Study)
Reprinted from: *Int. J. Environ. Res. Public Health* **2022**, 20, 778, doi:10.3390/ijerph20010778 . . . 107

Michele C. Toledo, Janice S. Lee, Bruno L. Batista, Kelly P. K. Olympio and Adelaide C. Nardocci
Exposure to Inorganic Arsenic in Rice in Brazil: A Human Health Risk Assessment
Reprinted from: *Int. J. Environ. Res. Public Health* **2022**, 19, 16460, doi:10.3390/ijerph192416460 . 123

Fairah Barrozo, Gilmar Alves de Almeida, Maciel Santos Luz and Kelly Polido Kaneshiro Olympio
A Low-Cost Method Shows Potentially Toxic Element Levels in Dust Correlated with Elevated Blood Levels of These Chemicals in Children Exposed to an Informal Home-Based Production Environment
Reprinted from: *Int. J. Environ. Res. Public Health* **2022**, *19*, 16236, doi:10.3390/ijerph192316236 . **141**

Joyce Aparecida Tavares Miranda, Fabíola Helena S. Fogaça, Sara C. Cunha, Mariana Batha Alonso, João Paulo M. Torres and José Oliveira Fernandes
Agrochemical Residues in Fish and Bivalves from Sepetiba Bay and Parnaiba River Delta, Brazil
Reprinted from: *Int. J. Environ. Res. Public Health* **2022**, *19*, 15790, doi:10.3390/ijerph192315790 . **155**

Camila Vitorino dos Santos and Helena Ribeiro
Potential Transformation of Contaminated Areas into Public Parks: Evidence from São Paulo, Brazil
Reprinted from: *Int. J. Environ. Res. Public Health* **2022**, *19*, 11933, doi:10.3390/ijerph191911933 . **169**

Armando Meyer, Aline Souza Espindola Santos, Carmen Ildes Rodrigues Froes Asmus, Volney Magalhaes Camara, Antônio José Leal Costa and Dale P. Sandler et al.
Acute Kidney Failure among Brazilian Agricultural Workers: A Death-Certificate Case-Control Study
Reprinted from: *Int. J. Environ. Res. Public Health* **2022**, *19*, 6519, doi:10.3390/ijerph19116519 . . . **189**

Rogério Adas Ayres de Oliveira, Bruna Duarte Pinto, Bruno Hojo Rebouças, Daniel Ciampi de Andrade, Ana Claudia Santiago de Vasconcellos and Paulo Cesar Basta
Neurological Impacts of Chronic Methylmercury Exposure in Munduruku Indigenous Adults: Somatosensory, Motor, and Cognitive Abnormalities
Reprinted from: *Int. J. Environ. Res. Public Health* **2021**, *18*, 10270, doi:10.3390/ijerph181910270 . **201**

Joeseph William Kempton, André Reynaldo Santos Périssé, Cristina Barroso Hofer, Ana Claudia Santiago de Vasconcellos, Paulo Victor de Sousa Viana and Marcelo de Oliveira Lima et al.
An Assessment of Health Outcomes and Methylmercury Exposure in Munduruku Indigenous Women of Childbearing Age and Their Children under 2 Years Old
Reprinted from: *Int. J. Environ. Res. Public Health* **2021**, *18*, 10091, doi:10.3390/ijerph181910091 . **221**

Paulo Cesar Basta, Paulo Victor de Sousa Viana, Ana Claudia Santiago de Vasconcellos, André Reynaldo Santos Périssé, Cristina Barroso Hofer and Natalia Santana Paiva et al.
Mercury Exposure in Munduruku Indigenous Communities from Brazilian Amazon: Methodological Background and an Overview of the Principal Results
Reprinted from: *Int. J. Environ. Res. Public Health* **2021**, *18*, 9222, doi:10.3390/ijerph18179222 . . . **245**

Jesem Douglas Yamall Orellana, Giovanna Gatica-Domínguez, Juliana dos Santos Vaz, Paulo Augusto Ribeiro Neves, Ana Claudia Santiago de Vasconcellos and Sandra de Souza Hacon et al.
Intergenerational Association of Short Maternal Stature with Stunting in Yanomami Indigenous Children from the Brazilian Amazon
Reprinted from: *Int. J. Environ. Res. Public Health* **2021**, *18*, 9130, doi:10.3390/ijerph18179130 . . . **277**

Rafaela Waddington Achatz, Ana Claudia Santiago de Vasconcellos, Lucia Pereira, Paulo Victor de Sousa Viana and Paulo Cesar Basta
Impacts of the Goldmining and Chronic Methylmercury Exposure on the Good-Living and Mental Health of Munduruku Native Communities in the Amazon Basin
Reprinted from: *Int. J. Environ. Res. Public Health* **2021**, *18*, 8994, doi:10.3390/ijerph18178994 . . . **291**

Jamila Alessandra Perini, Mayara Calixto Silva, Ana Claudia Santiago de Vasconcellos, Paulo Victor Sousa Viana, Marcelo Oliveira Lima and Iracina Maura Jesus et al.
Genetic Polymorphism of Delta Aminolevulinic Acid Dehydratase (*ALAD*) Gene and Symptoms of Chronic Mercury Exposure in Munduruku Indigenous Children within the Brazilian Amazon
Reprinted from: *Int. J. Environ. Res. Public Health* **2021**, *18*, 8746, doi:10.3390/ijerph18168746 . . . **309**

Ana Claudia Santiago de Vasconcellos, Gustavo Hallwass, Jaqueline Gato Bezerra, Angélico Nonato Serrão Aciole, Heloisa Nascimento de Moura Meneses and Marcelo de Oliveira Lima et al.
Health Risk Assessment of Mercury Exposure from Fish Consumption in Munduruku Indigenous Communities in the Brazilian Amazon
Reprinted from: *Int. J. Environ. Res. Public Health* **2021**, *18*, 7940, doi:10.3390/ijerph18157940 . . . **321**

Júlia Alves Menezes, Ana Paula Madureira, Rhavena Barbosa dos Santos, Isabela de Brito Duval, Pedro Regoto and Carina Margonari et al.
Analyzing Spatial Patterns of Health Vulnerability to Drought in the Brazilian Semiarid Region
Reprinted from: *Int. J. Environ. Res. Public Health* **2021**, *18*, 6262, doi:10.3390/ijerph18126262 . . . **337**

About the Editors

Rejane C. Marques

She holds a degree in Nursing from the Federal University of Rondônia (1993), a Bachelor's degree in Nursing and Obstetrics from the Federal University of Rondônia (1993), a Master's degree in Tropical Diseases from the Federal University of Pará (2002), and a PhD in Biological Sciences (Biophysics) from the Federal University of Rio de Janeiro (2007). She was a professor at the Federal University of Rio de Janeiro-Campus Macaé (2010 to 2020), working on the Undergraduate Nursing and Midwifery course and the Graduate Program in Environmental Sciences and Conservation (PPG-CiAC). She was a professor at the Federal University of Rondônia (1997 to 2010), working on the Undergraduate Nursing course and the Graduate Program in Teaching Health Sciences. She is a Visiting Extension Scholarship holder at UFRGS (2022-2023), acting as a supervisor in the Health with Agent Project (CONASEMS/UFRGS/MS).

José Dórea

He graduated from the Federal Rural University of Pernambuco (1968) and the University of Massachusetts (USA) with an MSc (1971) and PhD (1975) in Nutritional Biochemistry. He gained teaching experience at University of Brasília (2014), alongside Professor Emeritus, and the University of Hawaii (USA) (1988) and UNICAMP (1989). He carried out extensive research in Nutrition and Ecotoxicology on the following topics: human milk, biomarkers, endocrine-active pollutants, mercury toxicology, and population health (urban and riverside in the Amazon).

Rafael Junqueira Buralli

He is a Doctor and Master of Public Health at the School of Public Health of the University of São Paulo (FSP/USP), with a sandwich doctorate at the University of California, Berkeley and the School of Public Health of the University of Chile. He is currently a post-doctoral researcher in environmental epidemiology and a FAPESP fellow at the Faculty of Medicine of the USP. He was a Technical Consultant at the Pan American Health Organization (OPS) in the General Coordination of Worker's Health Surveillance, of the Brazilian Ministry of Health (CGSAT/SVS/MS), working on various topics of health surveillance, environmental health, occupational health, and public health emergencies. He graduated in physiotherapy, gaining experience in orthopedic rehabilitation and lecturing in higher education. He was a substitute professor at the Federal University of Espírito Santo (UFES) and the University of Brasília (UnB). He is part of the Executive Committee of the Latin American and Caribbean Chapter of the International Society for Environmental Epidemiology (ISEE-LAC) and the Little Things Matter (LTM) project for scientific communication. He is a reviewer for international scientific journals and a collaborator in several research projects. He has a special interest in topics related to environmental and worker health, epidemiology, health surveillance, and scientific communication.

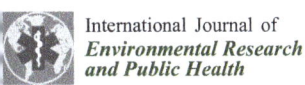

Article

Mercury Exposure in Women of Reproductive Age in Rondônia State, Amazon Region, Brazil

Thayssa C. S. Bello [1,*], Rafael J. Buralli [2], Mônica P. L. Cunha [3], José G. Dórea [4], Fredi A. Diaz-Quijano [5], Jean R. D. Guimarães [6] and Rejane C. Marques [1]

1. Programa de Pós-Graduação em Ciências Ambientais e Conservação, Universidade Federal do Rio de Janeiro (UFRJ), Macaé 27965-045, Brazil; rejanecorreamarques@gmail.com
2. Departamento de Medicina Preventiva, Faculdade de Medicina, Universidade de São Paulo (FMUSP), São Paulo 01246-903, Brazil; rafael.buralli@gmail.com
3. Programa de Pós-Graduação em Desenvolvimento Regional e Meio Ambiente, Universidade Federal de Rondônia (UNIR), Porto Velho 76801-058, Brazil; monicaplcunha@gmail.com
4. Departamento de Nutrição, Universidade de Brasília (UnB), Brasília 70970-000, Brazil; jg.dorea@gmail.com
5. Departamento de Epidemiologia, Faculdade de Saúde Pública, Universidade de São Paulo (USP), São Paulo 01246-904, Brazil; frediazq@msn.com
6. Instituto de Biofísica Carlos Chagas Filho, Universidade Federal do Rio de Janeiro (UFRJ), Rio de Janeiro 21941-170, Brazil; jeanrdg@biof.ufrj.br
* Correspondence: thayssa_bello@hotmail.com

Abstract: Environmental contamination by mercury (Hg) is a problem of global scale that affects human health. This study's aim was to evaluate Hg exposure among women of reproductive age residing in the Madeira River basin, in the State of Rondônia, Brazilian Amazon. This longitudinal cohort study used linear regression models to assess the effects on Hg levels of breastfeeding duration at 6 months, and of breastfeeding duration and number of new children at 2-year and 5-year. Breastfeeding duration was significantly associated with maternal Hg levels in all regression models (6 months, 2 years and 5 years) and no significant association was observed between the number of children and the change in maternal Hg levels in the 2-year and 5-year models. This longitudinal cohort study evaluated Hg levels and contributing factors among pregnant women from different communities (riverine, rural, mining and urban) in Rondônia, Amazon Region, for 5 years. A well-coordinated and designed national biomonitoring program is urgently needed to better understand the current situation of Hg levels in Brazil and the Amazon.

Keywords: Amazon; environmental contamination; mercury; women; breastfeeding

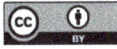

1. Introduction

Environmental contamination by mercury (Hg) is a problem of global scale that affects human health in high-income countries, such as Sweden, Canada, Japan, the United States of America and Finland [1–4], as well as in lower- and middle-income countries (LMIC), such as Brazil, China, Venezuela, Colombia and Iraq [1,5–7].

In the late 1970s, the Amazon experienced an intense gold rush, and the Madeira River was one of its most active areas, with hundreds of illegal barges excavating bottom sediment to obtain gold by amalgamation with Hg. The recent surge in gold prices in international markets provided a renewed push to the activity [8], and illegal gold mining exploded worldwide. In Brazil, this was dramatically amplified during the Bolsonaro presidency (2019–2022) that dismantled the legal framework underlying environmental surveillance activities and strongly reduced the material support to all institutions involved. The result, among so many others, is that tens of thousands of gold miners invaded indigenous territories, such as the Ianomamis in Roraima and the Mundurukus on the Tapajos River, causing irreversible socio-environmental impacts during these 4 years of total official laxism.

In addition to the Hg emissions from gold mining, the Madeira River carries an important load of natural Hg from the soil erosion of the Andes and deforested areas [9–11]. In 2017, the Minamata Convention on Mercury—an international treaty to reduce Hg use and emissions—came into force. It is the result of negotiations involving 140 countries under the United Nations Environment Programme (UNEP) [12]. To date, the Convention has 128 signatories, including Brazil [12], though the country signed the convention only a few months before the start of the Bolsonaro period. The convention aims to protect human health and the environment from anthropogenic emissions and releases of Hg and its compounds, especially vulnerable populations, women and children, and through them, the future generations [12,13].

As these groups are the most vulnerable and sensitive to possible long-term effects, there is a general recommendation that pregnant women, children and women of childbearing age should avoid exposure to Hg [14]. By modulating the endocrine system, Hg causes a decrease in luteinizing hormone (LH), estradiol, progesterone and prolactin, and an increase in menstrual disorders [15]. These hormones are essential for the maintenance of the female reproductive cycle, and a disorder can cause adverse reproductive outcomes. Given the adverse effects of Hg compounds, it is imperative to assess exposure so that early predictive effects of toxicity can be detected, especially in vulnerable populations [16].

Mercury is usually released in inorganic form and transformed by aquatic bacteria into methylmercury, a potent neurotoxin that biomagnifies along the food chain. As a result, human exposure to mercury is strongly dependent on fish intake frequency. Therefore, lifestyle and diet play an important role in Hg exposure [17]. Kirk et al. [18] found that, due to its neurotoxic potential, Hg exposure through seafood generates a cost of approximately EUR 10 billion per year for the European Union. Consumption of fish with high concentrations of Hg by pregnant women can cause serious problems in the neurological development of the offspring [19]. Dórea and Marques [20] reported that prenatal exposure to this metal may be associated with adverse effects on pregnancy, birth and child development. Lee et al. [21] showed that in late pregnancy, high levels of Hg in maternal blood are associated with an increased risk of newborns with low birth weight.

Xue et al. [22] reported an increased risk of preterm births associated with low to moderate Hg exposure. Women who gave birth before 35 weeks of pregnancy had hair Hg concentrations above the 90th percentile (greater than 0.55 $\mu g \cdot g^{-1}$) compared to women who gave birth to term babies (37 to 41 weeks and six days). Dallaire et al. [23] found a negative correlation between cord blood Hg levels and gestational age at birth.

Hg levels in hair are strongly correlated with MeHg intake in an individual's diet [20]. Therefore, the concentration of Hg in hair has been used in many studies as a bioindicator of human exposure [20,24] because it is easy to collect, store and manipulate [25,26]. In addition, its chemical stability facilitates retrospective studies [24,27]. In Brazil, many studies conducted in the Amazon region have used hair as a biomarker of Hg exposure [28–32] among different exposed populations.

Knowing the real influence of Hg exposure on women's health is a matter of great relevance to public health. The development and implementation of appropriate public policies and actions to mitigate the associated risks is fundamental. To the health sector, this context represents a challenge that forces it to constantly review the situation of environmental deterioration and its repercussions on the quality of life.

This study's aims were to evaluate Hg exposure among women of reproductive age residing in the Madeira River basin, in the State of Rondônia, Brazilian Amazon, prior to the ratification of the Minamata Convention, and to investigate possible associated factors. It is hoped that the results can serve as a baseline for evaluating the effectiveness of the implementation of the convention.

2. Materials and Methods

This longitudinal cohort study with a quantitative and analytical approach evaluated 1433 women of reproductive age who lived in the area covered by the Jamari, Madeira and

Mamoré rivers, in the Rondônia State, Brazilian Amazon. All women who were pregnant between 2006 and 2007 were invited to participate in the study. We invited 1668 pregnant mothers; 215 women dropped out within the first semester of the study and 20 during the first year. In the subsequent evaluations, there were no dropouts. All women who agreed to participate were selected according to the following criteria: healthy women during pregnancy, absence of congenital malformations, and residing for at least five years in the study area. Participants were classified as groups of interest derived from rural, urban, riverine and mining areas, according to their place of residence (community). The mining area is located in Bom Futuro, on the banks of the Jamari River, affluent of the Madeira River. It is legal mining, extracting tin from cassiterite, and its activity does not result in any direct Hg emission; it was included in the sampling because it is an important economic activity of the region. Figure 1 shows the study area, which covers more than 733 km along the Madeira River basin and tributaries.

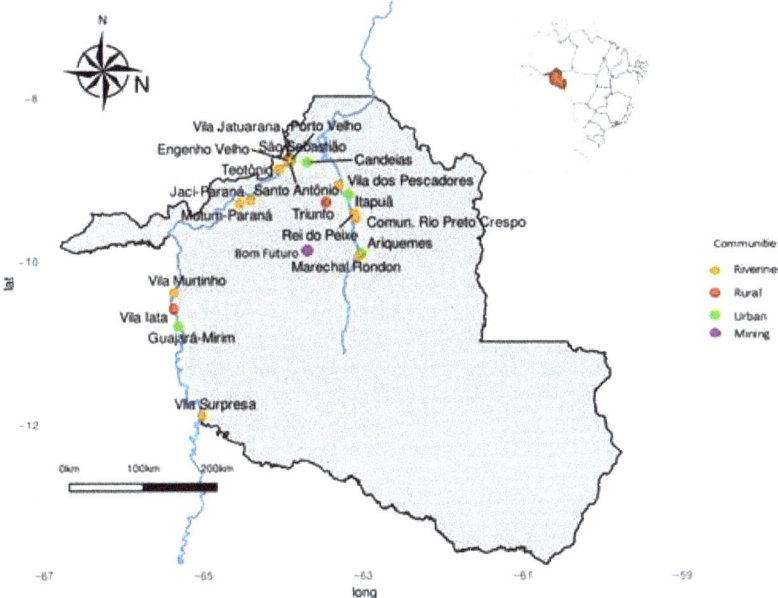

Figure 1. Study locations. Source: adapted from Marques et al. [26].

Participants' data were obtained through questionnaires after written authorization. The questionnaire contained open and closed questions in order to obtain participants' information on socio demographic data, eating habits and health status. A questionnaire was applied at the time of inclusion in the study, and a hair sample was collected from each participant. At scheduled home visits (6 months postpartum, 2 years and 5 years), a new questionnaire was applied, women were asked about their daily intake of fish and breastfeeding practices, and hair samples were collected. The study was approved by the Research Ethics Committee of the Federal University of Rondônia (REC/NUSAU/UNIR, file number: 012/CEP/NUSAU).

2.1. Determination of Total Hg Concentrations

Total Hg concentrations were checked in hair samples (five to ten grams) collected from the occipital region of the mothers, close to the scalp. Samples were placed in transparent plastic bags and properly identified, stored at room temperature and taken for analysis to the Laboratorio de Radioisotopos, Instituto de Biofisica Carlos Chagas Filho, Universidade Federal do Rio de Janeiro.

Hair samples were washed with a 0.01% EDTA solution, rinsed with ultrapure water and dried in an oven at 50 °C. Then, they were fractionated as much as possible with stainless steel scissors for better homogenization and increased efficiency of the acid digestion [33]. After being weighed, they were digested with 5 mL of HNO3 and H_2SO_4 (1:1) and 4 mL of 5% KMnO4 using a digester block at 80 °C for 40 min. Total Hg was determined by cold vapor generation atomic absorption spectrophotometry (CV-AAS) on a Perkin-Elmer® FIMS-400 apparatus (Waltham, MA, USA). The results were expressed in $\mu g \cdot g^{-1}$. Precision and accuracy of Hg determinations were assured by the use of internal standards, triplicate analyses of samples and certified reference materials (IAEA-085 and 086, Vienna, Austria) with recoveries of 92%. All glassware used was washed clean, rinsed with 5% (w/v) EDTA and double distilled water and left to rest in 5% (w/v) HNO_3 overnight. Before use, it was rinsed again in double-distilled water and dried at 100 °C for 12 h.

2.2. Statistical Analysis

Differences between groups of interest (rural, urban, riverine and mining) were analyzed. The following variables were considered: maternal age; number of children in each period; years of education; family income; number of cohabitants; type of residence (wood, brick, mixed, straw); household situation (owned, rented, from relatives, borrowed); water supply (piped, well, river, piped/well, public tap, piped/river); energy supply (yes/no); gestational period (in weeks); breastfeeding duration (in months); place of delivery (hospital, residence); type of delivery (normal, cesarean); newborn's sex (female, male); fetal maturity (pre-term, term, post-term); number of children (prenatal, 2 years, 5 years); maternal fish consumption (days per week), and levels of total Hg.

The analyses were performed with software R® (RStudio, Version 1.2.5001, 2019, Boston, MA, USA), and Stata 12 (StataCorp, 2011, College Station, TX, USA). Shapiro–Wilk test was used to verify data distribution. Since data did not present a normal distribution, non-parametric procedures were used. Participants' characteristics and differences between groups of interest were presented as median, minimum, maximum and percentiles (P25–P75%). Correlations between Hg levels and exposure variables (number of children, breastfeeding duration and fish consumption) were performed using the Kendall test to assess the degree of association between them.

Based on a DAG model (Figure 2), two versions were established to guide the model adjustments for covariates: (a) Hg levels at 6 months (outcome), considering that the '*number of children*' had minimal variability and, therefore, was naturally adjusted; (b) 2 years and 5 years, in which the variable '*number of children*' was included as an independent variable (births in the period). The DAG's (Figure 2) testable independence implications were evaluated using linear regression models and were not rejected ($p > 0.05$ for all tests), which was interpreted as an indicator of consistency between data and DAG [34].

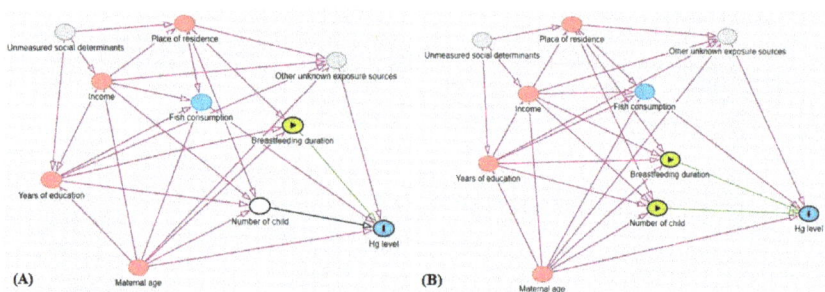

Figure 2. DAG models: (**A**) 6-month period, including only breastfeeding duration as independent variable; (**B**) 2 years and 5 years period, including number of children and breastfeeding duration as independent variables.

Linear regression models of Hg levels in each period (in $\mu g \cdot g^{-1}$) on breastfeeding duration at 6 months, and on breastfeeding duration and number of new children at the 2 and 5 years follow-up were performed, adjusting for family income, years of education, maternal age and place of residence (groups of interest). In the 2 years and 5 years models, when the total number of children was equal to or less than that reported at the beginning of the study, an increment value of zero children was allocated assuming reduced breastfeeding possibility. This happened only in 18 (1.26%) and 11 participants (0.77%), in 2 years and 5 years analyses, respectively. A term of interaction between *'number of new children'* (final-initial) and *'breastfeeding duration'* obtained by multiplying those variables, was tested in the multiple model but was not significant. Thus, this interaction was not considered in the final model.

3. Results

Participants' age ranged from 13 to 43 years (median 21 years), and 267 participants (18.6%) were aged less than 18 years. Mean family income was BRL 651.19 per month, which is about USD 130. The national monthly minimum wage was BRL 380 in Brazil when the participants' socioeconomic data were collected for the study (2007). Participants almost doubled their number of children in 5 years. Median number of children was two per woman at the beginning of the study, and four per woman after five years of follow-up (Table 1). Median education was 5 years of study, ranging from 0 to 17 years. Median number of residents per household was six individuals, ranging from 2 to 16 cohabitants. Most participants owned their houses (54.57%), which were mostly made of wood (63.64%), had well water (48.88%) or river water (20.46%). Most participants had electricity (71.24%) (Table 1).

Table 1. Socioeconomic and demographic characteristics of studied women (n = 1433), Rondônia State, Brazilian Amazon.

Variables	Median (Min–Max)	P25–P75%
Age (in years)	21 (13–43)	18–26
Number of child (at enrolment)	2 (0–12)	1–3
Number of child (at 2 y follow-up)	3 (1–13)	2–4
Number of child (at 5 y follow-up)	4 (1–13)	3–5
Years of education	5 (0–17)	4–8
Family income (BRL)	560 (50–4500)	400–800
Number of cohabitants	6 (2–16)	4–8
Type of residence	n	%
Wood	912	63.64
Brick	263	18.35
Mixed	230	16.05
Straw	28	1.95
Household situation		
Owned	782	54.57
Rented	207	14.45
From relatives	280	19.53
Borrowed	164	11.44
Water supply		
Piped	273	19.06
Well	700	48.88
River	293	20.46
Piped/well	146	10.19
Public tap	14	0.97
Piped/river	6	0.42
Energy supply		
Yes	1021	71.24
No	412	28.76
Fish consumption		
Yes	1342	93.64
No	91	6.36

Notes: Min = minimum; Max = maximum; P25–75% = 25th and 75th percentile; y = years; n = number

Participants delivered at 39.09 weeks of pregnancy (median), that is, 90.09% at normal fetal maturity (37 to 42 weeks). Birth environment was hospital for most participants (74.80%), with 58.47% of women having normal delivery (Table 2). Regarding the newborns' sex, 50.52% were girls and 49.48% boys (Table 2). Considering all groups, breastfeeding duration ranged from 0 to 24 months (median 6 months), and was longer among riverine and rural communities (median 6 months), and shorter among the tin mining community (Tables 2 and 3). Riverine and rural groups had the highest number of children at all assessed time periods (Table 3). About 93.64% of participants reported fish consumption, with the highest rates among riverine communities (median 5 days per week) (Table 1), followed by rural (median 3 days per week). Lower fish consumption was observed among mining and urban communities (Table 3).

Table 2. Birth and duration of breastfeeding characteristics of studied women (n = 1433), Rondônia State, Brazilian Amazon.

Variables	Median (Min–Max)	P25–P75%
Gestation period (in weeks)	39 (32–43)	38–40
Breastfeeding duration (in months)	6 (0–24)	3–9
Place of delivery	n	%
Hospital	1072	74.80
Residence	361	25.19
Type of delivery		
Normal	838	58.47
Cesarean	595	41.53
Newborn sex		
Female	724	50.52
Male	709	49.48
Fetal maturity		
Preterm	84	5.86
Term	1291	90.09
Post-term	58	4.04

Notes: Min = minimum; Max = maximum; P25–75% = 25th and 75th percentile.

Table 3. Number of children, breastfeeding duration, total Hg levels (in $\mu g \cdot g^{-1}$), fish consumption frequency, according to place of residence of studied women (n = 1433), Rondônia State, Brazilian Amazon.

Variables	Tin Mining (n = 294)		Riverine (n = 396)		Rural (n = 67)		Urban (n = 676)	
	Median (Min–Max)	P25–P75%	Median (Min–Max)	P25–P75%	Median (Min–Max)	P25–P75%	Median (Min–Max)	P25–P75%
Number of children								
Prenatal	2 (0–5)	1–2	2 (0–12)	1–3	2 (0–10)	1–3	2 (0–8)	1–3
After 2 y	3 (1–7)	2–4	3 (1–13)	2–4	3 (1–11)	2–4	3 (1–9)	2–4
After 5 y	3 (1–7)	3–4	4 (2–13)	3–5	4 (2–11)	3–5	4 (1–10)	3–5
Breastfeeding duration (in months)	5 (1–24)	3–7	6 (0–24)	5–11	6 (1–24)	4–10	5 (0–24)	2–10
Hg ($\mu g \cdot g^{-1}$)								
Prenatal	4.45 (1.53–11.94)	3.4–5.51	12.11 (1.02–130.72)	7.22–18.09	7.82 (2.56–41.10)	6.23–9.89	5.36 (0.22–24.14)	3.84–6.84
After 6 months	3.07 (0.88–9.66)	2.33–4.12	11.33 (0.70–125.21)	6.83–17.33	7.09 (2.64–41.75)	5.91–9.15	4.66 (0.50–19.59)	3.47–6.11
After 2 y	3.92 (1.04–9.14)	3.20–4.94	11.50 (0.87–129.15)	6.49–17.76	7.73 (1.91–42.34)	5.70–9.46	5.28 (0.49–29.72)	3.85–6.94
After 5 y	3.75 (0.68–9.88)	3.13–4.95	12.22 (0.56–146.87)	8.10–18.98	7.34 (1.53–44.86)	5.14–9.88	5.36 (0.55–15.84)	3.76–7.50
Fish consumption (days per week)	1 (0–2)	1–2	5 (0–7)	3–7	3 (1–7)	2–5	2 (0–7)	1–3

Notes: Min = minimum; Max = maximum; P25–75% = 25th and 75th percentile; y = years; n = number.

In general, higher Hg levels were found among riverine, followed by rural communities, while lower concentrations were observed among mining communities (Table 3).

In the correlation analysis, fish consumption was significantly related to Hg levels in all groups throughout all assessed periods, except in the tin mining community, where fish consumption is the lowest (Table 4). On the other hand, breastfeeding duration was significantly associated with maternal Hg levels in all regression models (6 months, 2 years and 5 years), after adjusting for family income, years of education, maternal age and place of residence (groups of interest). Each month of breastfeeding was associated with a Hg decrease of 0.053 µg·g^{-1} for the 6-month period, 0.037 µg·g^{-1} for the 2 y period and 0.053 µg·g^{-1} for the 5 years period. No significant association was observed between the number of children and the change of maternal Hg levels in the 2 years and 5 years models (Table 5).

Table 4. Correlation between Total Hg levels (in µg·g^{-1}) and number of children, breastfeeding duration and fish consumption in the prenatal period, after 6 months, 2 and 5 years of studied women (n = 1433), according to the place of residence, Rondônia State, Brazilian Amazon.

Variables	Mining (n = 294)	Riverine (n = 396)	Rural (n = 67)	Urban (n = 676)
	(tau) p-Value	*(tau) p-Value*	*(tau) p-Value*	*(tau) p-Value*
** Number of children and Hg levels prenatal	(0.041) 0.337	(0.046) 0.202	(−0.020) 0.821	(0.004) 0.864
Number of children and Hg levels at 2 y	(−0.028) 0.513	(0.056) 0.121	(−0.052) 0.561	(−0.020) 0.476
Number of children and Hg levels at 5 y	(−0.063) 0.142	(0.060) 0.099	(−0.007) 0.933	(0.002) 0.941
Breastfeeding duration and Hg levels prenatal	(0.045) 0.268	(0.077) **0.028 ***	(0.152) 0.081	(0.042) 0.109
Breastfeeding duration and Hg levels at 6 m	(−0.007) 0.848	(0.073) **0.037 ***	(0.080) 0.325	(−0.002) 0.927
Breastfeeding duration and Hg levels at 2 y	(0.009) 0.812	(0.021) 0.548	(0.133) 0.127	(0.028) 0.281
Breastfeeding duration and Hg levels at 5 y	(−0.005) 0.891	(−0.013) 0.713	(0.064) 0.460	(−0.002) 0.940
Fish consumption and Hg levels prenatal	(0.024) 0.596	(0.663) **<0.001 ***	(0.418) **<0.001 ***	(0.541) **<0.001 ***
Fish consumption and Hg levels at 6 months	(0.025) 0.590	(0.676) **<0.001 ***	(0.455) **<0.001 ***	(0.495) **<0.001 ***
Fish consumption and Hg levels at 2 y	(0.002) 0.960	(0.687) **<0.001 ***	(0.393) **<0.001 ***	(0.263) **<0.001 ***
Fish consumption and Hg levels at 5 y	(−0.001) 0.982	(0.686) **<0.001 ***	(0.470) **<0.001 ***	(0.426) **<0.001 ***

Notes: Tau: Kendall's correlation coefficient; * $p < 0.05$; ** At the six-month assessment, it was assumed that number of children was constant, as all participants had only one child from the study enrolment until six-month follow-up. y = years; m = months

Table 5. Linear regression of total Hg levels (in µg·g^{-1}) on breastfeeding duration and number of children among studied women (n = 1433), Rondônia State, Brazilian Amazon, Brazil.

	Coefficient *	95% Confidence Interval	
6 months Breastfeeding duration #	−0.0531607	−0.0981262	−0.0081952
2 years Breastfeeding duration #	−0.0372642	−0.0658661	−0.0086623

Table 5. Cont.

	Coefficient *	95% Confidence Interval		p-Value
Number of children $^\Psi$ 5 years	−0.3023673	−0.7058452	0.1011105	0.14
Breastfeeding duration #	−0.0535429	−0.0896773	−0.0174084	0.004 **
Number of children $^\Psi$	−0.1050237	−0.3999480	0.1899007	0.49

Breastfeeding duration in months; $^\Psi$ Number of children increment, compared to last period; * Models were adjusted for income, years of education, maternal age and place of residence; 2-year and 5-year models also considered the number of children as an independent variable; ** $p < 0.05$.

4. Discussion

This study evaluated pre-Minamata Convention Hg levels among women of reproductive age from the Rondônia State, Brazilian Amazon, and investigated associated factors. Participants are among the population segment most sensitive to Hg toxicity. In the gestational and puerperal period, women can expose their children to Hg through placental transfer and breastfeeding [1,20]. Considering the safe reference levels of 6 µg·g^{-1} for women of reproductive age [1], this study points to elevated Hg levels among women in Rondônia, especially among riverine and rural communities (ranging from 1.02 to 146.80 µg·g^{-1}).

Many factors can influence the body's Hg burden, and some are especially relevant in this study: the global Hg deposition; Hg exposure due to gold mining activities in the Madeira River basin; and exposure to natural Hg present in the Amazonian soils, lixiviated to waterways due to unsustainable soil use practices. All these Hg sources contribute to fish contamination and consequently, the humans who eat them. There is already sufficient evidence that the fish-based diet of the inhabitants of this region is contaminated with methylmercury (MeHg). Barbosa et al. [35] compared populations in the Brazilian Amazon exposed to Hg by different routes (artisanal gold mining vs. fish consumption) and showed that, in general, hair levels were a more reliable descriptor for Hg exposure from fish (mainly MeHg) than for Hg vapor from artisanal gold mining activities.

Brazilian women, especially those from the Amazon, are exposed to high levels of Hg contamination. Hacon et al. [36] evaluated women from Alta Floresta, in the southern Amazon basin, exposed to Hg through work activities (mining) and diet (fish consumption), and found hair Hg levels ranged between 0.05 and 8.2 µg·g^{-1}. In urban areas of the Amazon with relatively low fish consumption, a significant correlation was found between Hg levels in mothers and newborns [27,37]. Compared to urban mothers, traditional riverine mothers had significantly higher Hg levels in hair [31,37] and milk [31], which may be explained by higher fish consumption.

Comparing this study results with previous research, similar Hg levels were found with other communities in the Amazon region [30,31,36,38–41] and in South America [42–46], all exceeding internationally accepted safety levels for total Hg in hair [1].

In this study, a difference in Hg levels was found between the analyzed groups, with the riverine and rural communities having the highest levels. The correlation analysis reinforced hair Hg as a reliable biomarker of Hg levels from fish intake as advocated by [2]. These populations with high Hg levels are characterized by remote dwellings, far from major centers, and by having fishing as an important part of their livelihood.

Alves et al. [46] and Baldewsingh et al. [47] found higher levels of Hg among rural than urban communities, as a result of less diverse diet patterns. Drouillet-Pinard et al. [48] and Sakamoto et al. [49] also found that hair Hg levels are mainly associated with fish consumption. Vejrup et al. [50] observed that about 88% of Hg concentration comes from diet, corroborating the MercuNorth study, which found high Hg levels due to elevated fish consumption [51].

The Madeira River basin communities have been strongly impacted by predatory activities related to the region's economic development for at least four decades. In addition to the unbridled search for gold, deforestation, forest burning, opening of roads, and construction of hydroelectric dams triggered intensive migrations to the region. The migration caused socioeconomic and lifestyle changes among the local population [20,52,53], resulting in cultural differences, changes in eating habits, and the search for other nutritional sources, which may partially explain the differences found in the analyzed groups. In general, the differences observed between the studied groups reflected these changes in the Amazonian populations. When analyzing the mining community of Garimpo de Bom Futuro, which receives immigrants from other regions of Brazil, one can see how much the cultural component influences the population consumption habits. In these women, the diet included few weekly meals with fish, while rural and riverine women maintain traditional habits of high fish consumption.

Elevated Hg levels among rural and riverine women appear to be almost entirely due to their diet rich in fish, probably those with higher trophic level and predatory fish, which are known to accumulate significant Hg levels in their tissues [32]. This exposure route among the study women is supported by the collected data, indicating high frequency of fish consumption.

It should be noted that in 2011, a joint committee of the Food and Agriculture Organization (FAO) of the United Nations and the World Health Organization (WHO) stated that the health benefits associated with omega-3 fatty acids from fish outweighed the possible adverse neurological effects of ingesting Hg contained in fish [54]. Recommendations for decreased fish consumption in women of childbearing age, pregnant and lactating women are aimed to decrease risks on maternal reproduction and on infant growth and development. On the other hand, fish consumption offers benefits that may provide neuroprotection in children because it is rich in selenium and omega-3 [55,56].

In the Amazon region, fish is an important dietary item that is introduced at a very early age in the diet of the riverine group. Dorea [57] showed that the highly starchy manioc-flour diet is complemented mainly by protein provided by fish consumption. Fish are an exceptional source of nutritional and functional substances. They are a rich source of sulphur amino-acids and bioavailable iodine. These are crucial, on the one hand, to counterbalance cassava compounds that interfere in iodine uptake, and on the other, the iodine paucity in foods derived from the typically iodine-depleted soils of tropical rain forests. In addition to being a good source of selenium and other essential nutrients, Amazonian fish also enhance absorption of zinc and iron from plant foods in the human diet [57].

This study's participants reported a median breastfeeding time of six months, ranging between 0 and 24 months, and the breastfeeding duration was significantly associated with maternal Hg levels, which may have a negative impact on infants' health. On the other hand, Cunha et al. [58] demonstrate that even in the face of the transfer of Hg by breast milk, breastfeeding has well-defended benefits that offset the adverse effects of Hg. The ability of MeHg to be transferred via breastfeeding is well known. However, it is not possible to define exactly how much MeHg absorbed by the child is excreted through human milk [59]. Bakir et al. [5] and Greenwood et al. [60] found that Hg levels in lactating women were lower than in non-breastfeeding women, indicating the excretion of the metal through milk.

In contrast, Barbosa and Dórea [61] found that placental transfer has a higher rate of Hg transfer than breast milk in an Amazonian population, even when breastfeeding occurred for a long period of time. Barbosa et al. [38] also observed a decrease of up to 20% of maternal hair Hg levels from the first to third trimester of pregnancy, with a return to pre-pregnancy levels in the first trimester after delivery, reinforcing the importance of placental vertical transfer and suggesting that the Hg transfer through breast milk has less relevance.

Furthermore, a negative association (although non-significant) was observed between the number of children and mothers' Hg levels, which may indicate an effect of mercury loss from vertical transmission from mother to fetus during pregnancy. When comparing the participants' prenatal Hg levels and at six months after birth, a decrease was observed in all groups, reinforcing previous findings on placental transfer and breastfeeding. However, after 2 years and 5 years of follow-up, this pattern was not repeated in all groups. In riverine and rural communities, where there is greater fish consumption, Hg levels are much higher compared to urban and tin mining locations, since the protein sources in the diet of these populations is more diversified.

Considering the heterogeneity of the assessed communities, this study's findings on Hg levels of women from the Rondônia State can support the establishment of Hg background levels prior to the Minamata Convention. After five years of follow-up, the mean Hg level was still above the acceptable limit in an important proportion of women, with potential risk of fetal exposure if these women became pregnant. For this reason, monitoring Hg levels in women of reproductive age is of paramount importance, particularly for women who are more susceptible due to high contaminated-fish consumption.

In this sense, the successful implementation of the Minamata Convention depends on adequate scientific research, policy and decision making. In the case of Brazil, since the signature of the Convention, we saw little research and policy, and decision making strongly stimulated Hg use and emission and not the opposite. The Hg risks to human health, especially for women of childbearing age, are multifactorial, and the complexity of social and cultural aspects of the Amazonian communities must be taken into account. However, it is clear that the Bolsonaro period combined all factors that can lead to increased, rather than reduced, Hg exposure in the Amazon, in obvious and frontal opposition with the Minamata Convention's declared objectives.

This study has some limitations that need to be disclosed. Firstly, breastfeeding duration was evaluated in the 2 years follow-up considering the period since the study began, without data on the duration of breastfeeding in subsequent pregnancies. Some participants have breastfed for a long period (up to 24 months), which may have overestimated the effect of breastfeeding on mothers' Hg levels. Still, estimates of the effect of breastfeeding on Hg level changes were consistent across the different follow-up intervals (6 months, 2 years and 5 years). It is also important to highlight that some pregnant and lactating women in the Amazon region have the cultural habit of avoiding eating predatory/top-of-chain fish during the puerperium [62], which may have contributed to the Hg reduction observed. Moreover, the low variability in the number of children born in the study period, especially in the 2 years follow-up may be underestimating the effects of this variable on mothers' Hg levels. In this sense, a follow-up to evaluate this effect for a longer period is recommended. Finally, the existence of residual confounding cannot be ruled out, although the DAG-guided covariate adjustment model was consistent with the data (considering testable implications) and observed associations were consistent across the different analyses.

Lastly, the assessment of children's Hg levels and exactly how much is displaced from mothers during pregnancy and breastfeeding was not the subject of this study, but it is essential knowledge and should be addressed by future research.

5. Conclusions

This longitudinal cohort study evaluated Hg levels and contributing factors among pregnant women from different communities (riverine, rural, mining and urban) in Rondônia, Amazon Region, for 5 years. In general, Hg levels considerably above the limits considered safe by the WHO standards were observed among the participating women, especially those from riverine and rural communities, mainly due to the high consumption of contaminated fish. Moreover, a consistent (significant) association was observed between the reduction in maternal Hg levels and the duration of breastfeeding, in addition to a negative (non-significant) association with the number of children. It is important to highlight that mothers' Hg level is a balance between her ingestion/absorption and loss, especially through pregnancy and breastfeeding, in this case.

It is noteworthy that the Minamata Convention must be supported and enforced in Brazil, particularly in the Amazonian region. To this end, periodic management and Hg monitoring are essential, as that would help in assessing whether risk management actions are effectively translating into decreased Hg exposure. In addition, a well-coordinated and designed national biomonitoring program is urgently needed to better understand the current situation of Hg levels in Brazil and the Amazon.

Author Contributions: T.C.S.B., R.C.M. and J.G.D. contributed to study design, data collection/analysis and manuscript drafting. R.J.B. contributed to study design, data analysis and manuscript drafting. M.P.L.C. contributed to data collection and manuscript drafting. F.A.D.-Q. contributed to data analysis. J.R.D.G. contributed to manuscript drafting. All authors have read and agreed to the published version of the manuscript.

Funding: This study was supported by CNPq/MCT grant (project-555516/2006-7; project-575573/2008-2) and CAPES (Finance Code 001). FADQ was granted a fellowship for research productivity from the Brazilian National Council for Scientific and Technological Development (CNPq), process number: 312656/2019-0.

Institutional Review Board Statement: The study was approved by the Research Ethics Committee of the Federal University of Rondônia (REC/NUSAU/UNIR, file number: 012/CEP/NUSAU).

Informed Consent Statement: Informed consent was obtained from all subjects involved in the study.

Data Availability Statement: The data presented in this study are available on request from the corresponding author.

Acknowledgments: We greatly appreciate the mothers' participation, and the support of the University of Rondônia students and staff. We are also grateful to the Rondônia State Health Secretariat staff, especially the community health professionals.

Conflicts of Interest: The authors declare no conflict of interest.

References

1. World Health Organization (WHO). *Environmental Health Criteria 101—Methylmercury*; WHO: Geneva, Switzerland, 1990; 99p.
2. von Rein, K.; Hylander, L.D. Experiences from phasing out the use of mercury in Sweden. *Reg. Environ. Chang.* **2000**, *1*, 126–134. [CrossRef]
3. Legrand, M.; Feeley, M.; Tikhonov, C.; Schoen, D.; Li-Muller, A. Methylmercury blood guidance values for Canada. *Can. J. Public Health* **2010**, *101*, 28–31. [CrossRef] [PubMed]
4. Mozaffarian, D.; Shi, P.; Morris, J.S.; Spiegelman, D.; Grandjean, P.; Siscovick, D.S.; Willett, W.C.; Rimm, E.B. Mercury exposure and risk of cardiovascular disease in two U.S. cohorts. *N. Engl. J. Med.* **2011**, *364*, 1116–1125. [CrossRef] [PubMed]
5. Bakir, F.; Damluji, S.F.; Amin-Zaki, L.; Murtadha, M.; Khalidi, A.; Al-Rawi, N.Y.; Tikriti, S.; Dahahir, H.I.; Clarkson, T.W.; Smith, J.C.; et al. Methylmercury poisoning in Iraq. *Science* **1973**, *181*, 230–241. [CrossRef]
6. Malm, O. Gold mining as a source of mercury exposure in the Brazilian Amazon. *Environ. Res.* **1998**, *77*, 73–78. [CrossRef]
7. Wang, X.; Sun, X.; Zhang, Y.; Chen, M.; Villanger, G.D.; Aase, H.; Xia, Y. Identifying a critical window of maternal metal exposure for maternal and neonatal thyroid function in China: A cohort study. *Environ. Int.* **2020**, *139*, 105696. [CrossRef]
8. Cleary, D. *Anatomy of the Amazon Gold Rush*, 1st ed.; University of Iowa Press: Iowa City, IA, USA, 1990; p. 287.
9. Roulet, M.; Saint-Aubin, M.; Tran, S.; Rhéault, I.; Farella, N.; da Silva, E.J.; Dezencourt, J.; Passos, C.J.S.; Soares, G.S.; Guimarães, J.R.; et al. The geochemistry of mercury in the central Amazonian soils developed on the Alter do Chao formation of the lower Tapajós River Valley, Pará State, Brazil. *Sci. Total Environ.* **1998**, *223*, 1–24. [CrossRef]
10. Akagi, H.; Naganuma, A. Human exposure to mercury and the accumulation of methylmercury that is associated with gold mining in the Amazon Basin, Brazil. *J. Health Sci.* **2000**, *46*, 323–328. [CrossRef]
11. Roulet, M.; Lucotte, M.; Guimarães, J.R.; Rheault, I. Methylmercury in water, seston, and epiphyton of an Amazonian river and its floodplain, Tapajós River, Brazil. *Sci. Total Environ.* **2000**, *261*, 43–59. [CrossRef]
12. United Nations Environment Programme (UNEP). *Minamata Convention on Mercury*; United Nations: Geneva, Switzerland, 2019; 72p, Available online: http://www.mercuryconvention.org/Portals/11/documents/Booklets/COP3-version/Minamata-Convention-booklet-Sep2019-EN.pdf (accessed on 6 February 2023).
13. Camara Dos Deputados. *Decreto nº 9.470, de 14 de Agosto de 2018*; Diário Oficial da República Federativa do Brasil; Poder Executivo: Brasília, Brasil, 2018; Seção 1; p. 65.

14. European Food Safety Authority (EFSA). Statement on the benefits of fish/seafood consumption compared to the risks of methylmercury in fish/seafood. *EFSA J.* **2015**, *13*, 3982. [CrossRef]
15. Henriques, M.C.; Loureiro, S.; Fardilha, M.; Herdeiro, M.T. Exposure to mercury and human reproductive health: A systematic review. *Reprod. Toxicol.* **2019**, *85*, 93–103. [CrossRef]
16. Ruggieri, F.; Majorani, C.; Domanico, F.; Alimonti, A. Mercury in Children: Current state on exposure through human biomonitoring studies. *Int. J. Environ. Res. Public Health* **2017**, *14*, 519. [CrossRef]
17. Schoeman, K.; Bend, J.R.; Hill, J.; Nash, K.; Koren, G. Defining a lowest observable adverse effect hair concentration of mercury for neurodevelopmental effects of Prenatal Methylmercury exposure through maternal fish consumption: A systematic review. *Ther. Drug Monit.* **2009**, *31*, 670–682. [CrossRef]
18. Kirk, L.E.; Jørgensen, J.S.; Nielsen, F.; Grandjean, P. Public health benefits of hair-mercury analysis and dietary advice in lowering methylmercury exposure in pregnant women. *Scand. J. Public Health* **2017**, *45*, 444–451. [CrossRef]
19. Schoeman, K.; Tanaka, T.; Bend, J.R.; Koren, G. Hair mercury levels of women of reproductive age in Ontario, Canada: Implications to fetal safety and fish consumption. *J. Pediatr.* **2010**, *157*, 127–131. [CrossRef]
20. Dórea, J.G.; Marques, R.C. Mercury levels and human health in the Amazon Basin. *Ann. Hum. Biol.* **2016**, *43*, 349–359. [CrossRef]
21. Lee, B.E.; Hong, Y.C.; Park, H.; Ha, M.; Koo, B.S.; Chang, N.; Roh, Y.M.; Kim, B.N.; Kim, Y.J.; Kim, B.M.; et al. Interaction between GSTM1/GSTT1 polymorphism and blood mercury on birth weight. *Environ. Health Perspect.* **2010**, *118*, 437–443. [CrossRef]
22. Xue, F.; Holzman, C.; Rahbar, M.H.; Trosko, K.; Fisher, L. Fischer, Maternal fish consumption, mercury levels, and risk of preterm delivery. *Environ. Health Perspect.* **2007**, *115*, 42–47. [CrossRef]
23. Dallaire, R.; Dewailly, E.; Ayotte, P.; Forget-Dubois, N.; Jacobson, S.W.; Jacobson, J.; Muckle, G. Exposure to organochlorines and mercury through fish and marine mammal consumption: Associations with growth and duration of gestation among Inuit newborns. *Environ. Int.* **2013**, *54*, 85–91. [CrossRef]
24. Castro, N.S.S.; Lima, M.O. Hair as a Biomarker of Long Term Mercury Exposure in Brazilian Amazon: A Systematic Review. *Int. J. Environ. Res. Public Health* **2018**, *15*, 500. [CrossRef]
25. Airey, D. Mercury in human hair due to environment and diet: A review. *Environ. Health Perspect.* **1983**, *52*, 303–316. [CrossRef] [PubMed]
26. Marques, R.C.; Bernardi, J.V.E.; Dórea, J.G.; Brandão, K.G.; Bueno, L.; Leão, R.S.; Malm, O. Fish consumption during pregnancy, mercury transfer, and birth weight along the Madeira River Basin in Amazonia. *Int. J. Environ. Res. Public Health* **2013**, *10*, 2150–2163. [CrossRef] [PubMed]
27. Marques, R.C.; Dórea, J.G.; Bastos, W.R.; Rebelo, M.F.; Fonseca, M.F.; Malm, O. Maternal mercury exposure and neuro-motor development in breastfed infants from Porto Velho (Amazon), Brazil. *Int. J. Hyg. Environ. Health* **2007**, *210*, 51–60. [CrossRef] [PubMed]
28. Marques, R.C.; Dórea, J.G.; Bernardi, J.V.E.; Bastos, W.R.; Malm, O. Data relating neurodevelopment of exclusively breastfed children of urban mothers and pre- and post-natal mercury exposure. *Data Brief* **2019**, *25*, 104283. [CrossRef] [PubMed]
29. Marques, R.C.; Dórea, J.G.; Cunha, M.P.L.; Bello, T.C.S.; Bernardi, J.V.E.; Malm, O. Data relating to maternal fish consumption, methylmercury exposure, and early child neurodevelopment in the traditional living of Western Amazonians. *Data Brief* **2019**, *1*, 104153. [CrossRef]
30. Corvelo, T.C.O.; Oliveira, E.A.F.; de Parijós, A.M.; de Oliveira, C.S.B.; de Loiola, R.S.P.; de Araújo, A.A.; da Costa, C.A.; Silveira, L.C.L.; Pinheiro, M.C.N. Monitoring mercury exposure in reproductive aged women inhabiting the Tapajós River Basin, Amazon. *Bull. Environ. Contam. Toxicol.* **2014**, *93*, 42–46. [CrossRef]
31. Vieira, S.M.; de Almeida, R.; Holanda, I.B.B.; Mussy, M.H.; Galvão, R.C.F.; Crispim, P.T.B.; Dórea, J.G.; Bastos, W.R. Total and methyl-mercury in hair and milk of mothers living in the city of Porto Velho and in villages along the Rio Madeira, Amazon, Brazil. *Int. J. Hyg. Environ. Health* **2013**, *216*, 682–689. [CrossRef]
32. Dórea, J.G.; Barbosa, A.C.; Ferrari, I.; de Souza, J.R. Mercury in hair and in fish consumed by Riparian women of the Rio Negro, Amazon, Brazil. *Int. J. Environ. Health Res.* **2003**, *13*, 239–248. [CrossRef]
33. Malm, O.; Pfeiffer, W.C.; Souza, C.M.M. Utilização do acessório de geração de vapor frio para análise de mercúrio em investigações ambientais por espectrofotometria de absorção atômica. *Cien. Cult.* **1989**, *41*, 88–92.
34. Textor, J.; van der Zander, B.; Gilthorpe, M.S.; Liskiewicz, M.; Ellison, G.T. Robust causal inference using directed acyclic graphs: The R package 'dagitty'. *Int. J. Epidemiol.* **2016**, *45*, 1887–1894. [CrossRef]
35. Barbosa, A.C.; Boischio, A.A.; East, G.A.; Ferrari, I.; Gonçalves, A.; Silva, P.R.M.; da Cruz, T.M.E. Mercury contamination in the Brazilian Amazon. Environmental and occupational aspects. *Water Air Soil Pollut.* **1995**, *80*, 109–121. [CrossRef]
36. Hacon, S.S.; Yokoo, E.; Valente, J.; Campos, R.C.; da Silva, V.A.; de Menezes, A.C.; de Moraes, L.P.; Ignotti, E. Exposure to mercury in pregnant women from Alta Floresta- Amazon basin, Brazil. *Environ. Res.* **2000**, *84*, 204–210. [CrossRef]
37. Marques, R.C.; Bernardi, J.V.E.; Dórea, J.G.; Leão, R.S.; Malm, O. Mercury transfer during pregnancy and breastfeeding: Hair mercury concentrations as biomarker. *Biol. Trace Elem. Res.* **2013**, *154*, 326–332. [CrossRef]
38. Barbosa, A.C.; Silva, S.R.; Dórea, J.G. Concentration of mercury in hair of indigenous mothers and infants from the Amazon basin. *Arch. Environ. Contam. Toxicol.* **1998**, *34*, 100–105. [CrossRef]
39. Oliveira, R.C.; Dórea, J.G.; Bernardi, J.V.; Bastos, W.R.; Almeida, R.; Manzatto, A.G. Fish consumption by traditional subsistence villagers of the Rio Madeira (Amazon): Impact on hair mercury. *Ann. Hum. Biol.* **2010**, *37*, 629–642. [CrossRef]

40. Faial, K.; Deus, R.; Deus, S.; Neves, R.; Jesus, I.; Santos, E.; Alves, C.N.; Brasil, D. Mercury levels assessment in hair of riverside inhabitants of the Tapajós River, Pará State, Amazon, Brazil: Fish consumption as a possible route of exposure. *J. Trace Elem. Med. Biol.* **2015**, *30*, 66–76. [CrossRef]
41. Vega, C.; Orellana, J.D.Y.; Oliveira, M.W.; Hacon, S.S.; Basta, P.C. Human mercury exposure in Yanomami indigenous villages from the Brazilian Amazon. *Int. J. Environ. Res. Public Health* **2018**, *15*, 1051. [CrossRef]
42. Peplow, D.; Augustine, S. Community-led assessment of risk from exposure to mercury by native Amerindian Wayana in Southeast Suriname. *J. Environ. Public Health* **2011**, *2012*, 674596. [CrossRef]
43. Alcala-Orozco, M.; Caballero-Gallardo, K.; Olivero-Verbel, J. Mercury exposure assessment in indigenous communities from Tarapaca village, Cotuhe and Putumayo Rivers, Colombian Amazon. *Environ. Sci. Pollut. Res. Int.* **2019**, *26*, 36458–36467. [CrossRef]
44. Valdelamar-Villegas, J.; Olivero-Verbel, J. High Mercury Levels in the Indigenous Population of the Yaigojé Apaporis National Natural Park, Colombian Amazon. *Biol. Trace Elem. Res.* **2020**, *194*, 3–12. [CrossRef]
45. Díaz, S.M.; Palma, R.M.; Muñoz, M.N.; Becerra-Arias, C.; Niño, J.A.F. Factors Associated with High Mercury Levels in Women and Girls from The Mojana Region, Colombia, 2013–2015. *Int. J. Environ. Res. Public Health* **2020**, *17*, 1827. [CrossRef] [PubMed]
46. Baldewsingh, G.K.; Hindori-Mohangoo, A.D.; van Eer, E.D.; Covert, H.H.; Shankar, A.; Wickliffe, J.K.; Shi, L.; Lichtveld, M.Y.; Zijlmans, W.C.W.R. Association of Mercury Exposure and Maternal Sociodemographics on Birth Outcomes of Indigenous and Tribal Women in Suriname. *Int. J. Environ. Res. Public Health* **2021**, *18*, 6370. [CrossRef] [PubMed]
47. Alves, M.F.A.; Fraiji, N.A.; Barbosa, A.C.; de Lima, D.S.N.; Souza, J.R.; Dórea, J.G.; Cordeiro, G.W.O. Fish consumption, mercury exposure and serum antinuclear antibody in Amazonians. *Int. J. Environ. Health Res.* **2006**, *16*, 255–262. [CrossRef] [PubMed]
48. Drouillet-Pinard, P.; Huel, G.; Slama, R.; Forhan, A.; Sahuquillo, J.; Goua, V.; Thiébaugeorges, O.; Foliguet, B.; Magnin, G.; Kaminski, M.; et al. Prenatal mercury contamination: Relationship with maternal seafood consumption during pregnancy and fetal growth in the 'EDEN mother–child' cohort. *Br. J. Nutr.* **2010**, *104*, 1096–1100. [CrossRef] [PubMed]
49. Sakamoto, M.; Kubota, M.; Murata, K.; Nakai, K.; Sonoda, I.; Satoh, H. Changes in Mercury concentrations of segmental maternal hair during gestation and their correlations with other biomarkers of fetal exposure to methylmercury in the japanese population. *Environ. Res.* **2008**, *106*, 270–276. [CrossRef]
50. Vejrup, K.; Brantsæter, A.L.; Knutsen, H.K.; Magnus, P.; Alexander, J.; Kvalem, H.E.; Meltzer, H.M.; Hougen, M. Prenatal Mercury exposure and infant birth weight in the Norwegian mother and child cohort study. *Public Health Nutr.* **2014**, *17*, 2071–2080. [CrossRef]
51. Adlard, B.; Lemire, M.; Bonefeld-Jørgensen, E.C.; Long, M.; Ólafsdíttir, K.; Odland, J.O.; Rautio, A.; Myllynen, P.; Sandanger, T.M.; Dudarev, A.A.; et al. MercuNorth—Monitoring mercury in pregnant women from the Arctic as a baseline to assess the effectiveness of the Minamata Convention. *Int. J. Public Health* **2021**, *80*, 1881345. [CrossRef]
52. Fearnside, P.M. Brazil's Samuel dam: Lessons for hydroelectric development policy and the environment in Amazonia. *Environ. Manag.* **2005**, *35*, 1–19. [CrossRef]
53. Fearnside, P.M.; Laurance, W.F.; Cochrane, M.A.; Bergen, S.; Sampaio, P.D.; Barber, C.; D'Angelo, S.; Fernandes, T. O futuro da Amazônia: Modelos para prever as consequências da infraestrutura futura nos planos plurianuais. *Novos Cad. NAEA (Online)* **2012**, *15*, 25–52. [CrossRef]
54. Food and Agriculture Organization; World Health Organization (FAO/WHO). *Report of the Joint FAO/WHO Expert Consultation on the Risks and Benefits of Fish Consumption*; FAO: Rome, Italy; WHO: Geneva, Switzerland, 2011; 50pp, Available online: http://www.fao.org/3/ba0136e/ba0136e00.pdf (accessed on 20 October 2022).
55. Bramante, C.T.; Spiller, P.; Landa, M. Fish consumption during pregnancy: An opportunity, not a risk. *JAMA Pediatr.* **2018**, *172*, 801–802. [CrossRef]
56. Taylor, C.M.; Emmett, P.M.; Emond, A.M.; Golding, J. A review of guidance on fish consumption in pregnancy: Is it for purpose? *Public Health Nutr.* **2018**, *21*, 2149–2159. [CrossRef]
57. Dorea, J.G. Cassava cyanogens and fish mercury are high but safely consumed in the diet of native Amazonians. *Ecotoxicol. Environ. Saf.* **2004**, *57*, 248–256. [CrossRef]
58. Cunha, M.P.L.; Marques, R.C.; Dórea, J.G. Influence of Maternal Fish Intake on the Anthropometric Indices of Children in the Western Amazon. *Nutrients* **2018**, *10*, 1146. [CrossRef]
59. Grandjean, P.; Jørgensen, P.J.; Weihe, P. Human milk as a source of methylmercury exposure in infants. *Environ. Health Perspect.* **1994**, *102*, 74–77. [CrossRef]
60. Greenwood, M.R.; Clarkson, T.W.; Doherty, R.A.; Amin-Zaki, L.; Elhassani, S.; Majeed, M.A. Blood clearance half-times in lactating and nonlactating members of a population exposed to methymercury. *Environ. Res.* **1978**, *16*, 48–54. [CrossRef]
61. Barbosa, A.C.; Dórea, J.G. Indices of mercury contamination during breast feeding in Amazon Basin. *Environ. Toxicol. Pharmacol.* **1998**, *6*, 71–79. [CrossRef]
62. Matos, M.L.; Arruda, L.C. O uso da memória para investigação de ritos no parto e "resguardo" em Santarém (PA). *Percursos* **2016**, *2*, 10–22. [CrossRef]

Disclaimer/Publisher's Note: The statements, opinions and data contained in all publications are solely those of the individual author(s) and contributor(s) and not of MDPI and/or the editor(s). MDPI and/or the editor(s) disclaim responsibility for any injury to people or property resulting from any ideas, methods, instructions or products referred to in the content.

A Multi-Pollutant and Meteorological Analysis of Cardiorespiratory Mortality among the Elderly in São Paulo, Brazil—An Artificial Neural Networks Approach

Luciana Leirião, Michelle de Oliveira, Tiago Martins * and Simone Miraglia

Institute of Environmental, Chemical and Pharmaceutical Sciences, Federal University of Sao Paulo (UNIFESP), Diadema 09913030, Brazil
* Correspondence: tdmartins@unifesp.br

Abstract: Traditionally, studies that associate air pollution with health effects relate individual pollutants to outcomes such as mortality or hospital admissions. However, models capable of analyzing the effects resulting from the atmosphere mixture are demanded. In this study, multilayer perceptron neural networks were evaluated to associate PM_{10}, NO_2, and SO_2 concentrations, temperature, wind speed, and relative air humidity with cardiorespiratory mortality among the elderly in São Paulo, Brazil. Daily data from 2007 to 2019 were considered and different numbers of neurons on the hidden layer, algorithms, and a combination of activation functions were tested. The best-fitted artificial neural network (ANN) resulted in a MAPE equal to 13.46%. When individual season data were analyzed, the MAPE decreased to 11%. The most influential variables in cardiorespiratory mortality among the elderly were PM_{10} and NO_2 concentrations. The relative humidity variable is more important during the dry season, and temperature is more important during the rainy season. The models were not subjected to the multicollinearity issue as with classical regression models. The use of ANNs to relate air quality to health outcomes is still very incipient, and this work highlights that it is a powerful tool that should be further explored.

Keywords: air pollution; health effects; multi-pollutant model; artificial neural network

1. Introduction

Air pollution is the first environmental risk factor for the world's population [1]. According to the Global Burden of Disease (GBD), in 2019, there were 6.67 million excess deaths due to exposure to particulate matter pollutants [2]. Other authors argue that the world's mortality due to particulate matter exposure may be even greater if other death causes behind the ones considered by the GBD were computed. Burnett et al. [3], for instance, calculate that particulate matter with a diameter of 2.5 µm or less ($PM_{2.5}$) could have been responsible for 8.5 million deaths in 2015 worldwide.

The literature concerning the harmful effects of air pollution exposure has been increasing since 2011 [4]. Although the majority of the studies associate the pollutant concentrations with respiratory diseases, chronic diseases, and cardiovascular diseases [5–8], recent research has emerged suggesting that air pollution may be associated with mental disorders and other diseases, such as DNA methylation changes, inflammatory disease, skin disease, and abortion [4,9].

The effects of air pollution are not the same across the population; the elderly, children, and people with chronic diseases are the main risk group [4]. Studies point to higher risks in the elderly compared to the rest of the population, probably as a consequence of pre-existing disease complications, and the main pollutant affecting this group is particulate matter [10–12]. Temperature and relative humidity increases also appear to play a fundamental role in mortality [13–15].

Several authors around the world have aimed to understand the health effects among the elderly of an increase of 10 µg/m^3 or 50 µg/m^3 in the daily concentration of pollutants such as particulate matter (PM) and sulfur dioxide (SO_2). The most discussed outcomes are hospitalizations related to the respiratory system or chronic obstructive pulmonary disease and deaths from respiratory causes [16–21]. Studies aiming to associate elderly mortality with pollutant exposure are mainly single-pollutant analyses. In order to better understand the role of air pollution in the elderly, more investigations focusing on exposure to multi-pollutant mixtures are needed [11].

Despite the wide variety of studies around the world, they are mainly concentrated in countries with a temperate climate, being less frequent in countries with a tropical climate [22]. Among tropical countries, Brazil stands out as one of the most studied countries (along with India and Australia) [22]. Studying air pollution health effects jointly with temperature variation is important in these countries since the results found may be quite different from the ones obtained in temperate countries, given the lower temperature variation throughout the year [23].

Among the regions with a tropical climate, the municipality of São Paulo (Brazil) stands out in relation to studies that aim to estimate the health effects of air pollution exposure. The city is among the 10 most populous in the world, being the largest in Latin America with more than 12 million inhabitants [24]. According to a 2016 study, which so far is the most recent application of the official WHO methodology in São Paulo, about 5000 premature deaths annually can be associated with excess $PM_{2.5}$ in the atmosphere [25]. Vehicles are mainly responsible for the high concentration of pollutants in the atmosphere, and the official estimation is that there are almost 9 million vehicles in the municipality (8% of the national fleet in 0.17% of Brazil's territory) [26]. The city's status as a global economic hub (31% of Brazil's GDP [27]) attracts people with a typical profile that prefers using their car to public transportation. Thus, the emission of air pollutants and the large number of people exposed to these pollutants position São Paulo as a global challenge in terms of its environmental and public health issues.

Since the 1990s, several studies relating adverse health effects to pollutant concentrations have been carried out in São Paulo [28–31]. The most recent studies (from 2015 on) considered the particulate matter with a diameter of less than 10 µm (PM_{10}), nitrogen dioxide (NO_2), carbon monoxide (CO), ozone (O_3), and SO_2 pollutants, and several health outcomes. Bravo [32] investigated the relationship between PM_{10}, NO_2, SO_2, CO, and O_3 (individually analyzed) and non-accidental, cardiovascular, and respiratory deaths among city residents and found a positive relationship for all analyses, except between O_3 concentration and cardiovascular deaths. Abe et al. [33] demonstrated a positive relationship between PM_{10} concentration and cardiovascular and respiratory deaths. Finally, Santana et al. [34] demonstrated the positive relationship between pollutants PM, O_3, CO, SO_2, and NO_2 (individually analyzed) and hospitalizations due to respiratory diseases.

A few recent studies have focused on the health effects among the elderly population in São Paulo. Costa et al. [35] found that a 10 µg/m^3 addition to PM_{10} and NO_2 concentrations increased nonaccidental deaths among the elderly by 0.35% and 0.40%, respectively. According to the authors, the pollutant effects are even higher two days after the exposure (0.6% and 0.58% for PM_{10} and NO_2, respectively) [35]. Ferreira et al. [36] specifically analyzed the effect of particulate matter on hospital admissions among the elderly and concluded that the ionic composition of the pollutant (specifically the presence of SO_4^{2-} in PM_{10} and K^+ in $PM_{2.5}$) increases the health effects in this population. Finally, it is also highlighted that the elderly population of lower socioeconomic levels seems to be more affected in relation to air pollution in São Paulo [37].

Supported by scientific and technological development, São Paulo and several governments around the world have implemented actions aiming to reduce the concentration of pollutants in the atmosphere. These policies are mainly focused on particulate matter, which is the pollutant most frequently associated with health problems. However, the focus on single pollutants neglects the fact that the atmosphere is a complex mixture of substances subject to the action of physical and chemical processes and that individuals are not exposed to a single pollutant at a time but simultaneously to a mixture of them [38].

Scientific development aiming at understanding the joint effect of pollutants on human health has resulted in a series of models called multipollutant models (as opposed to the ones that consider only one pollutant at a time, called single pollutant models). One of the first studies of this type was carried out by Gold et al., in 1999, which considered the cumulative effect of $PM_{2.5}$ and O_3 on lung function [39]. According to Davalos et al. [40], the main models that have been adopted to analyze the joint effect of exposure to pollutants are additive main effects (AMEs); effect measure modification (EMM); unsupervised dimension reduction (UDR); supervised dimension reduction (SDR); and nonparametric methods. The lack of consensus on a specific model for this analysis is due to statistical challenges, such as the multicollinearity of the independent variables, and the interaction among components of the atmosphere [41].

The pollutants usually considered in multipollutant models are particulate matter ($PM_{2.5}$ or PM_{10}), nitrogen oxides (NO_x), and ozone (O_3) [40]. The health effects of exposure can be investigated by considering the pollutants simultaneously or in pairs. The results of several studies on the interaction of pollutants and their health effects are contradictory. While some authors describe additive effects, others describe independent or even antagonistic effects. In Colombia, Rodríguez-Villamizar et al. [42], through conditional negative binomial regression models, found an additive effect of NO_2 in relation to $PM_{2.5}$ when analyzing their association with cardiovascular hospitalizations. A similar result was found by Jiang et al. [43] in China regarding the addition of $PM_{2.5}$ to the O_3 effect. In this case, the authors used a generalized linear Poisson model. On the other hand, using the same statistical model, Zhang et al. [44] found a decrease in the association between NO_2 and cardiovascular mortality when the model was adjusted considering SO_2 and PM_{10} pollutants. More recently, Shin et al. [45] applied generalized additive over-dispersion Poisson regression models and described that the individual effects of O_3, NO_2, and $PM_{2.5}$ pollutants were not considered under or over-estimated when compared with multi-two or three pollutants models.

Health outcomes, in general, constitute a multifactorial problem. Thus, there is no medical consensus on the total number of variables and their importance in relation to these outcomes. The interaction between several variables (such as pollutant exposure, meteorological conditions, gender, life habits, age, etc.) is still unknown to medicine and this makes it difficult to explain the physiology of the phenomenon. Considering the statistical difficulty regarding the traditional models, artificial neural networks (ANNs) emerge as a powerful tool for this type of study. An ANN can manage a large complexity of information without the need to know the phenomenon itself (whether or not the variables are correlated). When interactions are so complex that it is difficult to separate one effect from another, ANNs can be a more interesting mathematical solution than simpler mathematical models that consider only one or a smaller number of variables.

ANNs are learning algorithms inspired by the nervous system of superior organisms [46]. So, they are based on simple processing units (neurons), which store experimental knowledge and make it available for use through a learning process [46]. In ANNs, neurons are distributed in one or more interrelated layers. Based on the existing data, the neurons are trained to estimate outputs from the input data. ANNs have been widely applied in air quality forecasting (mainly concerning particulate matter, nitrogen oxides, and ozone) based on meteorological variables, emissions, and traffic data [47,48]. Since they deal in a non-linear way with a large volume of data and have a high capacity to make generalizations, ANNs have a high potential to be explored to estimate health outcomes from air pollutant exposure [49].

São Paulo stands out in terms of the number of publications relating air pollution to health effects [22]. Although ANNs are still little applied in these studies around the world, some authors have used this approach in São Paulo. This allows comparisons and a margin for improvement. The comparison between the classical generalized linear model (GLM) and the artificial neural network in São Paulo revealed that the ANN shows better results when modeling the daily hospital admissions due to PM_{10} exposure and meteorological conditions [49]. In a multipollutant analysis, Miranda et al. [50] considered the monthly mean concentration of six air pollutants (PM_{10}, $PM_{2.5}$, O_3, CO, SO_2, and NO_2) to estimate hospitalizations for respiratory diseases. The best ANN found by the authors was able to estimate 85.5% of the experimental data, and the percentage errors (from 2% to 25%) were considered low [50]. Despite the good result, the study did not consider meteorological variables. In all previous studies, the best-fitted ANN had difficulties in estimating the highest and lowest values of the time series.

Bearing all this in mind and considering the difficulties and limitations inherent to the most traditional multipollutant models, this study aimed to use multilayer perceptron artificial neural networks to find a model able to associate PM_{10}, NO_2, and SO_2 concentrations and meteorological variables (temperature, wind speed, and relative air humidity) with cardiorespiratory mortality among the elderly population in São Paulo, Brazil.

2. Materials and Methods

2.1. Study Area, Data Sources, and Processing

The municipality of São Paulo is located in the Southeast region of Brazil, extends over 1521 km^2, and is estimated to have 12.3 million inhabitants [24]. Air quality is monitored by 18 monitoring stations controlled by the environmental company of the State of São Paulo (named CETESB—Companhia Ambiental do Estado de São Paulo), which are heterogeneously distributed (Figure 1). In 2019, the annual average concentration of PM_{10}, $PM_{2.5}$, and NO_2 pollutants in the municipality was, respectively, 28.66 µg/m^3, 16.41 µg/m^3, and 35.66 µg/m^3 [51]. These values were above the annual averages recommended by the World Health Organization, which are, respectively, 15 µg/m^3, 5 µg/m^3, and 10 µg/m^3 [52]. Even during 2020, when several services were paralyzed due to the COVID-19 pandemic, the annual concentrations of these pollutants were well above recommended levels (27.25 µg/m^3, 14.78 µg/m^3, and 30.77 µg/m^3 for PM_{10}, $PM_{2.5}$, and NO_2, respectively) [53].

To obtain the ANN proposed in this study, hourly air quality data were obtained from the CETESB database in all 18 monitoring stations from 1 January 2007 to 31 December 2019 (all data can be consulted on https://qualar.cetesb.sp.gov.br/qualar/home.do (accessed on 20 August 2022)). The data considered the concentration of PM_{10}, $PM_{2.5}$, O_3, NO_2, and SO_2 pollutants. Due to the existence of missing data in the database, $PM_{2.5}$ and O_3 data were disregarded. For the other pollutants, daily mean concentration was calculated considering only days with more than 75% of hourly data available.

For the calculation of the daily average concentration of the pollutants in the city of São Paulo, only the monitoring stations that had data for the entire time series were considered (Figure 1). So, the selection of the monitoring station respected only one criterion, which was the availability data for the entire time series. In relation to PM_{10}, the stations considered were: Cerqueira César, Congonhas, Grajaú, Nossa Senhora do Ó, and Parque D. Pedro II. For NO_2, the stations Cerqueira César, Congonhas, Ibirapuera, Parque D Pedro II, and Pinheiros were considered. Finally, for SO_2, the stations considered were Cerqueira Cesar and Congonhas.

The meteorological data considered in the investigation were daily means of air temperature, relative humidity, and wind speed. They were obtained from the Institute of Astronomy, Geophysics and Atmospheric Sciences of Sao Paulo University (IAG-Instituto de Astronomia, Geofísica e Ciências Atmosféricas da Universidade de São Paulo), which is located in the southern area of Sao Paulo municipality. The data are provided by completing a form on their website (http://www.estacao.iag.usp.br/sol_dados.php (accessed on 20 August 2022)).

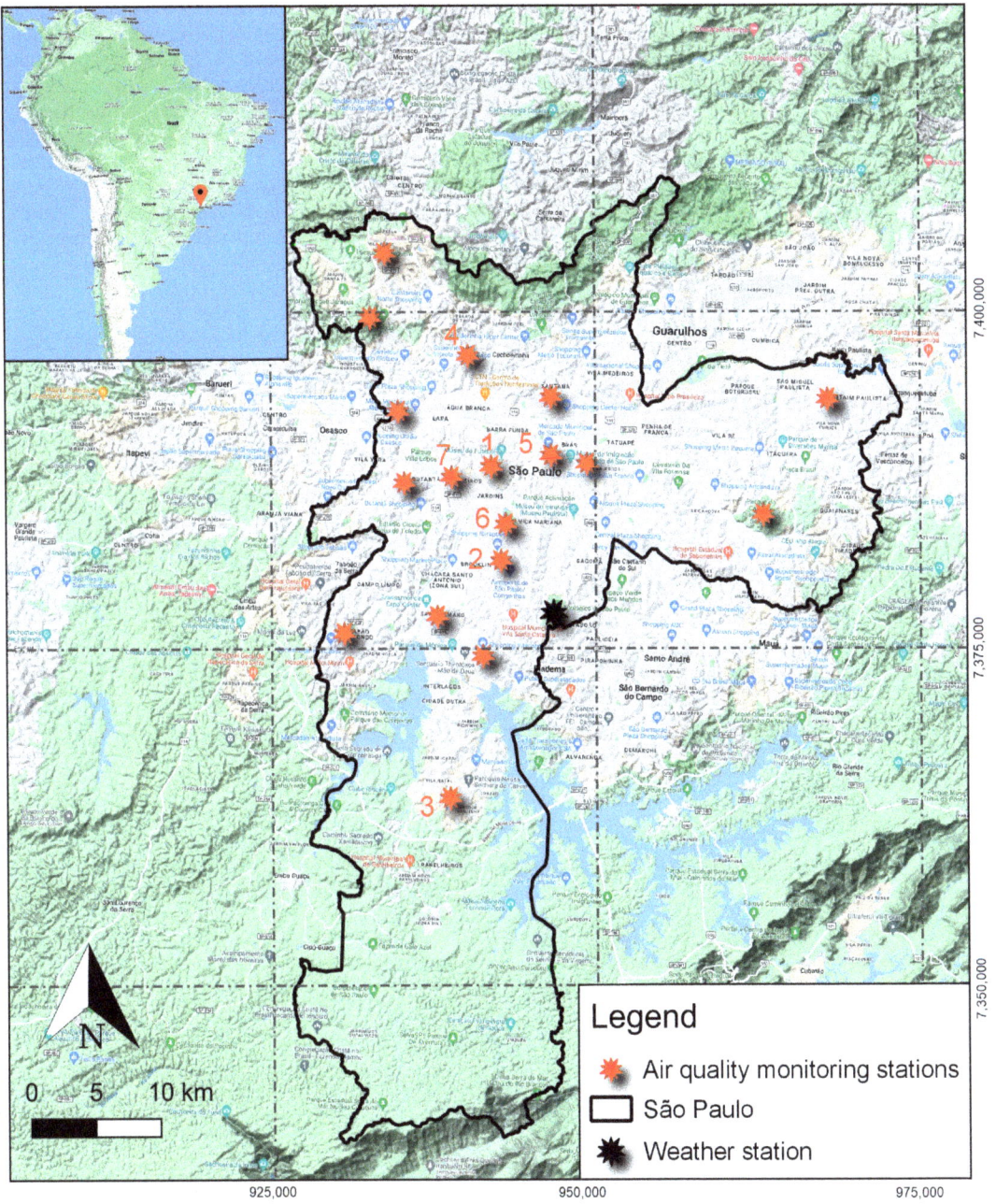

Figure 1. Map illustrating the Sao Paulo municipality and its 18 air quality monitoring stations. The numbers 1 to 7 indicate the following stations: Cerqueira César, Congonhas, Grajaú, Nossa Senhora do Ó, Parque D. Pedro II, Ibirapuera, and Pinheiros. Source: Elaborated by the authors on QGIS 2.18.20 software.

Daily mortality due to cardiorespiratory disease (chapters IX and X of ICD) data were obtained from the Informatics Department of the Brazilian Health System (named DATASUS). The data are open access and can be consulted on DATASUS website (https://datasus.saude.gov.br/informacoes-de-saude-tabnet/ (accessed on 20 August 2022)). The database contained all-age mortality and was filtered to consider only the deaths among the population older than 60 years. As the elderly population in the city grew by 36% during the analyzed period (from 1.2 million in 2007 to 1.9 million in 2019), the number of deaths was relativized by the total elderly population (>60 years) of each year. The population data for this relativization was consulted from the State of Sao Paulo System of Data Analysis (named Fundação SEADE) on the website https://municipios.seade.gov.br/ (accessed on 20 August 2022).

2.2. Artificial Neural Network

Using MATLAB programming language, several multilayer perceptron (MLP) neural networks were designed. The daily concentration of the three pollutants and meteorological variables were considered as inputs, and the respective cardiorespiratory mortality among the elderly population was considered as output (Figure 2).

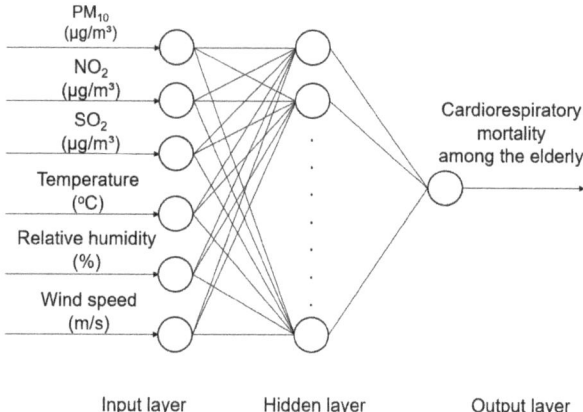

Figure 2. Schematic representation of ANN model with one hidden layer.

On MLPs, each neuron receives a synaptic weight, which represents the relative influence of the input data on the respective neuron. The result of the multiplication between the variable and its weight summed with a bias parameter results in an activation coefficient, as follows (Equation (1)):

$$\alpha_j = \sum_{i=1}^{z} w_{ij} x_i + b_j \quad (1)$$

where α_j is the activation value; z is the number of inputs; x_i is the neuron's input variable i; w_{ij} is the weight of the variable i on the neuron j; and b_j is the bias [46]. The neuron's output is then calculated by using an activation function over α_j, which can be linear or non-linear functions (such as hyperbolic tangent and sigmoidal).

The MLP uses an optimization algorithm to minimize an objective function (OF) that is related to the difference between the obtained output value and the expected one. This minimization is performed through a supervised learning technique to determine the weight and the bias of each neuron [46].

In this study, the MLP neural networks with one and two hidden layers were tested. Structures with 5, 10, 15, 20, 25, 30, and 35 neurons in the hidden layer were considered. More neurons were not used, because it would generate an overfitted model. Four different learning algorithms were used (Scaled Conjugate Gradient-trainscg, Levenberg–Marquardttrainlm, Powell–Beale conjugate gradient backpropagation-traincgb, and Bayesinan Regularization-trainbr), and the combinations of three activation functions (hyperbolic tangent sigmoid-tansig, linear-purelin, and logarithmic sigmoid-logsig) were tested. As we showed in previous studies, testing different learning algorithms, and the random separation of training and validation data, are important to achieve a good result. The main reason for including several ANN configurations was to increase the search for the configuration that leads to a good result. It totalized 420 ANN architectures. Each ANN configuration was trained 50 times. From the total obtained data, 70% was used for training, 15% for validation, and the remaining 15% for the test. Data division was randomly performed by the software. The validation step is performed at the same time as the training step, to prevent overfitting. The validation objective function is monitored during training, and the one stop criterion is the increase in this parameter when the training data objective function continues to decrease. Test data are used for an independent prediction after the training stopped.

The mean square error (MSE) was the objective function to be minimized. The errors of each of these steps were considered, and the network with the lower mean absolute percentage error (MAPE) was considered as the one with the best fit.

After determining the best ANN model, the importance (weight) of each variable to the cardiorespiratory mortality was calculated according to connection weight method [54]. For each variable i, we calculated the variable I_{ij} as follows (Equation (2)):

$$I_{ij} = w_{ij} \cdot w_{1j} \qquad (2)$$

where w_{ij} is the weight matrix of the hidden layer, being i input variables and j neurons in the hidden layer, and w_{1j} is the weight matrix of the output layer, being 1 output and j inputs (from the hidden layer). So, the importance of the input i (Imp_i) could be obtained by Equation (3):

$$Imp_i = \sum_j I_{ij} \qquad (3)$$

The seasonality behind all considered variables is widely described, with increases in pollutant concentrations and mortality during the dry season (from April to September) and reductions in the rainy season (from October to March) [53]. This characteristic hampers the neural networks from accurately estimating the highest and lowest values, as detected by Araujo et al. [49] and Miranda et al. [50]. For this reason, in this study, three models were developed. The first one (model I) considered all the collected data (4748 daily observations collected from 2007 to 2019). The second one (model II) considered only data from the rainy season (2369 daily observations considering only the months from October to March of the same year interval). Finally, the third model (model III) considered the data from the dry season (2379 daily observations considering only the months from April to September of the same year interval).

2.3. Generalized Linear Model

As the ANN approach is still little explored in investigating the relationship between air pollution or meteorological variables and health outcomes, the ANN models were validated by comparing the results with a traditional approach. Generalized linear models (GLMs) were originally defined by Nelder and Wedderburn in 1972 [55] as an extension of conventional linear models. GLMs are capable of dealing with distributions of the response variable different from the normal distribution and the relationship between input variables and output variables different from the linear [56].

In this study, a GLM with Gamma distribution was adopted due to the nature of the response variable (positive and continuous numbers). The link function adopted was of a loglink, resulting in the model represented by Equation (4):

$$\mu_i = exp(\beta_0 + \sum_1 \beta_1 x_i) \qquad (4)$$

where μ_i is the response variable; β is estimated by the model, and x_i is the independent variable.

Three models were developed using SPSS software. The first model (Model I') considered the entire database. The second (Model II') considered only the observations (daily measures) that occurred in the rainy season. Finally, the third (Model III') considered only the observations that occurred in the dry season.

As suggested by Conceição et al., for the construction of GLM models, a basic model was first built before adding the concentrations of pollutants [56]. In this basic model, the following explanatory variables were considered: month, year, day of the week, and meteorological variables (relative humidity, temperature and wind speed). Once the models with the best set of controls for seasonality and climate were defined, pollutant concentrations were included. So, Models I', II', and III' had as input variables the daily concentrations of PM_{10}, NO_2, and SO_2, and the variables considered as significative ($p < 0.05$) in the basic models. As response variables, we adopted cardiorespiratory mortality among the elderly (deaths per 100,000 elderly inhabitants).

The models were applied to estimate the response variable in all observations, and the MAPE was estimated. The distributions of MAPEs in the three models (Model I', Model II', and Model III') were compared with the distributions of MAPEs resulting from neural networks (Model I, Model II, and Model III).

3. Results

3.1. Descriptive Statistics

Over the years, there has been a decrease in the average concentration of the three pollutants considered in this study. The reduction was approximately 31.6% for PM_{10} (from 41.49 µg/m³ in 2007 to 28.35 µg/m³ in 2019), 31.3% for NO_2 (from 58.36 µg/m³ to 40.08 µg/m³), and 82.5% for SO_2 (from 9.66 µg/m³ to 1.68 µg/m³) (Figure 3).

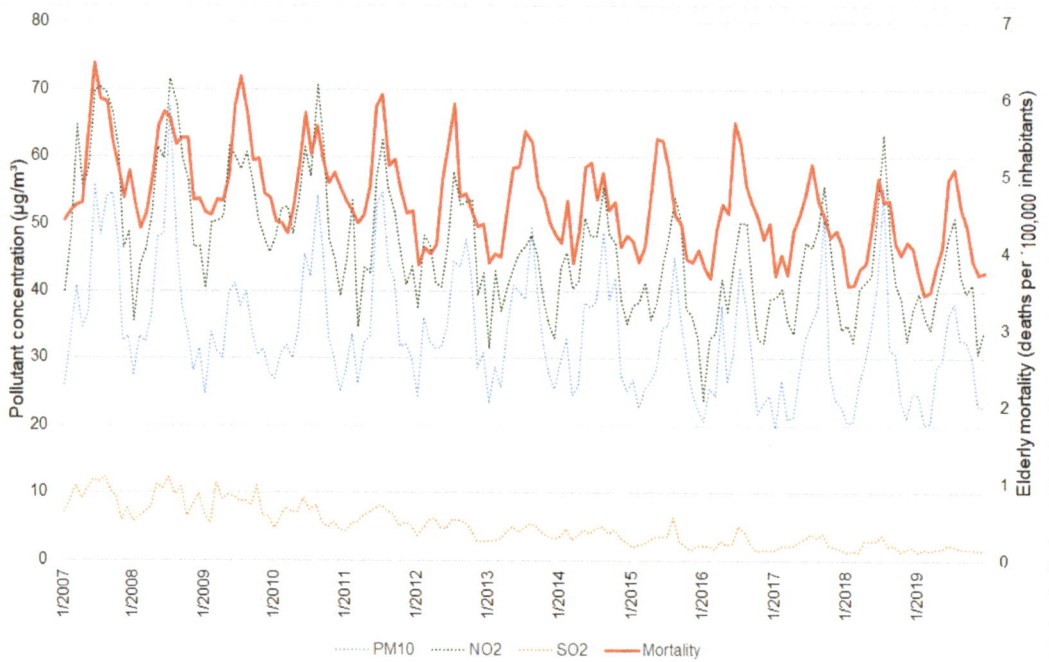

Figure 3. Line graph showing the daily variation of the concentrations of PM_{10}, NO_2, and SO_2 variables and elderly mortality between 2007 and 2019.

Regarding the meteorological variables, there were few changes over the analyzed period, except for the air relative humidity in 2014, which was considered an extremely dry year in the region of São Paulo [57]. It is observed that, in that year, the relative humidity was the lowest in the time series and that, during the rainy season, it was even lower than the one recorded during the dry season (76.5% during the rainy season versus 78.9% during the dry season) (Figure 4).

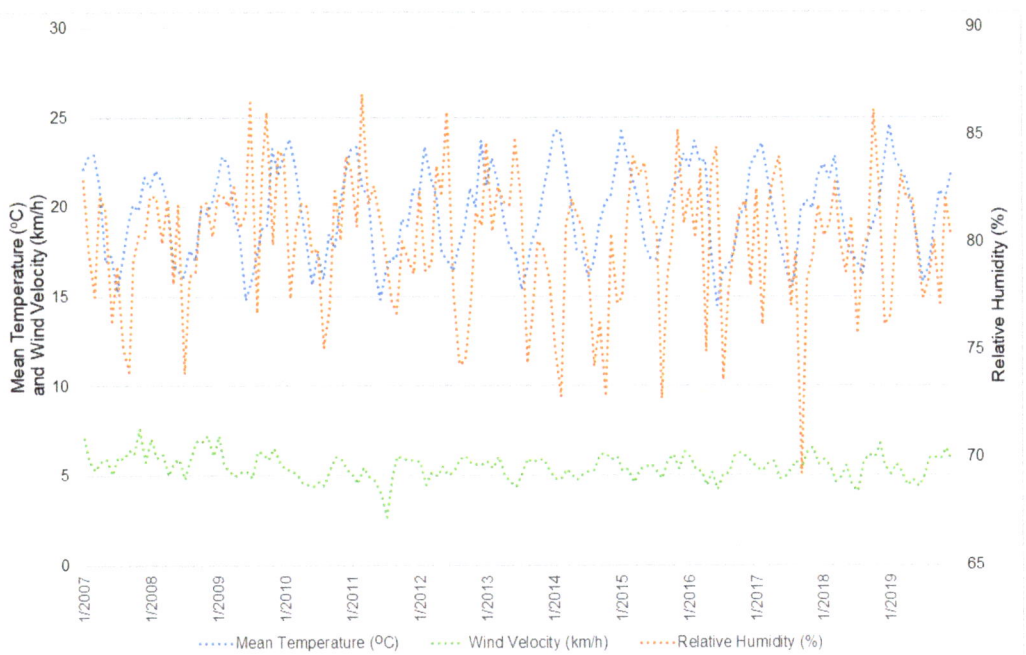

Figure 4. Line graph showing the daily variation of the mean temperature, wind velocity, and relative humidity variables between 2007 and 2019.

As well as the pollutants' concentrations, the daily mortality rate due to cardiorespiratory problems in the elderly decreased between 2007 and 2019 (from 5.2 to 4.08 per 100,000 inhabitants) (Figure 3). In both the pollutant concentrations and the cardiorespiratory mortality, is possible to clearly note the seasonality of the data, with peaks during the dry season (Figure 3).

3.2. Artificial Neural Networks

By analyzing the results of Model I (which considered all the available data for rainy and dry seasons), the ANN that best fitted the data had only one hidden layer and was composed of six input neurons, 25 neurons on the hidden layer, and one output neuron. The learning algorithm was trainlm, and the combination of activation functions was tansig and purelin. The value of the objective function was 0.614 for the training step, which is very low. The mean absolute percentage error (MAPE) of the ANN configuration was 13.46%. The mean errors of all ANN configurations ranged from 13.46% to 54.93%.

Based on this ANN, the estimated cardiorespiratory mortality (deaths per 10^5 elderly inhabitants) ranged between 0.59 and 6.29 while the real mortality ranged from 2.03 to 8.58. The errors of these estimates ranged between 0% and 131%. The biggest errors were concentrated in the estimates of the highest values of cardiorespiratory mortality (Figure 5).

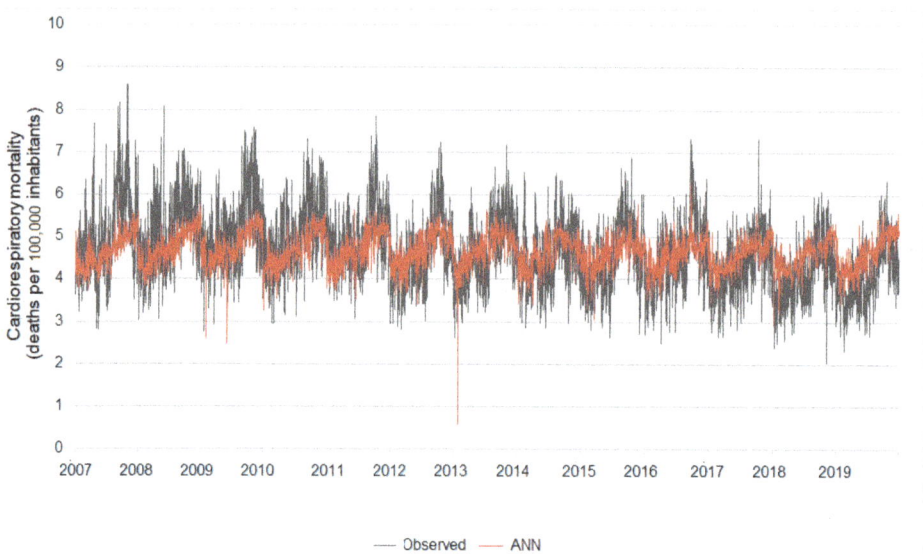

Figure 5. Real daily cardiorespiratory mortality versus that estimated by the Model I ANN. Results considering the ANN build from the entire database (considering rainy and dry seasons).

Considering Model II, in which only the data from the rainy season were used, the best ANN was the one hidden layer ANN composed of six input neurons, 30 neurons on the hidden layer, and one output neuron. The learning algorithm and the combination of activation functions were the same as the best ANN, considering the entire database (learning algorithm: trainlm; activation functions: tansig and purelin). The value of the objective function in the training step was equal to 0.375. and the MAPE was equal to 11.68%. The mean error of all ANN configurations ranged from 11.68% to 81.53%.

Based on this ANN, the estimated daily cardiorespiratory mortality ranged between 3.43 and 6.23 deaths per 10^5 elderly inhabitants. The real mortality considering only the data from the rainy season ranged from 2.30 to 8.09. The errors of these estimates ranged between 0% and 79% (Figure 6).

Finally, Model III, in which only data from the dry season were considered, the best-fitted ANN also had only one hidden layer. Its structure was six input neurons, 30 neurons in the hidden layer, and one output neuron. The learning algorithm was also trainlm, and the combination of activation functions, tansig and purelin. The value of the objective function of the training step was 0.452. The resulting mean absolute percentage was 11.07%. The mean error of all ANN configurations ranged from 11.07% to 58.55%.

Based on this ANN, the estimated cardiorespiratory mortality ranged between 3.64 and 8.60 deaths per 10^5 elderly inhabitants while the observed mortality ranged from 2.03 to 8.58. The errors of these estimates ranged between 0% and 144%. As observed in the results of the best-fitted ANN considering the entire database, the biggest errors were concerned with estimates of the lowest values of cardiorespiratory mortality (Figure 7).

The best structures of each one of the models were tested through 50 training iterations. The MSE distribution test is presented in Figure 8. For the models I, II, and III presented in the study, the MSE were 0.616, 0.375, and 0.452, respectively. The dispersion of the MSE presented a similar range for the three models (between 0.12 and 0.14).

The three models presented errors lower than 20% in more than 75% of the observations (Figure 9). Model I (considering the entire database) was the one with the highest MAPE (13%). By dividing the database according to season (rainy or dry), the MAPE was reduced to 11% in both models (I and II). This mean reduction was considered statistically significant (comparison between Models I and II: t test (7115) = 6.428; $p < 0.05$. Comparison between Models I and III: t test (7115) = 9.311; $p < 0.05$). The adoption of different models according to the season was also reflected in the reduction in outliers in the forecasts (Figure 9).

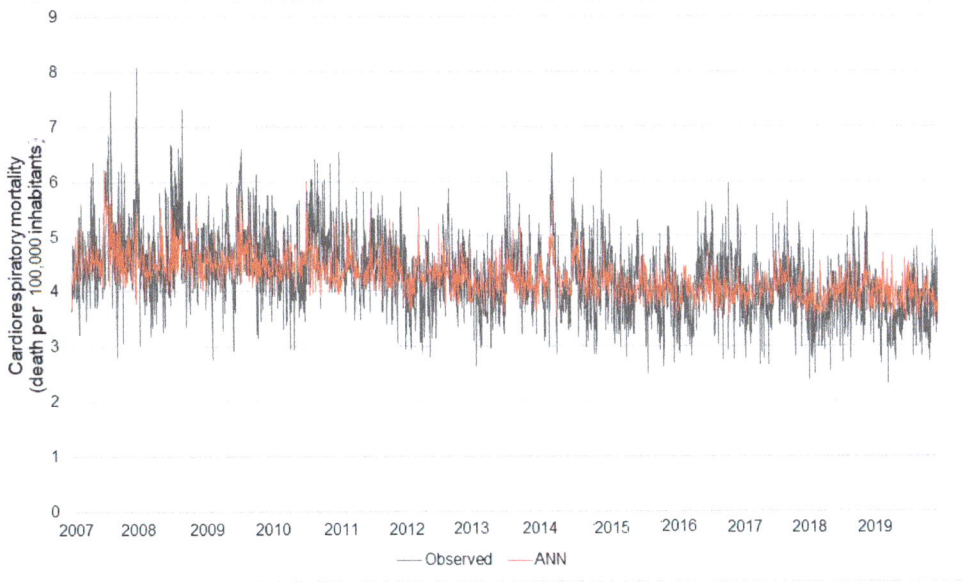

Figure 6. Real daily cardiorespiratory mortality versus that estimated by the Model II ANN. Results considering the ANN build from the rainy season database.

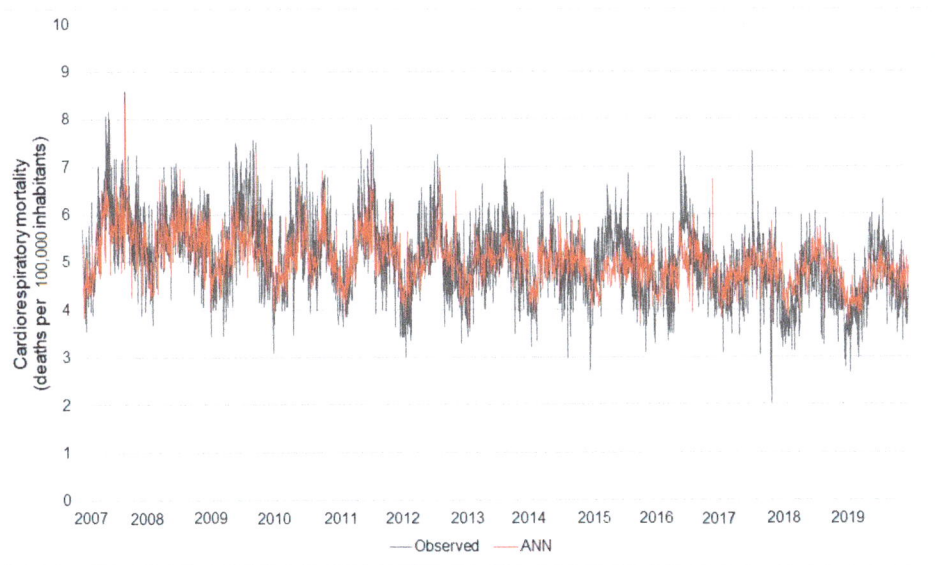

Figure 7. Real daily cardiorespiratory mortality versus that estimated by the Model III ANN. Results considering the ANN build from the dry season database.

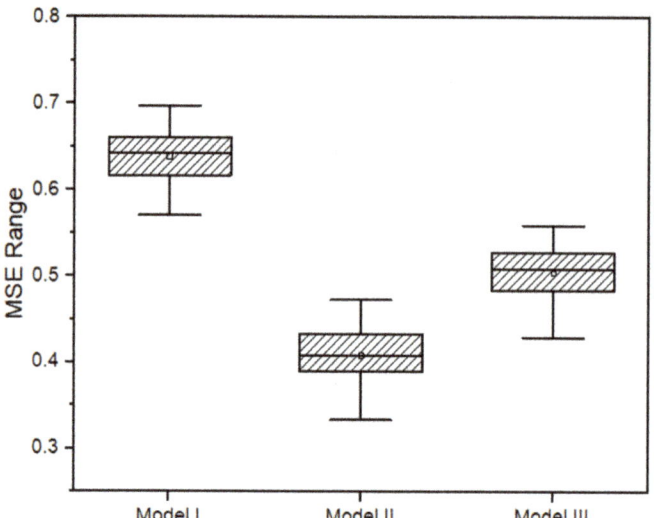

Figure 8. Boxplot indicating the MSE range from the training of the best ANN structure for each model. Vertical bars indicate the 1st and 4th quartiles. The dot inside the box indicates the mean value, and the horizontal bar indicates the median value.

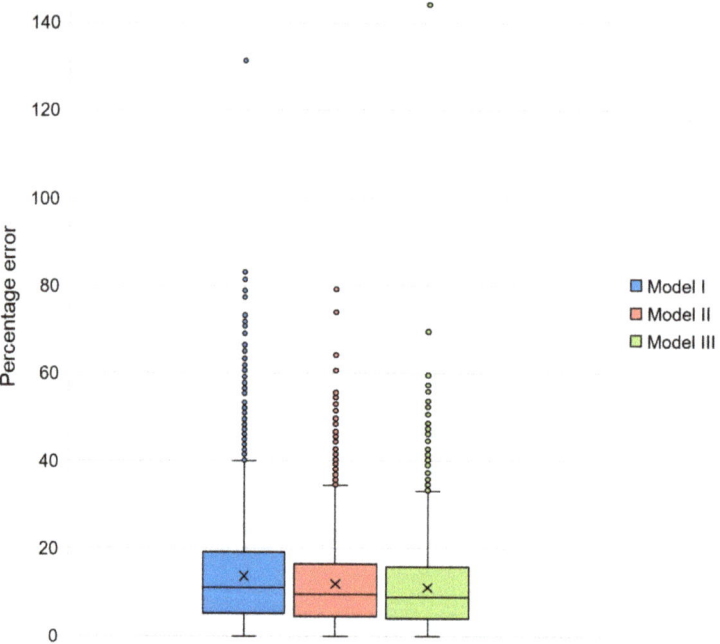

Figure 9. Boxplot indicating the MAPE distribution in Models I, II, and III. The box represents data between the 2nd and 3rd quartiles. Vertical bars indicate the 1st and 4th quartiles, and the circles represent the outliers. The × inside the box indicates the mean value, and the horizontal bar indicates the median value.

The structures of the best-fitted ANNs described above can be represented according to Equations (5) and (6):

Model I:

$$y_k = \sum_{j=1}^{25} w_{jk} \text{tansig} \left(\sum_{i=1}^{6} w_{ij} x_i + b_j \right)_j + b_k \quad (5)$$

Models II and III:

$$y_k = \sum_{j=1}^{30} w_{jk} \text{tansig} \left(\sum_{i=1}^{6} w_{ij} x_i + b_j \right)_j + b_k \quad (6)$$

where y_k is the desired output, w_{ij} and w_{jk} are the weights of the neurons in the hidden and output layers, respectively, and b_j and b_k are the bias of the neurons in the hidden and output layers, respectively. The weights and the bias for each model are given in the Supplemental Table S1.

After defining the best ANN for the three considered datasets, the determination of the influence of the inputs was obtained by using the connection weight method. The results are shown in Table 1. Among all the considered variables, for Model I, the results showed that SO_2 concentration was considered the most important variable, with 46.75% weight. When the rainy (Model II) and dry (Model III) seasons were separately analyzed, the PM_{10} concentration was revealed as the most important variable for both ANNs, with the importance of 68.34% and 29.07%, respectively. NO_2 concentration was presented as the second or third most influential variable in the models. Concerning the meteorological variables, wind speed is the least important variable in all three models. Temperature is more important during the rainy season, which comprises the summer (higher mean temperature), and relative humidity is more important during the dry season when the mean relative humidity is lower.

Table 1. Relative importance (%) of each variable for cardiorespiratory mortality. The importance is presented according to the three ANNs obtained: the first one considers all databases (Model I), the second considers only data from the rainy season (Model II), and the third considers the data from the dry season (Model III).

Variable	Importance (Position of Importance) (%)		
	Model I	Model II	Model III
PM_{10} concentration	12.32 (4)	68.34 (1)	29.07 (1)
NO_2 concentration	13.22 (3)	6.81 (3)	27.02 (2)
SO_2 concentration	46.75 (1)	3.01 (5)	16.51 (4)
Temperature	19.11 (2)	13.10 (2)	9.56 (5)
Relative humidity	4.80 (5)	6.10 (4)	16.67 (3)
Wind speed	3.80 (6)	2.64 (6)	1.17 (6)

3.3. ANN Validation by the Comparison with GLM Model

According to the basic model results, the whole set of variables was considered in Models I′ and III′, and only the wind speed was excluded from Model II′ ($p = 0.125$).

In Model I′, considering the entire database, all input variables except for PM_{10} concentration, temperature, and wind speed were considered relevant to cardiorespiratory mortality among the elderly ($p < 0.000$). As in the analysis of importance performed from Model I, in Model I′, the concentration of SO_2 showed a greater impact on the response variable than the concentration of the other pollutants analyzed ($\beta = -0.003$). Wind speed was excluded from Model II′ because it presented a p-value > 0.05 in the previous basic model. All other variables were considered significative in Model II′. In Model III′, wind speed was the only variable that did not present a p-value < 0.05. The parameter estimates for the pollutants in Models II′ and III′ were very similar to the ones estimated in Model I′ (Table 2).

Table 2. Estimated parameters for Models I', II', and III'. The generalized linear models were elaborated on SPSS software considering gamma distribution and a loglink equation.

	Model I'				Model II'				Model III'			
	β	95% CI		p-Value	β	95% CI		p-Value	β	95% CI		p-Value
(Intercept)	1.626	1.528	1.724	<0.000	1.168	1.021	1.315	<0.000	1.583	1.464	1.703	<0.000
PM$_{10}$	0.000	0.000	0.001	0.500	0.000	−0.001	0.001	0.753	0.001	0.000	0.002	0.008
NO$_2$	0.001	0.000	0.001	0.014	0.000	0.000	0.001	0.543	0.001	0.000	0.002	0.036
SO$_2$	−0.003	0.005	−0.001	0.003	−0.002	−0.005	0.000	0.104	−0.003	−0.006	0.000	0.035
Temperature	0.001	−0.002	0.003	0.648	0.011	0.007	0.015	<0.000	−0.008	−0.011	−0.005	<0.000
Relative humidity	−0.002	−0.003	−0.001	<0.000	−0.001	−0.002	0.000	0.009	−0.001	−0.002	0.000	0.035
Wind speed	−0.001	−0.004	0.002	0.570					0.002	−0.002	0.006	0.349

The separation of the database into two according to the season resulted in lower MAPEs for both Model II' (rainy season; t test (7115) = 4.323; $p < 0.000$) and Model III' (dry season; t test (7115) = 5.311; $p < 0.000$). Model I' presented a MAPE equal to 12.49%. and in Models II' and III', the MAPEs were equal to 11.08% and 10.76%, respectively. The MAPE distribution on each one of the models was very similar to the distribution resulting from the ANN models (Figure 10).

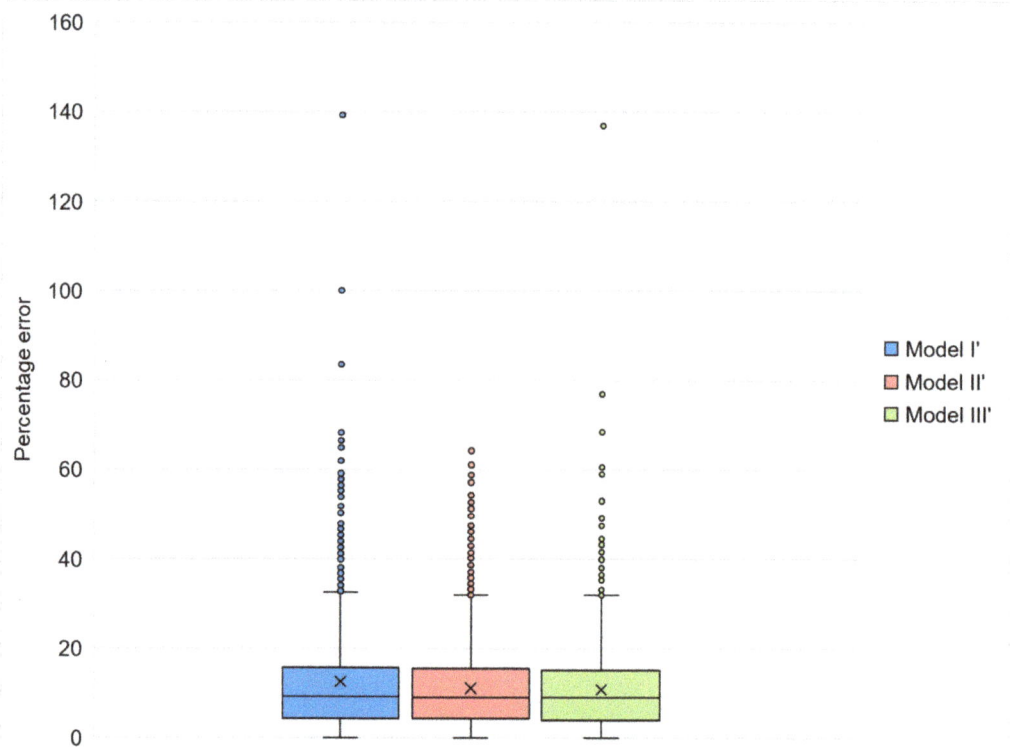

Figure 10. Boxplot indicating the MAPE distribution in Models I', II', and III'. The box represents data between the 2nd and 3rd quartiles. Vertical bars indicate the 1st and 4th quartiles, and the circles represent the outliers. The × inside the box indicates the mean value, and the horizontal bar indicates the median value.

4. Discussion

Air quality improvement in the city of São Paulo has been consistently observed over the last 30 years as a result of a series of environmental policies [58]. Throughout the 1990s, the city experienced an exit from industries, which settled in nearby regions in the interior of the state, and its economy began to be based on the services sector and business management [59]. As a consequence of industrial migration and the increase in the number of inhabitants from medium and high-income groups, mobile sources are the main factors responsible for air pollution [53,58]. Therefore, the main policies for the improvement in air quality observed since the 2000s are the no-drive day (in force since 1997) and a national program that imposes new technologies on vehicles and fuels, named PROCONVE [60,61]. Regarding PROCONVE, the mandatory use of catalysts in engines and the reduction in fuel sulfur content were responsible for the reduction in the CO, hydrocarbons, and SO_2 atmospheric concentrations [62–65]. In addition to these programs, more specific measures aimed at reducing heavy-duty vehicle emissions were adopted, such as the construction of a beltway road and driving restrictions for trucks in some corridors during the day time. These measures have contributed to reducing the concentration of pollutants such as NO_x and PM, bringing health improvements [66,67]. Despite the positive results attributed to these environmental policies, São Paulo continues to have air pollution levels above those recommended by the WHO, representing a constant risk to the health of the population [58]. So, studies aiming to model the health impacts of the air quality in Sao Paulo are still of great importance even with the reduction in the concentration of pollutants.

The seasonality observed in the concentration of pollutants is also followed by a seasonality in cardiorespiratory mortality among the elderly (see Figure 3). The annual variation in the concentration of pollutants is a consequence of the meteorological characteristics typically found in the two seasons of the year (rainy and dry), with the months between May and September being the most unfavorable to the pollutants' dispersion [53]. According to Sánchez-Ccoyllo and de Andrade [68], there is an increase in the concentration of particulate matter in the Metropolitan Region of São Paulo on days with high temperature, low relative humidity, absence of precipitation, and weak ventilation. Considering this, the worst pollution days tend to occur during the winter (between June and September), when these factors are more frequently associated [65]. In winter periods, the phenomenon of thermal inversion is also common in the municipality, which makes it difficult to disperse pollutants [69]. Air pollution is worse in the winter because colder and drier air traps more pollution. Added to this, long periods of drought in this season lead to occasional increases in the concentration, mainly of particulate matter [53]. Possibly, meteorological conditions are mainly responsible for the difference in the concentration of pollutants throughout the year, since it has already been demonstrated that the origin of particulate pollutants remains very similar during summer and winter [70]. In São Paulo, the winter is characterized by the driest period of the year. Thus, in addition to the greater amount of pollutants that penetrate the respiratory system, in this season, the elderly are also more susceptible to infections such as influenza and pneumonia, which are common during the winter and contribute to cardiorespiratory impairment [71,72]. The air pollution increment and the increased occurrence of respiratory diseases during the dry season explain the seasonality observed over the analyzed time series.

Unlike the models most frequently used to relate meteorological and pollution data with health outcomes, ANNs do not need prior adjustments due to the interaction between the input variables [73]. ANN models also do not require prior adjustments due to the seasonality of the data. In the application of the GLM, for example, the smoothing of seasonality must be undertaken considering explanatory variables related to this seasonality in the model or through techniques such as loess and cubic splines [56]. Thus, this work could simultaneously assess the effect of six variables on cardiorespiratory mortality among elderly people in São Paulo without previous data treatment. This possibility represents a great advance in relation to the linear models since these classical models are not efficient in managing interactions among the input variables [38]. In addition to the ability to manage multicollinearity, several studies that compared ANNs with other approaches pointed out that ANNs result in models with better precision [49,74,75].

By allowing the analysis of several variables regardless of the relationship among them, studies that apply ANNs to estimate the effects of air pollution on human health vary greatly in relation to the explanatory variables. Some studies, for instance, considered only pollutant concentrations [75,76]. Other studies included meteorological variables, days of the week, and traffic data as explanatory variables as well [77,78]. The presentation of the model's quality also varies among the studies, with indicators such as mean square error (MSE), mean error (ME), mean absolute percentage error (MAPE), and R-square (R^2). The diversity of variables and results constitutes an obstacle to the comparison of the results obtained in the studies.

Previous ANNs that related human health outcomes to pollutant concentrations in the São Paulo municipality reached higher MAPEs than the ones found in this work. Araujo et al. [49] considered PM_{10} concentration, temperature, relative humidity, days of the week, and holidays to estimate respiratory hospital admissions. They tested lags, and the best-fitted ANN reached a MAPE equal to 26%. Tadano et al. [78] considered the same input and output variables and obtained an ANN with a MAPE of 35%. Finally, Kachba et al. [77] considered CO, NO_x, O_3, SO_2, and PM concentrations and traffic data to infer respiratory hospital admissions and mortality and obtained a MAPE of 28% when analyzing the hospital admissions and 34% when analyzing the mortality.

Our model counted more input variables and a larger database (daily measures in a 12-year period), which could have improved the accuracy of the model resulting in a lower MAPE (11–13%). In addition, we considered data from several air quality monitoring stations, which could better represent the population exposure. According to Seo et al. (2022), by using data from multiple monitoring stations, the error associated with the ANN model can be lowered [79]. The previous studies conducted in São Paulo highlighted the great variability among the data, which may compromise the ability of the model to estimate the most extreme values [49,50]. In this work, the database was split into two seasons with specific meteorological characteristics (Models II and III) and proved to be an efficient way to deal with extreme values, reducing the MAPE to 11% (see Figure 8). The MAPE obtained in the present study is also low in comparison to the ones found in studies conducted in other cities. Polezer et al. [80], for instance, fitted $PM_{2.5}$ concentration, temperature, and relative humidity data in order to estimate respiratory hospital admissions. Their best-fitted ANN resulted in a MAPE of 29%.

Another factor that may have contributed to the results seen in this study is the focus of the analysis on the elderly population, which is the most affected by air pollutants.

The analysis of the most important variables in each of the models confirms that the data split into two seasons (rainy and dry), generating two distinct models, is a relevant strategy for estimating cardiorespiratory mortality as a function of the considered variables. In Model II, we considered the rainy period as our database. During this period, the relative humidity averaged 80% and, in just 1% of the days, it was below 60%. Keeping in mined indices considered healthy according to the WHO, the importance of this variable for the model was relatively low (6.10%). In other words, it can be inferred that, as the relative humidity remained in an interval considered healthy for almost the entire time series, it had little responsibility for the deaths that occurred on those days.

On the other hand, during the dry season, although the average relative humidity was similar to that of the rainy season (79%), 4% of the days recorded relative humidity below 60%. The greatest variance in the data is the result of days in which the relative humidity was much lower than that recommended by the WHO. In September, for example, relative humidities below 40% were recorded. The low relative humidity of the air, added to colder days, causes the drying of the respiratory surface mucosa, which can facilitate infections [81]. In addition, it decreases the activity of cilia that help remove particles from the air [82]. This impact of low relative humidity on health was captured by Model III, since in this model relative humidity reached an importance almost three times greater in relation to mortality among the elderly (16.67%).

A similar analysis can be performed regarding temperature. In São Paulo, summer occurs during the rainy season, and therefore, this season tends to register higher averages and higher temperature peaks. During the analyzed rainy season, 8.1% of the days had an average daily temperature above 25 °C. On those days, the temperature exceeded 30 °C, setting up possible heat waves. Studies have shown that the elderly are part of the group most affected by the occurrence of heat waves. This is because, with aging, responses to environmental conditions (which include thermoregulation) deteriorate [83]. According to the WHO, high temperatures directly contribute to cardiorespiratory mortality, especially among the elderly. In São Paulo, heat waves have already been associated with excess deaths related to both cardiovascular and respiratory systems. The cardiovascular system seems to be the most affected, and it is estimated that between 1985 and 2005, there were 6% excess deaths among elderly women and 2.5% among elderly men due to the occurrence of heat waves in São Paulo [84]. As in the rainy season, the temperature tends to be higher, and our Model II was able to detect the greater influence of temperature on cardiorespiratory mortality among the elderly. In this case, the importance was 13.1%, while during the dry period (Model III), when temperatures tend to be lower, the importance of temperature was lower (9.5%). According to Nguyen et al. [82], the high temperature associated with high humidity (which is very characteristic of the rainy season in São Paulo) requires an increase in the body's heat loss through the body surface. This is achieved through blood circulation, resulting in water loss and increased hemoconcentration. This phenomenon overloads the cardiovascular and respiratory systems, and may result in death [82].

In models II and III, PM_{10} and NO_2 pollutants are among the three most influential variables on elderly cardiorespiratory mortality. The annual mean concentrations registered for both pollutants between 2007 and 2019 were consistently higher than the WHO recommendations. For PM_{10}, the annual concentration ranged from 28.35 µg/m^3 to 41.49 µg/m^3, while the WHO recommendation is to not exceed 15 µg/m^3 [52]. For NO_2, the concentrations ranged from 38.25 µg/m^3 to 58.36 µg/m^3, while the WHO recommendation is below 10 µg/m^3 [52]. Considering the 24 h period, the WHO recommendation is to not exceed 45 µg/m^3 for PM_{10} and 25 µg/m^3 for NO_2 [52]. These values were surpassed in 19.8% of the days for PM_{10} and in 92.4% of the days for NO_2.

NO_2 concentration is of concern because is the most critical in relation to WHO recommendations, even though it is not the most important variable according to Models I and II. In São Paulo, vehicles are responsible for 65% of the NO_2 emissions and, despite the technological advances that have an effect on reducing emissions, the increase in the fleet and the high circulation of old vehicles are obstacles to improving air quality [58,61,85]. According to recent studies focused on limitations imposed on heavy-duty vehicles, these measures may be essential to maintain the NO_2 concentration within the standards recommended by WHO in São Paulo [66,86].

Exposure to NO_2 has already been associated with several respiratory symptoms, such as bronchoconstriction, increased bronchial reactivity, airway inflammation, and decreases in immune defense leading to enhanced susceptibility to respiratory infections [87]. All of these are exacerbated in susceptible populations, such as the elderly. According to Larrieu et al. [18], in a cohort study conducted in France between 200 and 2006, the 10 µg/m^3 enhancement in NO_2 concentration led to an excess relative risk of 12.3% for upper respiratory disease and 9% for lower respiratory disease among the elderly. The relative risk increase was higher for NO_2 than for PM_{10} and O_3 pollutants [18]. In addition to the direct health impacts from NO_2, it is important to emphasize that NO_2 concentration is closely related to the concentration of other pollutants, such as $PM_{2.5}$, O_3, and CO. So, it is unclear to what extent the impacts are due to only to NO_2 exposure or to the other pollutants too [87].

SO_2 was the pollutant whose reduction was the most significant in the last 30 years in São Paulo [58]. This reduction was mainly a consequence of the regulation of the stationary sources and of the sulfur content in diesel fuel [58]. The atmospheric concentration of this pollutant remained below the limits recommended by the WHO throughout the time series analyzed in this study. Even so, SO_2 concentration was identified as having high importance in the cardiorespiratory mortality of elderly people in São Paulo. This result reinforces the need for public policies aimed at reducing the concentration of all pollutants and not just $PM_{2.5}$. Moreover, considering the increase in the global proportion of elderly people among the population, understanding how small changes in air quality and weather conditions affect this group is fundamental to improving the quality of life [11,12].

The comparison between our ANN models with traditional GLMs revealed similar errors, validating the efficiency of ANN in modeling this type of data. It was also possible to observe (see Figures 9 and 10) that the distribution of errors in models constructed from ANNs is less variable than the distribution in GLMs. The superiority of neural networks in relation to other models has also been described by Araújo et al. In the case study carried out by the authors in São Paulo, the neural network presented a MAPE equal to 26%, while the MAPE of the GLM was 35% [49]. It is also important to emphasize that, unlike the most traditional model, an ANN is not subjected to multicollinearity issues. In our GLM models, evidence of multicollinearity is observed, such as negative β values describing relationships that should be directly related. In the ANN models, this problem is not present. According to Veaux and Ungar [88], due to the overparameterized aspect of the ANNs, they are insensitive to this problem and they can deal with multicollinear inputs without loss of precision.

Splitting the database into two according to seasons proved to be an efficient strategy in reducing errors for models built from ANNs and GLMs. The error difference found between Model I and Models II and II is probably because of the size of our database (n = 4748). When using the whole time series, the data pattern becomes too confusing for ANN to establish a pattern. When it is divided into the rainy and dry seasons, the pattern of the relationship between the variables becomes more constant.

As a gap that may be covered by further research, we suggest lag analyses. In this study, the efforts were focused on exploring the use of ANNs, which are still extremely underexplored in relating meteorological and pollution data to predict health outcomes. We also innovated by proposing the separation of the database as a strategy to reduce model error. Our analysis was limited to lag0, and it is known that although several physiological effects due to pollutants' presence in the organism occur within hours of exposure, death (especially cardiovascular) may take longer to occur [14,23]. The limitation of the study to lag 0 restricts but does not invalidate the analysis since mortality at lag 0 for both cardiovascular and respiratory causes has also been described by other authors [89–91].

As an artificial intelligence (AI) method, the use of ANNs has great potential to face typical challenges from low and middle-income countries, contributing to the achievement of health-related sustainable development goals [92]. Despite this potential, when it comes to the air pollution issue, most approaches have been aiming to forecast human exposure through air quality modeling [47]. Our work demonstrates that ANNs can be used to solve the problem inherent in common models used in multipollutant analysis and that the associated error can be very low.

5. Conclusions

This research took advantage of an artificial neural network approach to estimate elderly mortality due to cardiorespiratory issues as a function of the interaction of several air pollutants and meteorological variables. The method proved efficient in dealing with the classical model limitations and resulted in a MAPE of 13%, which is lower than the MAPEs presented in previous studies that applied ANN technics. Additionally, the strategy of splitting the database into two seasons was presented as an efficient strategy to improve the estimation of extreme values and reduce the MAPE. PM_{10} and NO_2 concentrations were among the most influential variables on cardiorespiratory mortality among the elderly in both models (rainy and dry seasons). The influence of relative humidity is higher during the dry season, and the influence of temperature is higher during the rainy season. Our results support a better understanding of the effect of the combination of air pollutants on human health. In addition, the resulting models have a low associated error, configuring a powerful tool for decision-makers in the evaluation of environmental public policies aimed at public health.

Supplementary Materials: The following are available online at https://www.mdpi.com/article/10.3390/ijerph20085458/s1, Table S1: The weights and the bias for 3 models.

Author Contributions: Conceptualization, L.L.; methodology, T.M.; validation, L.L., T.M. and S.M.; formal analysis, M.d.O.; investigation, L.L. and M.d.O.; data curation, L.L. and M.d.O.; writing—original draft preparation, L.L.; writing—review and editing, L.L., M.d.O., T.M. and S.M.; supervision, S.M.; project administration, S.M.; funding acquisition, L.L. and S.M. All authors have read and agreed to the published version of the manuscript.

Funding: This research was funded by the Coordenação de Aperfeiçoamento de Pessoal de Nível Superior, grant number 1808525, and by the Conselho Nacional de Desenvolvimento Científico e Tecnológico, grant number 161316/2021-2 and 308378/2021-0.

Institutional Review Board Statement: Not applicable.

Informed Consent Statement: Not applicable.

Data Availability Statement: No new data were created or analyzed in this study. Data sharing is not applicable to this article.

Conflicts of Interest: The authors declare no conflict of interest.

References

1. WHO. Ambient Air Pollution. Available online: https://www.who.int/teams/environment-climate-change-and-health/air-quality-and-health/ambient-air-pollution (accessed on 1 August 2021).
2. GBD 2019 Risk Factors Collaborators. Global Burden of 87 Risk Factors in 204 Countries and Territories, 1990–2019: A Systematic Analysis for the Global Burden of Disease Study 2019. *Lancet* **2020**, *396*, 1223–1249. [CrossRef]
3. Burnett, R.; Chen, H.; Fann, N.; Hubbell, B.; Pope, C.A.; Frostad, J.; Lim, S.S.; Kan, H.; Walker, K.D.; Thurston, G.D.; et al. Global Estimates of Mortality Associated with Long-Term Exposure to Outdoor Fine Particulate Matter. *Proc. Natl. Acad. Sci. USA* **2018**, *115*, 9592–9597. [CrossRef] [PubMed]
4. Sun, Z.; Zhu, D. Exposure to Outdoor Air Pollution and Its Human Health Outcomes: A Scoping Review. *PLoS ONE* **2019**, *14*, e0216550. [CrossRef]
5. Requia, W.J.; Adams, M.D.; Arain, A.; Papatheodorou, S.; Koutrakis, P.; Mahmoud, M. Global Association of Air Pollution and Cardiorespiratory Diseases: A Systematic Review, Meta-Analysis, and Investigation of Modifier Variables. *Am. J. Public Health* **2018**, *108*, S123–S130. [CrossRef] [PubMed]
6. Newell, K.; Kartsonaki, C.; Lam, K.B.H.; Kurmi, O.P. Cardiorespiratory Health Effects of Particulate Ambient Air Pollution Exposure in Low-Income and Middle-Income Countries: A Systematic Review and Meta-Analysis. *Lancet Planet. Health* **2017**, *1*, e360–e367. [CrossRef]
7. Krall, J.R.; Chang, H.H.; Waller, L.A.; Mulholland, J.A.; Winquist, A.; Talbott, E.O.; Rager, J.R.; Tolbert, P.E.; Sarnat, S.E. A Multicity Study of Air Pollution and Cardiorespiratory Emergency Department Visits: Comparing Approaches for Combining Estimates across Cities. *Environ. Int.* **2018**, *120*, 312–320. [CrossRef]
8. Seposo, X.; Ueda, K.; Sugata, S.; Yoshino, A.; Takami, A. Short-Term Effects of Air Pollution on Daily Single- and Co-Morbidity Cardiorespiratory Outpatient Visits. *Sci. Total Environ.* **2020**, *729*, 138934. [CrossRef] [PubMed]
9. Landrigan, P.J. Air Pollution and Health. *Lancet Public Health* **2017**, *2*, e4–e5. [CrossRef] [PubMed]
10. Makri, A.; Stilianakis, N.I. Vulnerability to Air Pollution Health Effects. *Int. J. Hyg. Environ. Health* **2008**, *211*, 326–336. [CrossRef] [PubMed]
11. Bentayeb, M.; Simoni, M.; Baiz, N.; Norback, D.; Baldacci, S.; Maio, S.; Viegi, G.; Annesi-Maesano, I. Adverse Respiratory Effects of Outdoor Air Pollution in the Elderly. *Int. J. Tuberc. Lung Dis.* **2012**, *16*, 1149–1161. [CrossRef] [PubMed]
12. Simoni, M.; Baldacci, S.; Maio, S.; Cerrai, S.; Sarno, G.; Viegi, G. Adverse Effects of Outdoor Pollution in the Elderly. *J. Thorac. Dis.* **2015**, *7*, 34–45. [CrossRef] [PubMed]
13. Koken, P.J.M.; Piver, W.T.; Ye, F.; Elixhauser, A.; Olsen, L.M.; Portier, C.J. Temperature, Air Pollution, and Hospitalization for Cardiovascular Diseases among Elderly People in Denver. *Environ. Health Perspect.* **2003**, *111*, 1312–1317. [CrossRef] [PubMed]
14. Kim, S.E.; Lim, Y.H.; Kim, H. Temperature Modifies the Association between Particulate Air Pollution and Mortality: A Multi-City Study in South Korea. *Sci. Total Environ.* **2015**, *524–525*, 376–383. [CrossRef]

15. Lepeule, J.; Litonjua, A.A.; Gasparrini, A.; Koutrakis, P.; Sparrow, D.; Vokonas, P.S.; Schwartz, J. Lung Function Association with Outdoor Temperature and Relative Humidity and Its Interaction with Air Pollution in the Elderly. *Environ. Res.* **2018**, *165*, 110–117. [CrossRef]
16. Schwartz, J. Short Term Fluctuations in Air Pollution and Hospital Admissions of the Elderly for Respiratory Disease. *Thorax* **1995**, *50*, 531–538. [CrossRef]
17. Medina-Ramón, M.; Zanobetti, A.; Schwartz, J. The Effect of Ozone and PM10 on Hospital Admissions for Pneumonia and Chronic Obstructive Pulmonary Disease: A National Multicity Study. *Am. J. Epidemiol.* **2006**, *163*, 579–588. [CrossRef] [PubMed]
18. Larrieu, S.; Lefranc, A.; Gault, G.; Chatignoux, E.; Couvy, F.; Jouves, B.; Filleul, L. Are the Short-Term Effects of Air Pollution Restricted to Cardiorespiratory Diseases? *Am. J. Epidemiol.* **2009**, *169*, 1201–1208. [CrossRef] [PubMed]
19. Franklin, M.; Zeka, A.; Schwartz, J. Association between PM2.5 and All-Cause and Specific-Cause Mortality in 27 US Communities. *J. Expo. Sci. Environ. Epidemiol.* **2007**, *17*, 279–287. [CrossRef]
20. Brunekreef, B.; Hoek, G.; Schouten, L.; Bausch-Goldbohm, S.; Fischer, P.; Armstrong, B.G.; Hughes, E.; Jerrett, M.; Beelen, R.; van den Brandt, P.A. Effects of Long-Term Exposure to Traffic-Related Air Pollution on Respiratory and Cardiovascular Mortality in the Netherlands: The NLCS-AIR Study. *Res. Rep. (Health Eff. Inst.)* **2009**, *139*, 5–71.
21. Dong, G.H.; Zhang, P.; Sun, B.; Zhang, L.; Chen, X.; Ma, N.; Yu, F.; Guo, H.; Huang, H.; Lee, Y.L.; et al. Long-Term Exposure to Ambient Air Pollution and Respiratory Disease Mortality in Shenyang, China: A 12-Year Population-Based Retrospective Cohort Study. *Respiration* **2012**, *84*, 360–368. [CrossRef]
22. Dominski, F.H.; Lorenzetti Branco, J.H.; Buonanno, G.; Stabile, L.; Gameiro da Silva, M.; Andrade, A. Effects of Air Pollution on Health: A Mapping Review of Systematic Reviews and Meta-Analyses. *Environ. Res.* **2021**, *201*, 111487. [CrossRef]
23. Yap, J.; Ng, Y.; Yeo, K.K.; Sahlén, A.; Lam, C.S.P.; Lee, V.; Ma, S. Particulate Air Pollution on Cardiovascular Mortality in the Tropics: Impact on the Elderly. *Environ. Health A Glob. Access Sci. Source* **2019**, *18*, 34. [CrossRef]
24. IBGE. Panorama São Paulo. Available online: https://cidades.ibge.gov.br/brasil/sp/sao-paulo/panorama (accessed on 20 October 2022).
25. Abe, K.C.; Miraglia, S.G.E.K. Health Impact Assessment of Air Pollution in São Paulo, Brazil. *Int. J. Environ. Res. Public Health* **2016**, *13*, 694. [CrossRef] [PubMed]
26. Ministério da Infraestrutura Frota de Veículos. 2021. Available online: https://www.gov.br/infraestrutura/pt-br/assuntos/transito/conteudo-Senatran/frota-de-veiculos-2021 (accessed on 20 October 2022).
27. SEADE PIB SP. Available online: https://www.seade.gov.br/produtos2/ (accessed on 10 April 2021).
28. Saldiva, P.H.N.; Lichtenfels, A.J.; Paiva, P.S.O.; Barone, I.A.; Martins, M.A.; Massad, E.; Pereira, J.C.R.; Xavier, V.P.; Singer, J.M.; Böhm, G.M. Association between Air Pollution and Mortality Due to Respiratory Diseases in Children in São Paulo, Brasil. *Environ. Res.* **1994**, *65*, 218–225. [CrossRef]
29. Saldiva, P.H.N.; Pope III, C.A.; Schwartz, J.; Dockery, D.W.; Lichtenfels, A.J.; Salge, J.M.; Barone, I.A.; Bohm, G.M. Air Pollution and Mortality in Elderly People: A Time-Series Study in Sao Paulo, Brazil. *Arch. Environ. Health Int. J.* **1995**, *50*, 159–163. [CrossRef] [PubMed]
30. Pereira, L.A.A.; Loomis, D.; de Conceição, G.M.S.; Braga, A.L.F.; Arcas, R.M.; Kishi, H.S.; Singer, J.M.; Böhm, G.M.; Saldiva, P.H.N. Association between Air Pollution and Intrauterine Mortality in Sao Paulo, Brazil. *Environ. Health Perspect.* **1998**, *106*, 325–329. [CrossRef]
31. Lin, C.A.; Martins, M.A.; Farhat, S.C.; Pope III, C.A.; de Conceição, G.M.S.; Anastácio, V.M.; Hatanaka, M.; Andrade, W.C.; Hamaue, W.R.; Böhm, G.M.; et al. Air Pollution and Respiratory Illness of Children in São Paulo, Brazil. *Paediatr. Perinat. Epidemiol.* **1999**, *13*, 475–488. [CrossRef]
32. Bravo, M.A.; Son, J.; De Freitas, C.U.; Gouveia, N.; Bell, M.L. Air Pollution and Mortality in São Paulo, Brazil: Effects of Multiple Pollutants and Analysis of Susceptible Populations. *J. Expo. Sci. Environ. Epidemiol.* **2016**, *26*, 150–161. [CrossRef] [PubMed]
33. Abe, K.C.; Dos Santos, G.M.S.; de Coêlho, M.S.Z.S.; Miraglia, S.G.E.K. PM 10 Exposure and Cardiorespiratory Mortality—Estimating the Effects and Economic Losses in São Paulo, Brazil. *Aerosol Air Qual. Res.* **2018**, *18*, 3127–3133. [CrossRef]
34. Santana, J.C.C.; Miranda, A.C.; Yamamura, C.L.K.; da Silva Filho, S.C.; Tambourgi, E.B.; Ho, L.L.; Berssaneti, F.T. Effects of Air Pollution on Human Health and Costs: Current Situation in São Paulo, Brazil. *Sustainability* **2020**, *12*, 4875. [CrossRef]
35. Costa, A.F.; Hoek, G.; Brunekreef, B.; de Leon, A.C.M.P. Air Pollution and Deaths among Elderly Residents of São Paulo, Brazil: An Analysis of Mortality Displacement. *Environ. Health Perspect.* **2017**, *125*, 349–354. [CrossRef] [PubMed]
36. Ferreira, T.M.; Forti, M.C.; de Freitas, C.U.; Nascimento, F.P.; Junger, W.L.; Gouveia, N. Effects of Particulate Matter and Its Chemical Constituents on Elderly Hospital Admissions Due to Circulatory and Respiratory Diseases. *Int. J. Environ. Res. Public Health* **2016**, *13*, 947. [CrossRef] [PubMed]
37. Martins, M.C.H.; Fatigati, F.L.; Véspoli, T.C.; Martins, L.C.; Pereira, L.A.; Martins, M.A.; Saldiva, P.H.N.; Braga, A.L.F. Influence of Socioeconomic Conditions on Air Pollution Adverse Health Effects in Elderly People: An Analysis of Six Regions in São Paulo, Brazil. *J. Epidemiol. Community Health* **2004**, *58*, 41–46. [CrossRef]
38. Dominici, F.; Peng, R.D.; Barr, C.D.; Bell, M.L. Protecting Human Health from Air Pollution: Shifting from a Single-Pollutant to a Multipollutant Approach. *Epidemiology* **2010**, *21*, 187–194. [CrossRef] [PubMed]
39. Gold, D.R.; Damokosh, A.I.; Pope, C.A.; Dockery, D.W.; McDonnell, W.F.; Serrano, P.; Retama, A.; Castillejos, M. Particulate and Ozone Pollutant Effects on the Respiratory Function of Children in Southwest Mexico City. *Epidemiology* **1999**, *10*, 470. [CrossRef]

40. Davalos, A.D.; Luben, T.J.; Herring, A.H.; Sacks, J.D. Current Approaches Used in Epidemiologic Studies to Examine Short-Term Multipollutant Air Pollution Exposures. *Ann. Epidemiol.* **2016**, *27*, 145–153.e1. [CrossRef]
41. Yu, L.; Liu, W.; Wang, X.; Ye, Z.; Tan, Q.; Qiu, W.; Nie, X.; Li, M.; Wang, B.; Chen, W. A Review of Practical Statistical Methods Used in Epidemiological Studies to Estimate the Health Effects of Multi-Pollutant Mixture. *Environ. Pollut.* **2022**, *306*, 119356. [CrossRef]
42. Rodríguez-Villamizar, L.A.; Rojas-Roa, N.Y.; Blanco-Becerra, L.C.; Herrera-Galindo, V.M.; Fernández-Niño, J.A. Short-Term Effects of Air Pollution on Respiratory and Circulatory Morbidity in Colombia 2011–2014: A Multi-City, Time-Series Analysis. *Int. J. Environ. Res. Public Health* **2018**, *15*, 1610. [CrossRef]
43. Jiang, Y.; Chen, J.; Wu, C.; Lin, X.; Zhou, Q.; Ji, S.; Yang, S.; Zhang, X.; Liu, B. Temporal Cross-Correlations between Air Pollutants and Outpatient Visits for Respiratory and Circulatory System Diseases in Fuzhou, China. *BMC Public Health* **2020**, *20*, 1131. [CrossRef]
44. Zhang, J.; Liu, Y.; Cui, L.L.; Liu, S.Q.; Yin, X.X.; Li, H.C. Ambient Air Pollution, Smog Episodes and Mortality in Jinan, China. *Sci. Rep.* **2017**, *7*, 11209. [CrossRef]
45. Shin, H.H.; Owen, J.; Maquiling, A.; Parajuli, R.P.; Smith-Doiron, M. Circulatory Health Risks from Additive Multi-Pollutant Models: Short-Term Exposure to Three Common Air Pollutants in Canada. *Environ. Sci. Pollut. Res.* **2023**, *30*, 15740–15755. [CrossRef] [PubMed]
46. Haykin, S. *Redes Neurais Princípios e Prática*, 2nd ed.; Grupo, A., Ed.; Pearson Education: Porto Alegre, Brazil, 2001.
47. Bellinger, C.; Mohomed Jabbar, M.S.; Zaïane, O.; Osornio-Vargas, A. A Systematic Review of Data Mining and Machine Learning for Air Pollution Epidemiology. *BMC Public Health* **2017**, *17*, 907. [CrossRef] [PubMed]
48. Cabaneros, S.M.; Calautit, J.K.; Hughes, B.R. A Review of Artificial Neural Network Models for Ambient Air Pollution Prediction. *Environ. Model. Softw.* **2019**, *119*, 285–304. [CrossRef]
49. Araujo, L.N.; Belotti, J.T.; Alves, T.A.; de Tadano, Y.S.; Siqueira, H. Ensemble Method Based on Artificial Neural Networks to Estimate Air Pollution Health Risks. *Environ. Model. Softw.* **2020**, *123*, 104567. [CrossRef]
50. Miranda, A.C.; Santana, J.C.C.; Yamamura, C.L.K.; Rosa, J.M.; Tambourgi, E.B.; Ho, L.L.; Berssaneti, F.T. Application of Neural Network to Simulate the Behavior of Hospitalizations and Their Costs under the Effects of Various Polluting Gases in the City of São Paulo. *Air Qual. Atmos. Health* **2021**, *14*, 2091–2099. [CrossRef]
51. CETESB. *Qualidade Do Ar No Estado de São Paulo 2019*; CETESB: São Paulo, Brazil, 2020.
52. WHO. *WHO Global Air Quality Guidelines*; WHO: Bonn, Germany, 2021.
53. CETESB. *Qualidade Do Ar No Estado de São Paulo 2020*; CETESB: São Paulo, Brazil, 2021.
54. Olden, J.D.; Jackson, D.A. Illuminating the "Black Box": Understanding Variable Contributions in Artificial Neural Networks. *Ecol. Modell.* **2002**, *154*, 135–150. [CrossRef]
55. McCullagh, P.; Nelder, J.A. *Generalized Linear Models*, 2nd ed.; Chapman and Hall: London, UK, 1989.
56. de Souza Conceição, G.M.; Saldiva, P.H.N.; da Motta Singer, J. Modelos MLG e MAG Para Análise Da Associação Entre Poluição Atmosférica e Marcadores de Morbi-Mortalidade: Uma Introdução Baseada Em Dados Da Cidade de São Paulo. *Rev. Bras. Epidemiol.* **2001**, *4*, 206–219. [CrossRef]
57. IAG—USP. *Boletim Climatológico Anual Da Estação Meteorológica Do Iag/Usp*; IAG—USP: São Paulo, Brazil, 2015.
58. de Fatima Andrade, M.; Kumar, P.; de Freitas, E.D.; Ynoue, R.Y.; Martins, J.; Martins, L.D.; Nogueira, T.; Perez-Martinez, P.; de Miranda, R.M.; Albuquerque, T.; et al. Air Quality in the Megacity of São Paulo: Evolution over the Last 30 Years and Future Perspectives. *Atmos. Environ.* **2017**, *159*, 66–82. [CrossRef]
59. Lencioni, S. Mudanças Na Metrópole de São Paulo (Brasil) e Transformações Industriais. *Rev. Dep. Geogr.* **1998**, *12*, 27–42. [CrossRef]
60. Martins, L.C.; do Rosário Dias de Oliveira Latorre, M.; Saldiva, P.P.H.N.; Braga, A.L.F. Relação Entre Poluição Atmosférica e Atendimentos Por Infecção de Vias Aéreas Superiores No Município de São Paulo: Avaliação Do Rodízio de Veículos. *Rev. Bras. Epidemiol.* **2001**, *4*, 220–229. [CrossRef]
61. Szwarcfiter, L.; Mendes, F.E.; La Rovere, E.L. Enhancing the Effects of the Brazilian Program to Reduce Atmospheric Pollutant Emissions from Vehicles. *Transp. Res. Part D Transp. Environ.* **2005**, *10*, 153–160. [CrossRef]
62. Boldt, T.; da Silva, A.W.; de Souza Leal, C. Uma Análise Físico-Química Dos Catalisadores Automotivos: Estudo Introdutório Das Propriedades e Eficiência Catalítica. In Proceedings of the 2o Simpósio de Integração Científica e Tecnológica do Sul Catarinense, Araranguá, Brazil, 21–22 October 2003; pp. 248–260.
63. do Carmo Rangel, M.; Carvalho, M.F.A. Impacto Dos Catalisadores Automotivos No Controle Da Qualidade Do Ar. *Quim. Nova* **2003**, *26*, 265–277. [CrossRef]
64. De Carvalho, R.N.; Vicentini, P.C.; de Sá, R.A.B.; Villela, A.C.S.; Botero, S.W. A Nova Gasolina S50 E O Proconve L6. In Proceedings of the XXI Simpósio Internacional de Engenharia Automotiva; 2014; pp. 184–193. [CrossRef]
65. Daemme, L.C.; Penteado, R.; Vicentini, P.C.; Errera, M.R. Impacto Da Redução Do Teor de Enxofre Da Gasolina S800 Para S50 Nas Emissões Da Frota Brasileira. In Proceedings of the XXVII Simpósio Internacional de Engenharia Automotiva, São Paulo, Brazil, 1 August 2019.
66. Pérez-Martínez, P.J.; de Fátima Andrade, M.; de Miranda, R.M. Heavy Truck Restrictions and Air Quality Implications in São Paulo, Brazil. *J. Environ. Manag.* **2017**, *202*, 55–68. [CrossRef] [PubMed]

67. He, J.; Gouveia, N.; Salvo, A. External Effects of Diesel Trucks Circulating Inside the São Paulo Megacity. *J. Eur. Econ. Assoc.* **2019**, *17*, 947–989. [CrossRef]
68. Sánchez-Ccoyllo, O.R.; de Andrade, M.F. The Influence of Meteorological Conditions on the Behavior of Pollutants Concentrations in São Paulo, Brazil. *Environ. Pollut.* **2002**, *116*, 257–263. [CrossRef]
69. Bourotte, C.; Forti, M.C.; Taniguchi, S.; Bícego, M.C.; Lotufo, P.A. A Wintertime Study of PAHs in Fine and Coarse Aerosols in São Paulo City, Brazil. *Atmos. Environ.* **2005**, *39*, 3799–3811. [CrossRef]
70. Castanho, A.D.A.; Artaxo, P. Wintertime and Summertime São Paulo Aerosol Source Apportionment Study. *Atmos. Environ.* **2001**, *35*, 4889–4902. [CrossRef]
71. Martins, L.C.; Latorre, M.D.R.D.D.O.; Cardoso, M.R.A.; Gonçalves, F.L.T.; Saldiva, P.H.N.; Braga, A.L.F. Air Pollution and Emergency Room Visits Due to Pneumonia and Influenza in São Paulo, Brazil. *Rev. Saude Publica* **2002**, *36*, 88–94. [CrossRef]
72. Francisco, P.M.S.B.; Donalisio, M.R.; Lattorre, M.D.R.D.D.O. Internações Por Doenças Respiratórias Em Idosos e a Intervenção Vacinal Contra Influenza No Estado de São Paulo Respiratory Disease Hospitalization in the Elderly in the State of São. *Rev. Bras. Epidemiol.* **2004**, *7*, 220–227. [CrossRef]
73. Larasati, A.; DeYong, C.; Slevitch, L. Comparing Neural Network and Ordinal Logistic Regression to Analyze Attitude Responses. *Serv. Sci.* **2011**, *3*, 304–312. [CrossRef]
74. Shakerkhatibi, M.; Dianat, I.; Asghari Jafarabadi, M.; Azak, R.; Kousha, A. Air Pollution and Hospital Admissions for Cardiorespiratory Diseases in Iran: Artificial Neural Network versus Conditional Logistic Regression. *Int. J. Environ. Sci. Technol.* **2015**, *12*, 3433–3442. [CrossRef]
75. Khojasteh, D.N.; Goudarzi, G.; Taghizadeh-Mehrjardi, R.; Asumadu-Sakyi, A.B.; Fehresti-Sani, M. Long-Term Effects of Outdoor Air Pollution on Mortality and Morbidity–Prediction Using Nonlinear Autoregressive and Artificial Neural Networks Models. *Atmos. Pollut. Res.* **2021**, *12*, 46–56. [CrossRef]
76. Kassomenos, P.; Petrakis, M.; Sarigiannis, D.; Gotti, A.; Karakitsios, S. Identifying the Contribution of Physical and Chemical Stressors to the Daily Number of Hospital Admissions Implementing an Artificial Neural Network Model. *Air Qual. Atmos. Health* **2011**, *4*, 263–272. [CrossRef]
77. Kachba, Y.R.; de Genaro Chiroli, D.M.; Belotti, J.T.; Alves, T.A.; de Souza Tadano, Y.; Siqueira, H. Influence of Vehicular Emission Variables To Morbidity and Mortality in the Largest Metropolis in South America. *Sustainability* **2020**, *12*, 2621. [CrossRef]
78. de Souza Tadano, Y.; Bacalhau, E.T.; Casacio, L.; Puchta, E.; Pereira, T.S.; Antonini Alves, T.; Ugaya, C.M.L.; Siqueira, H.V. Unorganized Machines to Estimate the Number of Hospital Admissions Due to Respiratory Diseases Caused by Pm10 Concentration. *Atmosphere* **2021**, *12*, 1345. [CrossRef]
79. Seo, S.; Min, C.; Preston, M.; Han, S.; Choi, S.H.; Kang, S.Y.; Kim, D. Ambient PM Concentrations as a Precursor of Emergency Visits for Respiratory Complaints: Roles of Deep Learning and Multi-Point Real-Time Monitoring. *Sustainability* **2022**, *14*, 2703. [CrossRef]
80. Polezer, G.; Tadano, Y.S.; Siqueira, H.V.; Godoi, A.F.L.; Yamamoto, C.I.; de André, P.A.; Pauliquevis, T.; de Andrade, M.F.; Oliveira, A.; Saldiva, P.H.N.; et al. Assessing the Impact of PM 2.5 on Respiratory Disease Using Artificial Neural Networks. *Environ. Pollut.* **2018**, *235*, 394–403. [CrossRef]
81. Air, I.; Munksgaard, B. Significance of Humidity and Temperature on Skin and Upper Airway Symptoms. *Indoor Air* **2003**, *13*, 344–352. [CrossRef]
82. Nguyen, J.L.; Schwartz, J.; Dockery, D.W. The Relationship between Indoor and Outdoor Temperature, Apparent Temperature, Relative Humidity, and Absolute Humidity. *Indoor Air* **2014**, *24*, 103–112. [CrossRef]
83. Guergova, S.; Dufour, A. Thermal Sensitivity in the Elderly: A Review. *Ageing Res. Rev.* **2011**, *10*, 80–92. [CrossRef]
84. Diniz, F.R.; Gonçalves, F.L.T.; Sheridan, S. Heat Wave and Elderly Mortality: Historical Analysis and Future Projection for Metropolitan Region of Sao Paulo, Brazil. *Atmosphere* **2020**, *11*, 933. [CrossRef]
85. Leirião, L.F.L.; Miraglia, S.G.E.K. Environmental and Health Impacts Due to the Violation of Brazilian Emissions Control Program Standards in Sao Paulo Metropolitan Area. *Transp. Res. Part D Transp. Environ.* **2019**, *70*, 70–76. [CrossRef]
86. Leirião, L.F.L.; Debone, D.; Pauliquevis, T.; do Rosário, N.; Miraglia, S. Environmental and Public Health Effects of Vehicle Emissions in a Large Metropolis: Case Study of a Truck Driver Strike in Sao Paulo, Brazil. *Atmos. Pollut. Res.* **2020**, *11*, 24–31. [CrossRef]
87. Costa, S.; Ferreira, J.; Silveira, C.; Costa, C.; Lopes, D.; Relvas, H.; Borrego, C.; Roebeling, P.; Miranda, A.I.; Paulo Teixeira, J. Integrating Health on Air Quality Assessment—Review Report on Health Risks of Two Major European Outdoor Air Pollutants: PM and NO_2. *J. Toxicol. Environ. Health Part B Crit. Rev.* **2014**, *17*, 307–340. [CrossRef]
88. De Veaux, R.D.; Ungar, L.H. Multicollinearity: A Tale of Two Nonparametric Regressions. In *Selecting Models from Data*; Cheeseman, P., Oldford, R.W., Eds.; Springer: New York, NY, USA, 1994; pp. 393–402.
89. Aga, E.; Samoli, E.; Touloumi, G.; Anderson, H.R.; Cadum, E.; Forsberg, B.; Goodman, P.; Goren, A.; Kotesovec, F.; Kriz, B.; et al. Short-Term Effects of Ambient Particles on Mortality in the Elderly: Results from 28 Cities in the APHEA2 Project. *Eur. Respir. J.* **2003**, *21* (Suppl. S40), 28–33. [CrossRef]
90. Chen, R.; Kan, H.; Chen, B.; Huang, W.; Bai, Z.; Song, G.; Pan, G. Association of Particulate Air Pollution with Daily Mortality: The China Air Pollution and Health Effects Study. *Am. J. Epidemiol.* **2012**, *175*, 1173–1181. [CrossRef] [PubMed]

91. Filleul, L.; Tertre, A.L.; Baldi, I.; Tessier, J.F. Difference in the Relation between Daily Mortality and Air Pollution among Elderly and All-Ages Populations in Southwestern France. *Environ. Res.* **2004**, *94*, 249–253. [CrossRef] [PubMed]
92. Schwalbe, N.; Wahl, B. Artificial Intelligence and the Future of Global Health. *Lancet* **2020**, *395*, 1579–1586. [CrossRef]

Disclaimer/Publisher's Note: The statements, opinions and data contained in all publications are solely those of the individual author(s) and contributor(s) and not of MDPI and/or the editor(s). MDPI and/or the editor(s) disclaim responsibility for any injury to people or property resulting from any ideas, methods, instructions or products referred to in the content.

Article

Acute Pesticide Poisoning in Tobacco Farming, According to Different Criteria

Neice Muller Xavier Faria [1,*], Rodrigo Dalke Meucci [2], Nadia Spada Fiori [1], Maria Laura Vidal Carret [1], Carlos Augusto Mello-da-Silva [3] and Anaclaudia Gastal Fassa [1]

1 Department of Social Medicine, Faculty of Medicine, Federal University of Pelotas, Pelotas 96030-000, Brazil
2 Faculty of Medicine, Federal University of Rio Grande, Rio Grande 96203-900, Brazil
3 Poison Information Center (CIT/RS), State Health Department, Porto Alegre 90610-000, Brazil
* Correspondence: neice@clinicagianisella.com.br

Abstract: Background: Brazil is one of the world's largest pesticide consumers, but information on pesticide poisoning among workers is scarce. Objective: To evaluate acute pesticide poisoning among tobacco growers, according to different criteria. Methods: This was a two-step cross-sectional study with 492 pesticide applicators. It used a 25 question pesticide-related symptoms (PRS) questionnaire and medical diagnosis for comparison with toxicological assessment. Associations were evaluated using Poisson regression. Results: 10.6% reported two or more PRS, while 8.1% reported three or more. Furthermore, 12.2% received a medical diagnosis of poisoning. According to toxicologists, possible cases accounted for 14.2% and probable cases for 4.3%. PRS increased during the period of greater exposure. Those exposed to dithiocarbamates, sulfentrazone, pyrethroids, fipronil and iprodione exhibited more PRS. The number of exposure types, multi-chemical exposure, clothes wet with pesticides and spillage on the body/clothes were associated with acute poisonings. All criteria showed sensitivity greater than 79% for probable cases but only greater than 70% for medical diagnosis when compared to possible cases, presenting substantial Kappa agreement. Conclusion: The prevalence of acute pesticide poisoning is much higher than officially recorded. Trained physicians can screen for pesticide poisoning. It is necessary to improve workers' education to reduce pesticide use and exposure to them.

Keywords: pesticide; poisoning; epidemiology; toxicology; tobacco; farmer

1. Introduction

For decades now, Brazil has been one of the world's largest consumers of pesticides [1,2]. Consumption of active ingredients per hectare of planted area increased from 2.9 kg/hectares in 2003 to 6.7 in 2014 [3]. According to the Brazilian Institute of Environment and Renewable Natural Resources (Instituto Brasileiro de Meio Ambiente—IBAMA), in 2021, a total of 720,869 tons of formulated pesticides were sold, which represents a 50% increase compared to 2012 [3]. This highly chemical agricultural production model has considerable impacts on the environment, such as soil and water contamination. Biocides also generate threats to living beings, especially pollinating insects, which contribute directly to agricultural production [4], in addition to negatively affecting birds and mammals, including humans.

Agricultural workers have frequent occupational and environmental exposure, often multi-chemical, and are at increased risk of pesticide poisoning and death. Estimates of acute poisoning prevalence vary depending on the source. According to the Notifiable Diseases Information System (Sistema de Informação de Agravos de Notificação—SINAN), in 2019 in Brazil, 7.7 cases of pesticide poisonings were reported per 100,000 inhabitants, including poisonings from products used in agriculture, public health, household pesticides, rodenticides and veterinary products [5].

Epidemiological studies indicate a much higher occurrence of pesticide poisoning among agricultural workers. Studies conducted in the Serra Gaúcha region with family farmers identified 2.0 to 3.8% who reported acute pesticide poisoning in the year before they were interviewed [6,7]. In addition, several studies have pointed to association between acute poisoning episodes and increased prevalence of chronic diseases, such as respiratory problems [8–11], hormonal disorders [12], neurological disorders [13] and mental disorders [14–19].

Records of pesticide poisoning are limited by difficulties in access to health services, especially in rural areas; failure to recognize cases and low adherence to case notification. Estimates of occurrence of pesticide poisoning in epidemiological studies are affected by the diversity of criteria used to identify and classify acute poisoning, with self-reported poisoning being the most frequently used. With the aim of increasing the comparability of findings, the World Health Organization (WHO) has proposed a methodology to classify acute pesticide poisonings as either possible cases or probable cases [20].

This study evaluates prevalence of acute pesticide poisoning among family farmers who applied pesticides, using a pesticide-related symptoms (PRS) questionnaire (developed according to the methodology proposed by the WHO), clinical physician diagnosis and toxicological assessment. The study also investigates occupational factors associated with acute pesticide poisoning.

2. Methods

2.1. Study Design and Participants

A cross-sectional study was carried out in São Lourenço do Sul, Rio Grande do Sul, the state that most produces tobacco in Brazil [21]. The study had three stages. The sample procedures took into account the sample size needed for the third stage, which addressed green tobacco sickness during harvest time and required the largest sample size. For sampling, 1100 of the 3852 tobacco sales invoices issued in 2009 were randomly selected. This article presents a subsample analysis of family tobacco growers aged 18 years or over, who applied pesticides, participated in the first and second stage of the study and worked in the 254 sampled farms in the Canta Galo and Santa Inês districts, which are the largest tobacco producers in the municipality of São Lourenço do Sul. The first stage occurred in the period of low exposure to pesticides, the second in the period of high exposure

The vast majority of farms (82%) were up to 40 hectares in size. The production context of the areas studied was detailed in previous publications [15,21,22]

2.2. Sociodemographic and Occupational Aspects

We investigated demographic aspects, i.e., gender and age; socioeconomic aspects, i.e., education in complete years of study and annual tobacco production in tons; behavioral aspects, i.e., smoking (never smoked, ex-smoker and smoker), alcohol consumption (in days/month) and Body mass index (BMI) (normal weight, overweight and obesity) [20].

2.3. Pesticide Exposure

Occupational exposure to pesticides in the month prior to the interview was characterized in number of days. Several forms of exposure were investigated in relation to the most recent contact with pesticides, such as applying herbicides or insecticides/fungicides, mixing/preparing mixture, cleaning equipment, washing contaminated clothing, having contact in transportation and storage, through wet clothing, reentering into the plantation without protection after application, and spilling on the body or on clothing. We also characterized the sum of the forms of pesticide exposure.

In order to gather information on what types of chemicals were used on the farms in the last 30 days, plastic cards were prepared with pictures of the main pesticides used in tobacco farming in the region, totaling 56 commercial formulations and more than 22 products (referred to as others). The date of most recent contact was also collected for each product reported. The chemical groups analyzed were organophosphorus compounds (organophosphates), neonicotinoids, pyrethroids, carbamates, benzoylurea, fipronil, clomazone, glyphosate, sulfentrazone, triazines, dithiocarbamates, metalaxyl, iprodione and copper compounds. The sum of the types of chemicals used was taken as an indicator of multi-chemical exposure.

The personal protective equipment (PPE) investigated were boots, masks and gloves to protect against chemicals, protective clothing, hat/headgear, characterizing the number of days they were used during work in the last 30 days. We also examined the sum of the PPE that each worker reported always using.

2.4. Pesticide Poisonings

In both stages, 25 symptoms common to pesticide poisonings that occurred in the last 15 days were investigated. Pesticide-related symptoms (PRS) were considered when they had appeared or worsened within 48 h after direct contact with these products. According to the classification proposed by the World Health Organization (WHO), a possible case of poisoning was considered to be when two or more PRS were present, while a probable case was considered to be when three or more PRS were present [20]. Medical assessment included standardized anamnesis and physical examination and was performed by clinical physicians trained by the study. The standardization of the medical evaluation instruments and the criteria to define whether or not the worker had acute pesticide poisoning were developed in a workshop on the subject with the participation of toxicologists and epidemiologists.

The toxicological assessment was performed by two toxicologists, and in case of disagreement, a third toxicologist also gave an opinion. The toxicological assessment took into consideration the PRS questionnaire, the medical assessment, and a set of complementary tests. Anthropometric data, vital signs, Gamma GT (GGT), and casual capillary blood glucose were collected. Plasma cholinesterase (Butyrylcholinesterase—BCHE) samples were also collected, whereby the measurement taken in the first stage was considered to be baseline BCHE, while the measurement taken in the second stage was considered to be measurement at high exposure. In cases of recent exposure to cholinesterase inhibitors, the BCHE measurement was considered in the toxicologists' diagnosis. In cases with decreased BCHE (at least a 20% reduction in relation to baseline BCHE) and/or altered GGT ($\geq$60 U/L), abdominal ultrasonography, liver function tests, and viral hepatitis serology were performed.

The toxicologists considered a probable case of poisoning to be when data were compatible with the expected clinical manifestations, considering the pesticides to which the tobacco grower was exposed in the period. They considered a possible case of poisoning to be when the data could be compatible with the expected clinical manifestations, considering the pesticides to which the tobacco grower was exposed in the period, but the available data did not allow other causes to be excluded (uncertainty about differential diagnoses).

2.5. Statistic Analysis

The data analysis described the study population, indicating the prevalence of pesticide poisoning in each population subgroup according to the different criteria studied. It then compared prevalence of PRS in the first and second stages, estimating the relative risk and confidence interval for the occurrence of the symptom in the second stage (high pesticide exposure) compared to the first stage (low exposure). It also examined whether there was a significant difference in the prevalence of symptoms among those exposed to each type of chemical evaluated when compared to those not exposed, using Pearson's chi-square test or Fisher's exact test for categories with numbers less than five.

Statistical analysis also included examining the factors associated with pesticide poisoning according to the different criteria by examining association using the chi-square test for categorical variables and the linear trend test for continuous variables. The adjusted analysis was performed using Poisson regression with robust variance. We used a hierarchical model containing demographic and socioeconomic aspects in the first level and behavioral aspects and occupational exposures to pesticides in the second level, keeping in the model variables with p-value less than or equal to 0.2. To avoid overlapping effects, occupational exposures to pesticides were examined one at a time, adjusting for the first level and behavioral variables.

Analysis of sensitivity, specificity, positive and negative predictive value was performed, taking the toxicological assessment as the gold standard. Agreement between the different diagnostic criteria in relation to the toxicologists' assessment as to possible case and probable case was examined using the Kappa test.

2.6. Ethical Issues

This study was approved by the Research Ethics Committee of the Medical School of the Federal University of Pelotas (Universidade Federal de Pelotas—UFPEL) as per letter number 11/2010. Eligible farm workers were informed about the research topic, the right to not take part, and the guarantee of confidentiality regarding individual information. Those who agreed to participate signed an informed consent form. Interviewees who were identified as having acute pesticide poisoning were referred for treatment in the public health system.

3. Results

3.1. Participants

A total of 492 tobacco growers who had applied pesticides in the previous year took part in the study. In the first stage, losses and refusals accounted for 5% in relation to those who were eligible, while in the second stage, they accounted for 4% in relation to the first stage. Ninety-eight percent were white, most were of German descent, 90% of whom belonged to the farm owner's family and the rest were tenants. Almost all (94.3%) had contact with pesticides in the last 20 days (data not shown).

3.2. Sociodemographic and Occupational Aspects

Among the tobacco growers, 26% were under 30 years old and 25.6% were 50 years old or over, 76.4% were male, 44% had 4 complete years or less of schooling, 29.5% consumed alcoholic beverages 8 days or more per month, 19.7% were smokers, and 12.6% were overweight. Among the farmers, 70.1% produced up to 9000 kg of tobacco per year. Regarding forms of exposure to pesticides, 74.7% prepared mixture, some 60% applied pesticide and/or cleaned equipment, 52.8% reported reentering into the plantation after pesticide application without using PPE, 45.3% washed contaminated clothes, 33.3% reported that their clothes got wet with pesticide while applying it, and 20.4% reported spilling pesticides on their bodies or clothes. Among the tobacco growers, 40.8% had 7 to 12 forms of exposure to pesticides, 32.5% were exposed to 5 or more types of chemicals, 24.6% were exposed for 5 days or more per month, and 37.2% always used four or five PPE items (Table 1).

Table 1. Acute Pesticide Poisoning according to criteria: Pesticide-Related Symptoms (PRS), medical diagnosis and toxicologists' assessment.

Variables	n (%)	2 or More PRS	3 or More PRS	Medical Diagnosis	Toxicologist Possible Case	Toxicologist Probable Case
Total sample	492 (100.0)	51 (10.6%)	39 (8.1%)	60 (12.2%)	70 (14.2%)	21 (4.3%)
Sex		▶$p = 0.001$	▶$p = 0.001$	▶$p = 0.11$	▶$p = 0.05$	▶$p = 0.03$
Male	376 (76.4)	30 (8.1)	22 (5.9)	41 (10.9)	47 (12.5)	12 (3.2)
Female	116 (23.6)	21 (19.3)	17 (15.6)	19 (16.5)	23 (19.8)	9 (7.8)
Age Group		▶$p = 0.83$	▶$p = 0.52$	▶$p = 0.20$	▶$p = 0.42$	$p = 0.74$ +
Up to 29 years	128 (26.0)	13 (10.3)	10 (7.9)	10 (7.9)	14 (10.9)	4 (3.1)
30–49 years	238 (48.4)	23 (10.0)	16 (7.0)	34 (14.3)	38 (16.0)	12 (5.0)
50 years and over	126 (25.6)	15 (12.1)	13 (10.5)	16 (12.7)	18 (14.3)	5 (4.0)
Schooling		▶$p = 0.70$	▶$p = 0.46$	▶$p = 0.49$	▶$p = 0.18$	$p = 0.16$ +
Up to 4 years	218 (44.3)	23 (10.6)	17 (7.9)	29 (13.4)	30 (13.8)	10 (4.6)
5–7 years	209 (42.5)	23 (11.6)	19 (9.5)	26 (12.4)	35 (16.7)	11 (5.3)
8 years and over	65 (13.2)	5 (7.8)	3 (4.7)	5 (7.8)	5 (7.7)	0 (0.0)

Table 1. Cont.

Variables	n (%)	2 or More PRS	3 or More PRS	Medical Diagnosis	Toxicologist Possible Case	Toxicologist Probable Case
Tobacco production		p = 0.01 *	►p = 0.05	p = 0.008 *	p = 0.08 *	p = 0.03 +
Up to 4000 kg	165 (34.1)	22 (13.8)	14 (8.8)	29 (17.8)	29 (17.6)	13 (7.9)
4001–9000 kg	178 (36.8)	23 (13.1)	20 (11.4)	20 (11.2)	25 (14.0)	4 (2.2)
Over 9000 kg	141 (29.1)	6 (4.4)	5 (3.7)	11 (7.8)	15 (10.6)	4 (2.8)
Alcohol consumption (Days/month)		p = 0.03 *	p = 0.02 *	p = 0.03 *	p = 0.07 *	p = 0.03 +
Does not drink	116 (23.6)	18 (15.8)	15 (13.2)	18 (15.5)	22 (19.0)	10 (8.6)
Up to 7 days/month	231 (47.0)	23 (10.2)	17 (7.6)	32 (14.0)	32 (13.9)	8 (3.5)
≥8 days/month	145 (29.5)	10 (7.1)	7 (5.0)	10 (6.9)	16 (11.0)	3 (2.1)
Tobacco smoking		►p = 0.68	p = 0.26 +	►p = 0.30	►p = 0.21	p = 0.53 +
No	307 (62.4)	33 (11.1)	28 (9.4)	35 (11.5)	45 (14.7)	15 (4.9)
Former smoker	88 (17.9)	10 (11.8)	7 (8.2)	15 (17.0)	16 (18.2)	4 (4.5)
Smoker	97 (19.7)	8 (8.2)	4 (4.1)	10 (10.3)	9 (9.3)	2 (2.1)
BMI		►p = 0.58	p = 0.46+	p = 0.14 *	►p = 0.13	p = 0.91 +
Normal weight	238 (48.4)	21 (9.1)	16 (7.0)	24 (10.1)	28 (11.8)	10 (4.2)
Overweight	192 (39.0)	23 (12.2)	19 (10.1)	26 (13.7)	35 (18.2)	9 (4.7)
Obese	62 (12.6)	7 (11.5)	4 (6.6)	10 (16.1)	7 (11.3)	2 (3.2)
Applying pesticides		►p = 0.01	►p = 0.03	►p = 0.09	►p = 0.07	►p = 0.07 +
No	196 (40.0)	12 (6.3)	9 (4.7)	18 (9.2)	21 (10.7)	4 (2.0)
Yes	294 (60.0)	39 (13.5)	30 (10.4)	42 (14.3)	49 (16.7)	17 (5.8)
Preparing mixture		►p = 0.05	►p = 0.16	►p = 0.10	►p = 0.05	p = 0.12 +
No	123 (25.3)	7 (5.8)	6 (5.0)	10 (8.1)	11 (8.9)	2 (1.6)
Yes	363 (74.7)	43 (12.1)	32 (9.0)	50 (13.9)	58 (16.0)	19 (5.2)
Washing contaminated clothing		►p = 0.03	►p = 0.03	►p = 0.02	►p = 0.13	►p = 0.01
No	268 (54.7)	21 (8.0)	15 (5.7)	24 (9.0)	32 (11.9)	6 (2.2)
Yes	222 (45.3)	30 (14.1)	24 (11.3)	35 (15.8)	37 (16.7)	15 (6.8)
Cleaning pesticide equipment		►p = 0.74	►p = 0.92	►p = 0.98	►p = 0.45	►p = 0.80
No	174 (35.4)	19 (11.3)	14 (8.3)	21 (12.2)	22 (12.6)	8 (4.6)
Yes	317 (64.6)	32 (10.3)	25 (8.1)	39 (12.3)	48 (15.1)	13 (4.1)
Reentering after application		►p = 0.01	►p = 0.01	►p = 0.22	►p = 0.78	►p = 0.97
No	230 (47.2)	16 (7.1)	11 (4.9)	24 (10.4)	32 (13.9)	10 (4.3)
Yes	257 (52.8)	35 (14.1)	28 (11.3)	36 (14.1)	38 (14.8)	11 (4.3)
Clothes wet during application		►p = 0.01	►p = 0.001	►p = 0.02	►p = 0.003	►p = 0.001
No	325 (66.7)	26 (8.2)	17 (5.3)	32 (9.9)	36 (11.1)	7 (2.2)
Yes	162 (33.3)	25 (15.8)	22 (13.9)	28 (17.4)	34 (21.0)	14 (8.6)
Spilling on body/clothing		►p < 0.001	►p < 0.001	►p = 0.047	►p < 0.005	►p < 0.001
No	389 (79.6)	31 (8.2)	22 (5.8)	42 (10.8)	47 (12.1)	8 (2.1)
Yes	100 (20.4)	20 (20.8)	17 (17.7)	18 (18.2)	23 (23.0)	13 (13.0)
Forms of exposure		p = 0.009 *	p = 0.005 *	p = 0.02 *	p = 0.002 *	p < 0.001 +
Up to 4 forms	128 (28.3)	6 (4.8)	5 (4.0)	10 (7.9)	9 (7.0)	0
5–6 forms	140 (30.9)	16 (11.7)	9 (6.6)	17 (12.1)	20 (14.3)	4 (2.9)
7–12 forms	185 (40.8)	26 (14.4)	23 (12.7)	31 (16.8)	36 (19.5)	16 (8.6)
Multi-chemical exposure		p < 0.001 *	p < 0.001 *	►p = 0.56	p = 0.01 *	p = 0.03 +
Used up to 2 types	143 (29.1)	9 (6.5)	6 (4.3)	16 (11.2)	14 (9.8)	2 (1.4)
Used 3–4 types	189 (38.4)	12 (6.5)	8 (4.3)	21 (11.1)	24 (12.7)	7 (3.7)
5 types or more	160 (32.5)	30 (19.2)	25 (16.0)	23 (14.6)	32 (20.0)	12 (7.5)
Frequency of exposure/month		p = 0.006 *	p = 0.003 *	►p = 0.86	p = 0.07 *	►p = 0.23
Up to 2 days/month	212 (43.8)	14 (6.8)	9 (4.3)	25 (11.8)	25 (11.8)	6 (2.8)
3–4 days/month	153 (31.6)	18 (12.0)	14 (9.3)	18 (11.8)	22 (14.4)	10 (6.5)
5 days/month or more	119 (24.6)	19 (16.4)	16 (13.8)	16 (13.7)	23 (19.3)	5 (4.2)
Always wear PPE		p = 0.01 *	p = 0.04 *	►p = 0.90	►p = 0.97	►p = 0.69
No/Uses one PPE	122 (24.8)	20 (17.2)	16 (13.8)	14 (11.5)	18 (14.8)	6 (4.9)
Two/three PPEs	209 (45.5)	19 (9.3)	13 (6.3)	27 (13.0)	30 (14.4)	7 (3.3)
Four/five PPEs	161 (37.2)	12 (7.6)	10 (6.3)	19 (11.8)	22 (13.7)	8 (5.0)

PRS = pesticide-related symptoms; BMI = body mass index; ► chi-square test; * linear trend test; + Fisher's exact test. Note: unknown data were excluded.

3.3. Acute Pesticide Poisonings Criteria

Among the tobacco growers, 10.6% reported two or more PRS, 8.1% reported three or more PRS, 12.2% received a medical diagnosis of acute pesticide poisoning. According to the toxicologists' assessment, 14.2% were classified as possible cases and 4.3% as probable cases of pesticide poisoning (Table 1). The prevalence of self-reported pesticide poisoning in the last year was 2% (data not shown).

3.4. Pesticide Related Symptoms—PRS

The symptoms that were significantly more frequent in the second stage when compared to the first stage were loss of appetite (RR/risk ratio 3.60); headache (RR 3.50); eye irritation (RR 3.29); salivation (RR 3.19); dyspepsia/difficult digestion (RR 2.82); blurred vision (RR 2.71); skin allergy (RR 2.38) and dizziness (RR 2.10) (Table 2).

Table 2. Pesticide-related symptoms (PRS) *—comparison between period of low and high exposure to pesticides ($n = 492$).

PRS *	Period of Pesticide Exposure		RR (95%CI)
	Low # n (%)	High & n (%)	
Total	492 (100.0)	492 (100.0)	
Loss of appetite	5 (1.0)	18 (3.7)	3.60 (1.35–9.62)
Headache	10 (2.0)	35 (7.1)	3.50 (1.75–6.99)
Irritated eyes	10 (2.0)	33 (6.7)	3.29 (1.64–6.59)
Salivation	5 (1.0)	16 (3.3)	3.19 (1.18–8.65)
Dyspepsia/digestion difficult	6 (1.2)	17 (3.5)	2.82 (1.12–7.08)
Blurred vision	7 (1.4)	19 (3.9)	2.71 (1.15–6.40)
Skin irritation/allergy	8 (1.6)	19 (3.9)	2.38 (1.05–5.38)
Dizziness	11 (2.2)	23 (4.7)	2.10 (1.03–4.25)
Skin burn	1 (0.2)	5 (1.0)	5.00 (0.59–42.64)
Tremors	2 (0.4)	8 (1.6)	3.99 (0.85–18.70)
Vomiting	3 (0.6)	10 (2.0)	3.34 (0.93–12.06)
Sweating	4 (0.8)	11 (2.2)	2.76 (0.88–8.60)
Paresthesia	6 (1.2)	15 (3.1)	2.51 (0.98–6.40)
Intense weakness	6 (1.2)	15 (3.1)	2.51 (0.98–6.39)
Cramps	2 (0.4)	5 (1.0)	2.51 (0.49–12.88)
Phlegm	4 (0.8)	9 (1.8)	2.25 (0.70–7.27)
Cough	4 (0.8)	8 (1.6)	2.10 (0.61–6.63)
Nausea/feeling sick	6 (1.2)	11 (2.2)	1.83 (0.68–4.92)
Shortness of breath	6 (1.2)	11 (2.2)	1.83 (0.68–4.92)
Palpitation	8 (1.6)	12 (2.4)	1.50 (0.62–3.64)
Tearing	4 (0.8)	6 (1.2)	1.50 (0.43–5.28)
Restlessness/irritability	16 (3.3)	20 (4.1)	1.25 (0.65–2.37)
Wheezing	4 (0.8)	5 (1.0)	1.25 (0.34–4.63)
Abdominal pain	5 (1.0)	6 (1.2)	1.20 (0.37–3.90)
Diarrhea	0	1 (0.4)	§

Note: RR—risk ratio (95%CI = 95% confidence interval); * In the last 15 days, has felt onset of symptoms or worsening symptoms up to 48 h after using pesticides; # Low pesticide exposure—first stage of the field work; & High pesticide exposure—second stage of the field work. § Risk Ratio Undefined.

3.5. Pesticide Chemical Types and PRS

The types of chemicals that farmer workers reported using the most with regard to insecticides were neonicotinoids (53.7%), organophosphates (48.6%) and pyrethroids (14,8%); with regard to weedkillers, they used clomazone (56.5%), glyphosate (30.5%) and sulfentrazone (25.6%); while with regard to fungicides, they used dithiocarbamates (38.2%), metalaxyl (30.3%) and iprodione (20.3%). Exposure to dithiocarbamates was significantly associated with an increase in nine PRS, exposure to sulfentrazone with an increase in eight PRS, exposure to pyrethroids with an increase in six PRS, exposure to iprodione and copper compounds with an increase in three PRS, and exposure to fipronil with an increase in two PRS (Table 3).

Table 3. Prevalence of Pesticide-Related Symptoms (PRS) according to chemical types used in the last month.

PRS Chemical Group	Total n (%)	Frequent Headache n (%)	Irritated Eyes n (%)	Dizziness n (%)	Restlessness/ Irritability n (%)	Skin Allergy n (%)	Blurred Vision n (%)	Loss of Appetite n (%)	Dyspepsia n (%)	Salivation n (%)	Paresthesia n (%)	Intense Weakness n (%)	Palpitation n (%)
Total sample	492 (100)	35 (7.1)	33 (6.7)	23 (4.7)	20 (4.1)	19 (3.9)	19 (3.9)	18 (3.7)	17 (3.5)	16 (3.3)	15 (3.1)	15 (3.1)	12 (2.4)
Neonicotinoids	264 (53.7)	16 (6.1)	20 (7.6)	12 (4.6)	12 (4.5)	9 (3.4)	13 (4.9)	9 (3.4)	11 (4.2)	9 (3.4)	7 (2.7)	10 (3.8)	6 (2.3)
Organophosphates	239 (48.6)	14 (5.9)	20 (8.4)	12 (5.0)	8 (3.3)	11 (4.6)	8 (3.3)	10 (4.2)	10 (4.2)	12 (5.0) *	4 (1.7) ° +	8 (3.4)	7 (2.9)
Pyrethroids	73 (14.8)	6 (8.2)	6 (8.2)	6 (8.3)	5 (6.8)	5 (6.8)	6 (8.2) *	3 (4.1) +	4 (5.5) +	6 (8.2) *	7 (9.6) ***	2 (2.7) +	3 (4.1) +
Carbamates	55 (11.2)	3 (5.5) +	5 (9.1)	2 (3.6) +	3 (5.5) +	4 (7.3) +	4 (7.3) +	2 (3.6) +	1 (1.8) +	2 (3.6) +	3 (5.5) +	0 (0.0) +	3 (5.5) +
Benzoylurea	55 (11.2)	3 (5.5) +	6 (10.9)	2 (3.6) +	3 (5.5) +	3 (5.5) +	3 (5.5) +	4 (7.3) +	3 (5.5) +	0 (0.0) +	3 (5.5) +	2 (3.6) +	1 (1.8) +
Fipronil	42 (8.5)	3 (7.1) +	2 (4.8) +	1 (2.4) +	3 (7.1) +	2 (4.8) +	1 (2.4) +	3 (7.1) +	4 (9.5) * +	1 (2.4) +	2 (4.8) +	3 (7.1) +	1 (2.4) +
Clomazone	278 (56.5)	19 (6.9)	18 (6.5)	9 (3.2) °	8 (5.3)	9 (3.2)	8 (2.9)	11 (4.0)	7 (2.5)	6 (2.2)	9 (3.2)	5 (1.8) °	6 (2.2)
Glyphosate	150 (30.5)	14 (9.3)	10 (6.7)	10 (6.7)	8 (5.3)	5 (3.3)	6 (4.0)	7 (5.6)	4 (2.7) +	9 (4.7)	6 (4.0)	6 (4.0)	4 (2.7) +
Sulfentrazone	126 (25.6)	12 (9.5)	12 (9.5)	9 (7.2)	8 (6.3)	7 (5.6)	9 (7.1) *	7 (5.6)	4 (2.7) +	6 (4.8)	7 (5.6) °	8 (6.3) **	3 (2.4) +
Triazines	39 (7.9)	5 (12.8)	1 (2.6) +	0 (0.0) +	1 (2.6) +	1 (2.6) +	0 (0.0) +	0 (0.0) +	2 (5.1) +	1 (2.6) +	1 (2.6) +	0 (0.0) +	0 (0.0) +
Dithiocarbamates	188 (38.2)	21 (11.2) **	20 (10.7) **	16 (8.5) **	14 (7.4) **	12 (6.4) *	11 (5.9) °	8 (4.3)	11 (5.9) **	11 (5.9) **	6 (3.2)	7 (3.7)	9 (4.8) **
Metalaxyl	149 (30.3)	15 (10.1)	15 (10.1) *	6 (4.0)	9 (6.0)	6 (4.0)	8 (5.4)	4 (2.7) +	5 (3.4)	6 (4.0)	3 (2.0) +	5 (3.4)	6 (4.0)
Iprodione	100 (20.3)	9 (9.0)	15 (15.0) ***	6 (6.0)	8 (8.0) *	4 (4.0) +	4 (4.0) +	3 (3.0) +	5 (5.0)	5 (5.0)	4 (4.0) +	3 (3.0) +	2 (2.0) +
Copper compounds	26 (5.3)	3 (11.5) +	3 (12.0) +	2 (7.7) +	0 (0.0) +	0 (0.0) +	0 (0.0) +	0 (0.0) +	0 (0.0) +	2 (7.7) +	3 (11.5) * +	0 (0.0) +	0 (0.0) +

PRS Chemical group	n (%)	Nausea/ Feeling Sick n (%)	Sweating n (%)	Shortness of Breath n (%)	Vomiting n (%)	Phlegm n (%)	Tremors n (%)	Cough n (%)	Abdominal Pain n (%)	Tearing n (%)	Cramps n (%)	Wheezing n (%)	Skin Burn n (%)	Diarrhea n (%)
Total		11 (2.2)	11 (2.2)	11 (2.2)	10 (2.0)	9 (1.8)	8 (1.6)	8 (1.6)	6 (1.2)	6 (1.2)	5 (1.0)	5 (1.0)	5 (1.0)	4 (0.8)
Neonicotinoids	264 (53.7)	6 (2.3)	2 (2.7) +	6 (2.3)	6 (2.3)	6 (2.3)	5 (1.9)	3 (1.1) +	4 (1.5)	4 (1.5)	3 (1.1) +	4 (1.5) +	4 (1.5) +	2 (1.1) +
Organophosphates	239 (48.6)	6 (2.5)	7 (2.9)	5 (2.1) °	5 (2.1)	5 (2.1)	4 (1.7) +	5 (2.1) +	3 (1.3) +	3 (1.3) +	2 (0.8) +	2 (0.8) +	2 (0.8) +	3 (1.3) +
Pyrethroids	73 (14.8)	4 (5.5) ° +	3 (4.1) +	4 (5.5) °	4 (5.5) * +	3 (4.1) +	4 (5.5) * +	1 (1.4) +	2 (2.7) +	2 (2.7) +	1 (1.4) +	2 (2.7) +	3 (4.1) * +	1 (1.4) +
Carbamates	55 (11.2)	3 (5.5) +	3 (5.5) +	3 (5.5) +	1 (1.8) +	3 (5.5) ° +	0 (0.0) +	2 (3.6) +	0 (0.0) +	2 (3.6) +	1 (1.8) +	1 (1.8) +	1 (1.8) +	0 (0.0) +
Benzoylurea	55 (11.2)	1 (1.8) +	0 (0.0) +	0 (0.0) +	0 (0.0) +	3 (5.5) ° +	0 (0.0) +	2 (3.6) +	0 (0.0) +	1 (1.8) +	1 (1.8) +	0 (0.0) +	2 (3.6) ° +	1 (1.8) +
Fipronil	42 (8.5)	2 (4.8) +	1 (2.4) +	3 (7.1) ° +	0 (0.0) +	0 (0.0) +	0 (0.0) +	0 (0.0) +	1 (2.4) +	0 (0.0) +	0 (0.0) +	0 (0.0) +	1 (2.4) +	0 (0.0) +
Clomazone	278 (56.5)	6 (2.2)	5 (1.8)	4 (1.4) +	6 (2.2)	6 (2.2)	3 (1.1) +	5 (1.8)	3 (1.1) +	4 (1.4) +	2 (0.7) +	2 (0.7) +	4 (1.4) +	2 (0.7) +
Glyphosate	150 (30.5)	6 (4.0) °	3 (2.0) +	5 (3.3) +	4 (2.7) +	4 (2.7) +	3 (2.0) +	5 (3.4) *	1 (0.7) +	2 (1.3) +	2 (1.3) +	3 (2.0) +	2 (1.3) +	1 (0.7) +
Sulfentrazone	126 (25.6)	5 (4.0)	4 (3.2) +	4 (3.2) +	6 (4.8) **	5 (4.0) **	5 (4.0) **	4 (3.2) +	3 (2.4) +	5 (4.0) ***	2 (1.3) +	4 (3.2) * +	4 (3.2) * +	2 (1.6) +
Triazines	39 (7.9)	0 (0.0) +	1 (2.6) +	0 (0.0) +	0 (0.0) +	0 (0.0) +	0 (0.0) +	0 (0.0) +	0 (0.0) +	0 (0.0) +	0 (0.0) +	0 (0.0) +	0 (0.0) +	0 (0.0) +
Dithiocarbamates	182 (37.0)	6 (3.2)	7 (3.7) °	9 (4.8) **	5 (2.7)	3 (2.0) +	4 (2.1) +	2 (1.3) +	3 (1.6) +	3 (1.6) +	1 (0.7) +	4 (2.1) ° +	1 (0.5) +	3 (1.6) +
Metalaxyl	149 (30.3)	4 (2.7) +	3 (2.0) +	6 (4.0) °	3 (2.0) +	3 (2.0) +	1 (0.7) +	2 (1.3) +	3 (1.6) +	0 (0.0) +	1 (0.7) +	3 (2.0) +	1 (0.7) +	1 (0.7) +
Iprodione	100 (20.3)	4 (4.0) +	5 (5.0) * +	2 (2.0) +	2 (2.0) +	1 (1.0) +	1 (1.0) +	0 (0.0) +	1 (1.0) +	1 (1.0) +	2 (2.0) +	1 (1.0) +	1 (1.0) +	1 (1.0) +
Copper compounds	26 (5.3)	0 (0.0) +	3 (11.5) * +	0 (0.0) +	1 (3.8) +	1 (3.8) +	0 (0.0) +	0 (0.0) +	2 (7.7) * +	1 (3.8) +	1 (4.0) +	0 (0.0) +	0 (0.0) +	1 (3.8) +

Note: ° $p \leq 0.10$; * $p \leq 0.05$; ** $p \leq 0.01$; *** $p \leq 0.001$ Chi-square test; + Fisher's exact test; PRS—pesticide-related symptoms.

3.6. Bivariate Analysis

In the bivariate analysis, women presented with 2.5 times more pesticide poisonings than men according to the PRS criterion and the toxicologists' assessment as probable cases. Among those whose tobacco production was up to 4000 kg, the frequency of the outcome was 2.5 times higher than those who produced more than 9000 kg according to the criteria of two or more PRS, medical diagnosis and probable case as per the toxicologists' assessment. Alcohol consumption was protective for poisoning, except for the criterion of possible case as per the toxicologists' assessment (Table 4). Age, schooling, BMI and smoking showed no association with any of the criteria.

Table 4. Association between socioeconomic factors and occupational exposure to pesticides with several criteria of acute pesticide poisoning—Crude analysis through Poisson Regression (n = 492).

Variables	2 or More PRS	3 or More PRS	Medical Diagnosis	Toxicologist Possible Case	Toxicologist Probable Case
Socioeconomic	Crude PR (CI)	Crude PR (CI)	Crude PR (CI)	Crude PR (CI)	Crude PR (CI)
Sex	▶p = 0.001	▶p = 0.002	▶p = 0.11	▶p = 0.05	▶p = 0.04
Male	1	1	1	1	1
Female	2.38 (1.42–3.98)	2.62 (1.45–4.76)	1.51 (0.92–2.50)	1.59 (0.99–1.17)	2.43 (1.05–5.63)
Tobacco production	p = 0.006 *	▶p = 0.07	p = 0.009 *	p = 0.08 *	▶p = 0.03
Up to 4000 kg	1	1	1	1	1
4001–9000 kg	0.94 (0.56–1.63)	1.29 (0.68–2.47)	0.63 (0.37–1.07)	0.80 (0.49–1.31)	0.29 (0.10–0.86)
Above 9000 kg	0.32 (0.13–0.76)	0.42 (0.15–1.13)	0.44 (0.23–0.85)	0.61 (0.34–1.08)	0.36 (0.12–1.08)
Alcohol consumption	p = 0.03 *	p = 0.02 *	p = 0.02 *	p = 0.08 *	p = 0.02 *
Does not drink	1	1	1	1	1
Up to 7 days/month	0.65 (0.37–1.15)	0.57 (0.30–1.11)	0.90 (0.53–1.53)	0.73 (0.45–1.20)	0.40 (0.16–0.99)
≥8 days/month	0.45 (0.22–0.94)	0.38 (0.16–0.90)	0.44 (0.21–0.93)	0.58 (0.32–1.06)	0.24 (0.07–0.85)
BMI	▶p = 0.58	▶p = 0.45	p = 0.13 *	▶p = 0.13	▶p = 0.88
Normal Weight	1	1	1	1	1
Overweight	1.34 (0.77–2.34)	1.45 (0.77–2.75)	1.36 (0.81–2.29)	1.55 (0.98–2.45)	1.12 (0.46–2.69)
Obese	1.26 (0.56–2.82)	0.95 (0.33–2.72)	1.60 (0.81–3.17)	0.96 (0.44–2.09)	0.77 (0.17–3.41)
Main Forms of Exposure to Pesticides					
Applying Pesticides	▶p = 0.02	▶p = 0.03	▶p = 0.10	▶p = 0.07	▶p = 0.06
No	1	1	1	1	1
Yes	2.14 (1.15–3.99)	1.98 (1.07–4.53)	1.55 (0.92–2.62)	1.56 (0.96–2.51)	2.83 (0.97–8.29)
Preparing mixture	▶p = 0.06	▶p = 0.17	▶p = 0.11	▶p = 0.06	▶p = 0.11
No	1	1	1	1	1
Yes	2.08 (0.96–4.49)	1.80 (0.77–4.21)	1.70 (0.89–3.26)	1.79 (0.97–3.29)	3.22 (0.76–13.62)
Washing contaminated clothing	▶p = 0.03	▶p = 0.03	▶p = 0.02	▶p = 0.14	▶p = 0.02
No	1	1	1	1	1
Yes	1.77 (1.05–3.00)	1.98 (1.07–3.68)	1.76 (1.08–2.87)	1.40 (0.90–2.16)	3.02 (1.19–7.65)
Reentering after application	▶p = 0.02	▶p = 0.01	▶p = 0.22	▶p = 0.78	▶p = 0.97
No	1	1	1	1	1
Yes	1.99 (1.14–3.50)	2.32 (1.18–4.55)	1.35 (0.83–2.20)	1.06 (0.69–1.64)	0.98 (0.43–2.28)
Clothes wet during application	▶p = 0.01	▶p = 0.002	▶p = 0.02	▶p = 0.004	▶p = 0.002
No	1	1	1	1	1
Yes	1.94 (1.16–3.24)	2.61 (1.42–4.76)	1.76 (1.10–2.82)	1.90 (1.23–2.91)	4.01 (1.65–9.75)
Spilling on body/clothing	▶p < 0.001	▶p < 0.001	▶p = 0.05	▶p = 0.005	▶p < 0.001
No	1	1	1	1	1
Yes	2.55 (1.53–4.28)	3.05 (1.69–5.53)	1.68 (1.01–2.79)	1.90 (1.22–2.98)	6.32 (2.69–14.83)
Forms of exposure [1]	p = 0.007 *	p = 0.008 *	p = 0.02 *	p = 0.002 *	
Up to 4 forms	1	1	1	1	(a)
5–6 forms	2.45 (0.99–6.07)	1.66 (0.57–4.81)	1.54 (0.73–3.24)	2.03 (0.96–4.30)	(a)
7 forms or more	3.02 (1.28–7.11)	3.20 (1.25–8.20)	2.14 (1.09–4.21)	2.77 (1.38–5.54)	(a)

Table 4. Cont.

Variables	2 or More PRS	3 or More PRS	Medical Diagnosis	Toxicologist Possible Case	Toxicologist Probable Case
Multi–chemical Exposure [2]	$p < 0.001$ *	$p < 0.001$ *	▶$p = 0.56$	$p = 0.01$ *	$p = 0.01$ *
Used up to 2 types	1	1	1	1	1
Used 3–4 types	1.00 (0.43–2.29)	1.00 (0.35–2.80)	0.99 (0.54–1.83)	1.30 (0.70–2.42)	2.65 (0.56–12.56)
Used 5 types or more	2.95 (1.45–5.99)	3.69 (1.56–8.72)	1.30 (0.72–2.36)	2.04 (1.14–3.67)	5.36 (1.22–23.55)
Frequency of use	$p = 0.006$ *	$p = 0.002$ *	▶$p = 0.86$	$p = 0.07$ *	▶$p = 0.25$
Up to 2 days/month	1	1	1	1	1
3–5 days/month	1.77 (0.91–3.45)	2.15 (0.95–4.83)	1.00 (0.57–1.76)	1.22 (0.72–2.08)	2.31 (0.86–6.22)
>5 days/month	2.42 (1.26–4.67)	3.17 (1.45–6.95)	1.16 (0.65–2.08)	1.64 (0.98–2.76)	1.49 (0.46–4.76)
Always wear PPE	$p = 0.001$ *	▶$p = 0.04$	▶$p = 0.90$	▶$p = 0.97$	▶$p = 0.69$
No/One PPE	1	1	1	1	1
Two/three PPEs	0.54 (0.30–0.97)	0.46 (0.23–0.92)	1.14 (0.62–2.08)	0.97 (0.57–1.67)	0.68 (0.23–1.98)
Four/five PPEs	0.44 (0.22–0.87)	0.46 (0.22–0.97)	1.03 (0.54–1.97)	0.93 (0.52–1.65)	1.01 (0.36–2.84)

Note: ▶ p-value of the Wald heterogeneity test; * p-value of linear trend test; [1] Sum of the 12 forms of exposure; [2] Sum of the types of chemicals used; (a) not possible to perform regression (zero category); PRS—pesticide-related symptoms; PPE—personal protective equipment; PR—prevalence ratio; CI—95% confidence interval.

As for the forms of exposure, having clothes wet with pesticide during application and suffering pesticide spillage on the body or clothes were associated with the outcome, with risks higher than 68% according to all criteria, reaching a risk of 300% for clothes wet with pesticide and 500% for spillage on the body or clothes according to the probable case criterion. Applying pesticides and going back into the plantation without PPE were associated with an almost two-fold increase in pesticide poisoning according to the two or more PRS and three or more PRS criteria. Washing contaminated clothing was associated with the outcome with risks ranging from 76% to 200% using the different criteria, except for the possible case criterion, for which there was no association (Table 4).

The number of forms of worker exposure showed significant direct association with the outcome (linear trend p-value less than 0.01), except for the probable diagnosis criterion, which did not have statistical power to perform the calculation. The same occurred with the number of types of chemicals used, except for the medical diagnosis criterion. The number of days of pesticide use showed direct association and the number of PPEs always used showed inverse association with the outcome according to the two or more PRS and three or more PRS criteria (Table 4).

3.7. Multivariate Analysis—Poisson Regression

The multivariate analysis was adjusted for gender, tobacco production and alcohol consumption. Alcohol consumption and washing contaminated clothes lost their association with the outcome, while being female and the number of days of pesticide use also became associated according to the possible case criterion as per the toxicologists' assessment. Pesticide poisoning was almost double among those exposed to pesticide solution preparation according to the two or more PRS and possible case criteria. Multi-chemical exposure not only remained associated with the PRS and toxicological criteria but also showed increased strength of association in those exposed to five or more types of pesticides. The other associations remained similar to those of the bivariate analysis (Table 5).

Table 5. Association between socioeconomic factors and occupational exposure to pesticides with several criteria of acute pesticide poisoning—adjusted analysis through Poisson regression ($n = 492$).

Variables	2 or More PRS	3 or More PRS	Medical Diagnosis	Toxicologist Possible Case	Toxicologist Probable Case
Socioeconomic	Adjusted PR (CI)	Adjusted PR (CI)	Adjusted PR (CI)	Adjusted PR (CI)	Adjusted PR (CI)
Sex	▶$p = 0.001$	▶$p = 0.002$	▶$p = 0.12$	▶$p = 0.04$	▶$p = 0.04$
Male	1	1	1	1	1
Female	2.31 (1.39–3.85)	2.57 (1.43–4.61)	1.48 (0.91–2.42)	1.60 (1.02–2.51)	2.34 (1.03–5.29)

Table 5. Cont.

Variables	2 or More PRS	3 or More PRS	Medical Diagnosis	Toxicologist Possible Case	Toxicologist Probable Case
Tobacco production	$p = 0.04$ *	$p = 0.08$ *	$p = 0.03$ *	$p = 0.25$ *	$p = 0.04$ *
Up to 4000 kg	1	1	1	1	1
4001–9000 kg	0.95 (0.56–1.62)	1.30 (0.69–2.46)	0.64 (0.38–1.08)	0.81 (0.50–1.32)	0.29 (0.10–0.87)
Above 9000 kg	0.33 (0.14–0.79)	0.43 (0.16–1.17)	0.45 (0.23–0.86)	0.62 (0.35–1.10)	0.37 (0.13–1.11)
Alcohol consumption	▶$p = 0.73$	▶$p = 0.69$	▶$p = 0.12$	▶$p = 0.60$	▶$p = 0.26$
Does not drink	1	1	1	1	1
Up to 7 days/month	0.93 (0.49–1.79)	0.85 (0.38–1.89)	1.02 (0.55–1.88)	0.83 (0.47–1.46)	0.48 (0.16–1.46)
≥8 days/month	0.73 (0.32–1.68)	0.64 (0.23–1.79)	0.50 (0.22–1.15)	0.70 (0.35–1.40)	0.29 (0.06–1.39)
Main Forms of Exposure to Pesticides					
Applying pesticides	▶$p = 0.02$	▶$p = 0.03$	▶$p = 0.17$	▶$p = 0.09$	▶$p = 0.06$
No	1	1	1	1	1
Yes	2.11 (1.16–3.86)	2.20 (1.10–4.43)	1.45 (0.86–2.44)	1.51 (0.94–2.44)	2.80 (0.98–7.99)
Preparing mixture	▶$p = 0.03$	▶$p = 0.08$	▶$p = 0.07$	▶$p = 0.03$	▶$p = 0.06$
No	1	1	1	1	1
Yes	2.33 (1.10–4.93)	2.09 (0.91–4.83)	1.80 (0.95–3.44)	1.93 (1.06–3.52)	3.81 (0.95–15.31)
Washing contaminated clothing	▶$p = 0.45$	▶$p = 0.33$	▶$p = 0.16$	▶$p = 0.74$	▶$p = 0.11$
No	1	1	1	1	1
Yes	1.24 (0.71–2.19)	1.40 (0.71–2.73)	1.45 (0.87–2.42)	1.09 (0.65–1.82)	2.23 (0.84–5.89)
Reentering after application	▶$p = 0.03$	▶$p = 0.02$	▶$p = 0.23$	▶$p = 0.75$	▶$p = 0.90$
No	1	1	1	1	1
Yes	1.86 (1.07–3.22)	2.17 (1.13–4.19)	1.35 (0.83–2.18)	1.07 (0.70–1.66)	0.95 (0.41–2.18)
Clothes wet during application	▶$p = 0.01$	▶$p = 0.002$	▶$p = 0.02$	▶$p = 0.002$	▶$p = 0.002$
No	1	1	1	1	1
Yes	1.94 (1.16–3.25)	2.65 (1.44–4.89)	1.72 (1.08–2.75)	1.99 (1.29–3.07)	4.11 (1.69–10.04)
Spilling on body/clothing	▶$p < 0.001$	▶$p < 0.001$	▶$p = 0.02$	▶$p = 0.002$	▶$p < 0.001$
No	1	1	1	1	1
Yes	2.76 (1.67–4.54)	3.44 (1.96–6.01)	1.82 (1.11–2.96)	1.99 (1.28–3.09)	6.52 (2.96–14.36)
Forms of exposure [1]	$p = 0.007$ *	$p = 0.007$ *	$p = 0.03$ *	$p = 0.02$ *	
Up to 4 forms	1	1	1	1	(a)
5–6 forms	2.17 (0.89–5.29)	1.47 (0.51–4.18)	1.37 (0.65–2.85)	1.80 (0.85–3.83)	(a)
7 forms or more	2.92 (1.26–6.78)	3.16 (1.24–8.01)	2.04 (1.03–4.03)	2.76 (1.36–5.58)	(a)
Multi–chemical exposure [2]	$p < 0.001$ *	$p < 0.001$ *	▶$p = 0.53$	$p = 0.005$ *	$p = 0.001$ *
Used up to 2 types	1	1	1	1	1
Used 3–4 types	1.16 (0.50–2.67)	1.19 (0.43–3.35)	1.08 (0.57–2.02)	1.38 (0.73–2.61)	3.23 (0.71–14.72)
Used 5 types or more	3.68 (1.77–7.65)	4.85 (2.03–11.59)	1.38 (0.73–2.60)	2.29 (1.25–4.19)	6.83 (1.65–28.33)
Frequency of pesticide use	$p = 0.003$ *	$p = 0.001$ *	▶$p = 0.78$	$p = 0.04$ *	▶$p = 0.20$
Up to 2 days/month	1	1	1	1	1
3–5 days/month	1.95 (1.01–3.76)	2.40 (1.08–5.34)	1.05 (0.60–1.84)	1.33 (0.78–2.27)	2.39 (0.91–6.30)
>5 days/month	2.46 (1.31–4.62)	3.24 (1.51–6.94)	1.23 (0.68–2.21)	1.73 (1.02–2.93)	1.52 (0.47–4.89)
Always wear PPE	$p = 0.01$ *	$p = 0.04$ *	▶$p = 0.94$	▶$p = 0.87$	▶$p = 0.45$
No/One PPE	1	1	1	1	1
Two/three PPEs	0.51 (0.28–0.91)	0.46 (0.22–0.93)	1.04 (0.57–1.88)	0.92 (0.54–1.56)	0.55 (0.19–1.57)
Four/five PPEs	0.42 (0.22–0.81)	0.45 (0.22–0.93)	0.94 (0.50–1.78)	0.86 (0.48–1.53)	0.94 (0.34–2.56)

Note: ▶p-value of the Wald heterogeneity test; * p-value of linear trend test; [1] Sum of the 12 forms of exposure; [2] Sum of the types of chemicals used; (a) not possible to perform regression (zero category); PRS—pesticide-related symptoms; PPE—personal protective equipment; PR—prevalence ratio; CI—95% confidence interval.

3.8. Sensitivity, Specificity, Predictive Value and Agreement

Table 6 shows the analysis of sensitivity, specificity, predictive value and agreement for two or more PRS, three or more PRS and medical diagnosis when comparing possible cases and probable cases of pesticide poisoning as per the toxicologists' assessment. All diagnostic criteria exhibited specificity above 95% for possible cases and above 90% for probable cases. The negative predictive value was greater than 90% for possible cases and 99% for probable cases. In the comparison with probable cases, the criteria that used PRS exhibited less than 50% sensitivity and a positive predictive value less than 61%, while medical diagnosis showed 73% sensitivity and an 85% positive predictive value. With regard to probable cases, sensitivity was greater than 79% for all criteria and positive predictive value was less than 39% for all criteria. Agreement as evaluated using the Kappa test was substantial for the comparison between medical diagnosis and possible cases (0.75) and moderate for three or more PRS compared with probable cases (0.49) and for medical diagnosis compared with probable cases (0.43).

Table 6. Sensitivity, specificity, positive/negative predictive value and agreement of PRS and medical diagnosis criteria for acute pesticide poisoning when compared with toxicology assessment. (Possible case = 14.2% and probable case = 4.3%).

Criterion	Sensitivity	Specificity	PPV	NPV	Kappa
Toxicology Assessment of Possible Case					
Two or more PRS	46.3%	95.2%	60.8%	91.6%	0.22 *
Three or more PRS	35.8%	96.2%	61.5%	90.2%	0.39 *
Medical Diagnosis	72.9%	97.9%	85.0%	95.6%	0.75 *
Toxicology Assessment of Probable Case					
Two or more PRS	79.0%	92.2%	29.4%	99.1%	0.19 *
Three or more PRS	79.0%	94.8%	38.5%	99.1%	0.49 *
Medical Diagnosis	90.5%	91.3%	31.7%	99.5%	0.43 *

Note: * Kappa Test p-value < 0.001; PPV—positive predictive value; NPV—negative predictive value; PRS—pesticide-related symptoms.

4. Discussion

The study indicates that the different criteria used result in variability in the estimates of acute pesticide poisoning, all of which are higher than self-reported information, which in turn, are higher than the official records that identified, at the most, 11 annual cases per 100,000 inhabitants [5,23]. In the Serra Gaúcha fruit growing, the prevalence of acute pesticide poisoning also varied according to the criterion used, being 3.8% in 12 months according to workers' self-reported information and 11% for probable cases according to the criterion of three or more PRS [7]. In the state of Espírito Santo, 7.5% of agricultural workers exhibited poisoning, based on self-reported previous medical diagnosis [19].

4.1. Pesticide-Related Symptoms-PRS

Questionnaires of PRS were used as a criterion for identifying pesticide poisoning in other studies, although with some differences in the list of symptoms [7,24–28] and in the criterion regarding the time between exposure and occurrence of symptoms, which varied from 24 h [25,26] to 48 h [24,28], or recent symptoms without specifying the period of time following pesticide use [7,27], or even presence of common poisoning symptoms without considering the time relationship with exposure [29]. Although all the PRS showed some degree of increase in the second stage (greater exposure to chemicals), the increase was only significant for some of the symptoms, possibly due to statistical power limitations. The symptoms assessed are common to several morbidities, but the exposure time criterion, according to the WHO methodology, suggests a link with occupational exposure, with some effects being caused by contact with chemicals, such as eye and skin symptoms, and others being systemic, such as neurological and digestive symptoms.

4.2. Pesticide Chemical Types

Among the types of chemicals that stood out in the associations with PRS, most are considered to have low acute toxicity, such as dithiocarbamates, sulfentrazone and iprodione, for example [30,31]. Most of these chemicals can cause skin and mucous membrane (respiratory, ocular and digestive) symptoms. Dithiocarbamate fungicides (especially mancozeb) are associated with acute poisoning; skin, respiratory system and ocular mucous membranes irritation, and with systemic effects, such as thyroid alterations, liver disease and kidney disease [32]. The weedkiller sulfentrazone, a lesser known pesticide, in addition to skin and mucous membrane symptoms, is linked to developmental and reproductive effects [31]. With regard to iprodione, studies with animals indicate that it has a carcinogenic effect and reproductive toxicity [33].

Pyrethroids are widely used insecticides, including in urban areas, and their acute allergic, respiratory and skin effects are well known, as well as systemic effects such as oxidative stress and neurotoxic, hepatotoxic and nephrotoxic symptoms, among others [34]. Fipronil is another increasingly used insecticide and can even be found in pet shops [35]. This insecticide is a GABA inhibitor (gamma-aminobutyric acid), which can produce neurological (headache, dizziness, paresthesia), ocular, gastrointestinal, respiratory and skin symptoms [36].

Occurrence of PRS can be due to either the individual effect or the combined effect of the various types of chemicals, as well as other components of the commercial formulation, such as surfactants and solvents. As such, multi-chemical exposure makes it difficult to identify the specific pesticide related to each symptom. It is possible that some associations (or the lack of them) may have been influenced by frequent exposure, by multi-chemical exposure and/or by limitations in the measurement of exposure. Toxicological research generally tests one product at a time and considers primarily the risk of death, assigning less toxicity to other effects. In addition to the paucity of information on the toxic effects of some types of chemicals on humans, there are fewer studies on the mild and moderate effects typical in the occupational context. The workers who exhibited PRS were active and displayed mild conditions with no need for referral to hospital or emergency services. For this reason, they may have shown some symptoms that are not among the main ones identified in severe cases.

4.3. Acute Pesticide Poisoning—Main Associated Factors

The higher prevalence of acute pesticide poisoning among women is consistent with other studies that have examined PRS among agricultural workers [7,25,26,37,38] but contrasts with official records in Brazil [5,23,39–41], in which pesticide poisonings are predominant among men. Official records may underestimate more the occurrence of poisoning among women, due to greater failure to investigate their occupation and/or exposure to pesticides, or by not considering common forms of female exposure, such as washing contaminated clothes. Hormonal mechanisms, smaller body area, lower adherence to PPE, and the fact that women report their health problems better may explain higher prevalence of poisoning among women [15]. Considering that pesticide application is a predominantly male task, this study assessed a particularly exposed subgroup of women, given that they had applied pesticides in the last year.

Inverse association between tobacco production and pesticide poisoning is consistent with the literature, which indicates that poorer socioeconomic conditions are related to poorer health conditions [42,43]. Farms with better economic indicators usually have a better level of technology, including pesticide application equipment, more adequate personal protection equipment, and better agricultural practices, implying a reduction in exposure. As it occurred in China [25], in our study there was no association between schooling and poisoning. This contrasted with previous studies in the Serra Gaúcha region that pointed to an inverse association between schooling and acute poisoning [6,7], as well as with other studies in which low schooling was associated with higher exposure to pesticides and unsafe practices during work involving pesticides [44]. There was limited statistical power to assess this association, especially since the vast majority (86.8%) of the workers studied had not completed elementary school.

In occupational exposure, the skin is the most important pesticide absorption route [28,45,46], and in hot climates, such as in tropical countries, absorption is even greater [25]. Several pesticides, such as organophosphorus compounds, carbamates and pyrethroids, demonstrate considerable cutaneous absorption [20,34,47,48]. In keeping with other studies [46,48,49], spilling pesticide on the body and wearing clothes wet from pesticides were associated with all criteria with great strength of association, especially the toxicological probable case criterion. Other studies indicated that poisoning was greater among workers who went back into the plantation without protection following spraying [28,49]. In our study, this aspect was associated with PRS. The direct association between number of chemical types and number of forms of exposure to pesticides with regard to all the poisoning criteria suggests that these may be indicators of exposure intensity.

4.4. Personal Protective Equipment—PPE

Some studies, especially clinical trials [45] focusing on PPE testing, point to their protective effect, while others question it [50,51]. Furthermore, some population-based studies [7] have not confirmed their protective effect, suggesting that it may be overestimated [52]. The inverse association between PPE use, found only with the PRS-based criteria and no significant association with the other criteria, led us to question the effectiveness of PPE. On the other hand, the lack of information concerning protection of the eyes, face and neck; the constancy, the adequacy and completeness of PPE used for specific forms of exposures; as well as the lack of information about PPE quality, PPE cleaning practices and PPE use in the different forms of exposure, limit evaluation of PPE. Although tobacco farmers report receiving frequent technical guidance, they do not always use PPE as recommended. Discomfort when using PPE in high temperatures, as well as its cost, are major factors for low adherence to PPE use [53].

4.5. Pesticide Poisoning Criteria Evaluation

The PRS questionnaire, considering three or more symptoms, has proven useful for probable case screening but does not adequately capture possible cases of pesticide poisoning. On the other hand, medical diagnosis by trained professionals, when compared to the toxicologists' assessment, has adequate sensitivity and agreement for screening both probable and possible cases, even without laboratory tests. It should be noted that the toxicologists' assessment, the other standard used, took into consideration all the other criteria and also presents a certain degree of subjectivity.

4.6. Limitations and Challenges

This study contained a representative sample of tobacco growers who applied pesticides, and the sample size was adequate for assessing prevalence of acute pesticide poisoning according to different criteria. However, there were limitations in the statistical power of the study to examine some associations, especially with the probable case outcome and in the comparison between the two stages. In addition, since all of them had applied pesticides in the previous year, there was little variability in some forms of exposure. Flumethralin (plant growth inhibitor), one of the most used chemical types, was not assessed because the period in which it is used had not started when the study fieldwork took place. It is also noteworthy that the forms of exposure were related to most recent contact with pesticides, which may have reduced the proportion of tobacco growers who reported doing certain tasks, such as washing contaminated clothes. The self-reported information about symptoms and pesticide exposure is valuable and easy to collect but can be imprecise and subjected to recall bias, in general, underestimating its prevalence. Since pesticide use has increased in Brazil, and given that there has not been much progress in investigating acute pesticide poisoning in the country, despite the study being conducted some time ago, it nevertheless presents relevant and conservative information in relation to the current situation [20].

The availability and cost of biomarkers in Brazil make their inclusion in epidemiological studies difficult, so our study only relied on BCHE testing. The use of cards with pictures of the most common pesticides reduced memory bias and, together with the detailing of exposure, ensured information quality. However, an expansion and improvement of laboratories for toxicological tests is needed to qualify clinical and epidemiological evaluations. The partnership with the Municipal Health Department and with Family

Health Strategy rural area health teams facilitated the logistics of the study and adherence of the tobacco farmers to the research. In return, the research provided training for health professionals in rural areas about acute pesticide and nicotine poisoning.

In order to obtain greater heterogeneity with regard to exposure, it is important for future studies to include all agricultural workers and not only those who applied pesticides in the previous year. This being a low-prevalence event, it is also essential to have a larger sample size, to enable more in-depth understanding of factors associated with probable cases. It is necessary to move forward with objective characterization of exposure by expanding the use of biomarkers. However, in the absence of biomarkers, it is important to prepare cards with pictures of the most commonly used pesticides in order to characterize their use. Moreover, when evaluating intense exposure, multi-chemical exposure and the number of forms of exposure can be used as indicators. The PRS questionnaire can be used in epidemiological studies to estimate probable cases. During the interviews, we noted that restlessness/irritability symptoms, although they are neurological symptoms, may indicate different neuropsychiatric problems and, therefore, should have been collected separately. For future studies we suggest replacing restlessness/irritability with restlessness/uneasiness and nervousness/irritability. PPE evaluation requires specific studies that allow a better understanding of the factors that reduce its protective role.

5. Conclusions and Recommendations

This study indicates an acute pesticide poisoning prevalence much higher than that officially recorded. Considering the high prevalence of poisoning, as well as the high and increasing use of these chemicals, public policies that seek to reduce exposure to pesticides should be encouraged, including the quest for sustainable agricultural production models [29], their replacement with less toxic products, as well as individual protection measures.

Among the main occupational associated factors, those with skin exposure stood out. Thus, special attention should be paid to reduce skin exposure through the implementation of occupational hygiene measures such as the quick removal of wet contaminated clothes, clean hands and skin with pesticide residues, caution when handling pesticides or when removing PPE and correct use of PPE. These approaches should go hand in hand with actions to educate workers about the toxicity of products, reading labels, product handling, forms of chemical exposure and the adoption of good agricultural practices.

This study indicates that the PRS questionnaire is an important tool to medical diagnosis and that trained physicians, even without laboratory tests, can screen for possible and probable cases of pesticide poisoning. Thus, these professionals should be trained to perform early detection, notification and clinical management of people who were poisoned. An open access site with information on the association of pesticides with acute poisoning and chronic effects, maintained by reputable public institutions, could be an important support for health professionals and researchers.

In addition, health teams need to be trained to guide agricultural workers and their families in preventing these forms of pesticide poisoning.

Author Contributions: Conceptualization, N.M.X.F., A.G.F. and R.D.M.; methodology, A.G.F. and N.M.X.F.; software, A.G.F., R.D.M. and N.S.F.; validation, N.M.X.F., A.G.F., R.D.M. and N.S.F.; formal analysis, N.M.X.F., R.D.M. and N.S.F.; investigation, N.M.X.F., A.G.F., R.D.M., N.S.F., M.L.V.C. and C.A.M.-d.-S.; resources, A.G.F., R.D.M. and N.S.F.; data curation, A.G.F., R.D.M. and N.S.F.; writing—original draft preparation, N.M.X.F. and A.G.F.; writing—review and editing, N.M.X.F., A.G.F., R.D.M., N.S.F., M.L.V.C. and C.A.M.-d.-S.; visualization, N.M.X.F., A.G.F., R.D.M. and N.S.F.; supervision, N.M.X.F., A.G.F., R.D.M., N.S.F. and M.L.V.C.; project administration, A.G.F.; funding acquisition, A.G.F., N.M.X.F. and R.D.M. All authors have read and agreed to the published version of the manuscript.

Funding: This research was funded by the National Council for Scientific and Technological Development (CNPq Process 483214/2009-4, 2009) and by the Research Support Foundation of the Rio Grande do Sul State (FAPERGS Process 09/0057.5, 2009).

Institutional Review Board Statement: The study was conducted according to the guidelines of the Declaration of Helsinki, and approved by the Research Ethics Committee of the Faculty of Medicine of the Federal University of Pelotas (protocol code 11/2010).

Informed Consent Statement: Informed consent was obtained from all subjects involved in the study.

Data Availability Statement: The data presented in this study are not publicly available due to ethical reasons.

Acknowledgments: Municipal Secretary of Health of São Lourenço do Sul, all participating staff (interviewers, support services, laboratory staff, technicians, physicians and toxicologists) and all participating tobacco growers.

Conflicts of Interest: The authors declare no conflict of interest.

References

1. Carneiro, F.F.; Augusto, L.G.d.S.; Rigotto, R.M.; Friedrich, K.; Burigo, A.C. Dossiê Abrasco: Um Alerta Sobre os Impactos dos Agrotóxicos na Saúde. EPSJV: Rio de Janeiro, Brazil; Expressão Popular: São Paulo, Brazil, 2015. Available online: https://www.abrasco.org.br/dossieagrotoxicos/wp-content/uploads/2013/10/DossieAbrasco_2015_web.pdf (accessed on 10 November 2022).
2. FAO. *Pesticides Use, Pesticides Trade and Pesticides Indicators–Global, Regional and Country Trends, 1990–2020*; FAOSTAT Analytical Briefs; Food and Agriculture Organization of the United Nations: Rome, Italy, 2022. Available online: https://www.fao.org/3/cc0918en/cc0918en.pdf (accessed on 25 November 2022).
3. IBAMA. *Relatórios de Comercialização de Agrotóxicos 2009–2020*; IBAMA-Ministério do Meio Ambiente_Instituto Brasileiro do Meio Ambiente e dos Recursos Naturais Renováveis: Brasília, Brazil, 2022. Available online: http://www.ibama.gov.br/agrotoxicos/relatorios-de-comercializacao-de-agrotoxicos#boletinsanuais (accessed on 10 November 2022).
4. Douglas, M.R.; Baisley, P.; Soba, S.; Kammerer, M.; Lonsdorf, E.V.; Grozinger, C.M. Putting pesticides on the map for pollinator research and conservation. *Sci. Data* **2022**, *9*, 571. [CrossRef] [PubMed]
5. Brasil, Ministério da Saúde, Secretaria de Vigilância em Saúde; Vigilância Epidemiológica. *SINAN Sistema de Informação de Agravos de Notificação*; TABNET-DATASUS; Ministério da Saúde (BR): Brasília, Brazil, 2022. Available online: http://tabnet.datasus.gov.br/cgi/deftohtm.exe?sinannet/cnv/Intoxbr.def (accessed on 10 November 2022).
6. Faria, N.M.; Facchini, L.A.; Fassa, A.G.; Tomasi, E. Rural work and pesticide poisoning. *Cad. Saude Publica* **2004**, *20*, 1298–1308. [CrossRef] [PubMed]
7. Faria, N.M.; Rosa, J.A.; Facchini, L.A. Poisoning by pesticides among family fruit farmers, Bento Goncalves, Southern Brazil. *Rev. Saude Publica* **2009**, *43*, 335–344. [CrossRef] [PubMed]
8. Baldi, I.; Robert, C.; Piantoni, F.; Tual, S.; Bouvier, G.; Lebailly, P.; Raherison, C. Agricultural exposure and asthma risk in the AGRICAN French cohort. *Int. J. Hyg. Environ. Health* **2014**, *217*, 435–442. [CrossRef]
9. Tual, S.; Clin, B.; Leveque-Morlais, N.; Raherison, C.; Baldi, I.; Lebailly, P. Agricultural exposures and chronic bronchitis: Findings from the AGRICAN (AGRIculture and CANcer) cohort. *Ann. Epidemiol.* **2013**, *23*, 539–545. [CrossRef]
10. Faria, N.M.; Facchini, L.A.; Fassa, A.G.; Tomasi, E. Pesticides and respiratory symptoms among farmers. *Rev. Saude Publica* **2005**, *39*, 973–981. [CrossRef]
11. Buralli, R.J.; Ribeiro, H.; Mauad, T.; Amato-Lourenço, L.F.; Salge, J.M.; Diaz-Quijano, F.A.; Leao, R.S.; Marques, R.C.; Silva, D.S.; Guimaraes, J.R.D. Respiratory Condition of Family Farmers Exposed to Pesticides in the State of Rio de Janeiro, Brazil. *Int. J. Environ. Res. Public Health* **2018**, *15*, 1203. [CrossRef]
12. Huang, H.S.; Lee, K.W.; Ho, C.H.; Hsu, C.C.; Su, S.B.; Wang, J.J.; Lin, H.J.; Huang, C.C. Increased risk for hypothyroidism after anticholinesterase pesticide poisoning: A nationwide population-based study. *Endocrine* **2017**, *57*, 436–444. [CrossRef]
13. Chuang, C.S.; Yang, K.W.; Yen, C.M.; Lin, C.L.; Kao, C.H. Risk of Seizures in Patients with Organophosphate Poisoning: A Nationwide Population-Based Study. *Int. J. Environ. Res. Public Health* **2019**, *16*, 3147. [CrossRef]
14. Cruzeiro Szortyka, A.L.S.; Faria, N.M.X.; Carvalho, M.P.; Feijo, F.R.; Meucci, R.D.; Flesch, B.D.; Fiori, N.S.; Fassa, A.G. Suicidality among South Brazilian tobacco growers. *Neurotoxicology* **2021**, *86*, 52–58. [CrossRef]
15. Faria, N.M.; Fassa, A.G.; Meucci, R.D.; Fiori, N.S.; Miranda, V.I. Occupational exposure to pesticides, nicotine and minor psychiatric disorders among tobacco farmers in southern Brazil. *Neurotoxicology* **2014**, *45*, 347–354. [CrossRef] [PubMed]
16. Koh, S.B.; Kim, T.H.; Min, S.; Lee, K.; Kang, D.R.; Choi, J.R. Exposure to pesticide as a risk factor for depression: A population-based longitudinal study in Korea. *Neurotoxicology* **2017**, *62*, 181–185. [CrossRef] [PubMed]
17. London, L.; Beseler, C.; Bouchard, M.F.; Bellinger, D.C.; Colosio, C.; Grandjean, P.; Harari, R.; Kootbodien, T.; Kromhout, H.; Little, F.; et al. Neurobehavioral and neurodevelopmental effects of pesticide exposures. *Neurotoxicology* **2012**, *33*, 887–896. [CrossRef]
18. Wesseling, C.; van Wendel de Joode, B.; Keifer, M.; London, L.; Mergler, D.; Stallones, L. Symptoms of psychological distress and suicidal ideation among banana workers with a history of poisoning by organophosphate or n-methyl carbamate pesticides. *Occup. Environ. Med.* **2010**, *67*, 778–784. [CrossRef]
19. Petarli, G.B.; Cattafesta, M.; Viana, M.C.M.; Bezerra, O.; Zandonade, E.; Salaroli, L.B. Depression in Brazilian farmers: Prevalence and associated factors. *J. Ment. Health* **2022**, *Online ahead of print*, 1–9. [CrossRef]

20. Thundiyil, J.G.; Stober, J.; Besbelli, N.; Pronczuk, J. Acute pesticide poisoning: A proposed classification tool. *Bull. World Health Organ.* **2008**, *86*, 205–209. [CrossRef]
21. Fassa, A.G.; Faria, N.M.; Meucci, R.D.; Fiori, N.S.; Miranda, V.I.; Facchini, L.A. Green tobacco sickness among tobacco farmers in southern Brazil. *Am. J. Ind. Med.* **2014**, *57*, 726–735. [CrossRef]
22. Fiori, N.S.; Fassa, A.G.; Faria, N.M.; Meucci, R.D.; Miranda, V.I.; Christiani, D.C. Wheezing in tobacco farm workers in southern Brazil. *Am. J. Ind. Med.* **2015**, *58*, 1217–1228. [CrossRef] [PubMed]
23. Carvalho, K.P.; Corassa, R.B.; Petarli, G.B.; Cattafesta, M.; Zandonade, E.; Salaroli, L.B. Exogenous pesticide poisoning in the state of Espirito Santo, Brazil, 2007-2016: Spatial distribution and temporal trend in the incidence rate and case fatality ratio of notified cases. *Epidemiol. Serv. Saude* **2022**, *31*, e2021424. [CrossRef] [PubMed]
24. Lee, W.J.; Cha, E.S.; Park, J.; Ko, Y.; Kim, H.J.; Kim, J. Incidence of acute occupational pesticide poisoning among male farmers in South Korea. *Am. J. Ind. Med.* **2012**, *55*, 799–807. [CrossRef]
25. Zhang, X.; Zhao, W.; Jing, R.; Wheeler, K.; Smith, G.A.; Stallones, L.; Xiang, H. Work-related pesticide poisoning among farmers in two villages of Southern China: A cross-sectional survey. *BMC Public Health* **2011**, *11*, 429. [CrossRef]
26. Kobashi, Y.; Srou, L.; Tsubokura, M.; Nishikawa, Y.; Laymithuna, N.; Hok, S.; Okawada, M. Vulnerable groups and protective habits associated with the number of symptoms caused by pesticide application in Kratie, Cambodia: A cross-sectional questionnaire study. *J. Rural. Med.* **2022**, *17*, 214–220. [CrossRef] [PubMed]
27. Neupane, D.; Jors, E.; Brandt, L. Pesticide use, erythrocyte acetylcholinesterase level and self-reported acute intoxication symptoms among vegetable farmers in Nepal: A cross-sectional study. *Environ. Health* **2014**, *13*, 98. [CrossRef]
28. Baldi, I.; Lebailly, P.; Bouvier, G.; Rondeau, V.; Kientz-Bouchart, V.; Canal-Raffin, M.; Garrigou, A. Levels and determinants of pesticide exposure in re-entry workers in vineyards: Results of the PESTEXPO study. *Environ. Res.* **2014**, *132*, 360–369. [CrossRef]
29. Buralli, R.J.; Ribeiro, H.; Iglesias, V.; Munoz-Quezada, M.T.; Leao, R.S.; Marques, R.C.; Almeida, M.M.C.; Guimaraes, J.R.D. Occupational exposure to pesticides and health symptoms among family farmers in Brazil. *Rev. Saude Publica* **2020**, *54*, 133. [CrossRef] [PubMed]
30. Roberts, J.R.; Reigart, J.R. *Recognition and Management of Pesticide Poisonings*, 6th ed.; EPA Environmental Protection Agency: Washington, DC, USA, 2013; 272p.
31. University, OS; Intertox. *Sulfentrazone*; WSDOT: Olympia, WA, USA, 2017. Available online: https://wsdot.wa.gov/sites/default/files/2021-10/Herbicides-factsheet-Sulfentrazone.pdf (accessed on 30 November 2022).
32. Dall'Agnol, J.C.; Ferri Pezzini, M.; Suarez Uribe, N.; Joveleviths, D. Systemic effects of the pesticide mancozeb A literature review. *Eur. Rev. Med. Pharmacol. Sci.* **2021**, *25*, 4113–4120. [CrossRef] [PubMed]
33. EFSA. Peer review of the pesticide risk assessment of the active substance iprodione. *EFSA J. Eur. Food Saf. Auth.* **2016**, *14*, 4609. Available online: https://efsa.onlinelibrary.wiley.com/doi/epdf/10.2903/j.efsa.2016.4609 (accessed on 2 December 2022).
34. Holynska-Iwan, I.; Szewczyk-Golec, K. Pyrethroids: How They Affect Human and Animal Health? *Medicina* **2020**, *56*, 582. [CrossRef] [PubMed]
35. Lee, S.J.; Mulay, P.; Diebolt-Brown, B.; Lackovic, M.J.; Mehler, L.N.; Beckman, J.; Waltz, J.; Prado, J.B.; Mitchell, Y.A.; Higgins, S.A.; et al. Acute illnesses associated with exposure to fipronil–surveillance data from 11 states in the United States, 2001–2007. *Clin. Toxicol.* **2010**, *48*, 737–744. [CrossRef] [PubMed]
36. EPA. *Fipronil*; Enviromental Protection Agency: Washington, DC, USA, 2022. Available online: https://ordspub.epa.gov/ords/pesticides/f?p=CHEMICALSEARCH:3::::21,3,31,7,12,25:P3_XCHEMICAL_ID:2377 (accessed on 5 December 2022).
37. Gyenwali, D.; Vaidya, A.; Tiwari, S.; Khatiwada, P.; Lamsal, D.R.; Giri, S. Pesticide poisoning in Chitwan, Nepal: A descriptive epidemiological study. *BMC Public Health* **2017**, *17*, 619. [CrossRef] [PubMed]
38. Jors, E.; Hay-Younes, J.; Condarco, M.A.; Condarco, G.; Cervantes, R.; Huici, O.; Baelum, J. Is gender a risk factor for pesticide intoxications among farmers in Bolivia? A cross-sectional study. *J. Agromedicine* **2013**, *18*, 132–139. [CrossRef] [PubMed]
39. Intoxicações exógenas por agrotóxicos no Estado de Santa Catarina-Relatório anual 2021. In *Saúde SdVe, editor. SUV–Superintendencia de Vigilância em Saúde—Programa*; VSPEA/SC: Florianópolis, Brazil, 2022.
40. Santana, V.S.; Moura, M.C.P.; Ferreira, F.; Lisboa, M.C. *Acidentes de Trabalho devido à Intoxicação por Agrotóxicos Entre Trabalhadores da Agropecuária 2000–2011, CCVISAT/UFBA, ed.*; UFBA: Salvador, BA, USA, 2012; Volume 4.
41. Freitas, A.B.; Garibotti, V. Characterization of notifications of exogenous pesticide poisoning in Rio Grande do Sul, Brazil, 2011-2018. *Epidemiol. Serv. Saude* **2020**, *29*, e2020061. [CrossRef] [PubMed]
42. Buendia, J.A.; Restrepo Chavarriaga, G.J.; Zuluaga, A.F. Social and economic variables related with Paraquat self-poisoning: An ecological study. *BMC Public Health* **2020**, *20*, 404. [CrossRef]
43. Tambe, A.B.; Mbanga, B.M.R.; Nzefa, D.L.; Nama, M.G. Pesticide usage and occupational hazards among farmers working in small-scale tomato farms in Cameroon. *J. Egypt. Public Health Assoc.* **2019**, *94*, 20. [CrossRef] [PubMed]
44. Veríssimo, G.; Kós, M.I.; Garcia, T.R.; Ramos, J.A.S.; Souza, C.C.; Moreira, J.C.; Meyer, A. Pesticide exposure among students and their families in Nova Friburgo, Rio de Janeiro. *Cienc. Saúde Coletiva* **2018**, *23*, 3903–3911. [CrossRef] [PubMed]
45. Lari, S.; Jonnalagadda, P.R.; Yamagani, P.; Medithi, S.; Vanka, J.; Pandiyan, A.; Naidu, M.; Jee, B. Assessment of dermal exposure to pesticides among farmers using dosimeter and hand washing methods. *Front. Public Health* **2022**, *10*, 957774. [CrossRef] [PubMed]
46. Damalas, C.A.; Koutroubas, S.D. Farmers' Exposure to Pesticides: Toxicity Types and Ways of Prevention. *Toxics* **2016**, *4*, 1. [CrossRef] [PubMed]

47. Faria, N.M.X.; Mello-da-Silva, C.A. Organofosforados e Carbamatos, Inseticidas inibidores da colinesterase. In *Emergências Toxicológicas: Princípios e Prática do Tratamento de Intoxicações Agudas*; Mello-da-Silva, C.A., Ed.; Editora Manole: São Paulo, Brazil, 2022; pp. 325–331.
48. Hudson, N.L.; Kasner, E.J.; Beckman, J.; Mehler, L.; Schwartz, A.; Higgins, S.; Bonnar-Prado, J.; Lackovic, M.; Mulay, P.; Mitchell, Y.; et al. Characteristics and magnitude of acute pesticide-related illnesses and injuries associated with pyrethrin and pyrethroid exposures–11 states, 2000-2008. *Am. J. Ind. Med.* **2014**, *57*, 15–30. [CrossRef]
49. Bureau, M.; Beziat, B.; Duporte, G.; Bouchart, V.; Lecluse, Y.; Barron, E.; Garrigou, A.; Devier, M.H.; Budzinski, H.; Lebailly, P.; et al. Pesticide exposure of workers in apple growing in France. *Int. Arch. Occup. Environ. Health* **2022**, *95*, 811–823. [CrossRef]
50. Leme, T.S.; Papini, S.; Vieira, E.; Luchini, L.C. Evaluation of personal protective equipment used by malathion sprayers in dengue control in Sao Paulo, Brazil. *Cad. Saude Publica* **2014**, *30*, 567–576. [CrossRef]
51. Veiga, M.M.; Duarte, F.J.d.C.M.; Meirelles, L.A.; Garrigou, A.; Baldi, I. A contaminação por agrotóxicos e os Equipamentos de Proteção Individual (EPIs). *Rev. Bras. Saúde Ocup.* **2007**, *32*, 57–68. [CrossRef]
52. Bresson, M.; Bureau, M.; Le Goff, J.; Lecluse, Y.; Robelot, E.; Delamare, J.; Baldi, I.; Lebailly, P. Pesticide Exposure in Fruit-Growers: Comparing Levels and Determinants Assessed under Usual Conditions of Work (CANEPA Study) with Those Predicted by Registration Process (Agricultural Operator Exposure Model). *Int. J. Environ. Res. Public Health* **2022**, *19*, 4611. [CrossRef] [PubMed]
53. Veiga, M.M.; Almeida, R.; Duarte, F. O desconforto térmico provocado pelos equipamentos de proteção individual (EPI) utilizados na aplicação de agrotóxicos. *Laboreal* **2016**, *12*, 83–94. [CrossRef]

Disclaimer/Publisher's Note: The statements, opinions and data contained in all publications are solely those of the individual author(s) and contributor(s) and not of MDPI and/or the editor(s). MDPI and/or the editor(s) disclaim responsibility for any injury to people or property resulting from any ideas, methods, instructions or products referred to in the content.

Article

Influence of Environmental Exposure to Steel Waste on Endocrine Dysregulation and *PER3* Gene Polymorphisms

Gilvania Barreto Feitosa Coutinho [1,*], Maria de Fátima Ramos Moreira [1], Frida Marina Fischer [2], Maria Carolina Reis dos Santos [1], Lucas Ferreira Feitosa [1], Sayonara Vieira de Azevedo [1], Renato Marçullo Borges [1], Michelle Nascimento-Sales [3,4], Marcelo Augusto Christoffolete [3], Marden Samir Santa-Marinha [1], Daniel Valente [1] and Liliane Reis Teixeira [1,*]

[1] Center for Studies on the Worker's Health and Human Ecology, Sergio Arouca National School of Public Health, Oswaldo Cruz Foundation, 1480 Leopoldo Bulhões St., Rio de Janeiro 21041-210, RJ, Brazil
[2] Department of Environmental Health, School of Public Health, University of São Paulo, São Paulo 01246-904, SP, Brazil
[3] Center for Natural and Human Sciences (CCNH), ABC Federal University (UFABC), Santo André 09210-580, SP, Brazil
[4] Centro de Ciências Biológicas e de Saúde (CBS), Universidade Cruzeiro do Sul (Unicsul), São Paulo 01506-000, SP, Brazil
* Correspondence: gil.aula.saude@gmail.com (G.B.F.C.); lilianeteixeira@ensp.fiocruz.br (L.R.T.)

Abstract: Objective: To evaluate the association between environmental exposure to the following chemical substances: cadmium (Cd), lead (Pb), nickel (Ni), manganese (Mn), benzene (BZN), and toluene (TLN), and Period Circadian Regulator 3 (*PER3*) gene variable number of tandem repeats (VNTR) polymorphisms, according to chronotype in a population living in a steel residue-contaminated area. Methods: This assessment comprises a study conducted from 2017 to 2019 with 159 participants who completed health, work, and Pittsburgh sleep scale questionnaires. Cd, Pb, Ni, Mn, BZN, and TLN concentrations in blood and urine were determined by Graphite Furnace Atomic Absorption Spectrometry (GFAAS) and Headspace Gas Chromatography (GC), and genotyping was carried out using Polymerase Chain Reaction (PCR). Results: A total of 47% of the participants were afternoon chronotype, 42% were indifferent, and 11% were morning chronotype. Insomnia and excessive sleepiness were associated with the indifferent chronotype, while higher urinary manganese levels were associated with the morning chronotype (Kruskal–Wallis chi-square = 9.16; $p < 0.01$). In turn, the evening chronotype was associated with poorer sleep quality, higher lead levels in blood, and BZN and TLN levels in urine ($\chi^2 = 11.20$; $p < 0.01$) in non-occupationally exposed individuals ($\chi^2 = 6.98$; $p < 0.01$) as well as the highest BZN ($\chi^2 = 9.66$; $p < 0.01$) and TLN ($\chi^2 = 5.71$; $p < 0.01$) levels detected in residents from the influence zone 2 (far from the slag). Conclusion: Mn, Pb, benzene, and toluene contaminants may have influenced the different chronotypes found in the steel residue-exposed population.

Keywords: steel industry; environmental exposure; endocrine disruptors; *PER3* gene polymorphism; chronotypes

1. Introduction

Human populations living near steel plants are environmentally exposed to residues [1–6]. The steel industry is characterized as a transformation industry for steel production because it involves the modification of raw materials such as charcoal or coke, sinter, and pellet iron ores. Other materials include quartz and limestone for the production of blast furnace gas, pig iron, steel slag, dust, and mud. This process generates steel slag as waste, containing calcium and metals such as silicon (Si), aluminum (Al), iron (Fe), manganese (Mn), magnesium (Mg), cadmium (Cd), chromium (Cr), lead (Pb), and nickel (Ni) [7,8].

In addition, benzene and toluene are two of the twenty most commonly used volatile organic compounds in industrial production [9,10], and they are utilized by the petrochemical and steel industries [8,11]. Exposure to these solvents can occur in two ways: when burning petroleum products or when industrial waste accumulates in deposits [12].

Such industrial waste pollutes the soil, air, surface and groundwater, and food, posing a health risk to those who are exposed. This is because these contaminants can harm many organs and systems, including the endocrine system, and thus affect their biological functions [4,13–16].

Long-term environmental exposure to low metal concentrations is the most common, and it is difficult to establish a cause–effect relationship because the effects of contamination take years to manifest and are generally nonspecific. Furthermore, each metal has its own toxicodynamic and toxicokinetic properties, such as molecular mimetism, oxidative damage, and bonds with DNA and proteins, which are also common toxicity mechanisms [17]. Lead toxicity primarily affects the nervous and hematopoietic systems, kidneys, and gastrointestinal tract in humans. It also has an impact on reproduction and development, as well as having a negative impact on the cardiovascular system. Ni inhalation induces cancer by affecting the respiratory system, nasal and mucosa cavity, kidneys, liver, and brain. Furthermore, Ni ingestion has been linked to gastrointestinal, hematological, hepatic, renal, and neurological problems, and dermal contact with Ni can cause dermatitis. In addition to being carcinogenic, hepatotoxic, and genotoxic, Cd causes hormonal dysfunctions and damages the kidneys, cardiovascular, respiratory, hematological, and nervous systems. Manganese is an essential element for humans, as it is involved in bone and tissue formation, reproductive functions, and carbohydrate and lipid metabolism. However, at high concentrations, such as those found in workplaces, it is neurotoxic [17].

Given the volatility and widespread use of benzene and toluene, inhalation is the most common route of exposure for these contaminants [18,19]. Human health consequences include central nervous system and auditory effects, changes in renal and dermatological functions, and, most importantly, changes in hormone levels [10,20–24]. Benzene primarily damages the bone marrow, which can result in a variety of hematological changes, including hypoplasia, dysplasia, and aplasia, as well as cancer [25]. Furthermore, rat studies have identified sleep disorders as one of the toluene and benzene exposure symptoms [23,26–29].

Aside from contaminating the environment, such toxics also act as Endocrine Disrupting Compounds (EDCs), as they can alter the endocrine system functions [15,17,30], which are considered the main organism interface with the environment [13,31]. As a result, hormonal disorders caused by endocrine gland dysfunction can result in a wide range of diseases caused by both acute and chronic exposure, including sleep disorders caused by the pineal gland's inappropriate release of melatonin. This one compound is the primary endocrine system hormone, which regulates circadian rhythms, including the rhythmicity of the sleep–wake cycle, among other functions [13].

The principal clock genes (*CLOCK, BMAL1, CRY1, CRY2, CKE, CKΣ, PER1, PER2*, and *PER3*) control the circadian rhythms in mammals. Changes in those genes can result in a variety of circadian genotypes, such as the morning/evening character, due mainly to interferences in melatonin expression and synthesis control [32–35], which cause rhythmicity disorders in the sleep–wake cycle [13]. Because the *PER3* gene VNTR polymorphism affects sleep–wake cycle synchronism [36], endocrine-disrupting substances (manganese, lead, benzene, and toluene) can modify the active sites in the central nervous system, where the pineal gland is located [37]. In addition, they may be neurotoxic through the hypothalamic–pituitary–adrenal axis, which stimulates the secretion of adrenocorticotropic hormone (ACTH), which is responsible for cortisol synthesis and secretion, besides initiating a melatonin inhibition or release response [38,39].

The association between environmental exposure to such substances and the sleep–wake cycle requires investigation. There are few studies on the subject, especially relating metals with *PER3* gene VNTR polymorphism. This study aimed to investigate the association between environmental exposure to chemical substances (Cd, Pb, Ni, Mn, benzene, and toluene) and *PER3* gene VNTR polymorphisms according to chronotype in a population residing in a steel residue-contaminated area.

2. Materials and Methods

A cross-sectional study was conducted in an adult population in Volta Redonda, Rio de Janeiro, Brazil. The study's subjects live near a steel waste dump. Furthermore, the condominium was built in an area that was previously used as a steel waste disposal site. The data were collected between July 2017 and January 2019. A convenience sample of the population was taken. Participants included 203 residents who had lived at the site for more than six months. Fourteen people who used medication for sleep disorders and thirty people who had some sleep disorders were excluded, leaving one hundred and fifty-nine people.

- Study area

The condominium was divided into two zones of influence (Figure 1), with each street's roundabout serving as the boundary between the two zones. Zone of influence 1 (near the slag) is near the steel slag wall, whereas Zone of Influence 2 (away from the slag) is near the main street (1043 St.). The distance between the wall and the roundabout is about 140 m, and the complementary space to the main street is about 252 m. The chosen location connects the condominium's internal regions and allows for population movement.

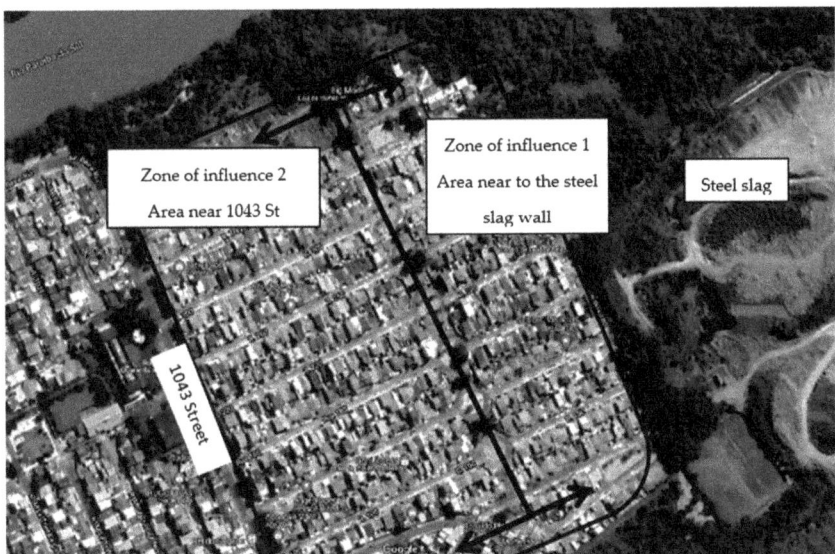

Figure 1. Delimitation of the influence zone concerning benzene and toluene exposure in the Volta Grande IV condominium.

- Data collection

During the first stage, the study participants answered two questionnaires: (1) a comprehensive questionnaire including information on working conditions and sociodemographic characteristics (age, marital status, education, and employment information, i.e., working time and chemical exposure to metals at work), lifestyles (use of tobacco, alcohol, and the consumption of other psychoactive substances), physical activity, familiar disease history, past and current health conditions. (2) The Pittsburgh Sleep Quality Index (SQI) scale developed by Buysse and collaborators [40] was also answered, comprising scores on quality and patterns of sleep.

- Biological samples

The second stage of the study comprised biological sample collection (urine and blood) to investigate Cr, Cd, Ni, Pb, Mn, benzene, and toluene exposures.

Urine samples were used for Cr, Ni, Cd, and Mn analysis. Whereas the collection process is non-invasive and thus more acceptable for obtaining samples, urine is one of the most-used biomarkers in the case of chronic exposure [41]. Cd accumulates in the kidneys and other tissues, and urinary Cd represents this total body content, reflecting a critical exposure [42]. Ni is an essential metal for human body physiology. However, there are currently no adequate exposure biomarkers. Because there is little correlation between environmental exposure and individual urine levels, group assessment is the most weighted way to estimate population risk [43]. Mn is also an essential element. Although it can be measured with high sensitivity in several biological compartments, including blood and urine, no adequate exposure biomarker exists [44]. Finally, Pb is stored in the bones, with less than 2% found in the blood. Although bone Pb is regarded as a chronic exposure biomarker, it is not uniformly distributed, accumulating in bone regions where calcification is most active during the exposure period. As a result, the most appropriate biomarker would be plasma Pb, which is directly related to lead in bone but is very difficult to measure due to hemolysis and its levels being close to the quantification limits of most analytical techniques. Given all these reasons, BPb remains the biomarker of choice for lead exposure around the world [45].

Metal determinations were carried out in two atomic absorption spectrometers, A Analyst 800 and 900 (Perkin Elmer, Norwalk, CT, USA), equipped with transverse electrothermal atomizers, longitudinal Zeeman background correctors, and AS-800 automatic samplers (Perkin Elmer, Norwalk, CT, USA). The methodologies used followed the previously established protocols by the Metals Sector in the Toxicology Laboratory (Cesteh/Ensp/Fiocruz). Whole blood was collected in heparinized vacutainer tubes for trace metal analyses, while urine was collected in previously decontaminated 50 mL containers. Cr, Ni, and Cd were determined in urine, Mn in urine and blood, and Pb in blood.

The determination of unmetabolized urinary benzene and toluene employed the solid phase microextraction technique (SPMT), an Agilent headspace gas chromatograph, and an autosampler. Ions 78 and 91 m/z were used for benzene and toluene quantification, respectively.

In the third stage, DNA was extracted from blood samples using the salting out method, according to Miller et al. [46]. After isolation, the genotyping of the number from the $PER3$ gene VNTR polymorphism associated with different chronotypes [33,47] was performed by conventional polymerase chain reaction (PCR) technique, according to Pereira et al. [34,47]. Reaction was carried out in MasterCycler thermocycler (Eppendorf AG, Hamburg, Germany) for 95 °C–2 min (HotStart), followed by 95 °C–15 s, 60 °C–25 s, and 72 °C–30 s for 35 cycles. We used 10 ng of DNA, 1× PCR Buffer, 0.2 mM dNTP mix, 0.33 µM primer mix and 5U Taq DNA Polymerase accordingly to manufacture (Sigma-Aldrich Inc., St Louis, MO, USA) standard protocol. Sense primer 5′-GAGCAGTCCTGCTACTACCG-3′ and antisense 5′-CTTGTACTTCCACATCAGTGCC-3′ were used. PCR products were submitted then to electrophoresis in Ethidium Bromide stained 1% agarose gel at 90 V for 1 h and image from the gel acquired with SmartView Pro Imager System (Major Science Co., Ltd., Taoyuan City, Taiwan). PCR products were 324 bp, 378 bp or both, corresponding to $PER3^{4/4}$ (evening), $PER3^{5/5}$ (morning) and $PER3^{4/5}$ (intermediate) chronotypes, respectively (Figure 2). For allelic frequency and Hardy–Weinberg equilibrium (HWE), all 4 repeats were considered as common allele (p) and 5 repeats were considered as rare allele (q).

- Statistical analyses

The descriptive data analysis first computed the means, standard deviations, and medians for all continuous variables, as well as the absolute and relative frequencies for categorical data. The data were then checked for normality (Shapiro–Wilk test). Because the data were not normally distributed, the Kruskal–Wallis chi-square test and the Wilcoxon test were used. A linear multivariate analysis was carried out controlled for potential confounders such as gender, age group, work exposure time, and/or residence time in a steel-residues contaminated area. It was not possible to control smoking and drinking habits, due to the small number of subjects. For Deviations from HWE in *PER3* VNTR polymorphism frequencies were assessed by goodness-of-fit χ^2 test, considering 3.841 as critical value, degree of freedom 1 and $\alpha = 0.05$. All analyses were set at a significance level of $p = 0.05$ and a confidence interval of 95% (CI = 95%). The Bar Charts with the median and the 95% confidence interval around this median were made. The Statistical Package for the Social Sciences 17.0 for Windows® software (SPSS Inc., Chicago, IL, USA) was used for all statistical assessments.

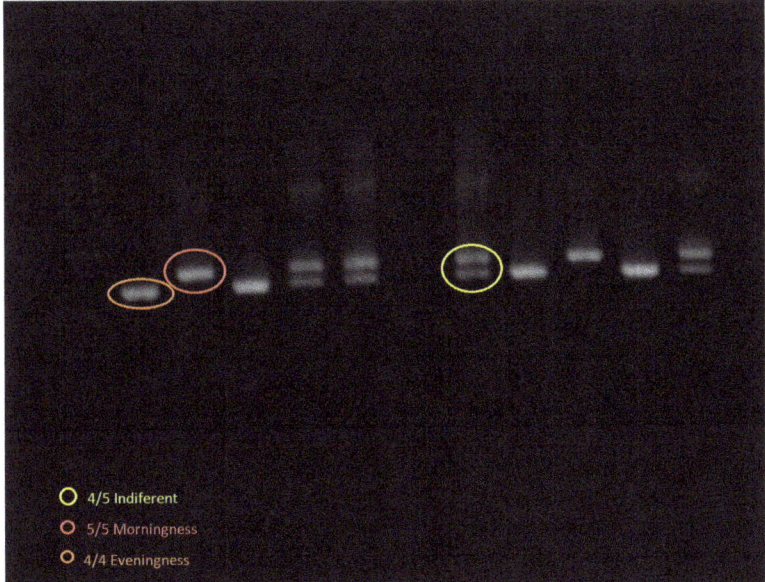

Figure 2. Image from the electrophoresis gel. PCR products corresponding to $PER3^{4/4}$ (evening), $PER3^{5/5}$ (morning), and $PER3^{4/5}$ (intermediate) chronotypes.

3. Results

3.1. Sociodemographic Aspects and PER3 Gene VNTR Polymorphism Frequencies

Of the 159 subjects, 69 (44%) were men and 90 (56%) were women, aged between 18 and 86 (median = 51 years old) and living in the condominium between 1 and 30 years (median = 14 years). The participants were mostly ex-smokers (18.5%), with only a small percentage (7.8%) claiming to be smokers. Regarding drinking habits, 37.6% drank only at social gatherings, and 4.8% had previously consumed alcohol. The study population included 43 people who reported doing domestic activities (23%), nine students (5%), and 19 retirees (10%). Of the 42 workers, all reported chemical or physical exposure at work (22.2%), with exposure periods ranging from 1 to 48 years (median = 10 years). Of 159 residents genotyped, 75 (46.9%) were $PER^{4/4}$, 67 (41.8%) were $PER^{4/5}$ and 17 (11.3%) $PER^{5/5}$. Allelic frequency for 4 repeats was 66.5% and for 5 repeats 33.5%. For HWE, $p^2 = 0.442$ (4 repeats, expected 70), $2pq = 0.446$ (expected 71) and $q^2 = 0.112$ (5 repeats, expected 18) Goodness-of-fit χ^2 test is 0.638, below 3.841 critical value, showing no deviation from HWE. The highest prevalence of the evening chronotype was observed for both men and women (women 48.4%, men 51.5%). The highest participation was of individuals over 50 (50.8%), 42.9% were between 22 and 50, and only 4.8% were under 21. The indiferent chronotype comprised 57.1% of ages below 21, while the evening chronotype included 54.4% of those over 50. According to habits, 41.7% of the afternoon chronotypes were smokers, and 57% did not drink alcohol.

3.2. Sleep–Wake Cycle According to PER3 Gene Polymorphism in the Population

The sleep patterns according to PER3 gene VNTR polymorphisms are in Table 1. Sleep latency in the morning chronotype group was lower (median = 10 min) when compared to the indifferent and evening (median = 15 min) chronotypes. When it came to bedtime, there were similarities between the morning, indifferent, and evening groups (median = 11 PM). The wake-up time was earlier for the morning group (median = 6 AM) than the other two groups (median = 6:30 AM). The sleep duration was slightly greater among the indifferent and evening groups (median = 8 h) compared to the morning group (median = 7 h). Excluding bedtime, morning chronotypes differed from the evening and indifferent groups for the other analyzed variables, albeit with no statistical significance.

Table 1. Sleep patterns according to PER 3 VNTR polymorphism.

Sleep Patterns/PER3	Evening			Indifferent			Morning		
	P_{25}	Median	P_{75}	P_{25}	Median	P_{75}	P_{25}	Median	P_{75}
Sleep latency (min)	5 min	15 min	30 min	8 min	15 min	40 min	7 min	10 min	20 min
Bedtime (PM)	10:00	11:00	12:00	10:00	11:00	12:00	11:00	11:00	11:45
Wake-up period (AM)	6:00	6:30	7:00	6:00	6:30	7:30	6:00	6:00	7:50
Sleep duration (h)	7 h	8 h	8:30 h	7 h	8 h	9 h	6:15 h	7 h	8 h

3.3. Sleep Complaints According to PER3 Gene VNTR Polymorphism in the Population

Table 2 shows sleep complaints according to PER3 gene polymorphisms. The indifferent group had a higher number of complaints about insomnia (58%) than the evening (32%) and morning (10%) groups (Friedman's chi-square = 154; $p < 0.01$). The same pattern was observed for excessive sleepiness (60%) in the indifferent group compared to the evening (36%) and morning (4%) groups (Friedman's chi-square = 158; $p < 0.01$). The evening group (55%) had more complaints about poor sleep quality than the indifferent (38%) and morning (7%) groups (Friedman's chi-square = 161; $p < 0.01$).

Table 2. Sleep complaints according to PER 3 VNTR polymorphism.

Variable	Categories	Chronotype		
		Evening N (%)	Indifferent N (%)	Morning N (%)
Insomnia	No	66 (54)	43 (35)	14 (11)
	Yes	10 (32)	18 (58)	3 (10)
Excessive sleepiness	No	69 (52)	49 (37)	15 (11)
	Yes	9 (36)	15 (60)	1 (4)
Quality of sleep	No	56 (47)	49 (41)	14 (12)
	Yes	23 (55)	16 (38)	3 (7)
Mood	No	60 (50)	48 (40)	11 (9)
	Yes	17 (43)	17 (43)	4 (15)

3.4. Lead, Manganese, Cadmium, and Nickel Levels in Blood and Urine According to PER 3 Gene VNTR Polymorphisms

Table 3 presents the concentrations of the metals investigated in blood and urine according to chronotypes. Tables 4 and 5 show lead and manganese levels in blood according to chronotype, stratified by age group, drinking habits, and chemical exposure at work. Figures 3–7 show median values for those metals according to subjects' chronotype.

Table 3. Lead and manganese in blood, and cadmium, nickel, and manganese in urine according to *PER3* gene VNTR polymorphisms.

Metal/Chronotype	Evening			Indifferent			Morning			Kruskal–Wallis χ^2	*p*-Value
	P_{25}	Median	P_{75}	P_{25}	Median	P_{75}	P_{25}	Median	P_{75}		
BPb ($\mu g\ dL^{-1}$)	1.27	2.05	2.72	1.27	1.56	2.13	1.00	1.52	2.00	5.62	0.06
BMn ($\mu g\ L^{-1}$)	5.85	6.88	8.84	5.58	7.06	9.61	5.66	7.36	8.39	0.49	0.79
UCd ($\mu g\ g^{-1}$ Creat)	0.23	0.39	0.81	0.19	0.41	0.92	0.16	0.33	0.66	0.61	0.74
UNi ($\mu g\ g^{-1}$ Creat)	1.24	2.55	4.40	1.38	1.96	4.64	1.43	3.51	7.62	1.41	0.49
UMn ($\mu g\ g^{-1}$ Creat)	0.28	0.44	0.92	0.22	0.35	0.49	0.37	0.64	1.79	9.16	0.01 *

* Statistically significant.

Table 4. Lead in blood ($\mu g\ dL^{-1}$) according to *PER3* VNTR polymorphism and stratified by age group, drinking habits, and chemical exposure at work.

Variable	Categories	Evening			Indifferent			Morning		
		P_{25}	Median	P_{75}	P_{25}	Median	P_{75}	P_{25}	Median	P_{75}
Sex	Female	1.36	1.85	2.19	1.31	1.47	1.73	096	1.18	1.27
	Male	1.83	2.27	2.70	1.52	1.66	2.13	1.61	1.90	3.03
Age group	<21	1.15	1.14	0.09	1.39	1.54	0.26	-	-	-
	22–50	1.92	1.96	0.65	1.59	1.59	0.57	1.78	1.52	1.26
	>50	2.55	2.26	1.66	1.85	1.60	0.82	1.79	1.54	0.95
Smoking habit	No	1.29	2.01	2.29	1.29	1.47	1.68	1.03	1.49	1.83
	Former smoker	1.86	2.40	2.92	1.39	2.45	2.70	-	-	-
	Yes	1.91	2.43	2.72	-	-	-	1.35	1.52	3.10
Current drinking habits	No	1.93	2.04	0.72	1.51	1.42	0.66	1.15	1.07	0.48
	Yes	2.96	2.60	2.06	1.84	1.58	0.81	2.45	2.00	1.20
Chemical exposure at work	No	2.17	2.15	1.22	1.65	1.54	0.72	1.76	1.80	0.92
	Yes	2.49	1.91	1.91	1.79	1.82	1.64	0.66	1.26	0.37

Table 5. Manganese in blood ($\mu g\ L^{-1}$) according to *PER3* gene VNTR polymorphisms stratified by sex, age group, smoking and drinking habits, and chemical exposure at work.

Variable	Categories	Evening			Indifferent			Morning			Test	*p*-Value
		P_{25}	Median	P_{75}	P_{25}	Median	P_{75}	P_{25}	Median	P_{75}		
Sex	Female	5.91	6.89	8.87	6.01	8.90	11.10	6.70	7.71	9.58	(W) = −2.39	0.02 *
	Male	5.74	6.78	8.77	5.23	6.41	8.52	4.90	5.59	7.30		
Age group	<21	8.64	9.61	10.43	6.41	7.85	9.26	-	-	-	χ^2 = 6.81	0.03 *
	22–50	6.20	7.58	8.56	6.46	8.37	10.48	7.36	7.72	8.96		
	>50	6.21	6.64	7.19	5.73	6.94	8.21	5.64	6.70	7.52		
Smoking habit	No	5.63	6.88	8.72	5.80	7.06	9.19	5.23	7.36	8.96	n.s.	
	Former smoker	5.78	6.48	7.98	4.77	7.52	9.74	7.14	7.42	-		
	Yes	5.10	8.71	13.01	4.61	5.70	7.38	4.90	7.78	-		
Current drinking habit	No	5.94	6.88	8.88	5.43	6.87	9.63	6.52	7.50	9.14	n.s.	
	Yes	5.02	6.55	8.15	5.90	7.52	8.96	4.91	7.14	7.78		
Chemical exposure at work	No	5.86	6.74	8.23	5.57	7.52	10.13	5.85	7.36	9.27	n.s.	
	Yes	5.76	7.64	8.94	5.61	6.94	8.58	4.90	5.49	-		

* Statistically significant; n.s. not significant.

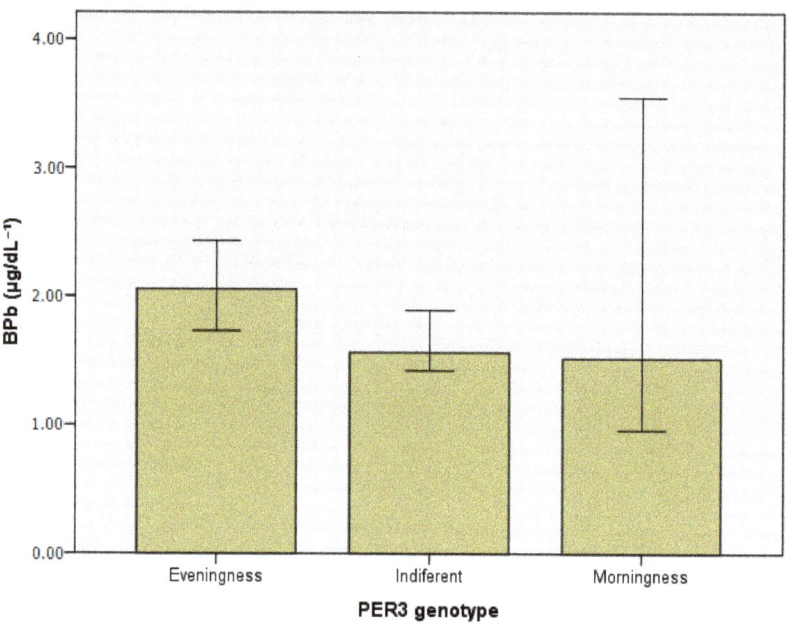

Figure 3. Lead in blood (μg/dL^{-1}) according to *PER3* gene VNTR polymorphisms.

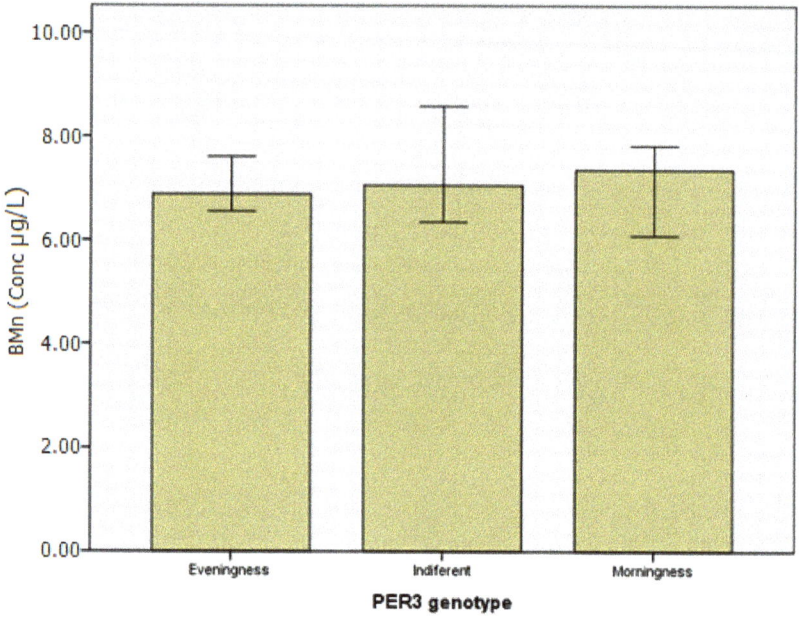

Figure 4. Manganese in blood (μg/L) according to *PER3* gene VNTR polymorphisms.

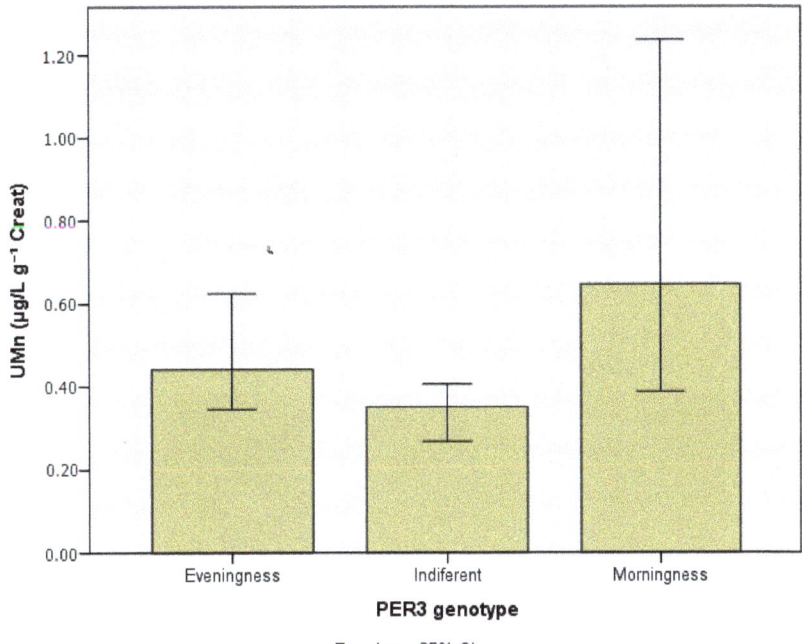

Figure 5. Manganese in urine (µg g^{-1} creat) according to *PER3* gene VNTR polymorphisms.

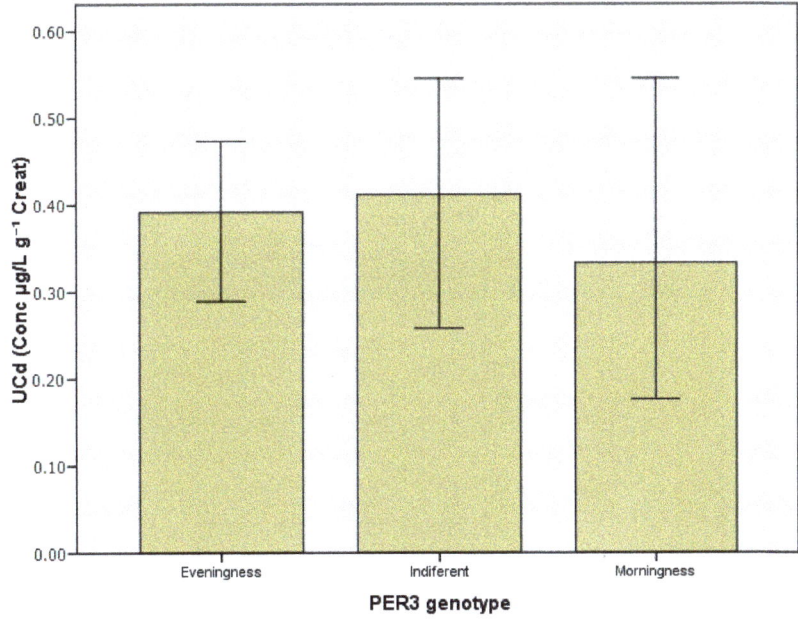

Figure 6. Cadmium in urine (µg g^{-1} creat) according to *PER3* gene VNTR polymorphisms.

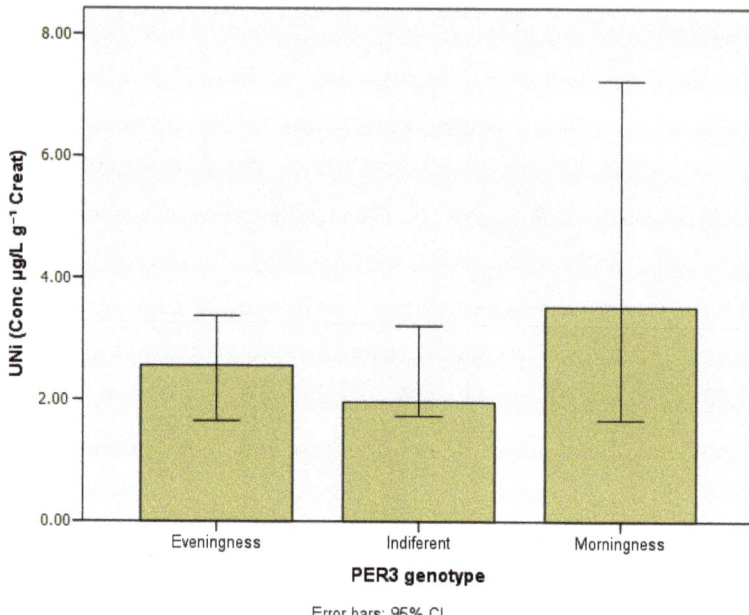

Figure 7. Nickel in urine (μg g^{-1} creat) according to *PER3* gene VNTR polymorphisms.

3.4.1. Lead in Blood (BPb)

Although BPb has borderline significance, concentrations in the evening group (2.05 μg dL^{-1}) were higher than in the indifferent and morning groups (Table 3). Concerning the age group and *PER3* gene polymorphisms (Table 4), BPb levels were higher in the evening group in individuals above 50 years. As for drinking habits, the highest BPb levels were detected in the evening group (2.26 μg dL^{-1}), especially among those who reported current drinking (2.60 μg dL^{-1}). For chemical exposure at work, BPb was higher in the evening group (1.91 μg dL^{-1}) and lower in the morning group (1.26 μg dL^{-1}).

3.4.2. Manganese in Blood (BMn)

Table 5 presents BMn according to chronotype for sex, age group, smoking and drinking habits, and chemical exposure at work.

Female subjects showed higher levels when compared to men (W = −2.39; *p* = 0.02), having the highest observed median level among indifferent group (8.90 μg L^{-1}). In terms of the subjects' ages, BMn levels decrease as they get older (Kruskal–Wallis χ^2 = 6.81; *p* = 0.03). Individuals under the age of 21 had the highest concentrations in the evening groups (9.61 μg L^{-1}), while those over the age of 50 had the lowest concentrations (6.64 μg L^{-1}). Smoking and drinking habits had increased BMn levels among morning subjects, yet with no statistical significance. Similarly, chemical exposure at work had no effect on the analyzed substance.

3.4.3. Cadmium, Nickel, and Manganese in Urine (UCd, UNi, UMn)

Cd levels in urine were comparable across *PER3* gene VNTR polymorphisms, with no statistical differences.

Despite having the highest Ni levels in the morning group, no statistical significance was found between groups.

Higher Mn concentrations in urine were observed in the morning group (0.64 μg g^{-1} creat) compared with the evening and indifferent groups (0.44 μg g^{-1} creat and 0.35 μg g^{-1} creat, respectively) (Kruskal–Wallis chi-square = 9.16; *p* < 0.01) (Figure 3).

3.4.4. Linear Regression Analysis According to PER 3 Gene VNTR Polymorphisms

The linear regression analysis indicated that Mn in urine was the only metal associated with the *PER3* gene VNTR polymorphism ($\beta = 0.39$ µg g^{-1} creat; CI > 0 and $p < 0.01$). According to the multivariate linear regression (Table 6), the highest Mn levels in urine were associated with the morning group. The linear regression analysis for the chronotypes control variables were sex, age, time of residence, and time of exposure at work. It was not possible controlling for smoking and drinking habits.

Table 6. Linear regression of the independent factors associated with chronotypes [1].

Coefficients	Non-Standardized Coefficients		Standardized Coefficients	t	Sig.	95.0% Confidence Interval for B	
Model	B	Standard Error	Beta			Lower Limit	Upper Limit
(Constant)	44.599	1.604		27.813	0.000 *	41.403	47.795
Mn (µg g^{-1} Creat)	0.798	0.224	0.387	3.564	0.001 *	0.352	1.244
Sex	1.137	0.571	0.215	1.990	0.050 *	−0.001	2.276
Age	−0.033	0.027	−0.137	−1.198	0.235	−0.087	0.022
Residence time	−0.048	0.053	−0.101	−0.892	0.375	−0.154	0.059
Exposure time at work	0.018	0.029	0.071	0.602	0.549	−0.041	0.076
Model Summary [2]							
Model	R	R Square	Adjusted R Square		Standard Error of the Estimate		
	0.449 [2]	0.202	0.147		2.450		

[1] Dependent Variable: *PER3* Genotype. [2] Predictors: (Constant), time and exposure at work, Mn (µg g^{-1} Creat) sex, residence time, age. * statistically significant.

3.5. Urinary Benzene e Toluene (µg L^{-1}) According to PER3 Gene Polymorphisms

Table 7 presents the concentrations of unmetabolized benzene and toluene in urine according to chronotype. When compared to the indifferent and morning groups, the evening group had the highest levels of unmetabolized benzene (179.04 µg L^{-1}) and toluene (148.58 µg L^{-1}) with statistical significance ($p < 0.01$). Figures 8 and 9 show the compounds median values according to subjects' chronotype.

Table 7. Concentrations of unmetabolized benzene and toluene in urine (µg L^{-1}) according to *PER3* gene VNTR polymorphism.

Benzene and Toluene/Chronotype	Evening			Indifferent			Morning			Friedman Test	p-Value
	P$_{25}$	Median	P$_{75}$	P$_{25}$	Median	P$_{75}$	P$_{25}$	Median	P$_{75}$		
Unmetabolized benzene (µg L^{-1})	128.88	179.04	336.66	99.67	106.57	169.87	87.42	90.02	-	21.00	<0.01 *
Unmetabolized toluene (µg L^{-1})	80.68	148.58	274.44	79.03	115.36	197.42	66.26	96.89	161.45	91.66	<0.01 *

* Statistically significant.

3.5.1. According to PER3 Gene VNTR Polymorphisms and Influence Zone

Table 8 displays the concentrations of unmetabolized benzene and toluene in the urine according to the *PER3* gene and the zone of influence. Benzene concentrations in individuals presenting the afternoon chronotype residing in zone 2 were higher (387.28 µg L^{-1}; $\chi^2 = 9.66$; $p < 0.01$) compared to those in zone 1. However, there was no association between toluene concentrations in resident individuals presenting the afternoon chronotype in the two zones, despite the higher levels detected in individuals presenting the afternoon chronotype in Zone 2 (164.00 µg L^{-1}; $\chi^2 = 5.71$; $p < 0.01$).

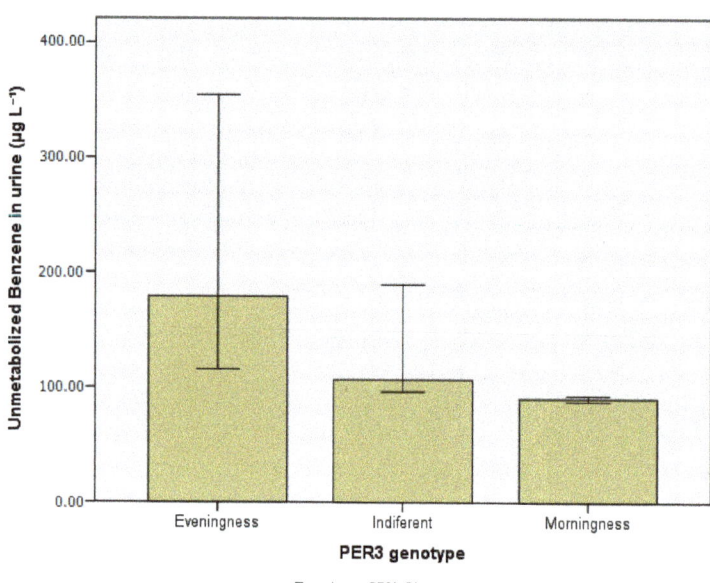

Figure 8. Unmetabolized benzene in urine (µg L^{-1}) according to *PER3* gene VNTR polymorphisms.

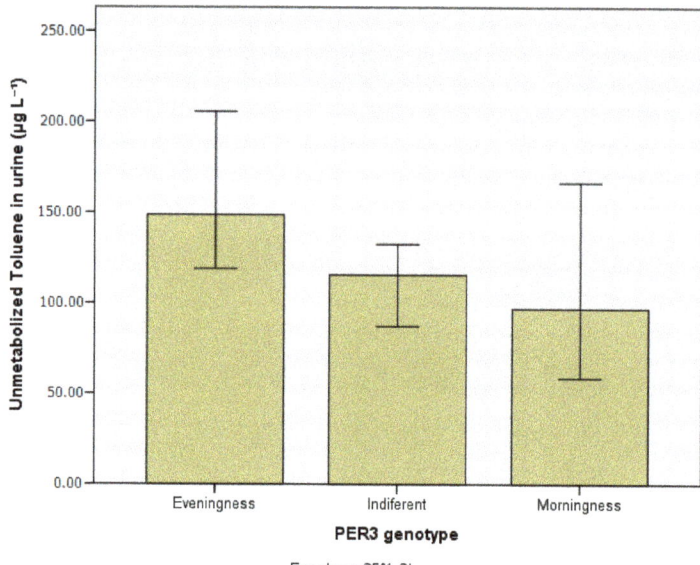

Figure 9. Unmetabolized toluene in urine (µg L^{-1}) according to *PER3* gene VNTR polymorphisms.

3.5.2. According to *PER3* Gene VNTR Polymorphisms and Occupational Exposure to Chemicals

The concentrations of unmetabolized benzene and toluene in urine (µg L^{-1}) are presented in Table 9 according to chronotype and occupational exposure. The benzene concentration (219.91 µg L^{-1}) was significantly higher in unexposed individuals with the afternoon chronotype than in those with exposure at work (115.51 µg L^{-1}) (Kruskal–Wallis $\chi^2 = 11.20$; $p < 0.01$), while there was no statistical significance for toluene.

Table 8. Unmetabolized benzene and toluene in urine (µg L^{-1}) according to *PER3* gene VNTR polymorphism and zone of influence.

Variables	Category	Evening P$_{25}$	Evening Median	Evening P$_{75}$	Indifferent P$_{25}$	Indifferent Median	Indifferent P$_{75}$	Morning P$_{25}$	Morning Median	Morning P$_{75}$	Kruskal–Wallis Test	p
Benzene (µg L^{-1})	Influence zone 2	233.03	387.28	510.54	104.00	128.53	179.57	-	-	-	9.66	0.05 *
	Influence zone 1	115.51	152.24	214.38	-	-	-	-	-	-		
Toluene (µg L^{-1})	Influence zone 2	114.22	164.00	293.69	68.55	105.63	175.15	56.22	120.91	166.47	5.71	0.34
	Influence zone 1	66.68	126.58	344.45	78.50	119.59	195.92	78.36	84.54	418.15		

* Statistically significant.

Table 9. Unmetabolized benzene and toluene in urine (µg L^{-1}) according to *PER3* gene polymorphisms and occupational exposure to chemicals.

Variables	Category	Evening P$_{25}$	Evening Median	Evening P$_{75}$	Indifferent P$_{25}$	Indifferent Median	Indifferent P$_{75}$	Morning P$_{25}$	Morning Median	Morning P$_{75}$	Kruskal–Wallis Test	p
Chemical Exposure at Work Benzene (µg L^{-1})	No	179.04	219.91	387.28	103.14	106.57	-	-	-	-	11.20	0.02 *
	Yes	65.78	115.51	155.03	-	-	-	-	-	-		
Chemical Exposure at Work Toluene (µg L^{-1})	No	80.82	142.60	271.45	86.61	127.23	207.09	58.60	84.54	166.47	6.98	0.14
	Yes	66.68	163.51	281.31	56.22	85.15	116.86	-	-	-		

* Statistically significant.

4. Discussion

Associations between the $PER3^{4/4}$ with higher BPb, and $PER^{5/5}$ with higher UMn were observed in the study population. The indifferent chronotype was associated with sleep complaints (insomnia and excessive sleepiness), while higher levels UMn were observed in the morning chronotypes. The evening chronotype was associated with poorer sleep quality and higher BPb, including in exposed workers over 50 years of age. We also observed an association of PER3 gene VNTR polymorphisms with higher levels of non-metabolized benzene and toluene in the urine of evening chronotype residents in zone 2 (distant from slag) and those unexposed at work.

4.1. Sociodemographic Aspects

In the present study, the PER3 polymorphism associated with the evening chronotype ($PER3^{4/4}$) was detected in approximately half of the study population, followed by the indifferent ($PER3^{4/5}$), and morning ($PER3^{5/5}$) chronotypes. The same association ($PER3\ ^{4/4}$) was observed in previous research [48–51] using a validated questionnaire. On the other hand, two studies assessing PER3 VNTR polymorphism [27] and a validated questionnaire [52], both concerning the Brazilian population, did not have results similar to a South African population [53,54]. Such discrepancies may be due to different latitudes, as photoperiod and ambient temperature variations in tropical countries throughout the year are low [55].

Due to the low participation rate of the resident population in the study, which made determining a significant association difficult, it is important to note that most participants have a social drinking habit, similar to a study of workers exposed to lead (Pb) in Taiwan, Asia [56], which reported a 38% alcohol consumption rate. However, the highest Pb concentrations were found among evening group drinkers, which was most likely due to a confounding variable. A similar finding was reported in a study [50], which also found associations between PER3 gene VNTR polymorphisms afternoon chronotypes and alcohol abuse.

4.2. Sleep–Wake Cycle According to PER3 Gene VNTR Polymorphisms in the Population

Although there was no statistical significance, the results found were similar to those in the literature for both sleep latency and wake-up time, while sleep duration was shorter in the morning chronotype group than the others. Some studies in different populations around the world found that clock gene polymorphisms are independently associated with circadian phenotypes. Those authors found PER3 gene VNTR polymorphism was associated with morning–evening tendencies [33,34]. Like our research, Carrier and collaborators found individuals identified as morningness prefer to wake up early in the morning compared to eveningness individuals [57]. Moreover, Taillard and colleagues found out late sleeping and waking especially on the weekends characterized eveningness individuals [58].

4.3. Sleep Complaints According to PER3 Gene VNTR Polymorphisms

Our study found statistical significance for insomnia complaints in people with an indifferent chronotype. In another study, conducted in Finland [59], insomnia complaints were observed for the afternoon chronotype. Because light sensitivity differs according to the PER3 gene VNTR polymorphism, with $PER3^{5/5}$ being more sensitive to light in the blue wavelength range than $PER3^{4/4}$ [60], those differences may be associated with different latitudes.

Several studies [15,56,59,60] investigated the effects of metal exposure on human health and found that environmental exposure to these contaminants can cause potentially toxic effects and insomnia-related disorders, among other findings. Some research has concluded that toluene exposure causes insomnia [27,29,61], as well as in chemical dependents exposed to both toluene and benzene [23]. Even at low levels of exposure, toxic effects can cause oxidative stress and subsequent DNA damage, according to studies [62–64].

In addition, an association with excessive sleepiness (60%) in indifferent chronotypes was also observed in our study. Researchers [52] identified higher rates of excessive sleepiness in individuals presenting the afternoon chronotype when applying a validated questionnaire, while another study [59] observed the same association when employing a non-validated questionnaire. However, excessive sleepiness is associated with other factors, such as sleep duration and working hours, making further assessments difficult. The worse reported sleep quality (55%) observed in this study was for the afternoon chronotype. Exposure to metals, including Cd, Pb, Ni, and Mn, has been reported as able to impair sleep quality [52,56]. Mohammadyan et al. [65], when adjusting the analysis for age, work experience, body mass index, and exposure to Pb as revealed by blood concentrations, detected a significant relationship with poorer sleep quality. Some studies have identified that benzene and toluene exposures can lead to sleep disorders with intense motor activity and, consequently, worse sleep quality [23,28,29]. The central nervous system is one of the first areas to account for the toxicity of those solvents [10,20–22,24].

4.4. Assessment of Manganese in Urine and Lead in Blood Levels According to PER3 Gene VNTR Polymorphism

Metals are well known endocrine-disrupting compounds [13,15,30,59]. Even with environmental and occupational regulations concerning exposure to those elements, low-levels exposure can also interfere with the endocrine system and circadian rhythm control and maintenance at a molecular level [55]. In this regard, melatonin and its metabolites act as metal-chelating agents and play an important role in inhibiting oxidative stress [37].

Although borderline significance between chronotypes, individuals presenting higher BPb belonged to the evening chronotype, according to our findings. However, when the subjects' ages were considered, Pb concentrations were higher in those over 50, since this toxic metal accumulates in blood [66].

Bone loss accelerates after menopause and bone demineralization may release bone lead into circulation. Osteoporosis and atherosclerosis may result from elevated homocysteine concentrations. In individuals over 50 years of age, BPb and homocysteine concentrations correlate as an increase in BPb leads to an increase in homocysteine levels [67]. In this way, some diseases, and physiological events, such as osteoporosis and menopause, may cause lead to be released from the bone into the blood [67,68].

Another result with borderline significance was that BPb decreased according to chronotype among workers who reported chemical exposure to metals, with higher levels found in subjects within the afternoon chronotype and lower levels found in subjects within the morning chronotype. In addition to communities living near industrial activities, occupational groups may face serious risks from exposure to that metal [13], as reported in another study that found an association between insomnia and Pb concentration in the urine of exposed workers [56]. The highest Pb levels are probably associated with the afternoon chronotype as the metal exhibits affinity to melatonin and can occupy its active site since a binding affinity exists between Pb and melatonin [38].

Elevated levels of manganese in urine were observed in the morning group in our study. Another research reported the same result even after controlling for sex, age, residence time, and work exposure time. Rats daily treated with Mn presented the first evidence that chronic Mn intoxication leads to activity and rest rhythm impairments in another study about metals and the endocrine disruption process [39].

Chuang et al. [55] reported higher UMn associated with decreased cortisol and serotonin levels in workers, important hormones related to the sleep–wake cycle. Serotonin is important in the melatonin synthesis cascade, which exhibits its acrophase in the middle of the night and remains lower during the day. Cortisol has its acrophase in the early hours of dawn and remains lower for the rest of the day. Therefore, metals such as Mn, playing a critical role in neuroendocrine functions, can initiate an adrenergic response or a stimulated cortisol release through the hypothalamic–pituitary–adrenal axis. Furthermore, xenobiotics linked to endocrine disruption may modify the active site of metals in the central nervous system. In addition, endocrine disruption may also be responsible for changes in the sleep–wake cycle rhythm, which involves a reduction in the synthesis of circulating melatonin and loss of serotonin. Thus, the chronic effects of metals and endocrine disruption can lead to two outcomes resulting from the same toxicological process [69]. In the case of Mn, high exposure levels may be associated with morning patterns due to its affinity to cortisol, presenting its acrophase in the early morning, which, in turn, may lead to an advancement of the waking phase in exposed individuals.

4.5. Urinary Benzene and Toluene Level Assessments

4.5.1. According to PER3 Gene VNTR Polymorphisms

Higher levels of non-metabolized benzene and toluene were observed in individuals presenting the afternoon chronotype. For many authors, those volatile organic compounds are toxic even at low concentrations [18–22]. Exogenous substances or their mixtures alter endocrine system function and behave as endocrine disruptors [30,70]. On the other hand, the central nervous system responds quickly to toluene and benzene toxicity [23,71,72]. Thus, both systems regulate and control all human body functions, including melatonin synthesis and hormone level alterations. Consequently, toluene and benzene exposure can lead to sleep disturbances [10,13,24,29].

4.5.2. According to PER3 Gene VNTR Polymorphisms and Influence Zone

Residents in influence zone 2 (far from the slag) exhibited the highest levels of unmetabolized benzene and toluene in their urine compared to those in influence zone 1, about 2-fold higher for benzene. The location of the collection points can explain this fact. Influence zone 2 was close to the main avenue of the condominium, which delimits it and makes its use mandatory. As it is the main street, the traffic of motor vehicles is high and, consequently, the burning of fossil fuels, mainly diesel and gasoline, is also elevated. Other studies confirmed the same results and proved the great influence of vehicular traffic on the levels of those contaminants in the environment. However, a concrete block factory located next to the sampling site, with several trucks carrying those blocks and burning fossil fuels, also contributed to the increase in detected levels [73–76].

The explanation for the detected values may be in the origin of those contaminants in the atmosphere. Usually, the presence of benzene is attributed to vehicular emissions, while other processes can also emit toluene due to volatilization [77,78]. The emission of those substances can also be attributed to stationary sources such as factories, industries, and gas stations [79–82]. In the steel industry, by-products such as benzene and toluene are generated in the coking step [83], an important source of widespread environmental exposure, given the volatilizing capacity of these substances.

4.5.3. According to PER3 Gene VNTR Polymorphisms and Occupational Chemical Exposure

Afternoon chronotype unexposed workers presented 2-fold higher benzene concentrations in urine ($\mu g\ L^{-1}$) compared to workers who reported occupational chemical exposure, in contrast with the results reported by Gore and collaborators [4]. In a review, the authors warned that occupational groups might also face exposure risks in addition to resident communities close to industrial activities [13].

The fact that the highest concentrations of urinary benzene were found in unexposed workers can be explained by workers omitting actual exposure for fear of losing their jobs at the steel company or related to the fact that 64% of afternoon chronotype workers reside in the zone of influence 2. It is important to highlight that exposure to benzene and toluene desynchronizes the sleep–wake cycle, affecting the monoaminergic response in brain areas related to sleep, which includes pineal gland function. The monoaminergic system is formed by noradrenaline, serotonin, and dopamine, which act in the modulation and integration of several cortical and subcortical activities, in turn regulating psychomotor activity, mood, appetite, and sleep [29]. Disorders related to chemical substance exposure, including benzene and toluene, are due to serotonergic transmission deficiency. As previously described, the neurotoxic consequences caused by benzene and toluene are no different from toxic metals such as Mn and Pb [10,19,24,39,61,72].

4.5.4. Study Limitations

Our study exhibits limitations that should be considered, such as a cross-sectional design, which allows only associations and long-term data collection (2017–2019), and not causality verifications. Even when applying a randomized sampling, low adherence to the study was noted, as many residents work or are related to workers in the local steel industry and were afraid of losing their jobs. Because of this, non-parametric tests were employed, which made it difficult to compare the results to population data. The data could also not be controlled for working conditions or smoking and drinking habits. Therefore, the findings reported herein may be applicable only to the specific population evaluated in this study.

5. Conclusions

To the best of our knowledge, this study is the first involving the investigation of an adult population living in a steel-contaminated area comprising a genetic analysis concerning chronotypes.

Chronobiological, toxic, and carcinogenic consequences were noted in the present study. So, we cannot rule out the hypothesis that Mn, Pb, benzene, and toluene may be responsible for changes in the sleep–wake cycle rhythm, which may have influenced the different chronotypes found in the steel residue-exposed population. Therefore, the condominium built on a steel residue-contaminated area is of concern, requiring the continuous monitoring of the local population. In addition, the *PER3* gene polymorphisms or the phenotypic chronotype can be used as a marker for endocrine changes and help in public policies related to the local health system and monitored environmental areas.

Author Contributions: All authors confirm having a part in this manuscript. Substantial contribution to the project and manuscript designs (conceptualization, methodology), data collecting, analysis, and interpretation: G.B.F.C., M.d.F.R.M., F.M.F., D.V., L.R.T., M.N.-S., M.A.C. and M.S.S.-M. Manuscript writing and/or revising: G.B.F.C., M.d.F.R.M., M.C.R.d.S., L.F.F., S.V.d.A. and R.M.B. Manuscript final version approval for publication: G.B.F.C., D.V., M.d.F.R.M., F.M.F. and L.R.T. All authors have read and agreed to the published version of the manuscript.

Funding: This research was funded by Carlos Chagas Filho Foundation for Research Support of the State of Rio de Janeiro (Fundação de Amparo à Pesquisa do Estado do Rio de Janeiro—FAPERJ)—n° E-26/203.263/2016; Coordination of Superior Level Staff Improvement (Coordenação de Aperfeiçoamento de Pessoal de Nível Superior—CAPES)—n° 88882.442921/2019-01; Center for Studies on Worker Health and Human Ecology, National School of Public Health Sergio Arouca, Oswaldo Cruz Foundation (Centro de Estudos da Saúde do Trabalhador e Ecologia Humana, Escola Nacional de Saúde Pública Sergio Arouca, Fundação Oswaldo Cruz—CESTEH/ENSP/FIOCRUZ). F.M.F. receives from CNPq a productivity grant 1A, number 306963/2021-3.

Institutional Review Board Statement: The project was approved by the Ethics Committee in Research, from ENSP, and followed the precepts of Ethics in Research with Human Beings (National Health Council, Resolution 466/2012), under CAAE no. 71369817.3.0000.5240.

Informed Consent Statement: Informed consent was obtained from all subjects involved in the study.

Data Availability Statement: The datasets generated and analyzed during the current study are not publicly available since personal data from subjects are protected according to the Ethics Committee but may be available from the corresponding author in aggregate form on reasonable request.

Conflicts of Interest: The authors declare no conflict of interest concerning the subject matter or materials discussed in this manuscript. Funders had no role in the design of the study; collection, analyses, or interpretation of data; in the writing of the manuscript; or in the decision to publish the results.

References

1. Kordas, K.; Casavantes, M.; Mendoza, C.; Lopez, P.; Ronquillo, D.; Rosado, J.L.; Vargas, G.G.; Stoltzfus, R.J. The Association Between Lead and Micronutrient Status, and Children's Sleep, Classroom Behavior, and Activity. *Arch. Environ. Occup.* **2007**, *62*, 105–112. [CrossRef] [PubMed]
2. Lambert, T.W.; Boehmer, J.; Feltham, J.; Guyn, L.; Shahid, R. Spatial Mapping of Lead, Arsenic, Iron, and Polycyclic Aromatic Hydrocarbon Soil Contamination in Sydney, Nova Scotia: Community Impact From the Coke Ovens and Steel Plant. *Arch. Environ. Occup.* **2011**, *66*, 128–145. [CrossRef] [PubMed]
3. Peña-Fernández, A.; González-Muñoz, M.J.; Lobo-Bedmar, M.C. Establishing the importance of human health risk assessment for metals and metalloids in urban environments. *Environ. Int.* **2014**, *72*, 176–185. [CrossRef] [PubMed]
4. Gore, A.C.; Chappell, V.A.; Fenton, S.E.; Flaws, J.A.; Nadal, A.; Prins, G.S.; Toppari, J.; Zoeller, R.T. EDC-2: The Endocrine Society's Second Scientific Statement on Endocrine-Disrupting Chemicals. *Endocr. Rev.* **2015**, *36*, E1–E150. [CrossRef] [PubMed]
5. Hu, Y.; Zhou, J.; Du, B.; Liu, H.; Zhang, W.; Liang, J.; Zhang, W.; You, L.; Zhou, J. Health risks to local residents from the exposure of heavy metals around the largest copper smelter in China. *Ecotoxicol. Environ. Saf.* **2019**, *171*, 329–336. [CrossRef]
6. Zierold, K.M.; Hagemeyer, A.N.; Sears, C.G. Health symptoms among adults living near a coal-burning power plant. *Arch. Environ. Occup.* **2019**, *75*, 289–296. [CrossRef]
7. Magalhães, M.O.L.; Amaral-Sobrinho, N.M.B.; Mazur, N. Uso de resíduos industriais na remediação de solo contaminado com cádmio e zinco. *Ciência Florest.* **2011**, *21*, 219–227. [CrossRef]
8. Pagliari, B.G.; Moreira, M.F.R.; Mannarino, C.F.; Santos, G.B. Risk of exposure to metals in soil contaminated by steel industry waste for a population in Volta Redonda, RJ. *Rev. Ambient. Água* **2021**, *16*, e2696. [CrossRef]
9. ATSDR (Agency for Toxic Substances and Disease Registry). *Toxicological Profile for Benzene*; U.S. Department of Health and Human Services: Washington, DC, USA, 2007.
10. ATSDR (Agency for Toxic Substances and Disease Registry). *Draft Toxicological Profile for Toluene*; Department of Health and Human Services: Washington, DC, USA, 2015.
11. Coutrim, M.X.; Carvalho, L.R.F.; Arcuri, A.S.A. Avaliação dos métodos analíticos para a determinação de metabólitos do benzeno como potenciais biomarcadores de exposição humana ao benzeno no ar. *Quim. Nova* **2000**, *23*, 653–663. [CrossRef]
12. Mcnally, S.; Sams, C.; Loizou, G.D.; Jones, K. Evidence for non-linear metabolism at low benzene exposures? A reanalysis of data. *Chem.-Biol. Interact.* **2017**, *278*, 256–268. [CrossRef]
13. Gore, A.C.; Crews, D.; Doan, L.L.; Merril, M.L.; Patisaul, H.; Zota, A. *Introduction to Endocrine Disrupting Chemicals (EDCs): A Guide for Public Interest Organizations and Policy-Makers*; Endocrine Society: Washington, DC, USA, 2014.
14. Jehan, S.; Khattak, S.A.; Muhammad, S.; Ali, L.; Rashid, A.; Hussain, M.L. Human health risks by potentially toxic metals in drinking water along the Hattar Industrial Estate, Pakistan. *Environ. Sci. Pollut. Res. Int.* **2020**, *27*, 2677–2690. [CrossRef]
15. Okereafor, U.; Makhatha, M.; Mekuto, L.; Uche-Okereafor, N.; Sebola, T.; Mavumengwana, V. Toxic Metal Implications on Agricultural Soils, Plants, Animals, Aquatic life and Human Health. *Int. J. Environ. Res. Public Health* **2020**, *17*, 2204. [CrossRef]
16. Chen, X.; Zhang, S.; Yi, L.; Liu, Z.; Ye, X.; Yu, B.; Shi, S.; Lu, X. Evaluation of Biodegradation of BTEX in the Subsurface of a Petrochemical Site near the Yangtze River, China. *Int. J. Environ. Res. Public Health* **2022**, *19*, 16449. [CrossRef] [PubMed]
17. Nordberg, G.F.; Fowler, B.A.; Nordberg, M. Toxicology of metals: Overview, definitions, concepts and trends. In *Handbook on the Toxicology of Metals*, 4th ed.; Academic Press: Cambridge, MA, USA, 2015; Volume 1, pp. 1–12.
18. Barata-silva, C.; Mitri, S.; Pavesi, T.; Saggioro, E.; Moreira, J.C. Benzeno: Reflexos sobre a saúde pública, presença ambiental e indicadores biológicos utilizados para a determinação da exposição. *Cad. Saúde Coletiva* **2014**, *22*, 329–342. [CrossRef]
19. Santos, M.V.C.; Figueiredo, V.O.; Arcuri, A.S.A.; Costa-Amaral, I.C.; Gonçalves, E.S.; Larentis, A.L. Aspectos toxicológicos do benzeno, biomarcadores de exposição e conflitos de interesses. *Rev. Bras. Saúde Ocup.* **2017**, *42*, 13. [CrossRef]
20. Depoortere, H.; Decobert, M.; Honoré, L. Drug effects on the EEG of various species of laboratory animals. *Neuropsychobiology* **1983**, *9*, 244–249. [CrossRef] [PubMed]
21. Compton, W.; Cottler, L.; Dinwiddeie, S.; Spitznagel, E.; Mager, D.; Asmus, C. Inhalant use: Characteristics and predictions. *Am. J. Addict.* **1994**, *3*, 263–272.
22. Halifeoglu, I.; Canatan, H.; Ustundag, B.; Ilhan, N.; Inanc, F. Effect of thinner inhalation on lipid peroxidation and some antioxidant enzymes of people working with paint thinner. *Cell Biochem. Funct.* **2000**, *18*, 263–267. [CrossRef]
23. Martinez, A.; Luna, G.; Calvo, J.M.; Valdés-Cruz, A.; Magdaleno-Madrigal, V.; Fernández-Mas, R.; Martínez, D.; Fernández-Guardiola, A. Análisis espectral (3D) electroencefalográfico de los efectos de la inhalación de compuestos orgánicos volátiles industriales sobre el sueño y la atención en el humano. *Salud Ment.* **2002**, *25*, 56–67.
24. Konjin, Z.N.; Azari, M.R.; Shekoohi, Y.; Seyedi, M. Efficacy of Urinary Hippuric Acid as a Biomarker of Low Level Exposure to Toluene in Petroleum Depot Workers. *Int. J. Occup. Hyg.* **2013**, *5*, 139–143.
25. Instituto Nacional de Câncer (INCA, National Cancer Institute). *Ambiente, Trabalho e Câncer: Aspectos Epidemiológicos, Toxicológicos e Regulatórios*; INCA: Rio de Janeiro, Brazil, 2021; 290p.
26. Yamawaki, S.; Segawa, T.; Sarai, K. Effects of acute and chronic toluene inhalation on behavior and (3H) serotonin binding in rat. *Life Sci.* **1982**, *30*, 1997–2002. [CrossRef] [PubMed]
27. Arito, H.; Tsuruta, H.; Nakagaki, K.; Tanaka, S. Partial insomnia, hyperactivity and hyperdipsia induced by repeated administration of toluene in rats: Their relation to brain monoamine metabolism. *Toxicology* **1985**, *37*, 99–110. [CrossRef] [PubMed]

28. Von Euler, G.; Fuxe, K.; Hansson, T.; Ogren, S.O.; Agnati, L.F.; Eneroth, P.; Härfstrand, A.; Gustafsson, J.A. Effects of chronic toluene exposure on central monoamine and peptide receptors and their interactions in the adult male rat. *Toxicology* **1988**, *52*, 3–26. [CrossRef]
29. Alfaro-Rodríguez, A.; Bueno-Nava, A.; González-Piña, R.; Arch-Tirado, E.; Vargas-Sánchez, J.; Avila-Luna, A. Chronic exposure to toluene changes the sleep-wake pattern and brain monoamine content in rats. *Acta Neurobiol. Exp.* **2011**, *71*, 183–192.
30. Zhou, X.; Yang, Z.; Luo, Z.; Li, H.; Chen, G. Endocrine disrupting chemicals in wild freshwater fishes: Species, tissues, sizes and human health risks. *Environ. Pollut.* **2018**, *244*, 462–468. [CrossRef] [PubMed]
31. European Commission on Environment. *Community Strategy for Endocrine Disruptors*, 4th ed.; EU: Brussels, Belgium, 2011.
32. Griefahn, B. The application of a questionnaire for circadian type in the assignment of a shift workplace. *Zarbwiss* **2002**, *54*, 142–149.
33. Archer, S.N.; Robilliard, D.L.; Skene, D.J.; Smits, M.; Williams, A.; Arendt, J.; von Schantz, M. A Length Polymorphism in the Circadian Clock Gene Per3 is Linked to Delayed Sleep Phase Syndrome and Extreme Diurnal Preference. *Sleep* **2003**, *26*, 413–415. [CrossRef]
34. Pereira, D.S.; Tufik, S.; Louzada, F.M.; Benedito-Silva, A.A.; Lopez, A.R.; Lemos, N.A.; Korczak, A.L.; D'Almeida, V.; Pedrazzoli, M. Association of the Length Polymorphism in the Human Per3 Gene with the Delayed Sleep-Phase Syndrome: Does Latitude Have an Influence Upon It? *Sleep* **2005**, *28*, 29–32.
35. Sabino, F.C.; de Oliveira, J.A.; Pedrazzoli, M. Per3 expression in different tissues of Cebus apella. *Sleep Sci.* **2016**, *9*, 262–265. [CrossRef]
36. Esquifino, A.I.; Cano, P.; Jiménez-Ortega, V.; Fernández-Mateos, P.; Cardinali, D.P. Neuroendocrine-immune correlates of circadian physiology: Studies in experimental models of arthritis, ethanol feeding, aging, social isolation, and calorie restriction. *Endocrine* **2007**, *32*, 1–19. [CrossRef]
37. Parmalee, N.L.; Aschner, M. Metals and Circadian Rhythms. In *Advances in Neurotoxicology*; Aschner, M., Costa., L.G., Eds.; Academic Press: Cambridge, MA, USA, 2017; pp. 119–130.
38. Limson, J.; Nyokong, T.; Daya, S. The interaction of melatonin and its precursors with aluminium, cadmium, copper, iron, lead, and zinc: An adsorptive voltammetric study. *J. Pineal Res.* **1998**, *24*, 15–21. [CrossRef] [PubMed]
39. Bouabid, S.; Fifel, K.; Benazzouz, A.; Lakhdar-Ghazal, N. Consequences of manganese intoxication on the circadian rest-activity rhythms in the rat. *Neuroscience* **2016**, *331*, 13–23. [CrossRef]
40. Buysse, D.J.; Reynolds, C.F.; Monk, T.H.; Berman, S.R.; Kupfer, D.J. The Pittsburgh sleep quality index: A new instrument for psychiatric practice and research. *Psychiatry Res.* **1989**, *28*, 193–213. [CrossRef]
41. Agency for Toxic Substances and Disease Registry (ATSDR). *Toxicological Profile for Chromium*; U.S. Department of Health and Human Services: Washington, DC, USA, 2012.
42. Vacchi-Suzzi, C.; Kruse, D.; Harrington, J.; Levine, K.; Meliker, J.R. Is Urinary Cadmium a Biomarker of Long-term Exposure in Humans? A Review HHS Public Access. *Curr. Environ. Health Rep.* **2016**, *3*, 450–458. [CrossRef] [PubMed]
43. Agency for Toxic Substances and Disease Registry (ATSDR). *Toxicological Profile for Nickel*; ATSDR's Toxicological Profiles: Atlanta, GA, USA, 2010.
44. Baker, M.G.; Simpson, C.D.; Stover, B.; Sheppard, L.; Checkoway, H.; Racette, B.A.; Seixas, N.S. Blood manganese as an exposure biomarker: State of the evidence. *J. Occup. Environ. Hyg.* **2014**, *11*, 210–217. [CrossRef] [PubMed]
45. Agency for Toxic Substances and Disease Registry (ATSDR). *Toxicological Profile for Lead*; U.S. Department of Health and Human Services: Washington, DC, USA, 2020.
46. Miller, S.A.; Dykes, D.D.; Polesky, H.F. A simple salting out procedure for extracting DNA from human nucleated cells. *Nucleic Acids Res.* **1988**, *16*, 1215. [CrossRef] [PubMed]
47. Ebisawa, T.; Uchiyama, M.; Kajimura, N.; Mishima, K.; Kamei, Y.; Katoh, M.; Watanabe, T.; Sekimoto, M.; Shibui, K.; Kim, K.; et al. Association of structural polymorphisms in the human period3 gene with delayed sleep phase syndrome. *EMBO Rep.* **2001**, *2*, 342–346. [CrossRef]
48. Barclay, N.; Eley, T.C.; Mill, J.; Wong, C.C.Y.; Zavos, H.M.S.; Archer, S.N.; Gregory, A.M. Sleep quality and diurnal preference in a sample of young adults: Associations with 5HTTLPR, PER3, and CLOCK 3111. *Am. J. Med. Genet. B.* **2011**, *156*, 681–690. [CrossRef]
49. Von Schantz, M.; Taporoski, T.; Horimoto, A.; Esteban, N.; Vallada, H.; Krieger, J.; Pereira, A. Distribution and heritability of diurnal preference (chronotype) in a rural Brazilian family-based cohort, the Baependi study. *Sleep Med.* **2015**, *16*, S43–S44. [CrossRef]
50. Mansour, H.A.; Wood, J.; Chowdari, K.V.; Tumuluru, D.; Bamne, M.; Monk, T.H.; Nimgaonkar, V.L. Associations between period 3 gene polymorphisms and sleep- /chronotype-related variables in patients with late-life insomnia. *Chronobiol. Int.* **2017**, *34*, 624–631. [CrossRef]
51. Maukonen, M.; Havulinna, A.S.; Männistö, S.; Kanerva, N.; Salomaa, V.; Partonen, T. Genetic Associations of Chronotype in the Finnish General Population. *J. Biol. Rhythm.* **2020**, *35*, 501–511. [CrossRef] [PubMed]
52. Tempaku, P.F.; Ramirez Arruda, J.; Mazzotti, D.R.; Mazzotti, D.R.; Gonçalves, B.S.B.; Pedrazzoli, M.; Bittencourt, L.; Tufik, S. Characterization of bimodal chronotype and its association with sleep: A population-based study. *Chronobiol. Int.* **2017**, *34*, 504–510. [CrossRef] [PubMed]
53. Kunorozva, L.; Stephenson, K.J.; Rae, D.E.; Roden, L.C. Chronotype and Period3 Variable Number Tandem Repeat Polymorphism in Individual Sports Athletes. *Chronobiol. Int.* **2012**, *29*, 1004–1010. [CrossRef] [PubMed]

54. Shawa, N.; Roden, L.C. Chronotype of South African adults is affected by solar entrainment. *Chronobiol. Int.* **2016**, *33*, 315–323. [CrossRef]
55. Galano, A.; Medina, M.E.; Tan, D.X.; Reiter, R.J. Melatonin and its metabolites as copper chelating agents and their role in inhibiting oxidative stress: A physicochemical analysis. *J. Pineal Res.* **2014**, *58*, 107–116. [CrossRef]
56. Chuang, H.C.; Su, T.Y.; Chuang, K.J.; Hsiao, T.C.; Lin, H.L.; Hsu, Y.T.; Pan, C.H.; Lee, K.Y.; Ho, S.C.; Lai, C.H. Pulmonary exposure to metal fume particulate matter cause sleep disturbances in shipyard welders. *Environ. Pollut.* **2018**, *232*, 523–532. [CrossRef]
57. Carrier, J.; Monk, T.H.; Buysse, D.J.; Kupfer, D.J. Sleep and morningness-eveningness in the 'middle' years of life (20–59 y). *J. Sleep Res.* **1997**, *3*, 289–294. [CrossRef]
58. Taillard, J.; Philip, P.; Bioulac, B. Morningness/eveningness and the need for sleep. *J. Sleep Res.* **1999**, *8*, 291–295. [CrossRef]
59. Merikanto, I.; Kronholm, E.; Peltonen, M.; Laatikainen, T.; Lahti, T.; Partonen, T. Relation of Chronotype to Sleep Complaints in the General Finnish Population. *Chronobiol. Int.* **2012**, *29*, 311–317. [CrossRef]
60. Pirtskhalava, M.V.; Javakhadze, R.D.; Mirtskhulava, M.B.; Chakvetadze, N.V. Environmental safety risk research. *Georgian Med. News.* **2011**, *192*, 70–75.
61. Thetkathuek, A.; Jaidee, W.; Saowakhontha, S.; Ekburanawat, W. Neuropsychological Symptoms among Workers Exposed to Toluene and Xylene in Two Paint Manufacturing Factories in Eastern Thailand. *Adv. Prev. Med.* **2015**, *2015*, 183728. [CrossRef] [PubMed]
62. Kawai, T.; Ukai, H.; Inoue, O.; Maejima, Y.; Fukui, Y.; Ohashi, F.; Okamoto, S.; Takada, S.; Sakurai, H.; Ikeda, M. Evaluation of biomarkers of occupational exposure to toluene at low levels. *Int. Arch. Occup. Environ. Health* **2008**, *81*, 253–262. [CrossRef]
63. Moro, A.M.; Brucker, N.; Charão, M.; Bulcão, R.; Freitas, F.; Baierle, M.; Nascimento, S.; Valentini, J.; Cassini, C.; Salvador, M.; et al. Evaluation of genotoxicity and oxidative damage in painters exposed to low levels of toluene. *Environ. Mutagen.* **2012**, *746*, 42–48. [CrossRef]
64. Anastasiou, M.; Chalandon, Y.; Anchisi, S. Hemolytic anemia in cancer. *Rev. Med. Suisse* **2018**, *14*, 1021–1027. [PubMed]
65. Mohammadyan, M.; Moosazadeh, M.; Borji, A.; Khanjani, N.; Moghadam, S.R. Exposure to lead and its effect on sleep quality and digestive problems in soldering workers. *Environ. Monit. Assess.* **2019**, *191*, 184. [CrossRef] [PubMed]
66. Wei, J.; Zhang, J.; Ji, J.S. Association of environmental exposure to heavy metals and eczema in US population: Analysis of blood cadmium, lead, and mercury. *Arch. Environ. Occup.* **2018**, *74*, 239–251. [CrossRef]
67. Khalil, N.; Wilson, J.W.; Talbott, E.O.; Morrow, L.A.; Hochberg, M.C.; Hillier, T.A.; Muldoon, S.B.; Cummings, S.R.; Cauley, J.A. Association of blood lead concentrations with mortality in older women: A prospective cohort study. *Environ. Health* **2009**, *8*, 15. [CrossRef] [PubMed]
68. Fan, Y.; Sheng, J.; Liang, C.; Yang, L.; Liu, K.; Wang, Q.; Zhang, D.; Ma, Y.; Li, X.; Xie, S.; et al. Association of Blood Lead Levels with the Risk of Depressive Symptoms in the Elderly Chinese Population: Baseline Data of a Cohort Study. *Biol. Trace Elem. Res.* **2020**, *194*, 76–83. [CrossRef]
69. Handy, R.D. Chronic effects of copper exposure versus endocrine toxicity: Two sides of the same toxicological process? *Comp. Biochem. Physiol. Part A Mol. Integr. Physiol.* **2003**, *135*, 25–38. [CrossRef]
70. Rattan, S.; Flaws, J.A. The epigenetic impacts of endocrine disruptors on female reproduction across generations. *Biol. Reprod.* **2019**, *101*, 635–644. [CrossRef]
71. Azevedo, F.A. *Breves Referências aos Aspectos Toxicológicos do Benzeno*; Fundação José Silveira: Salvador, Brazil, 1990.
72. Arnold, S.M.; Angerer, J.; Boogard, P.J.; Hughes, M.F.; O'Lone, R.B.; Robison, S.H.; Schnatter, A.R. The use of biomonitoring data in exposure and human health risk assessment: Benzene case study. *Crit. Rev. Toxicol.* **2013**, *43*, 119–153. [CrossRef]
73. Romano, J. *Avaliação de Benzeno; Tolueno; o-Xileno; m, p-Xileno e Etilbenzeno na Atmosfera da Estação de Monitoramento de Pinheiros*; Companhia Ambiental do Estado de São Paulo: São Paulo, Brazil, 2016.
74. Marć, M.; Bielawska, M.; Wardencki, W.; Namieśnik, J.; Zabiegała, B. The influence of meteorological conditions and anthropogenic activities on the seasonal fluctuations of BTEX in the urban air of the Hanseatic city of Gdansk, Poland. *Environ. Sci. Pollut. Res.* **2015**, *22*, 11940–11954. [CrossRef]
75. Rad, H.D.; Babaei, A.A.; Goudarzi, G.; Angali, K.A.; Ramezani, Z.; Mohammadi, M.M. Levels and sources of BTEX in ambient air of Ahvaz metropolitan city. *Air Qual. Atmos. Health* **2019**, *7*, 515–524. [CrossRef]
76. Thorsson, S.; Eliasson, I. Passive and active sampling of benzene in different urban environments in Gothenburg, Sweden. *Water. Air. Soil Pollut.* **2006**, *173*, 39–56. [CrossRef]
77. Khoder, M.I. Ambient levels of volatile organic compounds in the atmosphere of Greater Cairo. *Atmos. Environ.* **2007**, *41*, 554–566. [CrossRef]
78. Laurentino, L.S.; Marques, M.R.C.; Corrêa, S.M. Impacto ambiental de kartódromos situados na cidade do Rio de Janeiro: Monitoramento de BTEX no ar e do nível de ruído. *Quim. Nova* **2012**, *35*, 1865–1869. [CrossRef]
79. Liu, J.; Mu, Y.; Zhang, Y.; Zhang, Z.; Wang, X.; Liu, Y.; Sun, Z. Atmospheric levels of BTEX compounds during the 2008 Olympic Games in the urban area of Beijing. *Sci. Total Environ.* **2009**, *408*, 109–116. [CrossRef] [PubMed]
80. Baltrėnas, P.; Baltrėnaitė, E.; Šerevičienė, V.; Pereira, P. Atmospheric BTEX concentrations in the vicinity of the crude oil refinery of the Baltic region. *Environ. Monit. Assess.* **2011**, *182*, 115–127. [CrossRef] [PubMed]
81. Król, S.; Zabiegała, B.; Namieśnik, J. Measurement of benzene concentration in urban air using passive sampling. *Anal. Bioanal. Chem.* **2012**, *403*, 1067–1082. [CrossRef]

82. Miller, L.; Xu, X.; Wheeler, A.; Atari, D.O.; Grgicak-Mannion, A.; Luginaah, I. Spatial variability and application of ratios between BTEX in two Canadian Cities. *Sci. World J.* **2011**, *11*, 2536–2549. [CrossRef]
83. Figueiredo, I.P. *Avaliação de Emissões Atmosféricas na Indústria Siderúrgica sob a ótica do Controle e Monitoramento: O caso da CSN*; Universidade Federal do Rio de Janeiro: Rio de Janeiro, Brazil, 2016.

Disclaimer/Publisher's Note: The statements, opinions and data contained in all publications are solely those of the individual author(s) and contributor(s) and not of MDPI and/or the editor(s). MDPI and/or the editor(s) disclaim responsibility for any injury to people or property resulting from any ideas, methods, instructions or products referred to in the content.

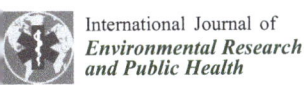

Article

Determinants of Exposure to Potentially Toxic Metals in Pregnant Women of the DSAN-12M Cohort in the Recôncavo Baiano, Brazil

Homègnon A. Ferréol Bah [1,2,*], Victor O. Martinez [3], Nathália R. dos Santos [2,3], Erival A. Gomes Junior [4], Daisy O. Costa [2,3], Elis Macêdo Pires [2], João V. Araújo Santana [2], Filipe da Silva Cerqueira [2] and José A. Menezes-Filho [1,2,3]

[1] Institute of Collective Health, Federal University of Bahia, Salvador 40110-040, Brazil
[2] Laboratory of Toxicology, College of Pharmacy, Federal University of Bahia, Salvador 40170-115, Brazil
[3] Graduate Program in Pharmacy, College of Pharmacy, Federal University of Bahia, Salvador 40170-115, Brazil
[4] Graduate Program in Food Science, College of Pharmacy, Federal University of Bahia, Salvador 40170-115, Brazil
* Correspondence: ferreol88@gmail.com; Tel.: +55-71-992-984-238

Abstract: Exposure to potentially toxic metals (PTM) threatens maternal and child health. We investigated the determinants of exposure to lead (Pb), cadmium (Cd), arsenic (As), and manganese (Mn) in 163 pregnant women from the Recôncavo Baiano, Brazil, enrolled in the DSAN-12M cohort. We measured these metals in biological samples (blood, toenails, and hair) and the Pb dust loading rates (RtPb) at their homes by graphite furnace atomic absorption spectrophotometry (GFAAS). Questionnaires were applied to collect sociodemographic and general habits data. Only 2.91% (n = 4) of the pregnant women had As levels above the detection limit. Few participants had levels above the recommended reference values for blood Pb (5.1; 95% CI: 2.1–10.1%), and Mn in hair or toenails (4.3; 95% CI: 2.3–10.1%). On the other hand, 61.1 (95% CI: 52.4–69.3%) had elevated blood Cd levels. After binary logistic regression, low socioeconomic status, domestic waste burning, being a passive smoker, multiparity, and renovating the house significantly increased the chances of having high levels of Mn, Pb, and Cd. We detected a worrying situation related to exposure to Cd, showing the urgency of implementing human biomonitoring in the general population, especially in situations of social vulnerability.

Keywords: environmental exposure; toxic metals; determinants; pregnancy; maternal health

1. Introduction

Environmental pollutants such as potentially toxic metals (PTM) have been associated with deleterious effects on human health depending on the magnitude of exposure [1]. Exposure to a high level of PTM such as lead (Pb), arsenic (As), cadmium (Cd) and the micronutrient manganese (Mn) have been the subject of several investigations in workers from the industrial and mining sector and in populations living in risk zones [2–6]. Over time, however, the neurotoxic potential of these metals, even at low exposure levels in children have been reported, [7–10] and there is a gap of knowledge regarding the toxicity of such contaminants in women [2]. In pregnant women, there is also a growing concern due to their vulnerability and the possibility of transferring PMT to the fetus; thus, compromising the child's development [10,11].

During the uterine phase and in childhood, the plasticity of the central nervous system (CNS), the immaturity of defense mechanisms, and fetal and child elimination mechanisms make them more susceptible than adults [12]. For example, low levels of exposure to Pb, As, and Cd have been associated with high blood pressure, changes in kidney function, and increased risk of preeclampsia for pregnant women, in addition to impairing the neurodevelopment of the fetus and child [13–15]. In the fetus, the immaturity of Mn elimination mechanisms explains its higher concentration when compared to the mother's in the umbilical cord, which may impair its cognitive development [10].

Studies have demonstrated possible interactions between PTM as a possible way to explain their toxicity in case of concomitant exposure [11,16–18]. Social or sociodemographic determinants may also favor exposure to these contaminants in vulnerable populations [19] in addition to acting conjointly with them to cause more exacerbated deleterious effects on health in general and to the CNS, specifically [20]. Although these metals have different physiological profiles, they show neurotoxic potential for children. Pb, As, and Cd are xenobiotics with no physiological role in the body and are considered threats to the kidney, liver, nervous system, and other organs [11,21]. Mn is an essential micronutrient whose excess has been associated with neurological damage, especially in children [9,22], while the occurrence of deleterious effects at low exposure levels is subject to inconsistency in the literature [23]. Therefore, there is a constant need for environmental and biological monitoring to detect possible sources of human exposure and raise awareness among populations about determinants and risk factors. Environmental components (water, soil, air) and biological matrices (blood, urine, nails, and hair) may serve that purpose [5,19,24].

These metals were chosen because they are naturally part of the environment, the need for more information on exposure in a population not occupationally exposed in the Brazilian context, and the health risk even at low levels. Also, PTM levels found in pregnant women are considered a proxy for intrauterine exposure. Previously, we reported moderate to high levels of PTM (Pb, Mn, and Cd) in the population (adults and school-age children of both sexes) of socially vulnerable communities in the same region [3–5,16,19,24]. However, although the PTM represents a threat during pregnancy, little is known about their real impact in socially vulnerable populations.

Considering women and fetus vulnerability during pregnancy when exposed to environmental contaminants, we carried out the study "Socioenvironmental Determinants of Child Neurodevelopment" (DSAN-12M), which is a birth cohort in the municipalities of Aratuípe and Nazaré das Farinhas in the Recôncavo Baiano, Brazil. The aims of this work are (i) to evaluate the exposure to PTM of the recruited pregnant women of the DSAN cohort, and (ii) to investigate the factors associated with such exposures.

2. Materials and Methods

2.1. Population and Study Design

This study is part of the DSAN-12M study in Aratuípe and Nazaré das Farinhas in the Recôncavo Baiano. These municipalities are inserted in a context of vulnerability due to unfavorable social conditions and the coexistence of some families with risky craft activities such as the production of lead-glazed ceramics, agricultural activities, and proximity to palm oil and soap factories, and quarries. The DSAN-12M assesses the impact of prenatal and postnatal environmental exposure to environmental contaminants (PTM, pesticides, and pathogens), maternal mental health and social factors that may impact children's neurodevelopment. In this cross-sectional study, we investigate the intensity of exposure to Pb, As, Cd, and Mn in a cohort of pregnant women, using environmental and biological matrices.

Field work started in July 2019 but stopped early March 2020 due to the COVID-19 pandemic. A second collection phase occurred between July 2021 thru September 2022.

Ethical issues: This project was approved by the research ethics committee of the Faculty of Pharmacy-UFBA through Resolution 466-CNS/2012, with approval No. 3246555.

2.1.1. Recruitment

Between 2006 and 2016, these two municipalities had an annual live birth average of 555 [25]. To invite as many pregnant women as possible, the field collection was carried out with the network of primary care units (PCU) of the Brazilian Public Health System (SUS is its acronym in Portuguese) in the municipalities of Nazaré (11 units) and Aratuípe (4 units) that carry out prenatal consultations. Considering the acceptance rate (70%)

in other surveys [19,26] in the same region, the expected number of participants was 390 pregnant women.

During the first prenatal consultation, the pregnant women in the first or second trimester were informed about the study aims and methods by the nurses and asked to meet with the field investigator staff. A detailed project explanation was presented during the visit to the participant's home. After the acceptance of the pregnant woman, the informed consent term was signed. In the case of a participant under 18 years, the legal guardian was asked to sign while the minor provided a written agreement.

As inclusion criteria, we selected pregnant women with a gestational age of fewer than 24 weeks who started their prenatal consultation at the PCU of the municipalities; lived in the region for at least one year before the pregnancy. Women with twin pregnancies under the prescription of medication potentially of neurotoxic risk for the fetus were excluded from the study.

2.1.2. Socioeconomic Data

Trained interviewers applied questionnaires to pregnant women. The socioeconomic level (SES), stratified into five categories from A to E, was defined based on the criteria of the Brazilian Association of Population Studies [27]. Data were collected on general daily habits, education level, diet, occupational history, work during pregnancy, parity, history of active or passive smoking, and proximity to probable sources of exposure to potentially toxic metals.

2.2. Assessment of Exposure to PTM

Pregnant women's exposures were measured using environmental and biological samples collected in the second trimester (between weeks 12 and 24). Domestic settled dust was used as an environmental indicator to estimate Pb exposure, which represents an indoor source. We calculated the Pb dust loading rate, while the biological samples used were blood (for Cd and Pb), hair (for Mn and As), and toenails (for Mn).

2.2.1. Assessment of Pb Dust Loading Rate (RtPb)

Details on the sampling method and Pb determination have been described elsewhere [19,28]. Briefly, in the participant's home, three disposable samplers (polyethylene Petri dishes) were installed on a support at a height of two meters in different rooms and left open for at least 30 days. After this period, the samplers were recovered and sent to the laboratory. The dust collected was solubilized in 40 mL of 7M ultrapure nitric acid and transferred to a volumetric flask of 50 mL and completed with ultrapure water. Pb analysis was performed by graphite furnace atomic absorption spectrophotometry (GFAAS) on an AA240Z, GTA-120 equipment (Varian®, Palo Alto, CA, USA). Pb levels were expressed as RtPb (μg Pb/m^2/30 days), following the methodology described in Menezes-Filho et al. [28].

2.2.2. Assessment of Biomarkers

Biological Sample Collection

Blood samples were collected by cubital venipuncture in vacuum tubes. Trace Elements Sodium Heparin tubes (Vacuette®, São Paulo, Brasil) were used for Pb and Cd determination. The samples were packed into isothermal boxes containing recyclable ice and transported to the Laboratory of Toxicology (Labtox) at the Faculty of Pharmacy of the Federal University of Bahia.

Occipital hair and toenail samples were collected with stainless steel tools (scissors and nail clipper). The first two centimeters of the hair tuft were used for Mn and As determinations as described by Menezes-Filho et al. [3]. The toenail polish was removed with an acetone-based solution before collection.

Blood Lead Level (PbB)

Blood samples were analyzed by GFAAS as described by Menezes-Filho et al. [29]. The Pb concentration was determined from the calibration curve obtained by diluting a standard Pb solution at 1000 µg/mL diluted in HNO_3 (2%). Samples in duplicates, calibrators and reference material for quality control were diluted (1 + 9). Samples from the Proficiency Program for Blood Lead Analysis at Instituto Adolfo Lutz were analyzed concomitantly to ensure the quality of the analytical method. The precision and accuracy obtained were 8.8% and 107.4%, respectively. The method's limit of detection (LOD) was 0.1 µg/dL. Samples with a PbB concentration below LOD were entered into the database with an LOD/2 value (i.e., 0.05 µg/dL).

Blood Cadmium Level (CdB)

CdB determinations were performed according to Kummrow et al. [30]. Briefly, 100 µL of the whole blood sample and certified reference material (Bio-Rad Lyphocheck®, Irvine, CA, USA) Whole Blood Metal Control Level 1) were transferred into Eppendorf® (Guangzhou, China) microtubes with 200 µL of 0.4% Triton X-100 solution and 100 µL of 3 M HNO_3. After mixing by vortex and centrifugation in a Sigma® (Osterode am Harz, Germany) microcentrifuge (at 15,183 g) for 15 min, the supernatant was analyzed by GFAAS. Quality control samples were reanalyzed every ten samples. The precision and accuracy obtained were 7.6% and 19.5%, respectively. The LOD was set at 0.1 µg/L, and results below this limit were entered into the dataset as LOD/2.

Hair and Toenail Mn (MnH and MnTn) and Hair As (AsH) Levels

Hair and toenail samples were cleansed with non-ionic detergent solution (Merck® (Darmstadt, Germany; Triton X-100; 1%) in an ultrasonic bath following the procedure reported by Dos Santos et al. [31]. The samples were dried at 60 °C for 3 to 4 h and approximately 50 mg were digested with 3 mL of spectroscopic grade concentrated nitric acid (JT Baker®, Deventer, The Netherlands) using the Mars-Express6 microwave (CEM, Dallas, Texas, USA). The digestion process was carried out according to the conditions specified by the manufacturer. Each digestion run was carried out with a reagent blank, and the certified reference materials under the same conditions as the samples to ensure the analytical quality of each run.

After complete digestion, the solution was transferred into graduated polypropylene centrifuge tubes (Corning®, St. Louis, MO, USA) and volume adjusted to 10 mL with ultrapure water.

MnH and MnTn: All samples were processed in duplicate while the reference material (IAEA-085 human hair) was analyzed in every twenty readings. Mn levels were determined by GFAAS. The results were expressed in µg of Mn/g of hair (MnH) or nails (MnTn). The LOD was set at 0.1 µg/L, and results from samples below this limit were included in the data set as LOD/2.

AsH: In the case of As, the process was the same as for Mn with the certified reference material, rice flour (SRM 1568b Rice Flour, NIST, Gaithersburg, MD, USA), used for quality assurance. The results were expressed in µg of As/g of hair. The LOD value was 0.09 µg/L, and results below this limit were included in the data set as LOD/2.

Analytical accuracy was estimated in the range of 100 and 104%. The intra- and inter-run precision was 1.5% and 3.3%, respectively.

2.3. Data Analysis

The absolute and relative frequencies of the main sociodemographic variables of the participants were presented. The distributions of continuous variables (such as age and PTM concentrations) were evaluated using the Kolmogorov–Smirnov (KS) or Shapiro–Wilk (SW) test, and they were described as mean (±standard deviation) and median (interquartile range).

The biomarker values were dichotomized for two purposes: first, to define the proportions (95%; confidence interval) of participants with PTM levels above the reference values recommended by official agencies or in the literature; then, the medians were used as a cut-off point to dichotomize the MnH, MnTn, and PbB used as dependent variables to define the determinants associated with values above the median (considered as high level in this study). In the case of CdB, the cut-off points considered were the reference values for non-smoking adult Brazilian women (0.6 μg/L), and smokers (1 μg/L) were maintained [32–34].

The Chi-square test (χ^2) was used to compare the frequencies of participants with high levels of biomarkers according to sociodemographic characteristics. Multivariate logistic regression (MLR) was used to investigate the relationship between the sociodemographic factors that showed association with the biomarkers of exposure to Mn (MnH and MnTn), Pb (PbB), and Cd (CdB) after dichotomization. Using Spearman's correlation analysis, possible correlations were estimated between biomarkers (considered continuous variables).

Variables such as maternal age, schooling, gestational age, municipality of residence, and pre-gestational BMI were considered confounders and adjusted in the MLR based on the literature [35,36]. SPSS software version 23 for Windows was used for statistical analysis, and the significance level was $p < 0.05$.

3. Results

Of the 327 pregnant invited, 187 (57.2%) agreed to participate in the study (Figure 1). Due to dropouts, address changes, and spontaneous miscarriage, we collected information and biological samples from 163 (87.2%) pregnant women. However, depending on the variables collected in the questionnaires and biological samples, we had additional losses due to the unavailability or fear of donating biological samples (such as blood or hair).

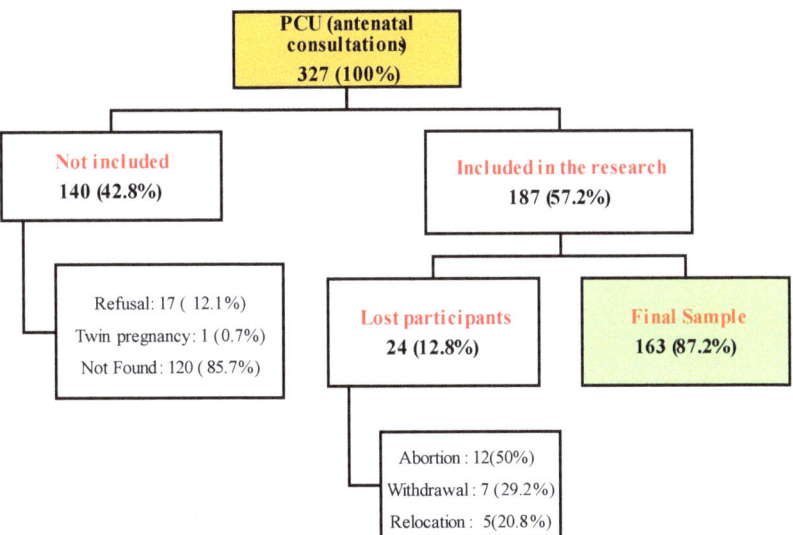

Figure 1. Selection flowchart of the population study.

3.1. Sociodemographic Characteristics of the Study Population

The sociodemographic data of the participants are presented in Table 1. The mean age of the participants was 27.0 (±6.1) years old, with an average of 18 weeks of pregnancy at the time of recruitment. Most pregnant women (94.5%) were self-declared as black or brown, and 43.6% were in their first pregnancy. More than two-thirds of the participants (68.2%) belong to a family with an income less than or equal to the minimum Brazilian wage (U$ 253), and 62.2% received assistance from the federal government.

Less than half of the participants (46.6%) completed high school, with only 9.6% having completed higher education. More than half (52.4%) were classified as low SES (classes D and E "low" and "lowest", respectively). Mean pre-gestational BMI was 25.1 kg/m², with 5.6% and 15.1% classified as "underweight" and obese, respectively. One-third (32.5%) of the families burned garbage, while 13.9% renovated their homes during pregnancy. Almost 20% of pregnant women live with a smoker (husband or other relatives); few pregnant women were active smokers, 10.1% (n = 15) before pregnancy and only 2.2% (n = 2) during pregnancy. The participants presented the same social characteristics regardless of their municipality of residence, although some variables had significantly different distributions.

Table 1. Sociodemographic and descriptive characteristics of the evaluated biomarkers of the study population.

Variables	Categories: n (%)			
Ethnicity	Black/Brown	154 (94.5)	White	9 (5.5)
Marital status	Married/Stable Union	89 (54.6)	Single/divorced	74 (45.4)
SES	D/E	77 (52.4)	C/B	70 (47.6)
Family income	Up to 1 salary	90 (68.2)	Above 1 salary	42 (31.8)
Government assistance	Yes	84 (62.2)	No	51 (37.8)
Education	Up to elementary school	87 (53.4)	High school and higher	76 (46.6)
Occupation	Housewife	51 (31.3)	Autonomous/other	112 (68.7)
House renovated	Yes	20 (13.9)	No	124 (86.1)
Passive smoker	Yes	32 (19.5)	No	112 (68.3)
Waste burning	Yes	53 (32.5)	No	110 (67.5)
First parity	Yes	71 (43.6)	No	92 (56.4)
	N		Mean ± SD	Median (Q1–Q3)
Age (years)	163		27.0 ± 6.1	26.8 (22.1–31.9)
Gestational age at inclusion (Weeks)	163		18.1 ± 5.3	18 (14.00–22.00)
Pre-gestational BMI (kg/m²)	126		25.1 ± 4.4	24.8 (22.1–28.03)
RtPb (µg/m²/30 days)	52		20.8 ± 22.2	13.0 (3.9–31.8)
PbB (µg/dL)	117		1.42 ± 2.23	0.9 (0.5–1.7)
MnH (µg/g)	131		0.4 ± 0.5	0.2 (0.1–0.5)
MnTn (µg/g)	105		0.9 ± 0.9	0.6 (0.4–1.1)
AsH (µg/g)	137		0.03 ± 0.02	0.02 (0.01–0.04)
CdB (µg/L)	126		0.8 ± 1.0	0.55 (0.1–0.9)

SD: Standard Deviation.

3.2. Descriptive of RtPb and Biomarkers

All the biomarkers and the RtPb (Table 1) showed a non-parametric distribution by the KS test and did not differ significantly according to the participant's origin. In general, the medians (Q1–Q3) of RtPb, PbB, AsH, CdB, MnH and MnTn were, respectively, 13.0 (3.9–31.8) µg/m²/30 days; 0.9 (0.5–1.7) µg/dL; 0.02 (0.01–0.04) µg/g; 0.55 (0.1–0.9) µg/L; 0.2 (0.1–0.5) µg/g, and 0.6 (0.4–1.1) µg/g.

3.3. The Proportion of Pregnant Women with Levels above the Reference Values

Table 2 presents the proportions (95%; confidence interval) of pregnant women with biomarker exposure levels above the reference values. No pregnant woman had an AsH level above 1.0 µg/g [37], while few had a higher exposure to Mn measured in hair or toenails (2 to 7%) [38,39] and Pb in blood (5.1%) [40]. However, the proportions of participants with CdB higher than the reference values were moderate to high, being 22.2% (15.6–30.0) for smokers (1.0 µg/L), 46% (37.5–54.7) and 61.1% (52.4–69.3), respectively for non-smoking Brazilian (0.6 µg/L) and US (0.4 µg/L) women [32–34,41].

Table 2. Proportion of pregnant women with PTM levels above the references.

	n	Freq. (prop. %)	(95% CI)	References
Cd				
CdB ≥ 0.4 µg/L	126	77 (61.1)	52.4–69.3	[41]
CdB ≥ 0.6 µg/L	126	58 (46.0)	37.5–54.7	[32,33]
CdB ≥ 1 µg/L	126	28 (22.2)	15.6–30.0	[34]
Mn				
MnH ≥ 1.2 µg/g	131	7 (4.3)	2.3–10.1	[38]
MnTn ≥ 4.14 µg/g	105	2 (1.9)	0.3–5.8	[39]
As				
AsH ≥ 1 µg/g	137	0 (0)	0–1.4	[37]
Pb				
PbB ≥ 3.5 µg/dL	117	6 (5.1)	2.1–10.1	[40]
PbB ≥ 2.0 µg/dL	117	23 (19.7)	13.2–27.5	[42]

Prop.: proportion.

3.4. Associations between Exposure Biomarkers

Spearman's correlation (Table 3) between exposure biomarkers showed a significant weak positive correlation between PbS and MnUp (rho = 0.240; p = 0.025).

Table 3. Spearman correlation matrix between environmental markers and exposure biomarkers.

	RtPb	MnH	MnTn	PbB	CdB
RtPb					
Rho	1.000	0.158	0.045	−0.216	0.012
P		0.268	0.776	0.159	0.938
N		51	42	44	46
MnH					
Rho		1.000	0.201 *	−0.063	0.010
P			0.044	0.486	0.911
N			101	126	116
MnTn					
Rho			1.000	0.240 *	0.121
P				0.025	0.245
N				87	94
PbB					
Rho				1.000	0.133
P					0.154
N					117
CdB					
Rho					1.000
P					
N					

* Correlation significant at 0.05 (bilateral).

3.5. Relationship between Exposure Biomarkers and Sociodemographic Variables

3.5.1. AsH

The values of AsH were undetectable, being only 2.91% (n = 4) of the samples with AsH concentration above the detection limit (0.09 µg/L) of the method. Therefore, it was not possible to interpret the results.

3.5.2. PbB

Only being primiparous was significantly associated (p = 0.018) with PbB concentrations. This relationship was confirmed by MLR (Table 4). Participants who had been pregnant in the past were 2.49 times more likely to have blood lead levels above the median.

Table 4. Determinants of PbB levels above the median after χ^2 and MLR test.

	PbS < 0.9 µg/dL n (%)	PbS ≥ 0.9 µg/dL n (%)	OR (95% CI)	p-Value
Education				
≤High school	26 (44.8)	32 (55.2)	Ref.	
≥Elementary school	33 (55.9)	26 (44.1)	0.59 (0.24–1.45)	0.245
Waste burning				
No	46 (53.5)	40 (46.5)	Ref.	
Yes	13 (41.9)	18 (58.1)	2.06 (0.76–5.58)	0.153
First parity				
Yes	31 (63.3)	18 (36.7)	Ref.	
No	28 (41.2)	40 (58.8)	2.49 (1.02–6.07)	0.045

Adjusted for BMI, municipality, age, gestational age, education.

3.5.3. Mn (MnH and MnTn)

Mn biomarkers showed significant associations with SES, education, being an active or passive smoker, monthly income, receiving government subsidies, and domestic waste burning. However, after MLR (Table 5), only SES and passive cigarette smoking maintained a significant association in the case of MnH. MnTn levels were influenced by exposure to waste burning and SES. All models showed statistical significance.

Table 5. Determinants of Mn biomarker levels above the median after χ^2 test and MLR analysis.

	MnUp < 0.6 µg/g n (%)	MnUp ≥ 0.6 µg/g n (%)	OR (95% CI)	p-Value
Active smoking				
No	51 (54.8)	42 (45.2)	Ref.	
Yes	2 (18.2)	9 (81.8)	2.62 (0.40–17.32)	0.318
SES				
C/B/A	35 (67.3)	17 (32.7)	Ref.	
D/E	16 (32.7)	33 (67.3)	4.23 (1.70–10.53)	0.002
Waste burning				
No	45 (58.4)	32 (41.6)	Ref.	
Yes	7 (26.9)	19 (73.1)	5.10 (1.43–17.69)	0.010
	MnC < 0.2 µg/g n (%)	MnC ≥ 0.2 µg/g n (%)	OR (95% CI)	
SES				
C/B/A	42 (67.7)	20 (32.3)	Ref.	
D/E	23 (35.9)	41 (64.1)	3.95 (1.79–8.73)	0.001
Passive smoking				
No	56 (58.3)	40 (41.7)	Ref.	
Yes	10 (34.5)	19 (65.5)	2.62 (1.004–6.835)	0.049

Adjusted for BMI, municipality, age, gestational age, education; SES: socioeconomic status.

3.5.4. CdB

The MLR analysis summarized in Table 6 shows that that pregnant women whose families burned domestic waste and renovated their houses during the gestational period were, respectively, 3.47 and 9.21 more likely to have CdB levels above 0.6 µg/L. Being exposed to cigarette smoke increases the likelihood of having CdB levels above 1.0 µg/L by four times.

Table 6. Determinants of CdB level above reference values based on χ^2 and MLR.

	CdS< 0.6 µg/L n (%)	CdS ≥ 0.6 µg/L n (%)	OR (95% CI)	p-Value
Passive smoking				
No	54 (58.7)	38 (41.3)	Ref.	
Yes	12 (40.0)	18 (60.0)	2.95 (0.98–8.85)	0.054
SES				
C/B/A	35 (60.3)	23 (39.7)	Ref.	
D/E	31 (49.2)	32 (50.8)	0.69 (0.23–2.05)	0.501
Waste burning				
No	54 (59.3)	37 (40.7)	Ref.	
Yes	13 (39.4)	20 (60.6)	3.47 (1.09–11.05)	0.035
House renovation				
No	59 (57.3)	44 (42.7)	Ref.	
Yes	5 (29.4)	12 (70.6)	9.21 (1.90–44.57)	0.006
	CdS < 1.0 µg/L n (%)	CdS ≥ 1.0 µg/L n (%)		
Passive smoking				
No	76 (82.6)	16 (17.4)	Ref.	
Yes	19 (63.3)	11 (36.7)	4.01 (1.24–13.038)	0.021
House renovation				
No	83 (80.6)	20 (19.4)	Ref.	
Yes	9 (52.9)	8 (47.1)	7.02 (1.78–27.37)	0.005

Adjusted for BMI, municipality, age, gestational age, education.

4. Discussion

In this exploratory study, we investigated the exposure to Pb, Cd, As, and Mn in biological samples (blood, hair, and toenails) of 163 pregnant women residing in two municipalities in the Recôncavo Baiano, Brazil. The exposure level to As was very low, with 98% of the participants having AsH below the method's LOD. However, 4.3 and 5.1% of the participants had biomarkers above the recommended reference values for Mn and Pb. We found a worrying situation regarding exposure to Cd, given that 22.2 to 61.1% of the pregnant women had high levels depending on the reference value considered. This work demonstrates the importance and urgency of implementing, as in developed countries, biomonitoring strategies in the general population, especially in those of vulnerable groups such as pregnant women and children living in impoverished regions. The low SES, domestic waste burning, passive smoking, being multiparous, and having renovated the house were some of the determinant factors of the high levels of Mn, Pb, and Cd in this population.

4.1. Lead

Considering the environmental sample, the median RtPb (13.0 µg/m^2/30 days) was much lower than the reference (431 µg/m^2) suggested by the US Agency for Environmental Protection [43]. As our methodology considered the duration (30 days) of dust deposition, we estimated for the period of gestation the range of exposure of our study population, using the minimum and maximum range found (0.57 to 89.9 µg/m^2/30 days). The results (5.13 to 802.71 µg/m^2 for nine months) showed a probable situation of risk for these pregnant women.

Compared with another study carried out with school-age children in the municipality of Aratuípe, in a community producing Pb glazed ceramics (Maragogipinho district, Bahia, Brazil) [19], the median level observed was lower than that found in the exposed (169 µg/m^2/30 days) or control (56.7 µg/m^2/30 days) group. In the case of other published works that used a methodology similar to this study, our average RtPb was identical to that found in homes (17 µg/m^2/30 days) in Germany [44] or daycare centers in Sydney, Australia (22 µg/m^2/30 days) [45]. This finding also corroborates with some of the reported geometric means of RtPb (between 19 and 63 µg/m^2/30 days) in elementary schools in Simões Filho, Bahia, Brazil [5].

PbB levels have been associated significantly with RtPb, as observed in several studies [19,45,46], showing evidence of the contribution of this matrix to human exposure. Although we found no correlation between RtPb and PbB, this possibility should be considered, as demonstrated by Ohtsu et al. [47].

The median (range) 0.95 (0.05–16.4) µg/dL of PbB was lower than the CDC recent reference value (3.5 µg/dL) [40,48]. Nonetheless, some participants presented a risky situation for themselves and their fetus, such as the participants with PbB levels above the reference value [40,42]. Also, considering only the limited number of pregnant women ($n = 9$) in the Maragogipinho district included in this research, the situation seems more worrying, since the median and mean PbB (3.07 and 1.9 µg/dL, respectively) were twofold higher than those found in the whole study population. It is essential to point out that these limits were not indicated as levels below which there are no toxic effects for humans, the pregnant woman, and the fetus [15,40,49].

In other studies, reporting exposure to low levels of Pb, the median found here was lower than the findings by Silver et al. [50], by La-Llave-León et al. [51], and Guy et al., [52] with a median (interquartile range) of 3.74 µg/dL (3.05–5.20). Despite the low level of PbB found by Guy et al. [52] in Benin, contrary to our investigation, almost half of the participants had PbB above the new CDC reference value. Few studies with pregnant women have reported levels lower than or similar to ours, such as Ohtsu et al. [47] in Japan, Wang et al. [53] and Perkins et al., ([54], in the USA). Despite this low level of PbB, Perkins et al. [54] reported the adverse effects of Pb on anthropometric outcomes in children born to pregnant women in their cohort. Some research has shown the negative CNS impacts of prenatal exposure to low levels of Pb in children. For example, Silver et al. [50] demonstrated an association of low levels of PbB with delayed maturation of the auditory and visual systems in neonates (with an average of two days of age), while Jedrychowski et al. [55] reported their association with low neurocognitive performance in a six-month-old baby.

Despite sufficient evidence in the literature on the relationship between socioeconomic factors and Pb exposure, only multiparity was associated with PbB levels above the median. The lack of relationship with other factors was also reported in other studies; for example, Ohtsu et al. [47] Taylor et al. [15] and Guy et al. [52] also found no association between PbB levels with factors such as exposure to cigarette smoking, SES, and the presence of peeling paint in the house. The low level of exposure, in addition to the absence of a specific exposure source, except for residents in Maragogipinho, maybe the reason, as reported by Taylor et al. [15].

Although only a significant influence of multiparity on PbB levels was detected, it is relevant to highlight the possible influences of some socioeconomic and environmental covariates. Passive smoking had a median PbB 1.28 times higher (1.02 vs. 0.80 µg/dL; $p = 0.786$) compared to those not exposed to cigarette smoke. Pregnant women from lower SES or education levels had higher medians when compared to another category of the same variable considered. In addition, considering only homes with peeling paint ($n = 67$), pregnant women who reported having a lot or moderate amount of peeling paint in their home had a median PbB (1.35 vs. 0.73 µg/dL; $p = 0.24$) 1.85 times higher than those with a little peeled amount. Taking into account the toxicity of Pb for the pregnant woman and the fetus and the existence of evidence in the literature, we suggest considering these factors in eventual awareness sessions for participants in our cohort and decision-makers in the respective municipalities.

4.2. Manganese

Few participants presented values of the Mn biomarkers above the reference values [38,39]. Ward et al. [39], suggested 4.14 µg/g as a cutoff point to distinguish welders exposed to Mn fumes from the control group of their study. Therefore, it is essential to consider that the reference values for these Mn biomarkers are also not related to the threshold compatible with the beneficial or deleterious effects of Mn. For the time being, there is little data on these matrices used as biomarkers either in the general population or in pregnant women [2,56,57]. Studies in populations with low levels are therefore essential to contribute to the correct definition of these reference values concerning possible effects; our cohort study has the final objective of estimating the impact of these exposures on children's neurodevelopment at 12 months.

Considering studies carried out with pregnant women, Mora et al. [58], found a geometric mean of 1.8 µg/g in pregnant women's hair in Costa Rica, while Rodrigues et al. [36], reported medians of 27.1 and 34.7 µg/g, respectively, in Pabna and Sirajdikhan (in Bangladesh). The difference is that these studies were conducted in areas close to sources of exposure (such as plantations using pesticides and drinking water from highly contaminated artesian wells), which could explain these levels above ours. Other studies carried out in children (15.2 µg/g) and in non-pregnant women (4.4 µg/g) in areas close to a ferromanganese alloy plant in Brazil also reported levels well above the ones reported here [3,4]. Even in the control group of their research, Menezes-Filho et al. [3] reported a median (1.76 µg/g) 8.8 times higher than those in this study. Regarding the evaluation of Mn in toenails, Signes-Pastor et al. [57] found in pregnant women a median (range) of 0.34 (0.17–0.72) µg/g, two times lower than that reported in this study. Our findings do not corroborate with those of Rodrigues et al. [36], probably due to the high levels of exposure.

Three factors associated with higher levels of Mn mainly stood out in the MLR: SES, waste burning, and passive exposure to cigarette smoke. However, most publications were carried out in populations with high exposure and mainly considered correlations or univariate analyzes [56], which makes comparisons difficult. Despite using hair and nails as matrices to estimate exposure to Mn, Viana et al. [4], found no correlation between Mn exposure and cigarette smoking or waste burning. Although Tasker et al. [10] used blood as a matrix in their investigation, the authors reported a relationship between second hand cigarette smoking and blood Mn levels (MnB) in the second trimester. Still, their finding was contrary to ours (lower levels of MnB in smokers). Contrary to our findings, Viana et al. [4] reported significantly higher median levels of MnH in individuals with less education.

Co-exposure to Pb and Mn: Of the metals evaluated, only Pb and Mn (PbB and MnTn) showed a correlation in their exposure dynamics. As the matrices (toenails and blood) do not suggest exposure simultaneously (7 to 12 months and 1-month window for toenails and blood [4,57], respectively), we suggest that this relationship is spurious and not related to any biological mechanism absorption of these metals.

4.3. Cadmium

CdB level is a biomarker of recent exposure to Cd, in addition to being a good proxy for chronic exposure to low levels; that is, even in a population not occupationally exposed, it is possible to find worrying levels [59,60]. The CdB values found in our study population point to a situation contrary to our expectations.

Mean and median values in this study exceeded CdB levels in workers and populations living close to areas with a source of exposure. Ferron et al. [6] reported in recycling sorting workers from São Paulo an arithmetic mean (0.47 µg/L) and median (0.44 µg/L) lower than our values (respectively, 0.81 and 0.55 µg/L). The control group of this study presented an average value 6.7 times lower than ours. Also worrying was the maximum value (7.61 µg/L), which is well above what was found by Ferron et al. [6] (2020) and Naka et al., [61]. In non-pregnant women residing in the industrial zone of the state of Amazonas [61], the authors also found a similar average (0.46 µg/L) while the control group presented a value (0.22 µg/L) 2.5 times lower.

Some studies conducted with general populations outside Brazil reported similar situations to ours. For example, Garner and Levallois [35] in Canada reported a geometric mean of 0.43 µg/L in non-pregnant women, similar to Sakellari et al. [62] in Greece and

Johntson et al. [60] from the USA. According to the authors [35,60], cigarette smoking may be the leading cause of the higher level of Cd. Indeed, as expected, passive exposure to cigarette smoke was significantly associated with a fourfold higher chance of having levels above 1 µg/L. Active smoking before pregnancy did not show a significant relationship with high levels of CdB, given the small number of observations. Passive cigarette smoking exposure is a relevant source of contamination of a multitude of compounds, which raises the importance of the shared responsibility of all residents in a home for the health of the pregnant woman and her fetus. Besides the pregnant woman stopping smoking, the other house residents would have to do the same or avoiding smoking indoors. Active or passive smoking status was self-reported by participants; the fact of not having evaluated cotinine, a biomarker of exposure to nicotine [60] may be a limitation of our study. Nevertheless, pregnancy is often a reason that leads many women to stop smoking or reduce their habit.

House renovation (or painting) was another determining factor that increased the likelihood of having CdB levels above 1 or 0.6 µg/L. We suggest that the type of paint used during the renovation could explain this finding. In fact, during our visits to the participants' homes, we noticed the reforms or changes in the residences to adjust for the arrival of the baby. Some works have shown the possibility of finding high levels of cadmium and other metals in paint pigments or building and renovation materials [63,64]. Other possible sources of exposure to Cd could be living close to or inside workshops or production units of palm oil, soap (some participants), or even a diet rich in shellfish or animal viscera. We have visited pregnant women whose homes were located in these environments. Regarding diet, data on food frequency is being processed.

None of the sociodemographic variables (SES, age, education, income, municipality) and the fact of not being primiparous were not associated with an increase in CdB above the reference values. Contrary to what was expected with alcohol consumption [35,60,65], no association was detected, probably because pregnant women stopped drinking when they were aware of their pregnancy.

4.4. Strengths and Limitations

As a cross-sectional study design, this work carries some limitations of this type of design, such as recall and nonresponse biases. For example, some biological samples were collected from only some participants; some refused to collect certain biological samples (blood or hair), while others were unavailable during the second semester. That may explain why there was no association in some statistical analyses. Despite the study design, our research was able to evaluate the current and chronic exposure to Mn as we evaluated its level in hair and toenails. Also, this work is one of the few carried out in developing countries with vulnerable populations; it adds evidence to sustain the urgency of implementing biomonitoring and vigilance of PTM exposure in Brazil.

5. Conclusions

Despite the low levels of exposure in general, this study showed worrying Cd exposure levels of most participants and reported the main risk factors of exposure to the PTM studied. Considering the evidence of the deleterious effects of low PTM levels on fetal development and the health of pregnant women, it is useful to investigate further. As a scientific community, there is a need to adopt a stronger position for implementing a biomonitoring policy in vulnerable populations.

Author Contributions: Conceptualization, H.A.F.B. and J.A.M.-F.; methodology and laboratory analysis, H.A.F.B., N.R.d.S., E.M.P., J.V.A.S. and F.d.S.C.; fieldwork, H.A.F.B., N.R.d.S., E.A.G.J., V.O.M., D.O.C., E.M.P., J.V.A.S. and F.d.S.C.; software, H.A.F.B. and J.A.M.-F.; validation, H.A.F.B.; formal analysis, H.A.F.B.; resources, E.M.P., J.V.A.S., F.d.S.C. and D.O.C.; data curation, H.A.F.B., E.A.G.J., V.O.M., D.O.C. and N.R.d.S.; writing—original draft preparation, H.A.F.B.; writing—review and editing, J.A.M.-F.; supervision, H.A.F.B., N.R.d.S., E.A.G.J., V.O.M. and D.O.C.; project administration, J.A.M.-F.; funding acquisition, J.A.M.-F., H.A.F.B., N.R.d.S., E.A.G.J., V.O.M. and D.O.C. All authors have read and agreed to the published version of the manuscript.

Funding: This study was supported by grants from the Fundação de Amparo à Pesquisa do Estado da Bahia (FAPESB-PPSUS Edital n° 2/2020, pedido n° 4393/2020) and the Conselho Nacional de Desenvolvimento Científico e Tecnológico (CNPq Universal Processo No. 421550/2018-0). H.A.F.B., J.V.A.S., and F.d.S.C. are recipients of scholarships from CNPq; N.R.d.S., V.O.M., and E.M.P. are recipient of scholarships from FAPESB; E.A.G.J is a recipient of a scholarship from Coordenação de Aperfeiçoamento de Pessoal de Nível Superior (CAPES).

Institutional Review Board Statement: This project was approved by the research ethics committee of the Faculty of Pharmacy-UFBA through Resolution 466-CNS/2012, with opinion No. 3246555 (approved on 4 May 2019).

Informed Consent Statement: Informed consent was obtained from all subjects involved in the study. Written informed consent has been obtained from the patient(s) to publish this paper.

Data Availability Statement: Not applicable.

Acknowledgments: The authors would like to thank to the volunteers (and their families) who agreed to participate in the study and acknowledge the support of the Health Secretariat of Aratuipe and Nazaré das Farinhas, including all health agents.

Conflicts of Interest: The authors declare no conflict of interest.

References

1. Tchounwou, P.B.; Yedjou, C.G.; Patlolla, A.K.; Sutton, D.J. Heavy metal toxicity and the environment. *Mol. Clin. Environ. Toxicol. Vol. 3 Environ. Toxicol.* **2012**, *101*, 133–164. [CrossRef] [PubMed]
2. Mergler, D. Neurotoxic exposures and effects: Gender and sex matter! Hänninen Lecture 2011. *Neurotoxicology* **2012**, *33*, 644–651. [CrossRef] [PubMed]
3. Menezes-Filho, J.A.; Paes, C.R.; Pontes, M.D.C.; Moreira, J.C.; Sarcinelli, P.N.; Mergler, D. High levels of hair manganese in children living in the vicinity of a ferro-manganese alloy production plant. *Neurotoxicology* **2009**, *30*, 1207–1213. [CrossRef] [PubMed]
4. Viana, G.F.D.S.; de Carvalho, C.F.; Nunes, L.S.; Rodrigues, J.L.; Ribeiro, N.S.; de Almeida, D.A.; Ferreira, J.R.D.; Abreu, N.; Menezes-Filho, J.A. Noninvasive biomarkers of manganese exposure and neuropsychological effects in environmentally exposed adults in Brazil. *Toxicol. Lett.* **2014**, *231*, 169–178. [CrossRef] [PubMed]
5. Rodrigues, J.L.; Bandeira, M.J.; Araújo, C.F.; dos Santos, N.R.; Anjos, A.L.S.; Koin, N.L.; Pereira, L.C.; Oliveira, S.S.; Mergler, D.; Menezes-Filho, J.A. Manganese and lead levels in settled dust in elementary schools are correlated with biomarkers of exposure in school-aged children. *Environ. Pollut.* **2018**, *236*, 1004–1013. [CrossRef]
6. Ferron, M.M.; Kuno, R.; De Campos, A.E.M.; De Castro, F.J.V.; Gouveia, N. Cadmium, lead and mercury in the blood of workers from recycling sorting facilities in São Paulo, Brazil. *Cad. Saude Publica* **2020**, *36*, e00072119. [CrossRef]
7. Heng, Y.Y.; Asad, I.; Coleman, B.; Menard, L.; Benki-Nugent, S.; Were, F.H.; Karr, C.J.; McHenry, M.S. Heavy metals and neurodevelopment of children in low and middle-income countries: A systematic review. *PLoS ONE* **2022**, *17*, e0265536. [CrossRef]
8. Betts, K.S. CDC Updates Guidelines for Children's Lead Exposure. *Environ. Health Perspect.* **2012**, *120*, a268. [CrossRef]
9. Aschner, M.; Guilarte, T.R.; Schneider, J.S.; Zheng, W. Manganese: Recent advances in understanding its transport and neurotoxicity. *Toxicol. Appl. Pharmacol.* **2007**, *221*, 131–147. [CrossRef]
10. Takser, L.; Lafond, J.; Bouchard, M.; St-Amour, G.; Mergler, D. Manganese levels during pregnancy and at birth: Relation to environmental factors and smoking in a Southwest Quebec population. *Environ. Res.* **2004**, *95*, 119–125. [CrossRef]
11. Dórea, J.G. Environmental exposure to low-level lead (Pb) co-occurring with other neurotoxicants in early life and neurodevelopment of children. *Environ. Res.* **2019**, *177*, 108641. [CrossRef]
12. Johnson, S.B.; Riis, J.L.; Noble, K. State of the Art Review: Poverty and the Developing Brain. *Pediatrics* **2016**, *137*, e20153075. [CrossRef]
13. Wang, B.; Liu, J.; Liu, B.; Liu, X.; Yu, X. Prenatal exposure to arsenic and neurobehavioral development of newborns in China. *Environ. Int.* **2018**, *121 Pt 1*, 421–427. [CrossRef]

14. Laine, J.; Ray, P.; Bodnar, W.; Cable, P.H.; Boggess, K.; Offenbacher, S.; Fry, R.C. Placental Cadmium Levels Are Associated with Increased Preeclampsia Risk. *PLoS ONE* **2015**, *10*, e0139341. [CrossRef]
15. Taylor, C.M.; Golding, J.; Hibbeln, J.; Emond, A.M. Environmental Factors Predicting Blood Lead Levels in Pregnant Women in the UK: The ALSPAC Study. *PLoS ONE* **2013**, *8*, e72371. [CrossRef]
16. Menezes-Filho, J.A.; Carvalho, C.F.; Rodrigues, J.L.G.; Araújo, C.F.S.; Dos Santos, N.R.; Lima, C.S.; Bandeira, M.J.; Marques, B.L.D.S.; Anjos, A.L.S.; Bah, H.A.F.; et al. Environmental Co-Exposure to Lead and Manganese and Intellectual Deficit in School-Aged Children. *Int. J. Environ. Res. Public Health* **2018**, *15*, 2418. [CrossRef]
17. Freire, C.; Amaya, E.; Gil, F.; Fernández, M.F.; Murcia, M.; Llop, S.; Andiarena, A.; Aurrekoetxea, J.; Bustamante, M.; Guxens, M.; et al. Prenatal co-exposure to neurotoxic metals and neurodevelopment in preschool children: The Environment and Childhood (INMA) Project. *Sci. Total. Environ.* **2018**, *621*, 340–351. [CrossRef]
18. Henn, B.C.; Coull, B.A.; Wright, R. Chemical mixtures and children's health. *Curr. Opin. Pediatr.* **2014**, *26*, 223–229. [CrossRef]
19. Bah, H.A.F.; Bandeira, M.J.; Gomes-Junior, E.A.; Anjos, A.L.S.; Rodrigues, Y.J.M.; Dos Santos, N.R.; Martinez, V.O.; Rocha, R.B.M.A.; Costa, R.G.; Adorno, E.V.; et al. Environmental exposure to lead and hematological parameters in Afro-Brazilian children living near artisanal glazed pottery workshops. *J. Environ. Sci. Health Part A* **2020**, *55*, 964–974. [CrossRef]
20. Tamayo, Y.; Ortiz, M.; Téllez-Rojo, M.M.; Trejo-Valdivia, B.; Schnaas, L.; Osorio-Valencia, E.; Coull, B.; Bellinger, D.; Wright, R.J.; Wright, R.O. Maternal stress modifies the effect of exposure to lead during pregnancy and 24-months old children's neurodevelopment. *Environ. Int.* **2017**, *98*, 191–197. [CrossRef]
21. Kort, S.A.R.; Wickliffe, J.; Shankar, A.; Shafer, M.; Hindori-Mohangoo, A.D.; Covert, H.H.; Lichtveld, M.; Zijlmans, W. The Association between Mercury and Lead Exposure and Liver and Kidney Function in Pregnant Surinamese Women Enrolled in the Caribbean Consortium for Research in Environmental and Occupational Health (CCREOH) Environmental Epidemiologic Cohort Study. *Toxics* **2022**, *10*, 584. [CrossRef] [PubMed]
22. Liu, W.; Xin, Y.; Li, Q.; Shang, Y.; Ping, Z.; Min, J.; Cahill, C.M.; Rogers, J.T.; Wang, F. Biomarkers of environmental manganese exposure and associations with childhood neurodevelopment: A systematic review and meta-analysis. *Environ. Health* **2020**, *19*, 104. [CrossRef] [PubMed]
23. Leonhard, M.J.; Chang, E.T.; Loccisano, A.E.; Garry, M.R. A systematic literature review of epidemiologic studies of developmental manganese exposure and neurodevelopmental outcomes. *Toxicology* **2019**, *420*, 46–65. [CrossRef]
24. Martinez, V.O.; Nunes, L.S.; Viana, G.S.; dos Santos, N.R.; Menezes-Filho, J.A. Biomarkers of cadmium exposure and renal function in estuarine adult villagers. *Int. Arch. Occup. Environ. Health* **2022**, *95*, 981–992. [CrossRef] [PubMed]
25. Sistema de Informações de Nascidos Vivos—(SINASC). Nascimentos por residência da mãe dos Municípios de Nazaré das Farinhas e Aratuípe e Ano do nascimento. DATASUS MS/SVS/DASIS. 2018.
26. Martinez, V.O.; Lima, F.W.D.M.; Rocha, R.B.A.; Bah, H.A.F.; Carvalho, C.F.; Menezes-Filho, J.A. Interaction of Toxoplasma gondii infection and elevated blood lead levels on children's neurobehavior. *Neurotoxicology* **2020**, *78*, 177–185. [CrossRef] [PubMed]
27. Associação Brasileira de Empresas de Pesquisa (ABEP). Critério de Classificação Econômica Brasil. 2018, pp. 1–3. Available online: https://www.abep.org/criterio-brasil (accessed on 4 February 2023).
28. Menezes-Filho, J.A.; de Souza, K.O.F.; Rodrigues, J.L.G.; dos Santos, N.R.; Bandeira, M.D.J.; Koin, N.L.; Oliveira, S.S.D.P.; Godoy, A.L.P.C.; Mergler, D. Manganese and lead in dust fall accumulation in elementary schools near a ferromanganese alloy plant. *Environ. Res.* **2016**, *148*, 322–329. [CrossRef]
29. Menezes-Filho, J.A.; Viana, G.F.D.S.; Paes, C.R. Determinants of lead exposure in children on the outskirts of Salvador, Brazil. *Environ. Monit. Assess.* **2012**, *184*, 2593–2603. [CrossRef]
30. Kummrow, F.; Silva, F.F.; Kuno, R.; Souza, A.L.; Oliveira, P.V. Biomonitoring method for the simultaneous determination of cadmium and lead in whole blood by electrothermal atomic absorption spectrometry for assessment of environmental exposure. *Talanta* **2008**, *75*, 246–252. [CrossRef]
31. Dos Santos, N.R.; Rodrigues, J.L.; Bandeira, M.J.; Anjos, A.L.D.S.; Araújo, C.D.F.S.; Adan, L.F.; Menezes-Filho, J.A. Manganese exposure and association with hormone imbalance in children living near a ferro-manganese alloy plant. *Environ. Res.* **2019**, *172*, 166–174. [CrossRef]
32. Kira, C.S.; Sakuma, A.M.; De Capitani, E.M.; de Freitas, C.U.; Cardoso, M.R.A.; Gouveia, N. Associated factors for higher lead and cadmium blood levels, and reference values derived from general population of São Paulo, Brazil. *Sci. Total Environ.* **2016**, *543 Pt A*, 628–635. [CrossRef]
33. Kuno, R.; Roquetti, M.H.; Becker, K.; Seiwert, M.; Gouveia, N. Reference values for lead, cadmium and mercury in the blood of adults from the metropolitan area of Sao Paulo, Brazil. *Int. J. Hyg. Environ. Health* **2013**, *216*, 243–249. [CrossRef]
34. Schulz, C.; Wilhelm, M.; Heudorf, U.; Kolossa-Gehring, M. Human Biomonitoring Commission of the German Federal Environment Agency. Update of the reference and HBM values derived by the German Human Biomonitoring Commission. *Int. J. Hyg. Environ. Health* **2011**, *215*, 26–35. [CrossRef]
35. Garner, R.; Levallois, P. Cadmium levels and sources of exposure among Canadian adults. *Health Rep.* **2016**, *27*, 10–18.
36. Rodrigues, E.G.; Kile, M.L.; Dobson, C.; Amarasiriwardena, C.J.; Quamruzzaman, Q.; Rahman, M.; Golam, M.; Christiani, D.C. Maternal-infant biomarkers of prenatal exposure to arsenic and manganese. *J. Expo. Sci. Environ. Epidemiol.* **2015**, *25*, 639–648. [CrossRef]
37. Agency for Toxic Substances and Disease Registry (ATSDR). *Toxicological Profile for Arsenic (Update)*; U.S. Department of Health and Human Services, Public Health Service: Atlanta, GA, USA, 2007.

38. Miekeley, N.; Carneiro, M.T.D.; Portodasilveira, C. How reliable are human hair reference intervals for trace elements? *Sci. Total Environ.* **1998**, *218*, 9–17. [CrossRef]
39. Ward, E.J.; Edmondson, D.; Nour, M.M.; Snyder, S.; Rosenthal, F.S.; Dydak, U. Toenail Manganese: A Sensitive and Specific Biomarker of Exposure to Manganese in Career Welders. *Ann. Work Expo. Health* **2017**, *62*, 101–111. [CrossRef]
40. Ruckart, P.Z.; Jones, R.L.; Courtney, J.G.; LeBlanc, T.T.; Jackson, W.; Karwowski, M.P.; Cheng, P.-Y.; Allwood, P.; Svendsen, E.R.; Breysse, P.N. Update of the Blood Lead Reference Value—United States, 2021. *MMWR. Morb. Mortal. Wkly. Rep.* **2021**, *70*, 1509–1512. [CrossRef]
41. Agency for Toxic Substances and Disease Registry (ATSDR). *Toxicological Profile for Cadmium*; U.S. Department of Health and Human Services, Public Health Service: Atlanta, GA, USA, 2012.
42. Gilbert, S.G.; Weiss, B. A rationale for lowering the blood lead action level from 10 to 2 µg/dL. *Neurotoxicology* **2006**, *27*, 693–701. [CrossRef]
43. US EPA. 40 Cfr Part 745. Lead; Identification of Dangerous Levels of Lead, 2001. Available online: http://www.gpo.gov/fdsys/pkg/FR-2001-01-05/pdf/01-84.pdf (accessed on 29 December 2022).
44. Meyer, I.; Heinrich, J.; Lippold, U. Factors Affecting Lead, Cadmium, and Arsenic Levels in House Dust in a Smelter Town in Eastern Germany. *Environ. Res.* **1999**, *81*, 32–44. [CrossRef]
45. Gulson, B.; Mizon, K.; Taylor, A.; Korsch, M.; Stauber, J.; Davis, J.M.; Louie, H.; Wu, M.; Swan, H. Changes in manganese and lead in the environment and young children associated with the introduction of methylcyclopentadienyl manganese tricarbonyl in gasoline—Preliminary results. *Environ. Res.* **2006**, *100*, 100–114. [CrossRef]
46. Gulson, B.; Mizon, K.; Taylor, A.; Korsch, M.; Davis, J.M.; Louie, H.; Wu, M.; Gomez, L.; Antin, L. Pathways of Pb and Mn observed in a 5-year longitudinal investigation in young children and environmental measures from an urban setting. *Environ. Pollut.* **2014**, *191*, 38–49. [CrossRef] [PubMed]
47. Ohtsu, M.; Mise, N.; Ikegami, A.; Mizuno, A.; Kobayashi, Y.; Nakagi, Y.; Nohara, K.; Yoshida, T.; Kayama, F. Oral exposure to lead for Japanese children and pregnant women, estimated using duplicate food portions and house dust analyses. *Environ. Health Prev. Med.* **2019**, *24*, 72. [CrossRef] [PubMed]
48. Ettinger, A.S.; Wengrovitz, A.M. Guidelines for the Identification and Management of Lead Exposure in Pregnant and Lactating Women. 2010. Available online: https://www.cdc.gov/nceh/lead/docs/publications/leadandpregnancy2010.pdf (accessed on 29 December 2022).
49. Taylor, C.M.; Kordas, K.; Golding, J.; Emond, A.M. Effects of low-level prenatal lead exposure on child IQ at 4 and 8 years in a UK birth cohort study. *Neurotoxicology* **2017**, *62*, 162–169. [CrossRef] [PubMed]
50. Silver, M.K.; Li, X.; Liu, Y.; Li, M.; Mai, X.; Kaciroti, N.; Kileny, P.; Tardif, T.; Meeker, J.D.; Lozoff, B. Low-level prenatal lead exposure and infant sensory function. *Environ. Health* **2016**, *15*, 65. [CrossRef] [PubMed]
51. La-Llave-León, O.; Méndez-Hernández, E.M.; Castellanos-Juárez, F.X.; Esquivel-Rodríguez, E.; Vázquez-Alaniz, F.; Sandoval-Carrillo, A.; García-Vargas, G.; Duarte-Sustaita, J.; Candelas-Rangel, J.L.; Salas-Pacheco, J.M. Association between Blood Lead Levels and Delta-Aminolevulinic Acid Dehydratase in Pregnant Women. *Int. J. Environ. Res. Public Health* **2017**, *14*, 432. [CrossRef]
52. Guy, M.; Accrombessi, M.; Fievet, N.; Yovo, E.; Massougbodji, A.; Le Bot, B.; Glorennec, P.; Bodeau-Livinec, F.; Briand, V. Toxics (Pb, Cd) and trace elements (Zn, Cu, Mn) in women during pregnancy and at delivery, South Benin, 2014–2015. *Environ. Res.* **2018**, *167*, 198–206. [CrossRef]
53. Wang, J.; Yang, Y.; Zhang, J.; Liu, N.; Xi, H.; Liang, H. Trends of Blood Lead Levels in US Pregnant Women: The National Health and Nutrition Examination Survey (2001–2018). *Front. Public Health* **2022**, *10*, 922563. [CrossRef]
54. Perkins, M.; Wright, R.O.; Amarasiriwardena, C.J.; Jayawardene, I.; Rifas-Shiman, S.L.; Oken, E. Very low maternal lead level in pregnancy and birth outcomes in an eastern Massachusetts population. *Ann. Epidemiology* **2014**, *24*, 915–919. [CrossRef]
55. Jedrychowski, W.; Perera, F.; Jankowski, J.; Rauh, V.; Flak, E.; Caldwell, K.L.; Jones, R.L.; Pac, A.; Lisowska-Miszczyk, I. Prenatal low-level lead exposure and developmental delay of infants at age 6 months (Krakow inner city study). *Int. J. Hyg. Environ. Health* **2008**, *211*, 345–351. [CrossRef]
56. Shilnikova, N.; Karyakina, N.; Farhat, N.; Ramoju, S.; Cline, B.; Momoli, F.; Mattison, D.; Jensen, N.; Terrell, R.; Krewski, D. Biomarkers of environmental manganese exposure. *Crit. Rev. Toxicol.* **2022**, *52*, 325–343. [CrossRef]
57. Signes-Pastor, A.J.; Bouchard, M.F.; Baker, E.; Jackson, B.P.; Karagas, M.R. Toenail manganese as biomarker of drinking water exposure: A reliability study from a US pregnancy cohort. *J. Expo. Sci. Environ. Epidemiol.* **2019**, *29*, 648–654. [CrossRef]
58. Mora, A.M.; Joode, B.V.W.D.; Mergler, D.; Córdoba, L.; Cano, C.; Quesada, R.; Smith, D.R.; Menezes-Filho, J.A.; Eskenazi, B. Maternal blood and hair manganese concentrations, fetal growth, and length of gestation in the ISA cohort in Costa Rica. *Environ. Res.* **2015**, *136*, 47–56. [CrossRef]
59. Kantola, M.; Purkunen, R.; Kröger, P.; Tooming, A.; Juravskaja, J.; Pasanen, M.; Saarikoski, S.; Vartiainen, T. Accumulation of Cadmium, Zinc, and Copper in Maternal Blood and Developmental Placental Tissue: Differences between Finland, Estonia, and St. Petersburg. *Environ. Res.* **2000**, *83*, 54–66. [CrossRef]
60. Johnston, J.E.; Valentiner, E.; Maxson, P.; Miranda, M.L.; Fry, R.C. Maternal Cadmium Levels during Pregnancy Associated with Lower Birth Weight in Infants in a North Carolina Cohort. *PLoS ONE* **2014**, *9*, e109661. [CrossRef]
61. Naka, K.S.; Mendes, L.D.C.D.S.; de Queiroz, T.K.L.; Costa, B.N.S.; de Jesus, I.M.; Câmara, V.D.M.; Lima, M.D.O. A comparative study of cadmium levels in blood from exposed populations in an industrial area of the Amazon, Brazil. *Sci. Total Environ.* **2019**, *698*, 134309. [CrossRef]

62. Sakellari, A.; Karavoltsos, S.; Kalogeropoulos, N.; Theodorou, D.; Dedoussis, G.; Chrysohoou, C.; Dassenakis, M.; Scoullos, M. Predictors of cadmium and lead concentrations in the blood of residents from the metropolitan area of Athens (Greece). *Sci. Total Environ.* **2016**, *568*, 263–270. [CrossRef]
63. Ogilo, J.K.; Onditi, A.O.; Salim, A.M.; Yusuf, A.O. Assessment of Levels of Heavy Metals in Paints from Interior Walls and Indoor Dust from Residential Houses in Nairobi City County, Kenya. *Chem. Sci. Int. J.* **2017**, *21*, 1–7. [CrossRef]
64. Apanpa-Qasim, A.F.I.; Adeyi, A.A.; Mudliar, S.N.; Raghunathan, K.; Thawale, P. Examination of Lead and Cadmium in Water-based Paints Marketed in Nigeria. *J. Health Pollut.* **2016**, *6*, 43–49. [CrossRef]
65. Martins, A.C.; Urbano, M.R.; Lopes, A.C.B.A.; Carvalho, M.D.F.H.; Buzzo, M.L.; Docea, A.O.; Mesas, A.E.; Aschner, M.; Silva, A.M.R.; Silbergeld, E.K.; et al. Blood cadmium levels and sources of exposure in an adult urban population in southern Brazil. *Environ. Res.* **2020**, *187*, 109618. [CrossRef]

Disclaimer/Publisher's Note: The statements, opinions and data contained in all publications are solely those of the individual author(s) and contributor(s) and not of MDPI and/or the editor(s). MDPI and/or the editor(s) disclaim responsibility for any injury to people or property resulting from any ideas, methods, instructions or products referred to in the content.

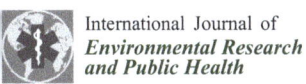

Article

Vocational Rehabilitation and Length of Stay at Work after Work-Related Musculoskeletal Disorders: A Longitudinal Study in Brazil

Cristiano Barreto de Miranda [1,*], João Silvestre Silva-Junior [2], Klauss Kleydmann Sabino Garcia [3], Flávia Nogueira e Ferreira de Sousa [3] and Frida Marina Fischer [1]

1. Department of Environmental Health and Graduate Program in Public Health, School of Public Health, University of São Paulo (FSP-USP), São Paulo 01246-904, Brazil
2. Department of Forensic Medicine, Bioethics, Occupational Medicine and Physical Medicine and Rehabilitation, University of São Palo Medicine School (FMUSP), São Paulo 01246-903, Brazil
3. General Coordinator of Occupational Health, Ministry of Health, Graduate Program in Tropical Medicine, University of Brasília (UnB), Brasília 70910-900, Brazil
* Correspondence: cristianobm@alumni.usp.br

Abstract: Vocational rehabilitation is an intervention to enhance the return to work and improve quality of life. The aim of this study was to evaluate sociodemographic and occupational factors associated with the length of stay at work among workers with work-related musculoskeletal disorders (WRMDs) who had undergone rehabilitation through the Brazilian public social security system. This was a longitudinal study among 680 workers with histories of disability due to WRMDs who returned to the formal job market after vocational rehabilitation between 2014 and 2018. Survival analysis was performed to identify the factors influencing permanence in work. Job dismissal occurred for 29.26% of the workers. The average duration of employment after returning to the formal job position was 56 months. The following factors were associated with shorter length of employment: living in the southeastern region (HR: 2.78; 95% CI 1.12–6.91) or southern region (HR: 2.68; 95% CI 1.04–6.90) of Brazil; working in transportation, storage or postal services (HR: 2.57; 95% CI 1.07–6.17); or working in financial activities, insurance or related services (HR: 2.70; 95% CI 1.05–6.89). These findings may contribute to the discussion about prevention of disability and interventions to ensure health care for workers with WRMD disabilities who undergo rehabilitation.

Keywords: vocational rehabilitation; return to work; work-related musculoskeletal disorders; occupational health

1. Introduction

Work-related musculoskeletal disorder (WRMD) is a term for injuries caused by repetitive tasks, intense exertion, mechanical compression, vibrations or sustained postures in occupational settings [1,2]. In addition to biomechanical risks, WRMDs are associated with organizational and psychosocial factors present in the work environment [3–5]. They are characterized by occurrences of several symptoms (which may or may not be concomitant), such as chronic pain, paresthesia, muscle discomfort and muscle fatigue, which are manifested mainly in the neck, shoulder girdle, upper limbs, lumbar spine region and knees [1,5].

WRMDs are the most significant cause of work-related illness in many countries. They negatively affect work capacity and quality of life, and are one of the main reasons for work disability [1,3]. In Brazil, data from the Information System on Notifiable Diseases (SINAN) of the Ministry of Health indicate that 104,665 cases of WRMD were reported between 2006 and 2021 [6]. It should be noted that, in Brazil, WRMDs are notifiable diseases that are monitored through a sentinel surveillance strategy, composed of healthcare units that identify, investigate and report WRMD cases.

Early diagnosis of WRMDs provides better results regarding the health of workers thus affected, especially when preventive treatment is implemented within the environment and work processes. On the other hand, non-preventive intervention and late diagnosis have been correlated with higher degrees of work disability and difficulties in returning to work [7,8].

Studies have shown that sociodemographic factors (gender, age and education) and occupational conditions (reduction in working hours and support from colleagues and bosses) can have an influence as facilitators or barriers to the effectiveness of returning to work after being away from work due to WRMDs [9–11].

When the disabling sickness evolves into a permanent condition and prevents workers from performing their usual functions, the Brazilian National Social Security Institute (INSS) may indicate placement in the vocational rehabilitation program. This public service offers educational assistance and professional adaptation (or readaptation) for insured individuals. During this rehabilitation, the disability aid is maintained until these individuals are considered to have achieved rehabilitation, such that they are able to perform an activity that ensures their subsistence. Otherwise, they are granted pensionable retirement on the grounds of permanent disability from which rehabilitation is impossible [12].

A previous study showed that the average cumulative incidence of rehabilitation was 57.4 per 1000 admissions to the Brazilian social security vocational rehabilitation program from 2007 to 2016 [13]. Although monitoring of rehabilitated workers who returned to work is recommended by social security, this practice is limited among vocational rehabilitation services, and information on rehabilitated workers reintegrated into work remains poor.

The main goal of the Brazilian vocational rehabilitation program is to enable workers with disabilities to qualify for a new work activity. Therefore, studies that investigate occupational factors such as the occupations and economic activity sectors that allow greater possibilities for reentry and permanence in work are fundamental for guiding actions that promote a sustained return to work in a highly competitive labor market. Knowledge of the occupations and economic activity sectors into which rehabilitated workers are placed while developing their work activity can help in understanding the occupational risks to which these workers are exposed. This can provide support for effective intervention strategies in the work environment that promote and protect the health of these workers.

In addition, there are few studies on returning to and remaining in work after vocational rehabilitation in Brazil. Knowledge of the factors associated with the length of stay at work after vocational rehabilitation can help identify workers who are more vulnerable to unemployment and support construction of strategies to facilitate a sustained return to work.

Therefore, the aim of this study was to evaluate sociodemographic and occupational factors associated with the length of stay at work among workers with disabilities due to WRMDs who had undergone rehabilitation through the Brazilian social security system.

2. Materials and Methods

2.1. Study Design and Population

This was a longitudinal study on workers with disabilities due to WRMDs who had undergone rehabilitation through the Brazilian Social Security system and who returned to the formal employment market between 2014 and 2018. The data referred to workers over 18 years old with an employment contract that was not time limited. Workers who had undergone rehabilitation and were holding more than one job, and workers with temporary employment were excluded from the study.

2.2. Data Sources

The 2018 Annual Social Information Report (RAIS) database, which contains retrospective information referring to previous years, was the primary data source. RAIS has nationwide coverage and provides information on formal employment relationships, with mandatory annual registration for public and private companies. RAIS is one of Brazil's main population databases for workers in the formal employment market [14]. RAIS does not provide data on diagnoses of work-related illnesses.

The Information System for Work Accident Communications (SISCAT) database records work-related accidents and illnesses notified by private companies that contribute to the degree of incidence of labor disability resulting from environmental risks at work [15]. This database was used to identify diagnoses of workers with WRMDs over the period from 2014 to 2018.

The RAIS and SISCAT databases were linked together using the method described by Garcia et al. (2022) [16]. This linkage was performed and provided by the General Coordination Office for Workers' Health of the Ministry of Health (CGSAT/MS) anonymously and without duplication, specifically for our study. Thus, we did not have access to any sensitive data on workers or companies.

Database linkage is a technique that enables correlations between different information sources in a single record [16]. A deterministic approach was used in this study: this identified pairs of completely concordant records through a standard identifier variable common to the different databases used [16]. The PIS (Social Integration Program) number was the key variable for making the linkage since it formed a unique identifier in the two databases studied.

Workers who had undergone rehabilitation through Social Security were identified by analyzing the variable "type of disability" in the RAIS database. This indicated whether a given worker currently presented a disability but was not participating in rehabilitation programs or whether this worker had completed the rehabilitation. The diagnosis of the WRMD was identified through the International Classification of Diseases version 10 (ICD-10), in chapter XIII, as codes M00 to M99 (from the SISCAT database). This information is not present in the RAIS database.

2.3. Study Variables

The dependent variable was "length of stay at work after returning", which was the total number of months that elapsed between the worker's date of admission to a job and the date of dismissal. The study period was 60 months from the date on which each rehabilitated worker returned to employment.

The following sociodemographic variables were analyzed: sex, age group, race/skin color, number of years of schooling and Brazilian macroregion of residence/work.

The following occupational variables were studied: average monthly salary range, company size, weekly working hours, occupation (classified based the Brazilian Classification of Occupations (CBO-2002)) and economic activity (classified based on the National Classification of Economic Activities (CNAE-2.0)). The CBO is the standardizing document for the recognition, naming and codification of the titles and contents of the occupations in the Brazilian labor market.

The CBO is structured in 10 major groups (one digit), 47 main subgroups (two digits), 193 subgroups (three digits), 596 occupation families (four digits) and 2666 occupations (six digits). For better data visualization, it was opted here to choose the occupation designated by the 10 major groups of the CBO. The CNAE is structured in 21 sections (one letter), 87 divisions (two digits), 286 groups (three digits), 673 classes (four digits) and 1302 subclasses (seven digits). For better data visualization, it was opted here to choose the economic activities designated by the 21 sections of the CNAE.

2.4. Statistical Analysis

A descriptive analysis on the distribution of the absolute and relative frequencies of all the variables studied was conducted. A survival analysis, in which cases of workers who were fired were considered to be "failures", was also conducted. The number of months between the date of job admission and the date of dismissal was recorded. Right censoring was undertaken the end of the follow-up, i.e., 60 months after the return to work, and in cases in which the dismissal occurred due to death or retirement.

Survival curves were constructed for the covariates using the Kaplan–Meier method [17]. To test whether the duration of employment differed between the categories of a given risk or protection factor (for example, between males and females), the log-rank test was used [18].

The Cox proportional hazards model was applied to the study variables in order to estimate the risk of dismissal from the job. Univariate analysis on each covariate was performed. In constructing the multiple model, variables in the univariate analysis that presented a significance level of $p < 0.20$ were included. The stepwise forward method was used, starting from the saturated model, until it was identified which model would explain most of the variance. The likelihood ratio of the proposed model in relation to the saturated model was used to assess the fit of the model (deviance analysis). For the final model, variables whose p-value was <0.05 were taken to be statistically significant. To evaluate the premise of the final model regarding the proportionality of risk, the Schoenfeld test was performed [19].

The hazard ratio expressed the association between the study variables and the outcome, with their respective 95% confidence intervals. A hazard ratio (HR) greater than one (HR > 1) denoted a greater risk of being dismissed from employment during the follow-up. HR < 1 denoted a lower risk of being dismissed from work during the study period [19].

2.5. Ethical Considerations

The Research Ethics Committee of the School of Public Health of the University of São Paulo (CAAE: 04267218.0.0000.5421, opinion number: 5113575) approved this study.

3. Results

Most of the 680 workers who underwent rehabilitation and then returned to the formal employment market between 2014 and 2018 were male (62.35%), had white skin color (52.79%), had up to 11 years of schooling (62.21%) and were living in the southeastern region of the country (41.18%). The workers' mean age was 44.68 years (SD = 8.30) and there was no statistical difference in the mean age between the sexes ($p = 0.459$) (Table 1).

Table 1. Sociodemographic characteristics of workers with disabilities due to WRMDs who had undergone rehabilitation through Social Security and then returned to the formal employment market. Brazil, 2014–2018 ($n = 680$).

Features	n (%)
Sex	
Male	424 (62.35)
Female	256 (37.65)
Age (in years)	
Up to 40	216 (31.76)
More than 40	464 (68.24)
Race/skin color	
White	359 (52.79)
Nonwhite	321 (47.21)
Number of years of schooling	
Up to 11	423 (62.21)
Above 11	257 (37.79)
Geographical region	
North	29 (4.26)
Northeast	188 (27.65)
Southeast	280 (41.18)
South	138 (20.29)
Center-west	45 (6.62)

Source: RAIS, 2018; SISCAT, 2016–2018.

Most of the rehabilitated workers (46.47%) had an average monthly remuneration in the range of 2.01 to 4 times the minimum wage (USD 400–800), were employed in a large company (44.41%) and worked for more than 40 h per week (80.29%). The most frequently observed occupational group was administrative service workers (70.44%) and the most frequently observed economic activity sector was transportation, storage and postal services (52.35%) (Table 2).

Table 2. Occupational characteristics of workers with disabilities due to WRMDs who had undergone rehabilitation through Social Security and then returned to the formal employment market. Brazil, 2014–2018 (n = 680).

Features	n (%)
Average monthly remuneration (times minimum wage)	
under 2	211 (31.03)
from 2 to 4	316 (46.47)
above 4	153 (22.50)
Company size	
Microenterprise	115 (16.91)
Small company	185 (27.21)
Medium company	78 (11.47)
Large company	302 (44.41)
Weekly working hours	
≤40	134 (19.71)
over 40	546 (80.29)
Occupation	
Administrative service workers	479 (70.44)
Workers within production of goods, industrial services, repair and maintenance	71 (10.44)
Midlevel technicians	41 (6.03)
Science and arts professionals	34 (5.00)
Service workers and sales workers in stores and markets	32 (4.71)
General managers	23 (3.38)
Economic activity	
Transportation, storage and postal services	356 (52.35)
Financial activities, insurance and related services	140 (20.59)
Processing industries	63 (9.26)
Other economic activities	40 (5.88)
Sale and repair of motor vehicles and motorcycles	39 (5.74)
Administrative activities and complementary services	22 (3.24)
Human health and social services	20 (2.94)

Source: RAIS, 2018; SISCAT, 2016–2018.

The most frequently observed musculoskeletal diagnosis was shoulder injury. This, together with synovitis, tenosynovitis and back pain, represented the majority (63.1%) of all musculoskeletal disorders (Table 3).

The median time spent in work was 56 months (SE: 0.04) (Figure 1).

Table 4 presents the results from univariate and multiple analyses on the associations between the length of time spent in work and the covariates studied. The variables selected for the multiple models were sex, race/skin color, number of years of schooling, geographical macroregion, company size, occupational group and economic activity group.

The final model was fitted according to the workers' sex, and the probability of agreement estimated through the model had a discriminatory or predictive value of 65.3%.

Thus, our findings showed that workers with disabilities due to WRMDs who returned to work after vocational rehabilitation, and who were living in the southeastern region (HR: 2.78; 95% CI 1.12–6.91) and southern region (HR: 2.68; 95% CI 1.04–6.90) were at higher risk of dismissal from work than workers in the northern region. Likewise, rehabilitated workers in the economic activity sectors of transportation, storage and postal services (HR: 2.57; 95% CI 1.07–6.17) or financial activities, insurance and related services (HR: 2.70;

95% CI 1.05–6.89) were at higher risk of dismissal than those in the manufacturing sector (Table 4).

Table 3. Distribution of workers who underwent rehabilitation through Social Security and then returned to the formal employment market, according to their primary clinical diagnoses of disability due to musculoskeletal disorders. Brazil, 2014–2018 (n = 680).

Clinical Diagnosis According to ICD-10 Chapter XIII, Codes M00-M99	n (%)
M75—Shoulder injuries	154 (22.65)
M65—Synovitis and tenosynovitis	141 (20.74)
M54—Back pain	134 (19.71)
M51—Other intervertebral disc disorders	63 (9.26)
M69—Other joint disorders not elsewhere classified	29 (4.26)
M23—Internal disorders of the knees	27 (3.97)
M77—Other enthesopathy	24 (3.53)
M50—Cervical disc disorders	18 (2.65)
M79—Other soft tissue disorders not elsewhere classified	12 (1.76)
M16—Coxarthrosis	11 (1.62)
Other musculoskeletal diseases	67 (9.85)

Source: RAIS, 2018; SISCAT, 2016–2018.

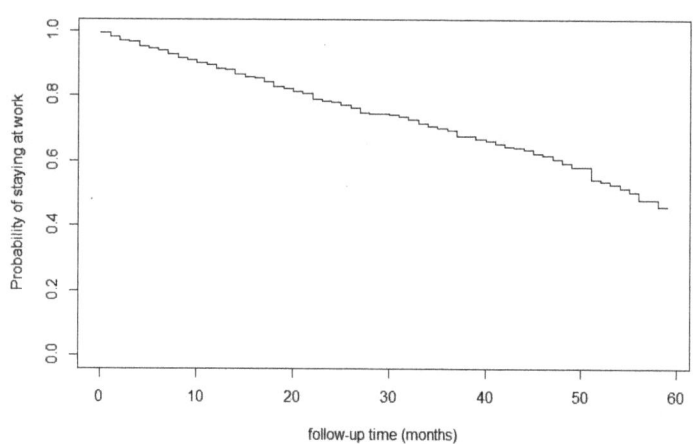

Figure 1. Probability of staying at work. Source: RAIS, 2018; SISCAT, 2016–2018.

Table 4. Univariate and multiple analyses (Cox regression) on the length at stay at work among workers who underwent rehabilitation through Social Security due to WRMD disabilities, who then returned to the formal employment market. Brazil, 2014–2018.

Features		Univariate		Multiple	
		HR	95% CI	HR	95% CI
Sex					
	Female	1.00	-	1.00	-
	Male	1.05	0.79–1.40	0.99	0.73–1.37
Age group					
	Up to 40 years	1.00	-		
	Over 40 years	0.98	0.73–1.32		
Race/skin color					
	White	1.00	-		
	Not White	0.82 [b]	0.62–1.90		

Table 4. Cont.

Features		Univariate		Multiple	
		HR	95% CI	HR	95% CI
Number of years of schooling					
	Up to 11 years	1.00	-		
	Over 11 years	1.47 [a]	1.11–1.95		
Geographical region					
	North	1.00	-	1.00	-
	Northeast	1.68	0.67–4.20	2.29	0.90–5.80
	Southeast	2.41 [b]	0.98–5.94	2.78 [a]	1.12–6.91
	South	2.08	0.82–5.28	2.68 [a]	1.04–6.90
	Center-west	2.15	0.78–5.91	2.41	0.87–6.72
Average monthly salary					
	Up to 2 times minimum wage	1.00	-		
	From 2.01 to 4 times minimum wage	0.79	0.57–1.08		
	Above 4 times minimum wage	0.87	0.60–1.28		
Company size					
	Microenterprise	1.00	-	1.00	-
	Small company	0.87	0.60–1.28	0.86	0.57–1.28
	Medium company	0.82	0.51–1.30	0.84	0.52–1.35
	Large company	0.41 [a]	0.28–0.61	0.60 [a]	0.38–0.92
Weekly working hours					
	Up to 40 h	1.00	-		
	Over 40 h	1.15	0.79–166		
Occupation					
	General managers	1.00	-	1.00	-
	Science and arts professionals	0.12 [a]	0.02–0.48	0.12 [a]	0.02–0.50
	Mid-level technicians	0.69	0.32–1.48	1.07	0.49–2.36
	Administrative service workers	0.56	0.30–1.03	0.61	0.30–1.23
	Service workers and salespeople in stores and markets	0.23 [a]	0.07–0.71	0.50	0.14–1.75
	Workers within production of goods, industrial services, repair and maintenance	0.26 [a]	0.11–0.58	0.69	0.25–1.94
Economic activity					
	Processing industries	1.00	-	1.00	-
	Sale and repair of motor vehicles and motorcycles	1.82	0.76–4.40	1.92	0.73–5.06
	Transportation, storage and postal services	2.92 [a]	1.50–5.60	2.57 [a]	1.07–6.17
	Financial activities, insurance and related services	3.47 [a]	1.74–6.94	2.70 [a]	1.05–6.89
	Administrative activities and complementary services	1.17	0.37–3.75	1.30	0.37–4.53
	Human health and social services	0.55	0.12–2.52	0.46	0.09–2.35
	Other economic activities	1.31	0.50–3.45	1.28	0.46–3.56

Adjusted for sex; [a], $p < 0.05$; [b], $p < 0.20$; HR: hazard ratio. Source: RAIS, 2018; SISCAT, 2016–2018.

On the other hand, rehabilitated workers employed in large companies were 60% more likely to remain in work than those employed in microenterprises. Being a rehabilitated worker in the occupational group of science and arts professionals also increased the chances of remaining employed for a longer time by 12%, compared with the occupational group of managers (Table 4).

4. Discussion

This study showed that seven out of ten workers who underwent rehabilitation due to WRMD disabilities between 2014 and 2018 remained employed. The results also showed that workers in the southeastern and southern regions who worked within the economic activity sectors of transportation, storage and postal services, or financial activities, insurance and related services, had shorter periods of formal employment after returning to work.

It is not possible to broadly compare our findings with those from other populations because of differences between countries' disability and return-to-work policies, along with methodological differences between studies. For example, a study comparing sustained return to work after two years of sick leave due to low back pain across six countries found a considerable difference in job retention, ranging from 22% among workers in a German cohort to 62% among workers in a Dutch cohort. Among the workers in the other four countries studied, the following results regarding permanence in employment were found: 31% in Denmark, 39% in Sweden, 49% in the USA and 49% in Israel [20].

In Brazil, rehabilitated workers who received social security benefits characterized as due to work-related sickness are entitled to job security for at least one year after the benefit ceases, according to social security legislation [12]. In addition, companies with 100 or more workers are legally required to fill 2% to 5% of their staff positions with rehabilitated professionals or people with disabilities [12].

In principle, the abovementioned legal measures favor permanence of rehabilitated employees in large companies, as seen in our results, which showed that the probability of remaining in the job in the first year after returning to work was greater than 80%. However, after this period, we observed that there was a constant decrease in the probability of remaining in work over the remainder of the months studied. This finding corroborates the results from a study by Vacaro and Pedroso (2011), which showed that there was a higher unemployment rate among workers who had undergone rehabilitation through the Brazilian social security vocational rehabilitation program one year after their return to work [21].

Sociodemographic characteristics such as sex, age group, race/skin color, income and number of years of schooling did not influence the sustainability of the return to work. Regarding sex, our findings do not corroborate previous studies that found that females were less likely to return to work [10,22]. However, when the duration of the sustained return to work was investigated, the influence of sex did not seem to be significant. A study carried out among workers with disabilities due to musculoskeletal disorders and mental disorders who were followed up for two years did not find any significant difference between men and women [23].

On the other hand, there is strong evidence that older individuals are less likely to return to work and stay at work [22–24]. Regarding the variables of number of years of schooling, race/skin color and income, the results available from previous studies were inconclusive, and divergences remain regarding the impact of these characteristics on reintegration into work [10,25,26].

Our findings also showed that living in the southeastern and southern regions of Brazil had a negative influence on staying at work. Although these regions have the best socioeconomic indicators in Brazil [27], the national economic crisis that began in 2015 has had a negative impact on this country's employment rates, such that the rates of unemployment and underutilization of the labor force in the southeastern and southern regions are now higher than in other Brazilian regions [28]. This context of a crisis in the labor market, with greater impact in these regions, may explain the results found in our study. Workers with work disabilities could possibly have greater difficulty in competing for employment, in terms of access and maintenance in the job, compared with others who are considered healthy. A previous study in Italy showed that almost a quarter of workers with work disabilities were fired after returning to work, within a scenario of neoliberal measures to make the labor market more flexible [29].

It is essential to point out that in the case of workers with a history of work disability, as in cases of WRMD, returning to work does not imply total pain control. The goal is for them to reach a state in which stability of the clinical condition is achieved, which thus favors the return to work [30].

However, in a context of intensification and precariousness of work, the chances of staying in the job are almost nil. The pace of work and the various abusive pressures tend to worsen the clinical picture of the illness, thereby further reducing the individual's ability to cope with the work [30]. Although the degree of disability among the rehabilitated patients was not evaluated in this study due to unavailability of this information in the databases investigated, a four-year cohort study conducted among nursing workers showed that nurses with impaired work ability were at higher risk of dismissal [31].

Regarding the relationship between the length of stay at work and the size of the company, it was found that rehabilitated workers in large companies stayed in the job for longer periods. This can be partly explained by the legal obligation mentioned above, in which large companies must allocate a percentage of vacancies to rehabilitated workers. Another explanation is that there is a greater possibility of finding compatible functions for rehabilitated workers in large companies.

Regarding occupational groups and the relationship with permanence in work, not many studies providing explanations about the occupations within which workers with disabilities due to musculoskeletal disorders would be at lower risk of remaining employed, in relation to economic activity sectors, could be found. However, evidence from previous studies has indicated that working in managerial and support activities that involve less interaction with the public presents a relationship with shorter times taken to return to work [32].

Our findings showed that rehabilitated workers engaged in "transportation, storage and postal service activities" and "financial activities, insurance and related services" remained employed for shorter times. This was possibly due to the characteristics of the activities involved in these areas, which particularly expose workers to a variety of occupational agents of a physical nature, such as noise and vibration; to ergonomic stressors at work, such as physical effort and load lifting; and to lower autonomy and control over productivity. Such jobs present higher stress levels and exacerbate these individuals' degree of incapacity [33]. Studies assessing the environmental characteristics of work, along with aspects of the context and content of work tasks, are needed.

The strength of the present study is that it presents external validity, given that it encompassed nationwide data with a longitudinal design in determining the outcome. Few Brazilian studies have evaluated the permanence of individuals in work after completing the vocational rehabilitation provided through social security. One limitation of the present study was the impossibility of identifying the date of leaving the rehabilitation program. Thus, it was unknown whether this was the first return to work after vocational rehabilitation. Another limitation was that this study did not include workers in the informal job market or workers with disabilities due to musculoskeletal diseases that were unrelated to work.

5. Conclusions

The length of stay at work among workers with histories of disability due to WMSDs who were reintegrated into formal employment through rehabilitation provided through the Brazilian social security system was influenced mainly by occupational factors related to the size of the company, type of occupation and sector of economic activity. It was found that workers in large companies and in the occupational group of "science and arts professionals" remained employed for longer than workers in microenterprises and in the occupational group of "general managers". Being a rehabilitated worker in the southeastern or southern region and carrying out economic activities of "transportation, storage and postal services" and "financial activities, insurance and related services" were factors that negatively influenced the length of stay in formal employment.

Although Brazilian legislation guarantees vacancies for rehabilitated workers, it is clear that this legislation needs to be more capable of broadly promoting these workers' inclusion. Despite the impossibility of ascertaining the degree of disability of the study subjects, the functional limitations of these rehabilitated workers meant that they were barred from performing some tasks that required certain skills. They were consequently at a disadvantage with regard to entering and staying in a highly competitive labor market in which formal employment is increasingly fragile.

We hope that the findings from this study can contribute to discussion and elaboration of more effective vocational rehabilitation measures, with a view to changing the limited approach in which workers are already incapacitated with regard to remaining in work activity. Early interventions are often more successful in relation to preventing harmful work conditions and promoting a sustainable return to work.

Author Contributions: Conceptualization, methodology, formal analysis and original draft preparation: C.B.d.M. Linkage method: K.K.S.G.; Editing and proofreading: C.B.d.M., J.S.S.-J., F.N.e.F.d.S. and K.K.S.G. Supervision, review, proofreading and acquisition of funding: F.M.F. All authors have read and agreed to the published version of the manuscript.

Funding: National Council for Scientific and Technological Development (Conselho Nacional de Desenvolvimento Científico e Tecnológico—CNPq), grant #423231/2018-9. Cristiano Barreto de Miranda received a CNPq doctoral grant, #140969/2017-9, and Frida Marina Fischer receives a CNPq research productivity grant, #306963/2021-3.

Institutional Review Board Statement: The Research Ethics Committee of the School of Public Health of the University of São Paulo (CAAE: 04267218.0.0000.5421, opinion number: 5113575) approved this study.

Informed Consent Statement: Participant consent was waived because this study used only information from institutional information systems.

Data Availability Statement: The data are not publicly available. A deidentified dataset can be obtained by contacting the first author.

Conflicts of Interest: The authors declare that there are no conflict of interest.

References

1. European Agency for Safety and Health at Work; Kok, J.; Vroonhof, P.; Snijders, J.; Roullis, G.; Clarke, M.; Peereboom, K.; Dorst, P.V.; Isusi, I. *Work-Related Musculoskeletal Disorders: Prevalence, Costs and Demographics in the EU*; European Agency for Safety and Health at Work: Bilbao, Spain, 2020. [CrossRef]
2. Friedenberg, R.; Kalichman, L.; Ezra, D.; Wacht, O.; Alperovitch-Najenson, D. Work-related musculoskeletal disorders and injuries among emergency medical technicians and paramedics: A comprehensive narrative review. *Arch. Environ. Occup. Health* **2019**, *77*, 9–17. [CrossRef]
3. Devereux, J.J.; Vlachonikolis, I.G.; Buckle, P.W. Epidemiological study to investigate potential interaction between physical and psychosocial factors at work that may increase the risk of symptoms of musculoskeletal disorder of the neck and upper limb. *Occup. Environ. Med.* **2002**, *59*, 269–277. [CrossRef] [PubMed]
4. Andersen, J.H.; Haahr, J.P.; Frost, P. Risk factors for more severe regional musculoskeletal symptoms: A two-year prospective study of a general working population. *Arthritis Rheum.* **2007**, *56*, 1355–1364. [CrossRef]
5. Tornqvist, E.W.; Hagberg, M.; Hagman, M.; Risberg, E.H.; Toomingas, A. The influence of working conditions and individual factors on the incidence of neck and upper limb symptoms among professional computer users. *Int. Arch. Occup. Environ. Health* **2009**, *82*, 689–702. [CrossRef]
6. DataSUS. *Tabnet Health Information*; Ministry of Health: Brasília, Brazil, 2022. Available online: http://www.datasus.gov.br (accessed on 15 November 2021).
7. Van Eerd, D.; Irvin, E.; Le Pouésard, M.; Butt, A.; Nasir, K. Workplace Musculoskeletal Disorder Prevention Practices and Experiences. *Inquiry* **2022**, *59*, 1–13. [CrossRef]
8. Stock, S.R.; Nicolakakis, N.; Vézina, N.; Vézina, M.; Gilbert, L.; Turcot, A.; Sultan-Taïeb, H.; Sinden, K.; Denis, M.A.; Delga, C.; et al. Are work organization interventions effective in preventing or reducing work-related musculoskeletal disorders? A systematic review of the literature. *Scand. J. Work Environ. Health* **2018**, *44*, 113–133. [CrossRef]
9. Burdorf, A.; Naaktgeboren, B.; Post, W. Prognostic factors for musculoskeletal sickness absence and return to work among welders and metal workers. *Occup. Environ. Med.* **1998**, *55*, 490–495. [CrossRef]
10. Lydell, M.; Grahn, B.; Månsson, J.; Baigi, A.; Marklund, B. Predictive factors of sustained return to work for persons with musculoskeletal disorders who participated in rehabilitation. *Work* **2009**, *33*, 317–328. [CrossRef]
11. Rashid, M.; Kristofferzon, M.-L.; Nilsson, A.; Heiden, M. Factors associated with return to work among people on work absence due to long-term neck or back pain: A narrative systematic review. *BMJ Open* **2017**, *7*, e014939. [CrossRef]
12. *Provides for Social Security Benefit Plans and Makes Other Provisions*; Law No. 8213 of 24 July 1991; Official Diary of the Union: Brasília, Brazil, 1991. Available online: https://www.planalto.gov.br/ccivil_03/leis/l8213cons.htm (accessed on 18 September 2021).
13. Miranda, C.B.; Silva-Junior, J.S.; Fernandes, G.A.; Fischer, F.M. Trends in the Cumulative Incidence of Vocational Rehabilitation Indicators in Brazil, 2007–2016. *Int. J. Environ. Res. Public Health* **2020**, *17*, 3952. [CrossRef]
14. Santana, V.S. Information Systems for Occupational Health. *Rev. Bras. Med. Trab.* **2019**, *17*, 34–35. [CrossRef]

15. *Infologo AEPS: Social Security Historical Database*; Ministry of Economy: Brasília, Brazil, 2022. Available online: http://www3.dataprev.gov.br/scripts10/dardoweb.cgi (accessed on 15 November 2021).
16. Garcia, K.K.S.; Miranda, C.B.; Sousa, F.N.E.F. Procedures for health data linkage: Applications in health surveillance. *Epidemiol. Serv. Saude* **2022**, *31*, e20211272. [CrossRef] [PubMed]
17. Kaplan, E.L.; Meier, P. Nonparametric estimation for incomplete observations. *J. Am. Stat. Assoc.* **1958**, *53*, 457–481. [CrossRef]
18. Miot, H.A. Survival analysis in clinical and experimental studies. *J. Vasc. Bras.* **2017**, *16*, 267–269. [CrossRef] [PubMed]
19. Carvalho, M.S.; Andreozzi, V.L.; Codeço, C.T.; Campos, D.P.; Barbosa, T.S.; Shimakura, S.E. *Survival Analysis: Theory and Applications in Health*, 2nd ed.; Editora Fiocruz: Rio de Janeiro, Brazil, 2011.
20. Anema, J.R.; Schellart, A.J.; Cassidy, J.D.; Loisel, P.; Veerman, T.J.; van der Beek, A.J. Can cross country differences in return-to-work after chronic occupational back pain be explained? An exploratory analysis on disability policies in a six country cohort study. *J. Occup. Rehabil.* **2009**, *19*, 419–426. [CrossRef] [PubMed]
21. Vacaro, J.E.; Pedroso, F.S. Performance of insured workers in the rehabilitation service at the National Institute for Social Security. *Acta Fisiátrica* **2011**, *18*, 200–205. [CrossRef]
22. Cancelliere, C.; Donovan, J.; Stochkendahl, M.J.; Biscardi, M.; Ammendolia, C.; Myburgh, C.; Cassidy, D. Factors affecting return to work after injury or illness: Best evidence synthesis of systematic reviews. *Chiropr. Man. Ther.* **2016**, *24*, 32. [CrossRef]
23. Kausto, J.; Pentti, J.; Oksanen, T.; Virta, L.J.; Virtanen, M.; Kivimaki, M.; Vahtera, J. Length of sickness absence and sustained return-to-work in mental disorders and musculoskeletal diseases: A cohort study of public sector employees. *Scand. J. Work Environ. Health* **2017**, *43*, 358–366. [CrossRef]
24. Valentin, G.H.; Pilegaard, M.S.; Vaegter, H.B.; Rosendal, M.; Ortenblad, L.; Vaeggemose, U.; Christensen, R. Prognostic factors for disability and sick leave in patients with subacute non-malignant pain: A systematic review of cohort studies. *BMJ Open* **2016**, *6*, e007616. [CrossRef]
25. Bültmann, U.; Franche, R.-L.; Hogg-Johnson, S.; Côté, P.; Lee, H.; Severin, C.; Vidmar, M.; Carnide, N. Health status, work limitations, and return-to-work trajectories in injured workers with musculoskeletal disorders. *Qual. Life Res.* **2007**, *16*, 1167–1178. [CrossRef]
26. Saldanha, J.H.S.; Pereira, A.P.M.; da Neves, R.F.; De Lima, M.A.G. Facilitating factors and barriers for returning to work in workers affected by Repetitive Strain Injury (RSI)/Work-Related Musculoskeletal Disorders (WMSDs). *Rev. Bras. Saúde Ocup.* **2013**, *38*, 122–138. [CrossRef]
27. *Classification of Company Size by Number of Workers*; Brazilian Institute of Geography and Statistics: Brasília, Brazil, 2006. Available online: www.igbe.gov.br (accessed on 11 June 2021).
28. De Oliveira, R.V.; Ladosky, M.H.; Rombaldi, M. The labor reform and its implications for the northeast: First reflections. *Cad. CRH* **2019**, *32*, 271–288. [CrossRef]
29. Galizzi, M.; Leombruini, R.; Pacelli, L. Successful return to work during labor market liberalization: The case of Italian injured workers. *J. Labour Mark. Res.* **2019**, *53*, 9. [CrossRef]
30. Maeno, M.; de Vilela, R.A.G. Occupational rehabilitation in Brazil: Elements for the development of public policy. *Rev. Bras. Saúde Ocup.* **2010**, *35*, 87–99. [CrossRef]
31. Martinez, M.C.; Fischer, F.M. Work ability as determinant of termination of employment: To resign or be dismissed? *J. Occup. Environ. Med.* **2019**, *61*, 272–281. [CrossRef]
32. Demou, E.; Smith, S.; Bhaskar, A.; Mackay, D.F.; Brown, J.; Hunt, K.; Vargas-Prada, S.; Macdonald, E.B. Evaluating sickness absence duration by musculoskeletal and mental health issues: A retrospective cohort study of Scottish healthcare workers. *BMJ Open* **2018**, *8*, e018085. [CrossRef]
33. *Regulatory Norm 04: Specialized Services in Safety Engineering and Occupational Medicine*; Ordinance MTb No. 3214 of 8 June 1987; Official Gazette of the Union, Ministry of Labor and Social Security: Brasília, Brazil, 1978.

Disclaimer/Publisher's Note: The statements, opinions and data contained in all publications are solely those of the individual author(s) and contributor(s) and not of MDPI and/or the editor(s). MDPI and/or the editor(s) disclaim responsibility for any injury to people or property resulting from any ideas, methods, instructions or products referred to in the content.

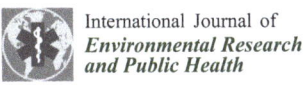

Article

Persistent Organic Pollutant Levels in Maternal and Cord Blood Plasma and Breast Milk: Results from the Rio Birth Cohort Pilot Study of Environmental Exposure and Childhood Development (PIPA Study)

Aline Souza Espindola Santos [1], Josino Costa Moreira [2], Ana Cristina Simoes Rosa [2], Volney Magalhães Câmara [1], Antonio Azeredo [1], Carmen Ildes Rodrigues Froes Asmus [3] and Armando Meyer [1,*]

[1] Occupational and Environmental Branch, Public Health Institute, Federal University of Rio de Janeiro, Rio de Janeiro 21941-598, Brazil
[2] Center for Studies of Human Ecology and Worker's Health, National School of Public Health, Oswaldo Cruz Foundation, Rio de Janeiro 21041-210, Brazil
[3] School of Medicine, Maternity School Hospital, Federal University of Rio de Janeiro, Rio de Janeiro 22240-000, Brazil
* Correspondence: armando@iesc.ufrj.br; Tel.: +55-21-973732000

Citation: Santos, A.S.E.; Moreira, J.C.; Rosa, A.C.S.; Câmara, V.M.; Azeredo, A.; Asmus, C.I.R.F.; Meyer, A. Persistent Organic Pollutant Levels in Maternal and Cord Blood Plasma and Breast Milk: Results from the Rio Birth Cohort Pilot Study of Environmental Exposure and Childhood Development (PIPA Study). *Int. J. Environ. Res. Public Health* **2023**, *20*, 778. https://doi.org/10.3390/ijerph20010778

Academic Editors: Rejane C. Marques, José Garrofe Dórea and Rafael Junqueira Buralli

Received: 7 November 2022
Revised: 23 December 2022
Accepted: 27 December 2022
Published: 31 December 2022

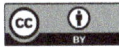

Copyright: © 2022 by the authors. Licensee MDPI, Basel, Switzerland. This article is an open access article distributed under the terms and conditions of the Creative Commons Attribution (CC BY) license (https://creativecommons.org/licenses/by/4.0/).

Abstract: Levels of polychlorinated biphenyls (PCB) and organochlorine pesticides (OCP) were evaluated in the breast milk and maternal and umbilical cord blood of pregnant women and their newborns in Rio de Janeiro, Brazil. The concentration of 11 PCB and 17 OCP were measured in 135 samples of maternal, and 116 samples of cord blood plasma, as well as 40, 47, and 45 samples of breast milk at 1st, 3rd, and 6th months after birth, respectively, using gas chromatography-mass spectrometry (GC-MS-MS). Women were asked to answer an enrollment questionnaire with reproductive, lifestyle, residential and sociodemographic questions. The most commonly detected OCPs and PCBs in the maternal and cord blood were 4,4′-DDE; β-HCH; γ-HCH; and PCB 28. 4,4′-DDE was also the most commonly detected OCP in breast milk samples. Although not statistically significant, ∑DDT levels were higher among women with pregestational BMI ≥ 30, and who were non-white and older (age > 40). Newborns with an Apgar score ≤ 8 at minute 5 of life showed significantly higher levels of ∑DDT in the cord blood. Persistent OCPs and PCBs were still detected in maternal and umbilical cord blood and breast milk, even after decades of their banishment in Brazil. They may pose a risk to maternal, fetal and children's health.

Keywords: organochlorine compounds; DDT; polychlorinated biphenyls; pregnant women; umbilical cord; breast milk; Brazil

1. Introduction

Organochlorine pesticides (OCP) and polychlorinated biphenyls (PCB) are classified as environmentally persistent organic pollutants due to their physical, chemical and toxicological properties, and pose a considerable threat to human health [1]. PCBs were used as flame retardants in industrial consumer products and old electrical devices, especially transformers and capacitors, which remain the primary source of these pollutants in urban areas of Brazil and around the world [2]. Brazil has prohibited their commercialization and manufacture through the Inter-Ministerial Ordinance No. 19, of 29 January 1981, with plans to eliminate these contaminants by 2028. OCPs were largely used in Brazil between the 1960s and mid-1980s in agricultural and public health campaigns [3]. In 1985, the use of OCPs as agricultural pesticides was prohibited in Brazil but allowed for other purposes, such as household pesticides, medicine to treat lice, wood preservatives and control of vector-borne diseases, until the early 2000s [3,4].

Despite this long-term prohibition, OCP and PCB residues are still found in the environment and food chain [5], representing Brazil's main pathway for human exposure [4]. Although OCP and PCB were banned in Brazil about 30–40 years ago, these substances are ubiquitous and stable; therefore, their reduction and elimination from the environment or food chain are prolonged. Several OCP, especially DDT metabolites, are reportedly found in highly consumed fish collected at Guanabara Bay, Rio de Janeiro, Brazil [6]. In addition, some of the pollutants found in Rio de Janeiro City air samples were DDT (median = 233 pg/m^3) and HCH (median = 340 pg/m^3) [7].

Due to their persistence and potential carcinogenicity, immunotoxicity, reproductive toxicity, neurotoxicity and endocrine-disrupting effects, OCP and PCB represent significant public health concerns [8]. These substances can cross the placental barrier and endanger the fetus' health [9]. Exposure to OCP and PCB during the first years of life is also impactful because the nervous and immune systems, as well as xenobiotic metabolic pathways, continue to develop until early childhood [10]. Studies have reported the presence of PCB and OCP or their metabolites in the blood of pregnant women [11], umbilical cord blood [12] and breast milk [13]. Other studies suggested that prenatal exposure to these substances is associated with adverse birth outcomes such as reduced size, weight and head circumference [14], and delayed neurodevelopment [15]. Some undesirable health effects have been found in descendants even after their grandmother's exposure to DDT [16].

In Brazil, only a few studies have examined the concentration of persistent organic pollutants in maternal and umbilical cord blood. We investigated the levels of 11 PCB and 17 OCP in the breast milk and blood of pregnant women, and their newborns' umbilical cords, enrolled in the pilot study of the Rio Birth Cohort (PIPA Study), in the city of Rio de Janeiro, Brazil. We also explored the relationship between the sociodemographic characteristics of the mothers and certain birth outcomes with the concentrations of the studied OCP and PCB.

2. Materials and Methods

2.1. Participants and Enrollment

PIPA is a hospital-based birth cohort study designed to examine the relationship between environmental exposure to several pollutants during pregnancy and any adverse effects upon delivery and the physiological development of the newborn from infancy to the age of 4. A pilot study was conducted from September 2017 through February 2018 and enrolled 142 pregnant women (Figure 1). In the current study, we described the levels of OCPs and PCBs in the maternal and umbilical cord blood of these women and their newborns [17].

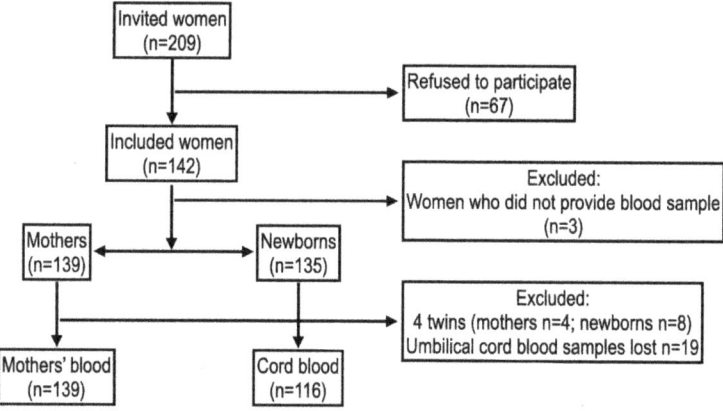

Figure 1. Flow diagram of the study population.

Pregnant women over 16 years of age and at the beginning of the third trimester of pregnancy were invited to participate in the Rio Birth Cohort pilot study during their visit to the Federal University of Rio de Janeiro's Maternity Hospital (UMH) in October and November of 2017. This hospital serves women living in low-income communities in the southern part of Rio de Janeiro City. High-risk pregnancies identified at any other medical unit in Rio de Janeiro may also be referred to the UMH.

2.2. Sampling

Out of 209 eligible pregnant women, 142 (67.9%) accepted the invitation to participate in the PIPA pilot study. A questionnaire containing socio-demographics, lifestyle (i.e., smoking, alcohol, physical activity), and prenatal questions was completed by all participants, but only 139 women (98%) authorized the use of blood samples for chemical analysis. Four samples showed insufficient amounts and were discarded.

A total of 135 deliveries occurred at UMH from October 2017 through February 2018. Samples of umbilical cord blood were collected from 126 (93%) of the newborns. The OCP were quantified in 135 (95%) maternal blood and 116 (86%) umbilical cord blood samples, as 10 of these samples showed hemolysis. Breast milk samples were collected from 40, 47, and 45 mothers at the 1st, 3rd, and 6th months of follow-up.

2.3. Analytical Methods

The OCP and PCB were analyzed through GC-MS/MS and included isomers of aldrin, dieldrin, endrin, DDT, DDD, DDE, HCH, HCB, mirex, endosulfan, chlordane, dicofol, heptachlor, methoxychlor, nonachlor pentachloroanisole, and the PCB congeners 28, 31, 52, 77, 101, 105, 118, 126, 128, 138, 153, 156, 169, 170 and 180. The analytical method has been adapted from Sarcinelli et al. [18].

Briefly, plasma samples were allowed to equilibrate at room temperature, and subsequently denatured and diluted with equal parts of methanol and water, then mixed and extracted on C18 solid-phase extraction (SPE) cartridges (JT Baker, Phillipsburg, NJ, USA). Each cartridge was dried and eluted with 7 mL of hexane. The eluate was applied to a florisil SPE cartridge, then eluted with petroleum ether: hexane (85:15) solution. The extracts were evaporated under a nitrogen atmosphere, and the volume was resuspended to 100 µL with hexane and analyzed by GC-MS/MS using 5 µL of 1,1'-biphenyl-4,4'dibromine at 1 µg mL^{-1} as the internal standard.

The GC-MS/MS analysis was performed using a Thermo Scientific, Waltham, MA, USA model TSQ 8000 EVO Pesticide Analyzer equipped with a Trace GC 1310 and an AS 1310 autosampler with a programmable temperature vaporization injector operating in the splitless mode using Thermo Fisher Xcalibur™ and TraceFinder™ software V.5. An Agilent DB-5MS phenylmethyl siloxane (30 m × 250 µm × 0.25 µm) column was used with ultrapure helium as the carrier gas at a constant flow rate of 1 mL min^{-1}. The injector temperature was 280 °C, and splitless injection occurred for 1 min. The flow was purged at 30 mL min^{-1} for 1.2 min and 2 µL of the sample was injected. The GC oven temperature ramp program mode was 50 °C (2 min) at 10 °C min^{-1} to 180 °C (0 min) at 3 °C min^{-1} to 230 °C (0 min) at 5 °C min^{-1} to 280 °C (0 min), and at 15 °C min^{-1} to 310 °C (7 min), for a total of 50.68 min. The detector temperature was set at 300 °C. Compounds were identified by selected reaction monitoring (SRM) adjusted for retention time. Spectrometric conditions were defined according to the National Institute of Standards and Technology (NIST) libraries included in the Tracefinder™ software, although some confirmations using Thermo AutoSRM were necessary; thus, the transitions were defined according to their high specificity combined with high abundance.

OCP concentrations were adjusted by concentrations of lipids in breast milk. For this, 9 mL of a mixture of hexane-acetone was added to a 1 mL milk sample. The mixture was vortexed for 1 min, then placed in ultrasound for 20 min and centrifuged at 4000 rpm ± 100 rpm for 15 min. The supernatant in previously weighed tubes was collected. The extraction was repeated. The supernatant solvent was evaporated under an N2 atmosphere until dry. The total fat was calculated by the weight difference of the tubes.

2.4. Quality Assurance and Quality Control for OCP and PCB Analysis

Spiked plasma were used to prepare calibration curves. Validation parameters (Table S1) included linearity, sensitivity, recovery tests, repeatability, the limit of detection (LOD) and limit of quantification (LOQ) based on the EPA 8081B method [19] and the Brazilian INMETRO Guide [20]. Eight-point calibration curves from 0.2 to 15 ng mL^{-1} were used to prepare the calibration curves by linear regression. Correlation coefficients ranged from 0.936 to 0.994, showing good linearity for both OCPs pesticides and PCBs. Sensitivity was calculated using the curve slope and varied from 111.655 to 212.082 for DDT and its isomers. The mean percentage recoveries ranged from 93% to 105% for OCP and from 87% to 107% for PCB, evaluated at 0.5, 5, and 15 ng mL^{-1}. LOD and LOQ were calculated from standard deviation multiplied by factor t (Student t) or per 10, respectively, for 7 replicates at 0.2 ng mL^{-1} lowest level. The factor t for 6 degrees of freedom at a 95% confidence interval was 1.943. The LOD was 0.015 ng mL^{-1} to 0.468 ng mL^{-1} for OCP and 0.2 ng mL^{-1} to 0.36 ng mL^{-1} for PCB. The LOQ was 0.045 ng mL^{-1} to 1.419 ng mL^{-1} for OCP pesticides and 0.05 ng mL^{-1} to 1.08 ng mL^{-1} for PCB. Repeatability at 2 ng mL^{-1} level ranged from 0.5 to 14.9% for within-day variability and from 0.8 to 8.6% for day-to-day variability.

To perform only one analysis per sample and obtain one chromatogram and SRM spectrum, analytical quality controls were performed for each batch using previously spiked plasma at 3 levels: 0.2, 0.5, and 1 ng mL^{-1} and blank. The control of sample results was made by monitoring the daily abundance values in spiked plasma at these 3 concentration levels and the slope for each batch control. If the variation between the last batches was greater than 20%, the batch was redone. Additionally, variations were <20% for two randomized samples, with extra available volume, done in duplicate in each batch.

The internal standard was added in all samples and controls to evaluate the injection and chromatographic batch conditions, being monitored over time by its area, and all analytes in a standard mixture with greater purity than 99%, at 1 µg mL^{-1} level. Solvent injections were also made every 10 samples to evaluate the carry-over effect and cleanness of the chromatographic system.

Three selective reaction monitoring transitions were exhaustively checked for each positive sample to avoid false positive results. The relative abundances of the three selected precursor ion–product ion transitions were obtained from high purity standards and monitored for each pesticide. Additionally, a very low variation in retention times was observed. Finally, each batch had its blank, quality control samples and a short calibration curve in spiked plasma, and sample levels were calculated by external standardization using linear regression.

2.5. Estimated Daily Intake and Hazard Quotient Calculations for Children

The EDI was estimated using the following equation: EDI = Cmilk × Cfat × Mingestion/BW; where EDI = estimated daily intake; Cmilk = pesticide concentration of pesticide in milk (ng/g of lipid); Cfat = milk fat content (%) in breastmilk; Mingestion = intake of breast milk [21]. The adopted values for EDI estimation were: 4% of lipid [22] and 700 g of human milk/day [23]. The HQ was calculated as the EDI divided by the reference dose (RfD) proposed by EPA (5 µg of ΣDDT/kg body wt./day) [24] and the provisional tolerable weekly intake (PTWI) adopted by FAO/WHO (10 µg of ΣDDT/kg body wt./day) [25–27]. HQ values higher than 1 mean that there is a risk associated with breast milk consumption.

2.6. Statistical Analysis

Descriptive analysis included frequency distribution of maternal characteristics such as age groups (16–19, 20–39, ≥40 years), ethnicity (white, nonwhite), monthly household income (R$ ≤ 1733.33, 1733.34–3000.00, and >3000.00), schooling (high school or less, higher education), BMI (<25, 25–29.9, ≥30), alcohol consumption (yes or no), smoking (never, before pregnancy, during pregnancy), exposure to second-hand smoke (yes or no) and gestational age (<37 or ≥37 weeks).

Newborn characteristics included sex, birth weight (<2500 or ≥2500 g), size for gestational age (small, appropriate, or large for gestational age) and Apgar at minute 5 (≤8 or >8).

The concentration of DDT and its metabolites, HCH isomers, all other OCPs and PCBs in the maternal and umbilical cord blood samples were described using the following parameters: LOD in ng/mL, distribution of frequencies, percent above LOD, geometric mean (GM), standard deviation, minimum, maximum and the 25th, 50th and 75th percentiles. In addition to the 11 PCBs and 17 OCPs, we also calculated these parameters for the sum of the concentrations of all persistent organic pollutants studied (OCPs + PCBs = $\sum$POP), OCPs ($\sum$OCPs), PCBs ($\sum$PCB), HCH isomers ($\sum$HCH) and DDT isomers/metabolites ($\sum$DDT). Blood concentrations below the LOD were excluded from the data set.

Frequency, GM, and its 95% confidence interval (95%CI) were also described for the sum of the compounds according to the mother's demographic variables and newborn birth characteristics. Since only 4,4'-DDE had a detection rate above 5% in the breast milk samples, only its GM was described in the 1st, 3rd and 6th follow-up months. We also described the 4,4'-DDE breast milk concentration for paired samples of mothers during at least two follow-ups of 3. Spearman correlation between DDE, $\sum$HCH, $\sum$DDT, $\sum$OCP and $\sum$OC in the maternal and cord blood and breast milk during the 1° and 3° months of follow-up were calculated.

Predictors of $\sum$DDT levels in maternal blood were estimated by linear regression models, crude and adjusted. Maternal age, BMI, education and ethnicity were used as independent variables, while the maternal blood levels of $\sum$DDT was the dependent one. We also used linear regression models to evaluated the association between $\sum$DDT levels in umbilical blood (independent variable) and birth outcomes, such as birth weight and length and Apgar score (dependent variables).

3. Results

The main characteristics of the sample population are presented in Table 1. The majority of pregnant women (82.7%) were between 20 and 39 years of age and non-white (73.6%). Approximately 45.2% reported an average household income between R$ 1733 and 3000 (USD 306–530), but 36% reported it to be below R$ 1733. Most of the participants (76.3%) had a high school degree or less. Regarding pre-gestational BMI, 47% of the mothers were normal weight, 33.3% were overweight, and 19.7% were obese. Alcohol consumption during pregnancy was reported by 46.6% of the women, while 10.9% reported smoking before pregnancy, and 9.3% smoked during pregnancy. In addition, 48.4% reported living with a person who smoked. Among the newborns, males were slightly more frequent (54.9%) than females. Seven percent of newborns had low birth weights (<2500 g), 9.8% of newborns were delivered before the 37th week of gestation and 19.5% showed an Apgar score below 8. Newborns appropriate, large, and small for gestational age accounted, respectively, for 81.5%, 10.7%, and 7.8% of the sample.

The concentrations of PCBs and OCPs in maternal and umbilical cord blood samples are shown in Table 2. The most abundant specific OCP compounds in maternal blood (in descending order) were 4,4'-DDE (22.2%), β-HCH (8.89%), and γ-HCH (7.41%), while in the umbilical cord blood samples, the most frequently detected substances were 4,4'-DDE (15.5%), beta-HCH (11.2%), 4,4'-DDT (10.3%), and 4,4'-DDD (7.8%). The frequency of the summed variables was similar in both types of sample, with $\sum$DDT (33;24.4%), and $\sum$HCH (13; 9.6%) in maternal blood samples, and $\sum$DDT (33; 28.5%), and $\sum$HCH (15; 12.9%) in umbilical cord blood samples. The concentration GM and range of the most commonly detected OCPs in maternal blood were 0.050–3.196 ng/mL (GM = 0.131) for 4,4'-DDE; 0.090–0.179 ng/mL (GM = 0.121) for β-HCH; 0.145–0.251 ng/mL (GM = 0.175) for γ-HCH; 0.030–3.249 ng/mL (GM = 0.136) for $\sum$DDT; and 0.090–0.430 ng/mL (GM = 0.230) for $\sum$HCH.

Table 1. Main characteristics of the studied population.

	N	%
Mothers' age (years)		
16–19	12	9.0
20–39	110	82.7
≥40	11	8.3
Ethnicity		
White	34	26.4
Non-white	95	73.6
Income *		
≤1733.33	36	31.3
1733.34–3000.00	52	45.2
>3000.00	27	23.5
Schooling		
High school or less	100	76.3
Higher education	31	23.7
Body Mass Index		
<25	55	47.0
25–29.9	39	33.3
≥30	23	19.7
Alcohol consumption		
Yes	61	46.6
No	70	53.4
Smoking		
Never	103	79.8
Before pregnancy	14	10.9
During pregnancy	12	9.3
Passive smoking		
Yes	62	48.4
No	66	51.6
Newborn sex		
Male	62	54.9
Female	51	45.1
Birth weight (g)		
<2500	8	7.0
≥2500	107	93.0
Size for gestational age		
Small for gestational age	8	7.8
Appropriate for gestational age	84	81.5
Large for gestational age	11	10.7
Gestational age (weeks)		
<37	10	9.8
≥37	92	90.2
Apgar 5th min		
≤8	22	19.5
>8	91	80.5

* Brazilian reais.

In the umbilical cord samples, these numbers were 0.052–5.440 ng/mL (GM = 0.150) for 4,4'-DDE, 0.023–0.169 ng/mL (GM = 0.071) for β-HCH, 0.050–0.477 ng/mL (GM = 0.099) for 4,4'-DDT, 0.030–0.226 ng/mL (GM = 0.066) for 4,4'-DDD, 0.030–6.231 ng/mL (GM = 0.151) for $\sum$DDT and 0.023–0.442 ng/mL (GM = 0.136) for $\sum$HCH (Table 2). The presence of 2,4'-DDT, 4,4'-DDD, 4,4'-DDT, dieldrin, endosulfan sulfate, methoxychlor, mirex, pentachloroanisole, and PCBs 28, 31, 52, 153 and 180 were detected in very few maternal blood samples (less than 5%), so their concentrations were not shown in the table. The same procedure was adopted for the description of concentrations of 2,4'-DDD, 2,4'-DDE, δ-HCH, endosulfan sulfate, dicofol, dieldrin, methoxychlor, mirex, pentachloroanisole and PCB 28, 31, 52, 101, 105, 118, 138, 128, 156 and 180 in umbilical cord blood samples. However, the levels of the compounds detected in less than 5% of the samples were included in ∑DDT, ∑HCH, ∑OCPs, and ∑POP.

Table 2. OCP and PCB concentrations in maternal and umbilical cord blood of the Rio Birth Cohort pilot study. Rio de Janeiro, Brazil, September 2017 to February 2018.

	LOD * ng/mL	Samples > LOD N (%)	GM ** (95%CI)	Min	25%	50%	75%	Max
Mothers' blood								
4,4′-DDE	0.045	30 (22.22)	0.131 (0.089–0.193)	0.050	0.069	0.087	0.198	3.196
∑DDT	-	33 (24.44)	0.136 (0.090–0.204)	0.030	0.067	0.085	0.215	3.249
β-HCH	0.02	12 (8.89)	0.121 (0.105–0.140)	0.090	0.102	0.119	0.144	0.179
γ-HCH	0.07	10 (7.41)	0.175 (0.150–0.205)	0.136	0.145	0.171	0.216	0.251
∑HCH	-	13 (9.63)	0.230 (0.173–0.306)	0.090	0.154	0.248	0.328	0.430
∑PCB [a]	-	11 (8.15)	0.110 (0.081–0.149)	0.064	0.068	0.097	0.160	0.255
∑OCPs [a]	-	41 (30.37)	0.187 (0.135–0.259)	0.030	0.080	0.171	0.308	3.249
∑POPs	-	46 (34.07)	0.190 (0.141–0.255)		0.084	0.169	0.305	3.249
Umbilical cord blood								
2,4′-DDT	0.02	8 (6.90)	0.133 (0.083–0.215)	0.065	0.082	0.183	0.206	0.254
4,4′-DDD	0.03	9 (7.76)	0.066 (0.037–0.118)	0.030	0.030	0.071	0.122	0.226
4,4′-DDE	0.05	18 (15.52)	0.150 (0.086–0.264)	0.052	0.065	0.110	0.266	5.440
4,4′-DDT	0.05	12 (10.34)	0.099 (0.059–0.168)	0.050	0.053	0.071	0.187	0.477
∑DDT	-	33 (28.45)	0.151 (0.100–0.227)	0.030	0.064	0.100	0.334	6.231
β-HCH	0.02	13 (11.21)	0.071 (0.047–0.105)	0.023	0.038	0.093	0.119	0.169
γ-HCH	0.07	6 (5.17)	0.157 (0.139–0.178)	0.138	0.140	0.157	0.177	0.178
∑HCH	-	15 (12.93)	0.136 (0.082–0.226)	0.023	0.073	0.178	0.289	0.442
PCB 153	0.02	6 (5.17)	0.076 (0.038–0.149)	0.021	0.043	0.080	0.155	0.204
∑PCB [b]	-	11 (9.48)	0.225 (0.118–0.430)	0.050	0.106	0.193	0.457	1.150
∑OCPs [b]	-	40 (34.48)	0.177 (0.124–0.252)	0.050	0.074	0.251	0.558	6.220
∑POP	-	41 (35.34)	0.192 (0.130–0.284)	0.050	0.074	0.247	0.734	6.270

* LOD—Detection limit; ** GM—Geometric mean; [a,b] ∑OCs and ∑PCBs included some organochlorines and congeners are not shown due to detection rates lower than 5%.

Table 3 shows that, in general, the concentrations of ∑DDT, ∑HCH, ∑OCPs, and ∑POP did not vary significantly as a function of maternal or newborns characteristics. Although not statistically significant, ∑DDT levels were slightly higher among non-white pregnant women, with an age > 40 and a pregestational BMI ≥ 30. On the other hand, newborns with an Apgar score of 8 or less showed significantly higher levels of ∑DDT in the umbilical cord blood.

Table 3. Levels of OCPs and PCBs according to maternal sociodemographic characteristics and birth variables. Rio Birth Cohort pilot study. Rio de Janeiro, Brazil, September 2017 to February 2018.

	ΣDDT	ΣHCH	ΣOCP	ΣPOP
		N; GM * (95%CI)		
Mothers				
Age				
16–19	2; 0.07 (0.02–0.25)	1; 0.27 (-)	4; 0.18 (0.04–0.70)	4; 0.18 (0.04–0.78)
20–39	22; 0.16 (0.10–0.25)	9; 0.21 (0.14–0.31)	29; 0.18 (0.12–0.26)	34; 0.18 (0.13–0.25)
≥40	9; 0.19 (0.06–0.61)	2; 0.12 (0.13–1.14)	8; 0.23 (0.07–0.69)	8; 0.23 (0.08–0.69)
Ethnicity				
White	13; 0.11 (0.07–0.20)	5; 0.29 (0.22–0.39)	15; 0.19 (0.12–0.30)	16; 0.19 (0.13–0.29)
Non-white	19; 0.15 (0.08–0.29)	8; 0.20 (0.13–0.31)	25; 0.19 (0.12–0.31)	29; 0.19 (0.12–0.29)
Income				
≤1733.33	4; 0.21 (0.02–2.32)	3; 0.24 (0.18–0.40)	6; 0.27 (0.08–0.89)	7; 0.25 (0.09–0.70)
1733.34–3000.00	10; 0.11 (0.07–0.17)	5; 0.24 (0.18–0.31)	14; 0.17 (0.12–0.24)	18; 0.17 (0.13–0.23)
>3000.00	13; 0.13 (0.06–0.30)	4; 0.19 (0.07–0.52)	14; 0.18 (0.09–0.38)	14; 0.19 (0.09–0.39)
Body Mass Index				
<25	11; 0.13 (0.07–0.26)	7; 0.28 (0.19–0.42)	16; 0.18 (0.11–0.30)	18; 0.19 (0.12–0.30)
25–29.9	12; 0.10 (0.05–0.23)	1; 0.28 (-) †	12; 0.14 (0.07–0.31)	13; 0.15 (0.07–0.29)
≥30	8; 0.25 (0.09–0.72)	3; 0.18 (0.02–0.68)	10; 0.30 (0.15–0.60)	10; 0.32 (0.16–0.64)
Newborns				
Sex				
Male	16; 0.18 (0.11–0.30)	9; 0.11 (0.05–0.23)	21; 0.19 (0.13–0.29)	22; 0.21 (0.13–0.33)
Female	16; 0.13 (0.06–0.27)	5; 0.17 (0.05–0.54)	17; 0.16 (0.08–0.34)	17; 0.18 (0.08–0.40)
Birth weight (g)				
<2500	3; 0.08 (0.05–0.13)	1; 0.25 (0.01–0.86)	4; 0.11 (0.04–0.27)	4; 0.11 (0.04–0.27)
≥2500	29; 0.17 (0.10–0.26)	14; 0.13 (0.08–0.22)	35; 0.19 (0.13–0.29)	36; 0.21 (0.14–0.33)
Gestational age (weeks)				
<37	4; 0.11 (0.04–0.34)	3; 0.17 (0.02–1.33)	5; 0.16 (0.05–0.55)	5; 0.17 (0.04–0.77)
≥37	23; 0.16 (0.09–0.28)	9; 0.08 (0.01–0.62)	28; 0.19 (0.12–0.30)	29; 0.20 (0.12–0.34)
Apgar 5th min				
≤8	6; 0.53 (0.11–2.51)	5; 0.08 (0.02–0.45)	7; 0.56 (0.16–1.98)	8; 0.54 (0.15–1.96)
>8	26; 0.12 (0.08–0.17)	10; 0.17 (0.12–0.25)	32; 0.14 (0.10–0.20)	32; 0.15 (0.11–0.22)

* Geometric Mean; † not a mean (n = 1).

The geometric mean of 4,4'-DDE concentrations in breast milk was lower in the 1st month of follow-up (n = 19; GM: 6.59; 95%CI: 3.33–13.05 ng/g) when compared with the 3rd (n = 22; GM: 15.12; 95%CI: 9.96–22.98 ng/g) and 6th (n = 6; GM: 11.41; 95% CI: 2.73–47.60 ng/g) months. ANOVA analysis showed no difference in 4,4'-DDE concentrations among the groups.

The calculated EDI varied from 5.98×10^{-6} to 1.17×10^{-3} μg of ΣDDT/kg body wt./day. The mean EDI was 0.21 μg of ΣDDT/kg body wt./day. The HQ values ranged from 5.98×10^{-3} and 1.20×10^{-2} to 1.17 and 2.34 according to EPA and FAO/WHO, respectively, and just one milk sample yielded an HQ value higher than 1.

Table 4 shows the correlation between DDE, ΣHCH, ΣDDT, ΣOCP, and ΣOC in the maternal and cord blood and breast milk during the 1° and 3° months of follow-up. Moderate correlations were observed between maternal ΣDDT and maternal ΣOCP (ρ = 0.709; p = <0.0001) and maternal ΣOC ρ = 0.684; p = <0.0001). ΣDDT in cord blood was most strongly correlated with ΣOCP (ρ = 0.913; p = <0.0001) and ΣOC (ρ = 0.911; p = <0.0001), whereas ΣOCP in cord blood was most strongly correlated with ΣOC ρ = 0.996; p = <0.0001) in cord blood. There were no correlations between DDE, ΣHCH, ΣDDT, ΣOCP, and ΣOC levels in the maternal and cord blood. Likewise, there were no correlations between DDE, ΣHCH, ΣDDT, ΣOCP and ΣOC levels in the maternal blood and breast milk.

Table 4. Spearman correlation table for detected POPs concentrations in maternal and cord blood and breast milk. Rio Birth Cohort pilot study, Rio de Janeiro, Brazil, September 2017 to February 2018.

		ΣDDT Mother	ΣDDT Cord	ΣOCP Mother	ΣOCP Cord	ΣOC Mother	ΣOC Cord	ΣHCH Mother	ΣHCH Cord	DDE Mother	DDE Cord	DDE BM 1° m *	DDE BM 3° m **
ΣDDT Mother	ρ	1.000	0.060	0.709	0.021	0.684	0.007	0.500	0.800	1.000	−0.500	0.286	0.257
	p		0.845	<0.0001	0.940	<0.0001	0.980	0.667	0.200		0.667	0.535	0.623
	n	33	13	32	15	32	15	3	4	2	3	7	6
ΣDDT Cord	ρ		1.000	−0.006	0.913	−0.029	0.911		0.500	−0.543	−0.700	0.500	−0.400
	p			0.983	<0.0001	0.911	<0.0001		0.667	0.266	0.188	0.667	0.600
	n		33	16	32	16	32	1	3	6	5	3	4
ΣOCP Mother	ρ			1.000	−0.051	0.964	−0.061	−0.400	−0.200	−0.543	0.029	0.429	0.517
	p				0.836	<0.0001	0.803	0.600	0.704	0.266	0.957	0.337	0.154
	n			41	19	43	19	4	6	6	6	7	9
ΣOCP Cord	ρ				1.000	−0.047	0.996		−0.800	−0.371	−0.500	0.400	−0.300
	p					0.847	<0.0001		0.200	0.468	0.391	0.600	0.624
	n				40	19	38	1	4	6	5	4	5
ΣOC Mother	ρ					1.000	−0.056	−0.200	0.071	−0.371	0.257	0.439	0.417
	p						0.819	0.747	0.879	0.468	0.623	0.337	0.265
	n					46	19	5	7	6	6	7	9
ΣOC Cord	ρ						1.00		−0.800	−0.393	−0.543	0.400	−0.300
	p								0.200	0.383	0.266	0.600	0.624
	n						40	1	4	7	6	4	5
ΣHCH Mother	ρ							1.000	0.500	0.600	1.000	−0.500	0.500
	p								0.667	0.285		0.667	0.667
	n							13	3	5	3	3	3
ΣHCH Cord	ρ								1.000	0.551	−0.086		
	p									0.257	0.872		
	n								15	6	6	1	1
DDE Mother	ρ									1.000	0.484	0.548	−0.042
	p										0.094	0.160	0.907
	n									30	13	8	10
DDE Cord	ρ										1.000	0.500	−0.300
	p											0.667	0.624
	n										18	3	5
DDE BM 1° m *	ρ											1.000	0.429
	p												0.337
	n											19	7
DDE BM 3° m **	ρ												1.000
	p												
	n												22

* BM 1° m: breast milk 1st month; ** BM 3° m: breast milk 3rd month.

Table 5 shows the results of the regression analysis for predictor factors of the ΣDDT levels in maternal blood. None of the analyses showed significant associations. Nevertheless, independently, age, BMI and being non-white showed trends in increasing maternal levels of ΣDDT, while having high school or higher education tended to decrease it. We also performed two adjusted models. The first one consisted of age as the main independent factor, adjusted for BMI. Although both variables still showed trends for increasing levels of maternal ΣDDT, their observed coefficients in the adjusted model were slightly lower than those in crude models. In the second adjusted model, we included ethnicity as an additional covariate. Age and BMI coefficients remained unchanged compared with model 1, and ethnicity's coefficient was slightly higher than observed in the independent model.

Umbilical blood level of ΣDDT was associated with a significant decrease in the Apgar score at the 5th minute in the studied newborns. ΣDDT levels in the umbilical cord also showed trends in decreasing birth weight and gestational length; however, it was not statistically significant. When adjusted for birth weight (model 1), the association between umbilical blood ΣDDT and Apgar score at the 5th minute remained practically unchanged.

Adding gestational length (model 2) led to a slight decrease in the β coefficient, but a significant confidence interval remained (Table 6).

Table 5. Regression models for maternal blood levels of ΣDDT predictors.

Independent Variables	Coefficient (95%CI)
Univariate models	
Age	0.037 (−0.012; 0.086)
BMI	0.024 (−0.044; 0.093)
Education (high school or more)	−0.082 (−0.989; 0.823)
Ethnicity (non-white)	0.131 (−0.748; 1.010)
Multivariate model 1	
Age	0.027 (−0.034; 0.089)
BMI	0.010 (−0.067; 0.086)
Multivariate model 2	
Age	0.027 (−0.037; 0.092)
BMI	0.010 (−0.070; 0.090)
Ethnicity (non-white)	0.183 (−0.748; 1.113)

Model 1: Dependent variable: ΣDDT levels in maternal blood; Independent variables: age and BMI. Model 2: Dependent variable: ΣDDT levels in maternal blood; Independent variables: age, BMI, and ethnicity.

Table 6. Regression analyses of the association between umbilical blood levels of ΣDDT and birth outcomes.

Dependent Variables	Coefficient (95%CI)
Univariate models	
Birth weight (grams)	−11.777 (−206.718; 183.164)
Gestational length (weeks)	−0.943 (−3.504; 1.618)
Apgar score 5th min	−0.441 (−0.645; −0.237)
Multivariate model 1	
Apgar score 5th min	−0.440 (−0.648; −0.233)
Multivariate model 2	
Apgar score 5th min	−0.405 (−0.651; −0.160)

Model 1: Dependent variable: Apgar score 5th min; Independent variables: ΣDDT levels in umbilical blood and birth weight. Model 2: Dependent variable: Apgar score 5th min; Independent variables: ΣDDT levels in umbilical blood, birth weight and gestational length.

4. Discussion

In this study, 4,4′-DDE, β-HCH, and γ-HCH were the most detected POPs in the blood of pregnant women; whereas, 4,4′-DDE; 4,4′-DDT and β-HCH were the most frequent OC detected in the umbilical cord blood of newborns. In a small number of cord blood samples, 4,4′DDT was identified. The presence of DDT in these samples can be related to the newborn difficulty in metabolizing 4,4′-DDT into 4,4′-DDE [28]. Although the presence and concentration of ΣDDT are decreasing with the age, some residues can be found even in some young mothers due to transference from parents and even grandparents [16]. In the present study, only one mother's blood sample presented 4,4′-DDT and 4,4′-DDE simultaneously, and yielded a high ratio of 4,4′-DDT/4,4′-DDE (13.1). We also detected 4,4′-DDT in one breast milk sample. In this case, the 4,4′-DDT/4,4′-DDE ratio was 0.16. Mekonen and colleagues [21] observed higher 4,4′-DDT/4,4′-DDE ratios (varying from 0.66 to 0.81, according to specific locations) in Ethiopian breast milk samples than those observed in the present study. According to Cohn et al. [29], this ratio could indicate recent commercial DDT exposure. Organochlorine pesticides (α- and β-endosulfan; 4,4′ and 4,4′DDD; 2,4′ and 4,4′-DDE, 2,4′-DDT; α-, β-, δ- and γ-HCH; cis-chlordane and trans-chlordane, mirex, methoxychlor, dieldrin and heptachlor) were measured in polyurethane foam (PUF) disks used as passive air samplers in 10 sampling sites surrounding the Guanabara Bay [7]. Surfaces of particulate matter, fine soil particles and resuspended dust represent important environmental exposure sources of pollutants to humans and could be integrated by exposed PUF disks as well as semi-volatile forms of OC. These environmental compartments could be sampled using PUF by diffusion according to the second Fick's Law of diffusion.

Our results demonstrated that elevated levels of ΣDDT were correlated positively with Apgar scores of 8 or less; while the mothers' age, BMI and race showed no correlations. The influence of prenatal exposure to DDT and DDE in children's neurodevelopmental development and the consequence of this exposure during childhood has been reported [15]. However, the influence of in utero exposure to DDT and DDE on Apgar scores is not fully understood.

Compared with similar studies, the concentration of 4,4'DDE found in this study was lower than that observed in pregnant women from Rio de Janeiro by Sarcinelli et al. [18], but similar to those reported by Bastos and colleagues [30]. However, the OCP concentrations reported by Sarcinelli et al. [18] were determined in blood samples collected from pregnant women between 1997 and 1998, when these substances were still being used in Brazil in campaigns for the control of vector-borne diseases. The study conducted by Bastos et al. [30] was conducted one decade later, after the prohibition of OCPs use in Brazil, and the women enrolled in their study were more likely exposed to levels of OCPs quite similar to those found currently.

A comparison with studies conducted in other countries, that did not correct the OCPs concentrations by the total blood lipid content, showed that the concentrations of 4,4'-DDE observed in our study were lower than those reported in the Arctic region of Russia, Salta and Ushuaia localities (North and South regions, respectively), Argentina, and in healthy pregnant women from Algarve region, South Portugal [31–33]. However, levels of 4,4'-DDT and 4,4'-DDD in the umbilical cord blood samples were higher in our study than those observed in studies conducted in Spain [28]. Overall, these results may suggest that the exposure of pregnant women and their newborns to DDT may be declining.

Similarly, in our study, β-HCH concentrations in maternal blood were lower than those observed in Argentina and Russia [31,32], but higher than those observed in Spain [28], while the concentration of γ-HCH was higher than that found in Russia [31]. In the umbilical cord blood samples, we observed β-HCH concentrations lower than those found in a study conducted in Canada [34], but higher than in Spain [28]. According to ATSDR [35], commercial lindane refers to products with more than 99% of γ-HCH. Among the HCH isomers, β-HCH presents slow-elimination kinetics and produces adverse effects such as red blood cell decrease, hemoglobin reduction and unconsciousness.

Due to the abandonment of large amounts of technical-grade HCH waste in the metropolitan area of Rio de Janeiro in the 60s, non-occupational exposure to organochlorines has been frequently reported [36]. Additionally, OCPs were used in public health campaigns to control leishmaniasis in endemic areas of Rio de Janeiro City until the 1990s [37]. Although, the majority of studies conducted in Rio de Janeiro did not describe the location of the participants' residences [4,30]. In our study, levels of ΣDDT, ΣHCH, ΣOCP, ΣPOP, and ΣPCB did not differ statistically regarding the mother's area of residence. These results may be due to the small number of samples with detectable levels of OCPs in this study. In the Rio Birth Cohort study, when 1000 pregnant women are expected to be enrolled, we may have enough statistical power to identify differences in organochlorine exposure based on the location of the mother's residence, which may help to identify possible sources of organochlorine exposure in the city of Rio de Janeiro.

In general, the concentrations of PCBs observed in the umbilical cord samples were similar to those observed in previous studies conducted in Rio de Janeiro; however, they were lower than those observed in a study conducted in the southern Brazilian city of Santa Maria [38]. PCB 138, 153, and 170 quantified in blood cord samples are congeners containing chlorine substitution at 2,2' positions, an important chemical property that decreases the enzymatic metabolism rate once compared with non-2,2' substituted PCB [38]. This characteristic also results in a higher trophic magnification observed in various studies worldwide. ATSDR [39] also points out that PCB 138 and 153 are the most prevalent congeners in human milk samples.

Socioeconomic and demographic characteristics have been positively correlated with OCP and PCB levels in maternal and umbilical cord blood in some epidemiological studies. For example, older pregnant women had the highest OCP concentration in several studies [31,32]. This study confirms this, as the level of DDT in blood, and its frequency, are proportional to age; older women (≥ 40 years) showed a higher incidence (77%) and higher levels of DDT in their blood. This result is expected because DDT was used extensively in Brazil until the 80s [4].

In the current study, participants with a BMI ≥ 30 also showed higher, though not statistically significant, concentrations of DDT in their blood. Few studies have evaluated robust associations between DDT and adiposity because the population's detection rate is generally low. La Merril and colleagues [40] observed DDT and their metabolites summed were significantly associated with increased adiposity in confounder-adjusted models. This study's detection rate for DDT and metabolites was above 90%. However, this association is inconsistent in birth cohort studies, and the differences in the detection rates among them may have impacted the estimates [41–44].

Generally, we observed that 4,4'-DDE concentration in breast milk in the 1st month was lower than in the 3rd and 6th-month follow-up. However, we observed an increase of 4,4'-DDE for 67% of mothers' paired samples with at least two follow-ups of three. In the same way, Lakind et al. [45] observed that in paired samples of breast milk for months 1–3 postpartum, concentrations of 4,4'-DDE inconsistently decreased during lactation, and increased for 71% of women. Yu et al. [46] found no differences between organochlorine levels in colostrum (obtained until the fifth day postpartum) and those in mature milk samples (after 14 days). There is no consensus on the relationship between educational level, income and blood concentrations of organochlorines. Controversial associations have been reported for food intake, especially seafood and fish, and high income and educational levels [47,48]. According to the Brazilian Institute of Geography and Statistics [49], the average household income in Brazil between 2017–2018 was approximately USD 1000 monthly (R$ 5500/month). In the current study, the majority of the families received less than the Brazilian minimum salary (currently about R$ USD 200/month); so, at least 32% of the studied pregnant women were classified as poor or very poor. Our results showed that the $\sum$DDT was higher among women with a monthly income lower than R$ 1733 (USD 315), but this difference was not statistically significant.

DDT residues and HQ have been calculated in breast milk samples in Brazilian studies. For example, Sant'ana et al. [50] analyzed human milk samples collected from rural and urban areas in Botucatu City, Brazil. The values expressed in whole milk varied from 1.0 to 101.2 µg of total DDT (expressed as op'-DDT+pp'-DDT+pp'-DDD)/L, and from 1.0 to 62.1 µg of total DDT (expressed as pp'-DDE)/L from mothers living in urban and rural areas, respectively. Once adjusted for 4% of lipid, these contamination values yielded HQ values varying from 0.14 in rural and urban areas to 14.168 for urban area mothers according to the FAO/WHO, and from 0.28 to 28.34 according to IRIS EPA calculations. It is important to highlight that the article was published in the 1980s, the same decade that DDT got banned in Brazil. Matuo et al. [51] analyzed colostrum obtained from 32 mothers living in Ribeirão Preto City, Brazil, in 1983 and 1984. The mean and higher total DDT obtained by the authors presented HQ values (3.5 and 9.52 according to FAO/WHO, and 7 and 19.4 according to IRIS EPA estimation, respectively) higher than one, and represented risk through breast milk consumption, also considering 4% of lipid in the whole milk. Other HQ values from studies around the world are shown in Table S2. In our study, the calculated HQ points out that milk consumption could not be considered safe for just one infant, and suggests that breastfeeding must be encouraged once breast milk is considered a safe and nutritionally appropriate food for children. Based on the contamination levels of $\sum$DDT in our analyzed milk samples, breastfeeding benefits outweigh the risks.

Our study observed positive and strong correlations between $\sum$DDT, $\sum$OCP, and $\sum$OC in maternal and cord blood samples. These results were expected, as the summation of OC and OCP included the sum of all DDT metabolites. However, there were no correlations between maternal and cord blood for all organochlorine metabolites that could indicate a substantial transfer of these substances by the placenta; although, studies have shown that the OCs transfer from the mother to the fetus [52,53]. Additionally, no correlations were found between maternal blood and breast milk samples, which could indicate the transfer of such compounds to infants by breastfeeding. However, correlation analyses were performed with a small sample size, and the results can be imprecise. In fact, we recognize the small sample size in our study as a limitation, as it could have affected most of bivariate and multivariate analyses, such as the regression ones.

The OCP and PCB concentrations in plasma samples were reported per unit volume of serum (ng/mL), not per unit volume of serum adjusted for the lipid content, and thus, comparisons of OCP and PCB concentrations were made possible, while other studies were limited to those that used the same unit of concentration.

5. Conclusions

Our results showed that pregnant women and their newborns are exposed to several persistent organic pollutants, even after decades of their banishment in Brazil. Although detection rates and concentrations of the majority of OCPs and PCBs were low, it is possible to state that pregnant women and their newborns living in a metropolitan area of Rio de Janeiro City are exposed to these substances, and the knowledge of their impact on childhood development is still a question to be solved.

Due to the potentially harmful effects of these substances on human reproduction and development, exposure to OCPs and PCBs, especially in vulnerable groups, such as pregnant women, women intending to conceive and newborns, need to be investigated in a larger population sample. Future results from the Rio Birth Cohort (PIPA study) certainly will allow us to confirm some associations observed in this pilot study, especially those between OCPs and age, BMI and Apgar score.

Supplementary Materials: The following supporting information can be downloaded at: https://www.mdpi.com/article/10.3390/ijerph20010778/s1, Table S1: Calibration parameters and limits for OCs and PCBs; Table S2: Estimated HQ from breast milk described in the literature. References [21–23,54–58] are cited in the supplementary materials.

Author Contributions: Conceptualization, A.M., C.I.R.F.A. and A.S.E.S.; methodology, A.M., A.S.E.S., C.I.R.F.A. and A.C.S.R.; formal analysis, A.M., J.C.M., A.A., A.C.S.R. and A.S.E.S.; investigation, A.M., C.I.R.F.A. and A.S.E.S.; data curation, A.M. and C.I.R.F.A.; writing—original draft preparation, A.M., J.C.M., A.A. and A.S.E.S.; writing—review and editing, A.M., A.S.E.S., C.I.R.F.A., J.C.M., A.A., V.M.C. and A.C.S.R.; supervision, A.M.; project administration, C.I.R.F.A., V.M.C., and A.M.; funding acquisition, C.I.R.F.A. All authors have read and agreed to the published version of the manuscript.

Funding: This research was funded by the Surveillance Health Secretary (Grant No. 733663/19-002), Science and Technology Department (Grant No. 404168/2019-1), CNPq—National Council for Scientific and Technological Development (Grant No. 409275/2018-2), and the Carlos Chagas Filho Foundation for Supporting Research in the State of Rio de Janeiro (Grant No. E-26/010.001894/2019).

Institutional Review Board Statement: The study was conducted in accordance with the Declaration of Helsinki and approved by the Ethics Committee of the Maternity School, Federal University of Rio de Janeiro (protocol 2.092.440).

Informed Consent Statement: Informed consent was obtained from all subjects involved in the study.

Data Availability Statement: Data supporting the reported results are stored with the corresponding author and is available upon request.

Conflicts of Interest: The authors declare no conflict of interest.

References

1. Longnecker, M.P.; Rogan, W.J.; Lucier, G. The human health effects of ddt (dichlorodiphenyltrichloroethane) and pcbs (polychlorinated biphenyls) and an overview of organochlorines in public health. *Annu. Rev. Public Health* **1997**, *18*, 211–244. [CrossRef] [PubMed]
2. Robertson, L.W.; Weber, R.; Nakano, T.; Johansson, N. PCBs risk evaluation, environmental protection, and management: 50-year research and counting for elimination by 2028. *Environ. Sci. Pollut. Res.* **2018**, *25*, 16269–16276. [CrossRef]
3. Brazil—Ministry of the Environment. *National Implementation Plan Brazil: Convention Stockholm*; Ministry of the Environment: Brasília, Brazil, 2015.
4. Delgado, I.F.; Barretto, H.H.; Kussumi, T.A.; Alleluia, I.B.; Baggio, C.D.A.; Paumgartten, F.J.R. Serum levels of organochlorine pesticides and polychlorinated biphenyls among inhabitants of Greater Metropolitan Rio de Janeiro, Brazil. *Cad. Saúde Pública* **2002**, *18*, 519–524. [CrossRef] [PubMed]
5. Ricking, M.; Schwarzbauer, J. DDT isomers and metabolites in the environment: An overview. *Environ. Chem. Lett.* **2012**, *10*, 317–323. [CrossRef]
6. Ferreira, V.B.; Estrella, L.F.; Alves, M.G.R.; Gallistl, C.; Vetter, W.; Silva, T.T.C.; Malm, O.; Torres, J.P.M.; Finco, F.D.B.A. Residues of legacy organochlorine pesticides and DDT metabolites in highly consumed fish from the polluted Guanabara Bay, Brazil: Distribution and assessment of human health risk. *J. Environ. Sci. Health Part B* **2020**, *55*, 30–41. [CrossRef] [PubMed]
7. Guida, Y.; de Carvalho, G.O.; Capella, R.; Pozo, K.; Lino, A.S.; Azeredo, A.; Carvalho, D.F.P.; Braga, A.L.F.; Torres, J.P.M.; Meire, R.O. Atmospheric Occurrence of Organochlorine Pesticides and Inhalation Cancer Risk in Urban Areas at Southeast Brazil. *Environ. Pollut.* **2021**, *271*, 116359. [CrossRef]
8. Ródio, G.R.; Rosset, I.G.; Brandalize, A.P.C. Pesticides exposure and consequences to human health. *Res. Soc. Dev.* **2021**, *10*, e43010817526. [CrossRef]
9. Bhatt, R.V. Environmental influence on reproductive health. *Int. J. Gynecol. Obstet.* **2000**, *70*, 69–75. [CrossRef]
10. Makri, A.; Goveia, M.; Balbus, J.; Parkin, R. Children's susceptibility to chemicals: A review by developmental stage. *J. Toxicol. Environ. Health Part B* **2004**, *7*, 417–435. [CrossRef]
11. Woodruff, T.J.; Zota, A.; Schwartz, J.M. Environmental Chemicals in Pregnant Women in the United States: NHANES 2003–2004. *Environ. Health Perspect.* **2011**, *119*, 878–885. [CrossRef]
12. Covaci, A.; Jorens, P.; Jacquemyn, Y.; Schepens, P. Distribution of PCBs and organochlorine pesticides in umbilical cord and maternal serum. *Sci. Total Environ.* **2002**, *298*, 45–53. [CrossRef]
13. Heck, M.; dos Santos, J.S.; Junior, S.B.; Costabeber, I.; Emanuelli, T. Estimation of children exposure to organochlorine compounds through milk in Rio Grande do Sul, Brazil. *Food Chem.* **2007**, *102*, 288–294. [CrossRef]
14. Sagiv, S.K.; Tolbert, P.E.; Altshul, L.M.; Korrick, S.A. Organochlorine Exposures During Pregnancy and Infant Size at Birth. *Epidemiology* **2007**, *18*, 120–129. [CrossRef] [PubMed]
15. Eskenazi, B.; Marks, A.R.; Bradman, A.; Fenster, L.; Johnson, C.; Barr, D.B.; Jewell, N.P. In Utero Exposure to Dichlorodiphenyltrichloroethane (DDT) and Dichlorodiphenyldichloroethylene (DDE) and Neurodevelopment Among Young Mexican American Children. *Pediatrics* **2006**, *118*, 233–241. [CrossRef] [PubMed]
16. Cirillo, P.M.; La Merrill, M.A.; Krigbaum, N.Y.; Cohn, B.A. Grandmaternal Perinatal Serum DDT in Relation to Granddaughter Early Menarche and Adult Obesity: Three Generations in the Child Health and Development Studies Cohort. *Cancer Epidemiol. Biomark. Prev.* **2021**, *30*, 1480–1488. [CrossRef]
17. Asmus, C.I.R.F.; Barbosa, A.P.; Meyer, A.; Damasceno, N.; Rosa, A.C.S.; Medronho, R.; Da Cunha, A.J.L.A.; Moreira, J.C.; Fernandes, T.V.R.D.B.; Martins, M.; et al. Rio Birth Cohort Study on Environmental Exposure and Childhood Development—PIPA Project. *Ann. Glob. Health* **2020**, *86*, 59. [CrossRef] [PubMed]
18. Sarcinelli, P.N.; Pereira, A.C.S.; Mesquita, S.A.; Oliveira-Silva, J.J.; Meyer, A.; Menezes, M.A.; Alves, S.R.; Mattos, R.C.; Moreira, J.C.; Wolff, M. Dietary and reproductive determinants of plasma organochlorine levels in pregnant women in Rio de Janeiro. *Environ. Res.* **2003**, *91*, 143–150. [CrossRef]
19. Environmental Protection Agency (EPA). *Method 8081B Organochlorine Pesticides by Gas Chromatography*; Revision; Environmental Protection Agency: Washington, DC, USA, 2007.
20. INMETRO. *Orientação sobre Validação de Métodos Analíticos. Documento de caráter orientativo, Pub. L. No. DOQ-CGCRE-008 Revisão*; National Institute of Metrology Standardization and Industrial Quality: Rio de Janeiro, Brazil, 2020.
21. Mekonen, S.; Ambelu, A.; Wondafrash, M.; Kolsteren, P.; Spanoghe, P. Exposure of infants to organochlorine pesticides from breast milk consumption in southwestern Ethiopia. *Sci. Rep.* **2021**, *11*, 22053. [CrossRef]
22. Azeredo, A.; Torres, J.P.; Fonseca, M.D.F.; Britto, J.L.; Bastos, W.R.; e Silva, C.E.A.; Cavalcanti, G.; Meire, R.O.; Sarcinelli, P.N.; Claudio, L.; et al. DDT and its metabolites in breast milk from the Madeira River basin in the Amazon, Brazil. *Chemosphere* **2008**, *73*, S246–S251. [CrossRef]
23. Souza, R.C.; Portella, R.B.; Almeida, P.V.N.B.; Pinto, C.O.; Gubert, P.; Da Silva, J.D.S.; Nakamura, T.C.; Rego, E.L.D. Human milk contamination by nine organochlorine pesticide residues (OCPs). *J. Environ. Sci. Health Part B* **2020**, *55*, 530–538. [CrossRef] [PubMed]
24. IRIS—Integrated Risk Information System. *p,p'-Dichlorodiphenyltrichloroethane (DDT) (CASRN 50-29-3)*; EPA—U.S. Environmental Protection Agency, National Center for Environmental Assessment: Washington, DC, USA, 1987.

25. Zhou, P.; Wu, Y.; Yin, S.; Li, J.; Zhao, Y.; Zhang, L.; Chen, H.; Liu, Y.; Yang, X.; Li, X. National survey of the levels of persistent organochlorine pesticides in the breast milk of mothers in China. *Environ. Pollut.* **2011**, *159*, 524–531. [CrossRef] [PubMed]
26. Lu, D.; Wang, D.; Ni, R.; Lin, Y.; Feng, C.; Xu, Q.; Jia, X.; Wang, G.; Zhou, Z. Organochlorine pesticides and their metabolites in human breast milk from Shanghai, China. *Environ. Sci. Pollut. Res.* **2015**, *22*, 9293–9306. [CrossRef]
27. Kuang, L.; Hou, Y.; Huang, F.; Hong, H.; Sun, H.; Deng, W.; Lin, H. Pesticide residues in breast milk and the associated risk assessment: A review focused on China. *Sci. Total Environ.* **2020**, *727*, 138412. [CrossRef]
28. Junqué, E.; Garcia, S.; Martínez, M.; Rovira, J.; Schuhmacher, M.; Grimalt, J.O. Changes of organochlorine compound concentrations in maternal serum during pregnancy and comparison to serum cord blood composition. *Environ. Res.* **2020**, *182*, 108994. [CrossRef]
29. Cohn, B.A.; Cirillo, P.M.; Christianson, R.E. Prenatal DDT Exposure and Testicular Cancer: A Nested Case-Control Study. *Arch. Environ. Occup. Health* **2010**, *65*, 127–134. [CrossRef] [PubMed]
30. Bastos, A.M.X.; De Souza, M.D.C.B.; Filho, G.L.D.A.; Krauss, T.M.; Pavesi, T.; Silva, L.E. Organochlorine compound levels in fertile and infertile women from Rio de Janeiro, Brazil. *Arq. Bras. Endocrinol. Metabol.* **2013**, *57*, 346–353. [CrossRef] [PubMed]
31. Bravo, N.; Grimalt, J.O.; Chashchin, M.; Chashchin, V.P.; Odland, J. Drivers of maternal accumulation of organohalogen pollutants in Arctic areas (Chukotka, Russia) and 4,4'-DDT effects on the newborns. *Environ. Int.* **2019**, *124*, 541–552. [CrossRef]
32. Bravo, N.; Hansen, S.; Økland, I.; Garí, M.; Álvarez, M.V.; Matiocevich, S.; Odland, J.; Grimalt, J.O. Influence of maternal and sociodemographic characteristics on the accumulation of organohalogen compounds in Argentinian women. The EMASAR study. *Environ. Res.* **2017**, *158*, 759–767. [CrossRef]
33. Lopes, B.; Arrebola, J.; Serafim, A.; Company, R.; Rosa, J.; Olea, N. Polychlorinated biphenyls (PCBs) and p,p'-dichlorodiphenyldichloroethylene (DDE) concentrations in maternal and umbilical cord serum in a human cohort from South Portugal. *Chemosphere* **2014**, *114*, 291–302. [CrossRef]
34. Walker, J.B.; Seddon, L.; McMullen, E.; Houseman, J.; Tofflemire, K.; Corriveau, A.; Weber, J.-P.; Mills, C.; Smith, S.; Van Oostdam, J. Organochlorine levels in maternal and umbilical cord blood plasma in Arctic Canada. *Sci. Total Environ.* **2003**, *302*, 27–52. [CrossRef]
35. *ATSDR: Toxicological Profile for Hexachlorocyclohexanes*; United States of America Department of Health and Human Services, Public Health Service, Agency for Toxic Substances and Disease Registry: Washington, DC, USA, 2005.
36. Asmus, C.I.R.F.; Alonzo, H.G.A.; Palácios, M.; da Silva, A.P.; Filhote, M.I.D.F.; Buosi, D.; Câmara, V.D.M. Assessment of human health risk from organochlorine pesticide residues in Cidade dos Meninos, Duque de Caxias, Rio de Janeiro, Brazil. *Cad. Saude Publica* **2008**, *24*, 755–766. [CrossRef] [PubMed]
37. Vieira, E.D.; Torres, J.P.; Malm, O. DDT Environmental Persistence from Its Use in a Vector Control Program: A Case Study. *Environ. Res.* **2001**, *86*, 174–182. [CrossRef]
38. Mohr, S.; dos Santos, J.S.; Schwanz, T.G.; Wagner, R.; Mozzaquatro, J.O.; Lorenzoni, A.S.; Costabeber, I.H. Polychlorinated biphenyls in umbilical cord serum of newborns from Rio Grande do Sul state, Brazil. *Clin. Chim. Acta* **2015**, *451*, 323–328. [CrossRef] [PubMed]
39. *ATSDR: Addendum to the Toxicological Profile for Polychlorinated Biphenyls*; United States of America Department of Health and Human Services, Public Health Service, Agency for Toxic Substances and Disease Registry: Washington, DC, USA, 2011.
40. La Merrill, M.A.; Johnson, C.L.; Smith, M.T.; Kandula, N.R.; Macherone, A.; Pennell, K.D.; Kanaya, A.M. Exposure to persistent organic pollutants (POPs) and their relationship to hepatic fat and insulin insensitivity among Asian Indian immigrants in the United States. *Environ. Sci. Technol.* **2019**, *53*, 13906–13918. [CrossRef]
41. Valvi, D.; Mendez, M.A.; Martinez, D.; Grimalt, J.; Torrent, M.; Sunyer, J.; Vrijheid, M. Prenatal Concentrations of Polychlorinated Biphenyls, DDE, and DDT and Overweight in Children: A Prospective Birth Cohort Study. *Environ. Health Perspect.* **2012**, *120*, 451–457. [CrossRef] [PubMed]
42. Warner, M.; Rauch, S.; Coker, E.S.; Harley, K.; Kogut, K.; Sjödin, A.; Eskenazi, B. Obesity in relation to serum persistent organic pollutant concentrations in CHAMACOS women. *Environ. Epidemiol.* **2018**, *2*, e032. [CrossRef]
43. Gladen, B.C.; Klebanoff, M.A.; Hediger, M.L.; Katz, S.H.; Barr, D.B.; Davis, M.D.; Longnecker, M. Prenatal DDT Exposure in Relation to Anthropometric and Pubertal Measures in Adolescent Males. *Environ. Health Perspect.* **2004**, *112*, 1761–1767. [CrossRef]
44. Cupul-Uicab, L.A.; Klebanoff, M.A.; Brock, J.W.; Longnecker, M.P. Prenatal Exposure to Persistent Organochlorines and Childhood Obesity in the U.S. Collaborative Perinatal Project. *Environ. Health Perspect.* **2013**, *121*, 1103–1109. [CrossRef]
45. LaKind, J.S.; Berlin, C.M.; Sjödin, A.; Turner, W.; Wang, R.Y.; Needham, L.L.; Paul, I.M.; Stokes, J.L.; Naiman, D.Q.; Patterson, D.G. Do Human Milk Concentrations of Persistent Organic Chemicals Really Decline During Lactation? Chemical Concentrations During Lactation and Milk/Serum Partitioning. *Environ. Health Perspect.* **2009**, *117*, 1625–1631. [CrossRef]
46. Yu, Z.; Palkovicova, L.; Drobna, B.; Petrik, J.; Kocan, A.; Trnovec, T.; Hertz-Picciotto, I. Comparison of organochlorine compound concentrations in colostrum and mature milk. *Chemosphere* **2007**, *66*, 1012–1018. [CrossRef]
47. Veyhe, A.S.; Hofoss, D.; Hansen, S.; Thomassen, Y.; Sandanger, T.M.; Odland, J.; Nieboer, E. The Northern Norway Mother-and-Child Contaminant Cohort (MISA) Study: PCA analyses of environmental contaminants in maternal sera and dietary intake in early pregnancy. *Int. J. Hyg. Environ. Health* **2015**, *218*, 254–264. [CrossRef] [PubMed]
48. Cao, L.-L.; Yan, C.-H.; Yu, X.-D.; Tian, Y.; Zhao, L.; Liu, J.-X.; Shen, X.-M. Relationship between serum concentrations of polychlorinated biphenyls and organochlorine pesticides and dietary habits of pregnant women in Shanghai. *Sci. Total Environ.* **2011**, *409*, 2997–3002. [CrossRef] [PubMed]

49. Brazil—Brazilian Institute of Statistics and Geography. *Family Budget Survey 2017–2018*; Brazilian Institute of Statistics and Geography: Rio de Janeiro, Brazil, 2019; ISBN 978-85-240-4505-9. Available online: https://biblioteca.ibge.gov.br/index.php/bibliotecacatalogo?view=detalhes&id=2101749 (accessed on 2 November 2022).
50. Sant'Ana, L.S.; Vassilieff, I.; Jokl, L. Levels of organochlorine insecticides in milk of mothers from urban and rural areas of botucatu, SP, Brazil. *Bull. Environ. Contam. Toxicol.* **1989**, *42*, 911–918. [CrossRef]
51. Matuo, Y.K.; Lopes, J.N.C.; Casanova, I.C.; Matuo, T. Organochlorine pesticide residues in human milk in the Ribeirão Preto region, state of São Paulo, Brazil. *Arch. Environ. Contam. Toxicol.* **1992**, *22*, 167–175. [CrossRef] [PubMed]
52. Zhang, X.; Wu, X.; Lei, B.; Jing, Y.; Jiang, Z.; Zhang, X.; Fang, X.; Yu, Y. Transplacental transfer characteristics of organochlorine pesticides in paired maternal and cord sera, and placentas and possible influencing factors. *Environ. Pollut.* **2018**, *233*, 446–454. [CrossRef] [PubMed]
53. Yin, S.; Zhang, J.; Guo, F.; Zhao, L.; Poma, G.; Covaci, A.; Liu, W. Transplacental transfer of organochlorine pesticides: Concentration ratio and chiral properties. *Environ. Int.* **2019**, *130*, 104939. [CrossRef]
54. Bedi, J.S.; Gill, J.P.S.; Aulakh, R.S.; Kaur, P.; Sharma, A.; Pooni, P.A. Pesticide residues in human breast milk: Risk assessment for infants from Punjab, India. *Sci. Total Environ.* **2013**, *463–464*, 720–726. [CrossRef]
55. Czaja, K.; Ludwicki, J.K.; Góralcyk, K.; Strucinski, P. Effect of age and number of deliveries on mean concentration of organochlorine compounds in human breast milk in Poland. *Bull. Environ. Contam. Toxicol.* **1997**, *59*, 407–413. [CrossRef]
56. Çoc, I.; Bilgili, A.; Özdemir, M.; Özbek, H.; Bilgili, N.; Burgaz, S. Organochlorine pesticide residues in human breast milk from agricultural regions of Turkey, 1996–1996. *Bull. Environ. Contam. Toxicol.* **1997**, *59*, 577–582. [CrossRef]
57. Rogan, W.J.; Gladen, B.C.; McKinney, J.D.; Carrera, N.; Hardy, P.; Thullen, J.; Tingelstad, J.; Tully, M. Polychlorinated biphenyls (PCBs) and dichlorodiphenyl dichloroethene in human milk: Effects on growth, morbity, and duration of lactation. *Am. J. Public Health* **1987**, *77*, 1294–1297. [CrossRef]
58. Bates, M.N.; Hannah, D.J.; Buckland, S.J.; Taucher, J.A.; van Maanen, T. Chlorinated organic contaminants in breast milk of New Zealand women. *Environ. Health Perspect.* **1994**, *102*, 211–217. [CrossRef] [PubMed]

Disclaimer/Publisher's Note: The statements, opinions and data contained in all publications are solely those of the individual author(s) and contributor(s) and not of MDPI and/or the editor(s). MDPI and/or the editor(s) disclaim responsibility for any injury to people or property resulting from any ideas, methods, instructions or products referred to in the content.

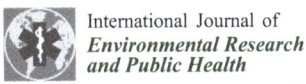

International Journal of *Environmental Research and Public Health*

Article

Exposure to Inorganic Arsenic in Rice in Brazil: A Human Health Risk Assessment

Michele C. Toledo [1,*], Janice S. Lee [2], Bruno L. Batista [3], Kelly P. K. Olympio [1] and Adelaide C. Nardocci [1]

1. School of Public Health, University of São Paulo, São Paulo 01246-904, Brazil
2. United States Environmental Protection Agency, Research Triangle Park, NC 27711, USA
3. Center for Natural and Human Sciences, Federal University of the ABC, Santo André 09210-580, Brazil
* Correspondence: michele.toledo@alumni.usp.br

Abstract: In certain populations, rice is the main source of exposure to inorganic arsenic (iAs), which is associated with cancer and non-cancer effects. Although rice is a staple food in Brazil, there have been few studies about the health risks for the Brazilian population. The objective of this study was to assess the risks of exposure to iAs from white rice and brown rice in Brazil, in terms of the carcinogenic and non-carcinogenic effects, and to propose measures to mitigate those risks. The incremental lifetime cancer risk (ILCR) and hazard quotient (HQ) were calculated in a probabilistic framework. The mean ILCR was 1.5×10^{-4} for white rice and 6.0×10^{-6} for brown rice. The HQ for white and brown rice was under 1. The ILCR for white and brown rice was high, even though the iAs concentration in rice is below the maximum contaminant level. The risk for brown rice consumption was lower, which was not expected. Various mitigation measures discussed in this report are estimated to reduce the risk from rice consumption by 5–67%. With the support of public policies, measures to reduce these risks for the Brazilian population would have a positive impact on public health.

Keywords: probabilistic risk assessment; hazard quotient; Monte Carlo; dietary exposure risk; mitigation measure; food contaminants

1. Introduction

Although arsenic exists in various chemical forms, it is mainly categorized, from a public health perspective, as organic or inorganic. These different forms occur naturally in the environment, and anthropogenic activities can substantially increase their concentration and bioavailability in soil and water, allowing them to be absorbed by plants in agricultural fields. Inorganic arsenic (iAs) is classified as a Group 1 carcinogen and is present in trace amounts in rocks, soil, air, food, and water [1,2]. Food and water are the most important sources of exposure to iAs, and rice (*Oryza sativa*) is the main source of exposure in some populations [3,4]. Rice is usually cultivated in flooded fields, where the anaerobic conditions increase iAs availability in soils. Arsenate is reduced to the more mobile arsenite, leading to a higher concentration of both forms close to the plant roots. Arsenate and arsenite are analogues of the plant micronutrients phosphate and silicic acid, respectively, therefore being easily taken up and stored by the plant. Fertilizers, pesticides, and the water used to irrigate the crops can also be sources of iAs [5,6].

Rice is a staple food for more than half of the world population, accounting for approximately 30% of the energy intake and 20% of the protein intake; it can, therefore, be a significant source of iAs and other metals [7–9]. The European Food Safety Authority has recognized rice as the main source of iAs for the European population [10]. In Asia, rice is also a staple food and tends to be the major source of iAs from food [11]. In a study conducted in China [12], the concentrations of iAs and other metals in rice were found to be above the maximum contaminant levels (MCLs) of 200 ng g^{-1} established by the United Nations Food and Agriculture Organization and the World Health Organization (FAO/WHO).

In Brazil, rice is one of the main components of daily meals and is consumed by the entire population, regardless of socioeconomic status. According to a national study conducted by the Brazilian Institute of Geography and Statistics, the average daily consumption of rice by adults is estimated to be 167 g [13], which is comparable to that reported for some locations in China [14]. Rice consumption accounts for 46–79% of the iAs ingested by the Brazilian population [15].

Epidemiological studies have shown that exposure to iAs is associated with cancer of the lung, bladder, kidney, skin, liver, and prostate [2]. The non-cancer effects from long-term oral exposure to iAs include dermal, cardiovascular, respiratory, and neurodevelopmental changes, and acute high-dose oral exposure has been associated with nausea, vomiting, diarrhea, and encephalopathy [16]. The susceptible life stages are pregnancy, infancy, and early childhood [4]. The Joint FAO/WHO Expert Committee on Food Additives recognizes iAs in rice as a public health concern [17], and quantitative risk assessment has been considered an important tool for risk management and to support decision-making in public health [18].

Only a few studies have evaluated exposure to iAs in rice in Brazil [15,19–24]. In the present study, we focused on a probabilistic analysis of the risk of exposure to iAs in polished (white) and husked (brown) rice from Brazil. Hypothetical scenarios of risk reduction were also assessed. Cancer and non-cancer risks were estimated using the slope factor and the U.S. Environmental Protection Agency (EPA) reference dose for iAs [25].

2. Materials and Methods

2.1. Average Daily Dose, Cancer Risk, and Hazard Quotient

The average daily dose by exposure pathway, which can account for differences between the age group of the exposed people regarding exposure factors such as body weight and eating habits, was estimated according to the following equation [26]:

$$ADD_j = \frac{[C \times IR_j \times ED_j \times EF_j]}{[BW_j \times AT]} \quad (1)$$

where ADD_j is the average daily dose in mg/kg-day estimated for the age group j; C is the concentration of iAs in raw rice (mg iAs/g rice); IR_j is the ingestion rate of rice (g rice/day) for the age group j; ED_j and EF_j are the exposure duration (years) and exposure frequency (days/year) for the age group j, respectively; BW_j is the body weight for the age group j; and AT is the average time, which is the $ED_j \times 365$ days.

As the exposure varies with age, the incremental lifetime cancer risk (ILCR) was estimated by summing the cancer risk in each age group [27], as follows:

$$ILCR = \sum_{j=1,n} (ADDj \times SF) \times \frac{ED_j}{LT} \quad (2)$$

where SF is the slope factor for oral iAs, which is 1.5 (mg/kg-day)$^{-1}$, LT is the lifetime, which is 70 years, and n is the number of age intervals. The ILCR estimates the incremental lifetime cancer risk for exposure to certain carcinogens. The result must be interpreted as a probability, represented as a value between 0 and 1. A risk of 10^{-5} indicates a probability of 1 chance in 100,000 of an individual developing cancer [26].

The risk of non-cancer effects (cardiovascular and dermal outcomes) was estimated by the hazard quotient (HQ) summing the fractional HQ of each age group, which is the $ADDj$ divided by the RfD weighted by exposure duration j:

$$HQ = \sum_{j=1,n} (\frac{ADD_j}{RfD}) \times \frac{ED_j}{LT} \quad (3)$$

where RfD is the reference dose for oral exposure to iAs, which is 0.003 mg/kg per day [25], and n is the number of age intervals. An HQ above 1 indicates that the average daily dose is higher than the reference dose, so there may be concern for potential noncancer effects.

The $ILCR$ and HQ calculations (Supplementary Material) were implemented in a probabilistic framework, with a Monte Carlo simulation of 100,000 iterations and with a confidence interval of 95%. The simulations were performed using distributions for the concentration of arsenic in rice. The probabilistic assessment was carried out in the open-source software YASAIw from the State of Washington Department of Ecology [28]. A limitation of this method is that the probabilistic analysis is an indirect measure of the risk.

2.2. Concentration of iAs in Brazilian Rice

The data related to the concentrations of iAs in white and brown rice (Supplementary Material) were obtained from a study conducted by Batista et al. [29], one of the few studies about iAs in rice from Brazil to which we had access. In that study, samples of raw rice were collected from different areas in Brazil, mainly the southern region, which is the largest rice-producing region in the country. There were 64 samples of white rice (all obtained from markets) and 90 samples of brown rice (69 from farms and 21 from markets). Firstly, the authors determined the total concentration of arsenic by microwave digestion of the rice samples, as described by Paniz et al. [30]. For this purpose, the samples were ground, sieved (<250 µm), and weighed (200 mg) in triplicate and then placed in 100-mL polytetrafluoroethylene vessels, where 4 mL of sub-distilled HNO_3 (20 vol%) and 1 mL of H_2O_2 (30 vol%) were added. The tubes were then placed in a microwave system (up to 35 bar). After cooling, ultrapure water was added to make up 50 mL, and then the samples were analyzed by inductively coupled plasma mass spectrometry (ICP-MS). Secondly, the concentration of arsenic chemical species was determined. The speciation analysis was performed as described by Batista et al. [19]. The samples, in two replicates, containing about 200-mg of ground and sieved (<250 µm) rice, were weighed into 50-mL conical tubes, treated with 10 mL of HNO_3 (2 vol%), and then stirred (100 rpm) for 24 h. In sequence, the tubes were heated (95 °C) in a water bath for 2.5 h. Finally, after cooling, the samples were analyzed using a high-performance liquid chromatography coupled to an ICP-MS. The concentration of iAs was considered the sum of the species arsenite and arsenate, and the concentration of organic arsenic was considered the sum of the species dimethyl arsenic and monomethyl arsenic. In this risk assessment, we only included iAs in the analysis.

2.3. Rice Consumption

The rice consumption for each age group, which includes only rice grain consumption (not rice-derived products, such as rice flour, present in certain kinds of food), was obtained from different sources, as also presented in Table S1 (Supplementary Material):

- From 4 months to 1 year and 5 to 10 years—the estimated rice consumption was based on the quantity recommended by the São Paulo Municipal Department of Education for consumption in schools and daycare centers [31,32]. Since we noticed that the recommended consumption was overestimated in comparison with the actual consumption for children 1 to 5 years of age (see below), we estimated that the actual rice consumption for children 4 months to 1 year and 5 to 10 years of age was 39.8% less than that. In the school diet, rice is served cooked (as a side dish, in soups, or as a dessert) and the quantities were registered in grams of raw rice. Students from 6 to 10 years of age have a part-time school period, having only one meal at school (lunch or dinner), and daily rice consumption for that age group was, therefore, estimated on the basis of the recommended quantity.
- From 1 to 5 years—data were obtained from a study involving 64 children at 2 daycare centers in the city of São Paulo [33], in which the portions of 24-h duplicate diet samples were recorded, including the food consumed at the daycare center and that consumed at home. The consumption of rice and soup containing rice was evaluated. Household measures (e.g., tablespoons) were converted to grams in accordance with nutrition guidelines [34,35].

- From 10 to 70 years—data were obtained from a study conducted by the Brazilian Institute of Geography and Statistics [13], in which the consumption of cooked rice in the last 48 h was determined on the basis of self-reports by interviewees in all Brazilian states, from 10 to 70 years.

Since there are no available data regarding daily consumption of brown rice in Brazil, the same rates were considered for white and brown rice.

2.4. Body Weight

Body weight was also obtained from the study conducted by the Brazilian Institute of Geography and Statistics [36]. Body weight was calculated by the weighted average of the male and female population, in relation to the total of interviewed individuals.

2.5. Exposure Frequency

Since rice is a staple food in Brazil, the exposure frequency (EF) for rice was considered to be 6 days/week (312.85 days/year).

2.6. Statistical Analysis

The statistical analysis was conducted with R software, version 3.5.0, and R studio, version 1.1.453 (The R Foundation for Statistical Computing, Vienna, Austria). We used the fitdistrplus package in order to fit the distribution of the iAs concentration datasets. The 64 white rice and 90 brown rice iAs concentrations from Batista et al. [29] were fit using the normal, lognormal and exponential distribution assumptions available in the fitdistrplus package. The distribution with the lowest Akaike information criterion value was selected. Pearson's correlation coefficient was calculated to identify a correlation between iAs and cadmium in rice as evidence of water management during rice cultivation.

Table S1 (Supplementary Material) summarizes the exposure parameters of body weight and rice dietary consumption rates for various age groups, obtained or estimated from the sources described above and adopted for the risk assessment.

The data for rice consumption and body weight did not have a good fit in any distribution, so to minimize the uncertainty, avoiding using mean values for the lifetime, the risk was assessed for age groups. The advantage of this approach is to obtain risk results for each age group, with it being possible to identify which is more vulnerable.

2.7. Hypothetical Scenarios of Risk Reduction

Adopting the same dose–response model for each of six different scenarios, we assessed hypothetical interventions intended to reduce the risk (Supplementary Material). The objective was to simulate the impact of different mitigation strategies, some of which were proposed by the U.S. Food and Drug Administration (FDA)—such as lowering the MCL or interrupting the exposure of infants and children—whereas others were based on our results.

3. Results

Figure 1 shows a box plot of iAs concentrations in white and brown rice. Table S2 shows the descriptive statistics (Supplementary Material). The normal distribution had the best fit for the white rice dataset (mean, 100.2 ± 44.6), whereas the log-normal distribution had the best fit for the brown rice data ($\mu = 4.1$; $\delta = 0.9$).

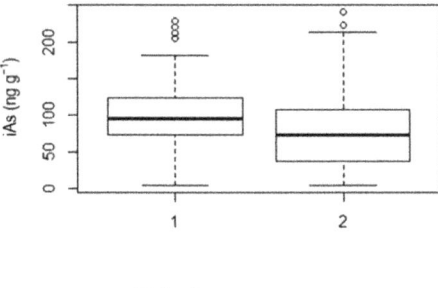

Figure 1. Box plot of inorganic arsenic (iAs) concentrations in polished (white) and husked (brown) rice.

3.1. Cancer Risk Associated with Exposure to iAs in Rice

Table 1 presents the results of cancer risk by age and ILCR, and Table S3 (Supplementary Material) presents the ADD by age. The mean and 95th percentiles of the total incremental lifetime cancer risk (ILCR) were 1.51×10^{-4} and 2.60×10^{-4} for white rice and 6.04×10^{-6} and 8.47×10^{-6} for brown rice. A limitation of this method is that it is not possible to determine the risk of a specific cancer, but the overall cancer related to exposure to iAs (liver, kidney, lung, bladder, and skin).

Table 1. Estimated incremental cancer risks and incremental lifetime cancer risk (means and 95th percentiles) associated with exposure to inorganic arsenic in polished (white) and husked (brown) rice.

Age (Years)	White Rice Cancer Risk and ILCR		Brown Rice Cancer Risk and ILCR	
	Mean	95th Percentile	Mean	95th Percentile
<1	1.62×10^{-6}	2.79×10^{-6}	6.47×10^{-8}	9.08×10^{-8}
1	9.19×10^{-6}	1.58×10^{-05}	3.66×10^{-7}	5.14×10^{-7}
2	7.39×10^{-6}	1.27×10^{-05}	2.95×10^{-7}	4.14×10^{-7}
3	7.23×10^{-6}	1.24×10^{-05}	2.88×10^{-7}	4.05×10^{-7}
4	7.02×10^{-6}	1.21×10^{-05}	2.80×10^{-7}	3.93×10^{-7}
5	5.52×10^{-6}	9.48×10^{-6}	2.20×10^{-7}	3.09×10^{-7}
6	5.09×10^{-6}	8.75×10^{-6}	2.03×10^{-7}	2.85×10^{-7}
7	4.52×10^{-6}	7.76×10^{-6}	1.80×10^{-7}	2.53×10^{-7}
8	4.07×10^{-6}	7.00×10^{-6}	1.62×10^{-7}	2.28×10^{-7}
9	3.56×10^{-6}	6.12×10^{-6}	1.42×10^{-7}	1.99×10^{-7}
10	3.12×10^{-6}	5.36×10^{-6}	1.24×10^{-7}	1.74×10^{-7}
11	2.77×10^{-6}	4.75×10^{-6}	1.10×10^{-7}	1.55×10^{-7}
12	2.45×10^{-6}	4.21×10^{-6}	9.76×10^{-08}	1.37×10^{-7}
13	2.21×10^{-6}	3.80×10^{-6}	8.82×10^{-08}	1.24×10^{-7}
14	2.06×10^{-6}	3.54×10^{-6}	8.21×10^{-08}	1.15×10^{-7}
15	1.92×10^{-6}	3.30×10^{-6}	7.66×10^{-08}	1.07×10^{-7}
16	1.85×10^{-6}	3.19×10^{-6}	7.40×10^{-08}	1.04×10^{-7}
17	1.79×10^{-6}	3.08×10^{-6}	7.15×10^{-08}	1.00×10^{-7}
18	1.75×10^{-6}	3.00×10^{-6}	6.96×10^{-08}	9.77×10^{-08}
19	1.79×10^{-6}	3.07×10^{-6}	7.13×10^{-08}	1.00×10^{-7}
20 to <25	8.58×10^{-6}	1.47×10^{-05}	3.42×10^{-7}	4.80×10^{-7}
25 to <30	8.20×10^{-6}	1.41×10^{-05}	3.27×10^{-7}	4.59×10^{-7}
30 to <35	8.05×10^{-6}	1.38×10^{-05}	3.21×10^{-7}	4.50×10^{-7}
35 to <45	1.59×10^{-05}	2.73×10^{-05}	6.32×10^{-7}	8.88×10^{-7}
45 to <55	1.57×10^{-05}	2.70×10^{-05}	6.27×10^{-7}	8.80×10^{-7}
55 to <65	1.46×10^{-05}	2.51×10^{-05}	5.82×10^{-7}	8.18×10^{-7}
65 to <70	3.46×10^{-6}	5.94×10^{-6}	1.38×10^{-7}	1.94×10^{-7}
ILCR	1.51×10^{-4}	2.60×10^{-4}	6.04×10^{-6}	8.47×10^{-6}

ILCR: incremental lifetime cancer risk.

3.2. Non-Cancer Risk of Exposure to iAs in Rice

The results of our analysis of the non-cancer risks of exposure to iAs in white and brown rice in Brazil, estimated by calculating the fractional HQ by age and the lifetime HQ, are presented in Table 2. The fractional and lifetime HQ for white and brown rice consumption were below 1 for individuals of all ages. The lifetime HQ found is 3.37×10^{-1} for white rice and 1.34×10^{-2} for brown rice. An HQ above 1 indicates that the dose ingested is higher than the reference dose and that there is a potential for adverse effects, in this context including cardiovascular and dermal effects [37].

Table 2. Estimated fractional hazard quotients by age and hazard quotient for a lifetime for exposure to inorganic arsenic in polished (white) and husked (brown) rice.

Age (Years)	White Rice Hazard Quotient		Brown Rice Hazard Quotient	
	Mean	95th Percentile	Mean	95th Percentile
<1	3.61×10^{-3}	6.20×10^{-3}	1.44×10^{-4}	2.04×10^{-4}
1	2.04×10^{-2}	3.51×10^{-2}	8.15×10^{-4}	1.15×10^{-3}
2	1.64×10^{-2}	2.82×10^{-2}	6.55×10^{-4}	9.27×10^{-4}
3	1.61×10^{-2}	2.76×10^{-2}	6.41×10^{-4}	9.07×10^{-4}
4	1.56×10^{-2}	2.68×10^{-2}	6.23×10^{-4}	8.81×10^{-4}
5	1.23×10^{-2}	2.11×10^{-2}	4.89×10^{-4}	6.92×10^{-4}
6	1.13×10^{-2}	1.94×10^{-2}	4.51×10^{-4}	6.38×10^{-4}
7	1.00×10^{-2}	1.73×10^{-2}	4.00×10^{-4}	5.67×10^{-4}
8	9.06×10^{-3}	1.56×10^{-2}	3.61×10^{-4}	5.11×10^{-4}
9	7.93×10^{-3}	1.36×10^{-2}	3.16×10^{-4}	4.47×10^{-4}
10	6.93×10^{-3}	1.19×10^{-2}	2.76×10^{-4}	3.91×10^{-4}
11	6.15×10^{-3}	1.06×10^{-2}	2.45×10^{-4}	3.47×10^{-4}
12	5.45×10^{-3}	9.35×10^{-3}	2.17×10^{-4}	3.07×10^{-4}
13	4.92×10^{-3}	8.45×10^{-3}	1.96×10^{-4}	2.77×10^{-4}
14	4.58×10^{-3}	7.86×10^{-3}	1.82×10^{-4}	2.58×10^{-4}
15	4.27×10^{-3}	7.34×10^{-3}	1.70×10^{-4}	2.41×10^{-4}
16	4.13×10^{-3}	7.09×10^{-3}	1.64×10^{-4}	2.33×10^{-4}
17	3.99×10^{-3}	6.85×10^{-3}	1.59×10^{-4}	2.25×10^{-4}
18	3.88×10^{-3}	6.67×10^{-3}	1.55×10^{-4}	2.19×10^{-4}
19	3.98×10^{-3}	6.83×10^{-3}	1.59×10^{-4}	2.24×10^{-4}
20 to <25	1.91×10^{-2}	3.28×10^{-2}	7.60×10^{-4}	1.08×10^{-3}
25 to <30	1.82×10^{-2}	3.13×10^{-2}	7.27×10^{-4}	1.03×10^{-3}
30 to <35	1.79×10^{-2}	3.07×10^{-2}	7.14×10^{-4}	1.01×10^{-3}
35 to <45	3.53×10^{-2}	6.06×10^{-2}	1.41×10^{-3}	1.99×10^{-3}
45 to <55	3.50×10^{-2}	6.01×10^{-2}	1.39×10^{-3}	1.97×10^{-3}
55 to <65	3.25×10^{-2}	5.58×10^{-2}	1.30×10^{-3}	1.83×10^{-3}
65 to <75	7.69×10^{-3}	1.32×10^{-2}	3.07×10^{-4}	4.34×10^{-4}
0 to <70	3.37×10^{-01}	5.78×10^{-01}	1.34×10^{-2}	1.90×10^{-2}

3.3. Exposure to iAs in Rice

In the present study, the mean concentration of iAs in white rice was found to be 100.1 ± 44.62 ng g^{-1}, which is lower than the MCL of 300 ng g^{-1} proposed by the BNMH for total arsenic [38]. That value is also lower than the MCL of 200 ng g^{-1} for iAs established by the Joint FAO/WHO Codex Committee on Contaminants in Foods [39], European Commission [40], and Chinese Ministry of Health [41]. Among the 64 samples of white rice evaluated in the present study, the concentration of iAs was above the FAO/WHO MCL (ranging from 200 ng g^{-1} to 220 ng g^{-1}, and thus in accordance with Brazilian MCL) in only 4 samples.

The mean concentration of iAs in brown rice was found to be 80.1 ± 55.5 ng g^{-1}. In Brazil, the MCL is the same (300.0 ng g^{-1}) for brown and white rice, although the

Joint FAO/WHO Codex Committee on Contaminants in Foods recommends an MCL of 350.0 ng g^{-1} for brown rice [42].

Many factors that can affect the concentration of iAs in rice can be associated with the location of the rice field [43]. Therefore, we conducted an analysis based on the location where the samples were collected, although we have that information only for the samples of brown rice obtained directly from farms. The samples of white rice were all obtained from markets, and the specific cultivation location was not noted on any of the labels [29]

Figure 2 shows a box plot of iAs concentrations in brown rice by cities where the farms were located [29]. Only cities with more than two samples were included, resulting in three of eight cities. The mean iAs concentration in samples from City 1 was 64.0 ± 19.0 ng g^{-1} ($n = 9$), 45.1 ± 43.0 ng g^{-1} ($n = 30$) from City 2, and 79.8 ± 22.0 ng g^{-1} ($n = 14$) from City 3. City 2 presented the highest variation, but on average, the three locations produced rice with concentration of iAs under 100 ng g^{-1}, suggesting that the studied farms produced rice with a low concentration of iAs.

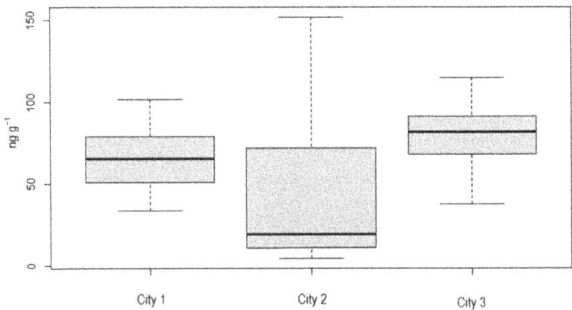

Figure 2. Box plot of inorganic arsenic (iAs) concentrations in brown rice from farms by city.

Figure 3 shows a box plot of iAs concentrations in brown rice by the origin of the samples (farms or markets), which were similarly processed [29]. The mean concentration of iAs for the samples obtained from markets ($n = 21$) of 154.91 ± 44.8 ng g^{-1} (range, 135.7–222.8 ng g^{-1}) was similar to that reported in the literature, but much higher than the 57.36 ± 34.6 ng g^{-1} (range, 45.1–79.7 ng g^{-1}) estimate from the samples obtained from farms ($n = 69$). That discrepancy influenced the overall mean iAs concentration in the dataset for brown rice. The farms where the brown rice was cultivated are located in two states in the southern region of Brazil—Rio Grande do Sul and Santa Catarina—the two main rice-producing states in the country, accounting for approximately 69% and 9% of the national rice production, respectively [44]. Of the brown rice samples purchased in markets, most were produced in Rio Grande do Sul or São Paulo, although the labels did not identify the specific cities, and 12 of the samples had labels that provided no information regarding the state in which the rice was grown. Possible explanations for the lower iAs concentrations in brown rice obtained from farms include the location and management of the farms, which receive support from the Brazilian Agency for Agricultural Research, a governmental agency linked to the Ministry of Agriculture, Livestock, and Food Supply. The mission of the agency is to improve agriculture practices, and one of its goals is to achieve food safety and food security, providing support for farmers to produce more food and food free of hazardous substances [45]. Adopting good agriculture practices, such as avoiding contamination sources and implementing water management, as well as monitoring soil and water quality, could indirectly result in lower iAs concentrations in rice.

In the southern region of Brazil, rice is usually cultivated in flooded fields. However, we hypothesized that rice farmers could be cultivating rice in unsaturated soils, which could explain the low concentration of iAs in rice, although it would also result in higher cadmium concentrations. Using cadmium concentration as an indicator, we found no linear correlation between arsenic and cadmium concentration in brown rice from farms (r = 0.049; p = 0.690), so there is no evidence that the rice was grown in unsaturated soils. Therefore, the low concentration of iAs is probably attributable to other factors.

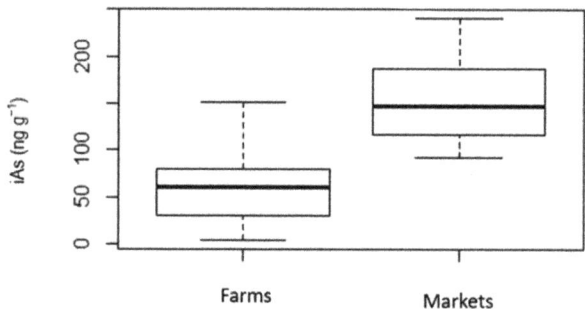

Figure 3. Box plot of inorganic arsenic (iAs) concentrations in husked (brown) rice from farms and markets.

3.4. Reducing the Risk

The concentration of arsenic in rice grains depends on the arsenic concentration in soil, its bioavailability, and the rice genotype (cultivar). Since some rice cultivars reportedly store less arsenic, selecting those cultivars could be a good strategy when the soil is known to contain bioavailable arsenic [46].

In the present study, we had information about brown rice varieties only for the samples collected directly from farms (i.e., not for those obtained from markets). Although there are four rice varieties, we had more than one sample for only two. The mean iAs concentration was 80.7 ± 22.35 ng g^{-1} for the Irga 424 variety ($n = 19$) and 46.6 ± 31.69 ng g^{-1} for the Puitá variety ($n = 48$), as shown in Figure 4. Adopting this rice variety could be an easy, effective strategy to reduce health risks for the population.

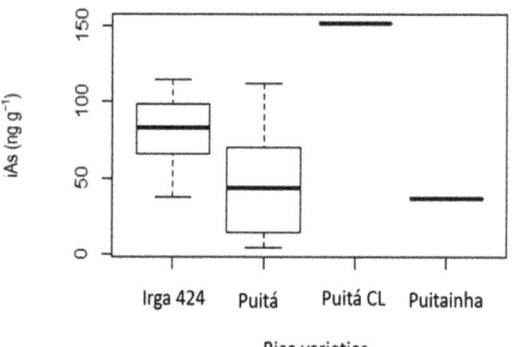

Figure 4. Box plot of inorganic arsenic (iAs) concentrations in four rice varieties.

The results of the present risk assessment describe the estimates of the incidence of cancer in the Brazilian population, based on the application of EPA's cancer slope and exposure scenarios adopted. By changing the inputs of the Monte Carlo analysis, we can simulate the likely impact of mitigation strategies [4]. We evaluated six different interventions aimed at reducing the cancer risk, calculating the risk for each of those interventions: scenario 1—consumption exclusively of brown rice from farms with low levels of iAs; scenario 2—consumption exclusively of brown rice of the Puitá variety, which was found to have the lowest iAs concentration (mean, 46.6 ng g^{-1}); scenario 3—adoption of a white rice MCL of 100 ng g^{-1}; scenario 4—adoption of a white rice MCL of 75 ng g^{-1}; scenario 5—adoption of a white rice MCL of 50 ng g^{-1}; and scenario 6—no consumption of white rice by infants and children ≤ 6 years of age (we chose white rice because it is the type of rice most widely consumed in Brazil). The U.S. FDA has proposed interventions similar to those evaluated here [4]. To calculate the risk for those hypothetical scenarios, any samples above the proposed limit were removed. For scenarios 1 and 2, the complete dataset was considered and the iAs limit was the maximum concentration found. Table 3 shows the parameters and the results of the risk assessment for each scenario.

Table 3. Estimated incremental lifetime cancer risk and parameters for hypothetical scenarios of interventions to reduce the cancer risk of exposure to inorganic arsenic in Brazil.

Scenario	iAs Limit (ng g^{-1})	N	iAs Concentration (ng g^{-1}) Mean; SD	Distribution (Mean; SD or μ; δ)	ILCR Mean	Reduction in ILCR 95th Percentile	(%)
1. Consumption of brown rice from farms with low iAs levels	151.9	69	57.36; 34.36	Log-normal (3.77; 0.87)	5.73×10^{-6}	8.13×10^{-6}	5.03
2. Consumption of brown rice of the Puitá variety	112	48	46.58; 31.68	Log-normal (3.51; 0.91)	5.38×10^{-6}	7.95×10^{-6}	10.85
3. Imposition of a white rice MCL of 100 ng g^{-1}	100	37	71.94; 22.47	Normal (71.94; 22.47)	1.10×10^{-4}	1.66×10^{-4}	27.29
4. Imposition of a white rice MCL of 75 ng g^{-1}	75	17	53.74; 21.15	Normal (53.74; 21.15)	8.27×10^{-05}	1.35×10^{-4}	45.39
5. Imposition of a white rice MCL of 50 ng g^{-1}	50	6	30.55; 16.85	Normal (30.55; 16.85)	4.88×10^{-05}	8.95×10^{-05}	67.79
6. No consumption of white rice ≤ 6 years of age	200	64	100.17; 44.62	Normal (100.17; 44.62)	1.17×10^{-4}	1.99×10^{-4}	22.67

iAs: inorganic arsenic; ILCR: incremental lifetime cancer risk; MCL: maximum contaminant level.

There is no guideline establishing an acceptable level of risk associated with exposure to arsenic in food. Some studies have used the EPA guideline for contaminated areas, which established an acceptable cancer risk ranging from 10^{-4} to 10^{-6} [12,47,48]. Scenario 2 presented the lowest ILCR, close to 10^{-6}, in which the MCL was 48 ng g^{-1}, more than 7 times lower than the MCL proposed by the FAO for white rice [39]. In this scenario, there is a reduction of almost 11% of the risk, compared with the risk of consuming brown rice. It is likely that polishing Puitá rice would further reduce the iAs content and, consequently, the risk.

Scenario 5 represents the adoption of an MCL of 50 ng g^{-1} for white rice, the kind of rice most widely consumed in Brazil, resulting in the highest decrease in ILCR, around 68% (compared with the risk from consumption of white rice) and third lowest ILCR. Excluding rice from the diet of infants and young children (scenario 6) is also a scenario proposed by the FDA [4], and it could reduce the ILCR by nearly 23%, although it would necessitate a substantial change in Brazilian culture, which is unlikely to happen. Daycare centers introduce rice into the diet of infants at four months of age, and that could be delayed, with another type of food—also rich in nutrients and unprocessed—being prioritized. The ILCR for scenario 6 is similar to that of reducing the MCL to 100 ng g^{-1} (scenario 3). In this context, Segura et al. [49] emphasized the need for crop-tracking, given that the iAs content in rice can vary significantly, even among samples from the same producer. That would allow the selection of grains with less iAs for consumption by vulnerable populations, such as infants and children.

4. Discussion

Rice consumption starts at an early age in Brazil. According to food consumption guidelines for daycare centers in the city of São Paulo, the consumption of rice and other kinds of solid food starts at 4 months of age [31]. Since the standard maternity leave in Brazil is 120 days [50], exclusive breastfeeding until 6 months of age, as recommended by the WHO [51], is a challenge. Measures to increase maternity leave in the country have recently been proposed. Since 2008, civil servants have had 180 days of maternity leave, and there are tax incentives for companies that grant 180 days of maternity leave to their employees [52]. However, the proportion of the workforce protected by labor laws that guarantee maternity leave has decreased [53].

The ILCR for exposure to iAs in white rice obtained in our study is lower than that reported for other countries where rice is also a staple food. In Saudi Arabia, Al-Saleh and Abduljabbar [12] found a mean ILCR of 5.8×10^{-2} (minimum of 1.2×10^{-2} and maximum of 2.6×10^{-1}). The authors used the concentrations of total arsenic but estimated that iAs represented 80–90% of the total. Another probabilistic risk assessment, conducted in China by Li et al. [14], found an average ILCR of 1.77×10^{-3}, higher than that found in the present study. Those authors evaluated the consumption of white rice and other foods, such as rice flour, coarse cereals, vegetables, fruit, meat, milk, eggs, and aquatic products. They found that the most relevant variable was the rate of ingestion of aquatic products, followed by the iAs concentration in rice. The ILCR varied among the different areas of the country, and the authors concluded that the risk was mainly explained by the kind of food consumed and the ingestion rate.

In Taiwan, Chen et al. [54] found the mean ILCR for exposure to iAs in white and brown rice to be 1.04×10^{-4} for males and 7.87×10^{-5} for females. The mean ILCR for exposure to iAs in white rice was reported to be 2.06×10^{-4} in Punjab, India [47]. These results are similar to the result found in our study.

A major risk assessment conducted in the United States by the FDA found a median ILCR of 3.4×10^{-5} for white rice (with 5% and 95% confidence limits of 0 and 6.9×10^{-5}, respectively) and 5.4×10^{-6} for brown rice (0 and 1.1×10^{-5} are the confidence limits of 5% and 95%, respectively) [4], both of which are lower than the values found in our study. That could be attributed to the fact that rice consumption is higher in Brazil. The authors of that study also calculated the risk associated with a higher—but still lower than that reported for Brazil—per serving (per eating occasion) dose level. On that basis, the median risk would be 1.36×10^{-4} for white rice (0 and 2.78×10^{-4} are the 5% and 95% confidence limits, respectively) and 1.64×10^{-4} for brown rice (0 and 3.38×10^{-4} are the 5% and 95% confidence limits, respectively).

The high ILCR values found in the present study are mainly associated with the elevated rice consumption in Brazil, which is on average for all age groups 156.6 g/day, compared with 17.1 g/day (including rice flour) in the United States [4]. According to Meharg [50], rice consumption is also very low (10.0 g/day) in the United Kingdom. However, rice consumption is much higher in most Asian countries, such as China, where the daily rice consumption can be as high as 218.64 g [55], as well as Bangladesh, Laos, and Myanmar, where it ranges from 400.0 g/day to 500.0 g/day [56].

Rice and beans make up 25% of the diet of the Brazilian population [13]. In Brazil, there are over ten popular dishes and desserts prepared with rice. The consumption of rice and beans is considered healthy compared with that of ultra-processed food, which are formulations of ingredients created by a series of industrial techniques and processes, such as packaged snacks, pre-prepared meat, pasta and pizza dishes, and others [57]. Rice and beans are rich in nutrients and calories, and their consumption can guarantee the daily ingestion of 50% of the recommended daily water intake. In Brazil, rice is also less expensive than is ultra-processed food and is accessible for people of all socioeconomic levels [58]. Approximately 83% of the Brazilian population consumes white rice, and about 4% consumes brown rice [13]. Given that the current population of Brazil is approximately 211 million, the population exposed to iAs in white and brown rice could be approximately 175 million and 8.4 million people, respectively.

The risk of consuming white rice is higher than is that of consuming brown rice, which is attributed to the lower concentration of iAs in brown rice. The Dietary Guidelines for the Brazilian Population established by the BNMH recommend the consumption of brown rice, rather than white rice, because of the composition, in terms of micronutrients and dietary fiber, of the former [58]. Jo and Todorov [59] reported that, as a result of the polishing process, white rice contains lower concentrations of phosphorus, potassium, manganese, and iron than does brown rice. Considering the results of the present risk assessment, we could conclude that brown rice is also a better option for human health. However, the sample size in this study does not allow for the conclusion that all Brazilian brown rice has less iAs than white rice. Further investigations of iAs in Brazilian rice are needed, given that the levels of arsenic in rice vary according to soil properties, type of irrigation, plant characteristics, and other factors. Samples of white and brown rice from the same location would be more appropriated for a comparative analysis.

Brown rice is typically reported to contain higher levels of arsenic than does white rice, because the arsenic is mainly stored in the external layers of the grain, which are partially removed when the grain is polished [60,61]. However, in the present study, the iAs concentration was found to be slightly lower in brown rice than in white rice, as confirmed by a hypothesis test (t-test, 95% confidence interval). The samples of brown and white rice came from different locations, and iAs concentration in rice can vary considerably according to the region of origin [43].

Regarding non-cancer risk, some studies have found HQ values above 1 for exposure to iAs in rice. In a study involving adults in Saudi Arabia, Al-Saleh et al. [12] found an HQ of 1.2 (SD = 0.4) for exposure to iAs in white rice. The authors assumed a daily rice consumption of 160 g/day to calculate the dose, and used the reference dose established by the EPA, as was used in the present study. In India, where arsenic in rice is a public health problem in some regions, Upadhyay et al. [62] estimated an HQ above 1 for all age groups and a correlation test suggested that the risk of arsenic poisoning is higher among infants and children than among adults. In a study conducted in Taiwan, Chen et al. [54] found an HQ below 1 for all individuals ≤ 65 years of age (between 0.08 and 0.3), although they adopted a 5-fold higher reference dose of 0.015 mg/kg per day. The same RfD was adopted by Lin et al. [63], which conducted a study of the non-cancer risk of exposure to total arsenic in rice for adults in 14 cities in China and found HQ values below 1 for all of the cities, between 0.07 and 0.3. In Punjab, India, Sharma et al. [47] found an HQ of 0.45 for exposure to total arsenic in specific rice varieties and an exposure period of 70 years, using the RfD proposed by EPA.

The risk results are affected by the concentration of iAs in rice, and similar concentrations have been found in other countries, including the United States and China. According to the FDA [4], the weighted mean concentration of iAs in 429 samples of different types of white rice based on the relative market-share estimates in the United States is 92.3 ng g^{-1} (standard error, 1.3). Considering different grain sizes, the mean concentration of iAs was 102.0 ng g^{-1} for long grain rice (n = 173), 81.5 ng g^{-1} for medium grain rice (n = 94), and 78.9 ng g^{-1} for short grain rice (n = 23). Similarly, in China, where rice is a staple food, Li et al. [14] reported an iAs concentration of 103.0 ng g^{-1} in 151 samples of white rice from published studies. Nevertheless, higher iAs concentrations, ranging from 290.0 ng g^{-1} to 950.0 ng g^{-1}, exceeding the WHO MCL and more than 9 times higher than the mean concentration found in our study, were found in white rice samples from India [62]. Lower levels were found in white rice from Taiwan, where rice is the primary staple food, the mean iAs concentration being 65.9 ng g^{-1} in 51 samples [54], and from Iran, a rice-producing country, the mean iAs concentration in 15 samples being 82.0 ng g^{-1} [64].

In Brazil, only a few studies have evaluated the concentration of iAs in white rice. One study assessed white rice purchased in local markets in the state of Minas Gerais, in the southeastern region of the country, and found an iAs concentration of 102.0 ng g^{-1} [15], comparable to that observed in the present study. Cerveira et al. [65] reported a mean iAs concentration of 94.2 ± 39.5 ng g^{-1} (range, 54.0–150.0 ng g^{-1}; $n = 7$), similar to our findings. Moreover, in the state of Minas Gerais, Corguinha et al. [66] found low concentrations of total arsenic, below the detection limit of 15.0 ng g^{-1}, which was attributed to a low concentration of arsenic in soil. In the present study, we have access to data of three samples from Minas Gerais and found iAs concentrations ranging from 105.0 ng g^{-1} to 132.0 ng g^{-1}, higher than the values reported in either of the studies cited above [29].

Higher mean concentrations of iAs were found in brown rice from Taiwan [54]: 103.9 ± 45.0 ng g^{-1} for arsenate and 2.2 ± 1.2 ng g^{-1} for mobile arsenite ($n = 13$). The U.S. FDA [4] reported a mean iAs concentration in brown rice of 156.5 ng g^{-1} (range, 34.0–249.0 ng g^{-1}), in 120 samples, as well as reporting a mean iAs concentration in 144 samples of jasmine, basmati, parboiled, and pre-cooked brown rice of 153.8 ± 3.2 ng g^{-1}. In contrast, Fu et al. [67] reported a mean predicted concentration of iAs in 282 samples of brown rice from Hainan, an island in China, of 57.0 ng g^{-1}, even lower than the concentration found in our study. That concentration was considered lower than or similar to that reported for other regions of China, which the authors suggested was attributed to soil properties (organic matter, phosphorus content, humic acid, and iron–manganese) and arsenic speciation in soil.

Other studies conducted in Brazil have reported concentrations of iAs in brown rice higher than those adopted in the present study, reported by Batista et al. [24]. Cerveira et al. [65] found concentrations ranging from 88.0 ng g^{-1} to 163.0 ng g^{-1} ($n = 4$), with a mean value of 131.0 ± 32.0 ng g^{-1}. Batista et al. [19] reported a mean iAs concentration of 188 ng g^{-1} (range, 176.0–202.0 ng g^{-1}) in samples of brown rice from the states of Rio Grande do Sul and São Paulo. Kato et al. [23] found significant variation in the levels of total arsenic in brown rice from the states of Rio Grande do Sul (235.0 ± 157.0 ng g^{-1}), Santa Catarina (157.0 ± 108.0 ng g^{-1}), and Mato Grosso (4.0 ± 2.0 ng g^{-1}), which was attributed to differences in water management and local features.

The concentration of iAs in rice can vary according to the presence of arsenic in soil or in water used for irrigation, natural or otherwise [68]; the current or past use of pesticides containing arsenic; anthropogenic sources of iAs, such as mining or industrial activities, near the rice paddies [5]; water management [69]; and rice variety [70,71]. In Brazil, some studies have identified significant variation in iAs concentrations and other non-essential elements in rice, even among rice grains from the same producer. Rice variety, microclimatic conditions, and geochemical properties are reported to be major factors affecting iAs concentration in rice [49,72].

Water management can influence arsenic concentration in rice. Rice cultivated under flooded conditions absorbs more arsenic than does that cultivated in unsaturated soils, while also absorbing less cadmium from soil [69]. Silva et al. [70] evaluated the iAs concentration in three different varieties of rice cultivated under different water conditions and during different phases of development. They found that water management had the greatest impact on iAs concentration during the reproductive period, in which cultivation in unsaturated soils resulted in the lowest arsenic accumulation in rice grains, as well as the highest accumulation of cadmium and lead. Both were below the acceptable levels established by the FAO/WHO [39].

Some types of fertilizers, pesticides, and soil acidity correctors, such as limestone, can be a source of arsenic in the environment. In another study conducted in Brazil, Avelar et al. [73] analyzed samples of limestone, a natural unprocessed mineral, and found an arsenic concentration of 11.74 ± 1.42 µg g^{-1}, similar to values reported for limestone in the United States, where the U.S. FDA has declared it a major source of arsenic in the soil, posing risks for humans and animals [4]. The anaerobic conditions in flooded fields favor pH correction, so no limestone is necessary. However, in some cases, rice seeds are sown directly onto dry soil, and the field is flooded 30 days later. Therefore, the recommendation is to use limestone only once every five years [74].

Phosphorus fertilizers can also be a source of arsenic in the environment. Avelar et al. [73] evaluated samples of phosphorus fertilizers in Brazil and found concentrations of total arsenic similar to or even lower than those reported for other countries around the world—11.74 ± 1.42 µg g^{-1}. Those concentrations were below the MCL established for Brazil, although Brazilian soils demand more phosphorus-rich fertilizers, because iron and aluminum are more likely to be adsorbed by soil particles than is phosphorus. In comparison with Europe, Brazil uses nearly 100 times more phosphorus fertilizer in agricultural fields (140 kg/ha). On average, 6.4 ± 1.2 g/ha of arsenic is added to the soil in Brazil every year. Although the arsenic concentrations in fertilizers do not pose a threat to human health in the short term, intensive medium- to long-term use of such fertilizers could lead to the accumulation of arsenic in soil, which can represent risks to human health, and soil monitoring is therefore necessary [75]. In a study conducted in the state of São Paulo, Campos [76] found that the intense use of phosphorus fertilizers for decades increased the soil concentrations of arsenic, as well as its mobility and availability, given that phosphorus, rather than arsenic, can be adsorbed by the soil. That increased the concentration of arsenic in groundwater and, consequently, in well water. In Rio Grande do Sul, the main rice-producing state in Brazil, contamination of soil and groundwater with arsenic, due to fertilizer factory activities, has been reported. In a study conducted in the Patos Lagoon Estuary, which is surrounded by rice paddies, Mirlean and Roisenberg [77] reported arsenic concentrations ranging from 7.5 µg g^{-1} to 27.5 µg g^{-1} in soil, exceeding the local background value (1.02 µg g^{-1}), and from 1.23 µg g^{-1} to 25.45 ng mL^{-1} in water, also exceeding the local background value (0.14 ng mL^{-1}). The authors concluded that the soil and water contamination are a result of precipitation from factory emissions, over a period of more than 40 years, accumulating total arsenic in the superficial horizon of the soil. Most studies of arsenic in the environment of Brazil, including those conducted in the states of Espírito Santo, Bahia, Rio de Janeiro, Paraná, and São Paulo [78–81], have attributed it to industrial or mining activities, which do not typically occur near rice paddies.

The rice cultivar is also an important factor for arsenic concentration in rice, as shown in Figure 3. In a study conducted in Punjab, India, Sharma et al. [47] investigated two rice varieties (PUSA1121 and PR122) and found that they may be suitable for cultivation in fields contaminated with arsenic. Another study conducted in India showed significant variability of arsenic concentration in five rice varieties [62]. In that study, the Ranjit variety showed a mean iAs concentration of 290 ± 0.021 ng g^{-1}, more than three times lower than the 950 ± 0.044 ng g^{-1} shown by the Gosai variety.

A number of measures for reducing the risk of iAs exposure associated with rice consumption have been proposed. Practices that can be adopted by the consumers, including rinsing, soaking, and some cooking methods, can remove part of the iAs. However, there are uncertainties regarding the effectiveness of such practices and the influence of the type of rice; in addition, the iAs content in the water used in cooking the rice can affect the final iAs concentration [4,82].

Sengupta et al. [83] reported that a method of washing and cooking rice, specific to India, removed up to 57% of the total arsenic from rice containing 203–540 ng g^{-1} of arsenic. Washing the rice approximately six times, until the water is clear, reduced the total arsenic concentration by approximately half, and cooking the rice at a rice-to-water ratio of 1:6, thereafter discarding the excess water, removed the remaining arsenic. A study conducted in Saudi Arabia showed that soaking rice for 20 min removed 98% of the total arsenic and that rinsing rice 3 times removed 97% [12]. In a study conducted in Japan, Naito et al. [84] observed that rinsing rice removed mainly iAs. Although rinsing and cooking practices can reduce the arsenic concentration in rice, such practices also reduce enriched iron, folate, thiamin, and niacin [4]. One study showed that rinsing rice before cooking had a minimal effect on arsenic concentration, while removing nutrients such as enriched iron, folate, thiamin, and niacin. Cooking rice in excess water proved to be more effective in reducing the iAs concentration in rice, removing 40–60% depending on the type of rice, while reducing those same nutrients by 50–70% [85]. Cooking the rice can also change the speciation of the arsenic to a form that is more toxic or less toxic, depending on the type of rice and its region of origin [43]. Preliminary estimates indicate that the reduction in iAs in rice from rinsing and cooking practices in water containing low levels of arsenic (<3 µg/L) ranges from 28% to 60%. Since there is substantial uncertainty in those estimates, there have been calls for further research to evaluate not only changes in total arsenic and iAs concentrations in rice but also the impact on nutritional content [4].

Nachman et al. [86] proposed actions that stakeholders (regulators, food producers, researchers, and health professionals) could take at each step of the supply chain to reduce the risk associated with dietary exposure to iAs. Brazil is committed to the Sustainable Development Goals of the United Nations, one of which, End Hunger, also calls for food safety and sustainable agriculture [87]. Investments in research are essential to assess best practices for reducing iAs concentrations in rice, and public policies could provide support to rice producers through education and by promoting the adoption of good agriculture practices.

Pedron et al. [88] evaluated polishing and washing rice for potential implementation in the food industry. Polishing the grain removed 13–54% of total arsenic, depending on the duration of the polishing, which ranged from 20 s to 60 s. In the case of brown rice, washing the grains removed approximately 38.8% of total arsenic. Jo and Todorov [59] found that polishing brown rice can remove 16–33% of iAs. However, these practices are known to reduce some nutrients, as reported by Pedron et al. [88], who found that washing and polishing rice reduced the concentrations of nutrients (manganese, iron, cobalt, copper, zinc, and selenium) by 33–95%.

Another potential arsenic mitigation strategy is using fungi from the rhizosphere of rice. Segura et al. [89] tested two genera of fungi and obtained promising results. The authors concluded that direct application of *Aspergillus* sp. in soils might be a good alternative for reducing iAs concentration in rice grains.

The Joint FAO/WHO Code of Practice for the Prevention and Reduction of Arsenic Contamination in Rice states that national authorities should consider the implementation of measures directed at the sources of iAs and the adoption of specific agricultural practices. Authorities could determine which measures are most appropriate for their countries. Such measures include the identification and avoidance of arsenic sources: water for irrigation, contaminated soil, atmospheric emissions and wastewater from industry, materials used in agricultural and livestock production (pesticides, veterinary medicines, feed, soil amendments, and fertilizers), and waste from other materials (e.g., timber treated with copper chrome arsenate). Specific agricultural measures include education programs for farmers and implementing aerobic conditions or intermittent flooding during rice production, although only if cadmium concentrations in rice are not a concern [5].

There is a need for additional studies aimed at determining which mitigation strategies are the most suitable, taking into consideration the complexity of aspects related to agriculture, daycare centers, schools, maternity leave, and culture. The same interventions proposed in the risk assessment conducted by the U.S. FDA produced results that were less significant, possibly because rice consumption is lower in the United States than in Brazil, or because the dose–response model was different. In their risk assessment of exposure to iAs in rice [4], eliminating rice from the diet of infants and children ≤ 6 years of age would reduce the ILCR by 6%, imposing an MCL of 100 ng g^{-1} would reduce the ILCR by 4.3–18.3%, imposing an MCL of 75 ng g^{-1} would reduce the ILCR by 20–37%, and imposing an MCL of 50 ng g^{-1} would reduce the ILCR by 44.5%.

5. Conclusions

An important finding is that the ILCR, as well as the cancer risk for each age or age group, associated with exposure to white rice in Brazil is high, even when the iAs concentration is under the MCLs proposed by the FAO/WHO and BNMH. That might be attributed to the high level of rice consumption in the country, and the MCL established by the BNMH does not seem to be appropriate in view of the exposure scenario. The incremental cancer risk is highest at 35–65 years of age, when rice consumption is high given the lower body weight at that age, resulting in a higher dose of iAs and, consequently, a higher incremental cancer risk. The results are influenced by the exposure parameters adopted and possibly by some uncertainties related to them. A more extensive exposure assessment is needed.

According to our findings, in Brazil, the risk associated with the consumption of brown rice appears to be lower than that associated with the consumption of white rice, given that we found the iAs concentration to be lower in brown rice. It is possible that the brown rice studied could be polished and sold as white rice. Thus, we can only conclude that samples of rice from some farms presented a lower concentration of iAs, and it is not specific to brown rice. Further studies are needed to verify our finding that some farms are producing rice with a lower concentration of iAs and, if verified, to implement interventions based on that understanding. We found some evidence that this low concentration of iAs could be explained by the variety of rice and by the practices adopted in rice fields.

The non-cancer risk associated with exposure to rice in Brazil is not concerning.

The actual ILCR is probably higher than that found in this study, because we did not consider the presence of rice in other foods, such as infant cereal and formula. On the other hand, this probabilistic analysis has inherent limitations and is an indirect measure of risk. In addition, we presented some potentially efficient options for mitigating the risk, each of which could have social, political, and economic effects. Those effects should be evaluated in future studies.

Supplementary Materials: The following supporting information can be downloaded at: https://www.mdpi.com/article/10.3390/ijerph192416460/s1. File S1: Probabilistic risk estimations of exposure to iAs in rice (white and brown). File S2: Hazard Quotient (HQ) calculations from exposure to iAs in rice. File S3: Inorganic As concentration in brown or white rice. File S4: Exposure to inorganic arsenic in rice in Brazil: A human health risk assessment. (Table S1. Parameters adopted for assessing the risk of exposure to inorganic arsenic in rice. Table S2. Descriptive statistics for inorganic arsenic (iAs) concentrations in samples of polished (white) and husked (brown) rice. Table S3. Estimated average daily dose (mg/kg-day) associated with exposure to inorganic arsenic in polished (white) and husked (brown) rice.). File S5: Probabilistic risk estimations of exposure to iAs in rice according 6 different scenarios of exposure to iAs in rice. References [13,29,31–33,36,90] is cited in the supplementary materials.

Author Contributions: Conceptualization, M.C.T. and A.C.N.; methodology, M.C.T., J.S.L. and A.C.N.; software, M.C.T.; validation, J.S.L. and A.C.N.; formal analysis, M.C.T.; investigation, M.C.T., J.S.L., B.L.B., K.P.K.O. and A.C.N.; resources, M.C.T. and A.C.N.; data curation, M.C.T., B.L.B. and K.P.K.O.; writing—original draft preparation, M.C.T.; writing—review and editing, M.C.T., J.S.L., B.L.B., K.P.K.O. and A.C.N.; visualization, M.C.T., J.S.L. and A.C.N.; supervision, A.C.N.; project administration, M.C.T. and A.C.N.; funding acquisition, M.C.T. and A.C.N. All authors have read and agreed to the published version of the manuscript.

Funding: This research was funded, in part, by the Brazilian Coordenação de Aperfeiçoamento de Pessoal de Nível Superior (CAPES, Office for the Advancement of Higher Education; Funding Code 001).

Data Availability Statement: The data presented in this study are available in the Supplementary Material.

Acknowledgments: We are grateful to Jeffrey Gift, Ingrid Druwe, and Allen Davis at USEPA for the technical support they provided.

Conflicts of Interest: The authors declare no conflict of interest.

References

1. IARC. *Arsenic and Arsenic Compounds Monograph*; IARC: Lyon, France, 2012; Volume 100C.
2. WHO. *List of Classifications*; WHO: Geneva, Switzerland, 2012; Volume 1–119.
3. EFSA Panel on Contaminants in the Food Chain. Statement on Tolerable Weekly Intake for Cadmium. *Off. J. Eur. Union* **2014**, *9*, 1975. [CrossRef]

4. U.S. FDA. *Arsenic in Rice and Rice Products Risk Assessment Report*; Center for Food Safety and Applied Nutrition, Food and Drug Administration, U.S. Department of Health and Human Services: College Park, MD, USA, 2016.
5. Joint FAO/WHO. *Code of Practice for the Prevention and Reduction of Arsenic Contamination in Rice*; Joint FAO/WHO: Geneva, Switzerland, 2017; Volume 1984.
6. Zhao, F.-J.; McGrath, S.P.; Meharg, A.A. Arsenic as a Food Chain Contaminant: Mechanisms of Plant Uptake and Metabolism and Mitigation Strategies. *Annu. Rev. Plant Biol.* **2010**, *61*, 535–559. [CrossRef]
7. Fu, Q.L.; Li, L.; Achal, V.; Jiao, A.Y.; Liu, Y. Concentrations of Heavy Metals and Arsenic in Market Rice Grain and Their Potential Health Risks to the Population of Fuzhou, China. *Hum. Ecol. Risk Assess.* **2015**, *21*, 117–128. [CrossRef]
8. Gross, B.L.; Zhao, Z. Archaeological and Genetic Insights into the Origins of Domesticated Rice. *Proc. Natl. Acad. Sci. USA* **2014**, *111*, 6190–6197. [CrossRef]
9. Ma, L.; Wang, L.; Tang, J.; Yang, Z. Arsenic Speciation and Heavy Metal Distribution in Polished Rice Grown in Guangdong Province, Southern China. *Food Chem.* **2017**, *233*, 110–116. [CrossRef]
10. EFSA. *Dietary Exposure to Inorganic Arsenic in the European Population*; EFSA: Parma, Italy, 2014.
11. Joint FAO/WHO. *Evaluation of Certain Food Additives and Contaminants*; Joint FAO/WHO: Geneva, Switzerland, 2011; Volume 14.
12. Al-Saleh, I.; Abduljabbar, M. Heavy Metals (Lead, Cadmium, Methylmercury, Arsenic) in Commonly Imported Rice Grains (Oryza Sativa) Sold in Saudi Arabia and Their Potential Health Risk. *Int. J. Hyg. Environ. Health* **2017**, *220*, 1168–1178. [CrossRef]
13. IBGE. Pesquisa de Orçamentos Familiares: 2008–2009. In *Análise Do Consumo Alimentar Pessoal No Brasil*; IBGE: Rio de Janeiro, Brazil, 2011.
14. Li, G.; Sun, G.X.; Williams, P.N.; Nunes, L.; Zhu, Y.G. Inorganic Arsenic in Chinese Food and Its Cancer Risk. *Environ. Int.* **2011**, *37*, 1219–1225. [CrossRef]
15. Ciminelli, V.S.T.; Gasparon, M.; Ng, J.C.; Silva, G.C.; Caldeira, C.L. Dietary Arsenic Exposure in Brazil: The Contribution of Rice and Beans. *Chemosphere* **2017**, *168*, 996–1003. [CrossRef]
16. ATSDR. *Toxicological Profile For Arsenic*; ATSDR: Atlanta, GA, USA, 2007.
17. JECFA. *Who Food Additives Series 64: Safety Evaluation of Certain Food Additives and Contaminants, Prepared by the Seventy-Third Meeting of JECFA Lead*; JECFA: Geneva, Switzerland, 2011.
18. FAO. *Guidance for Risk Management Options in Light of Different Risk Assessment Outcomes*; FAO: Kanagawa, Japan, 2015.
19. Batista, B.L.; Souza, J.M.O.; De Souza, S.S.; Barbosa, F. Speciation of Arsenic in Rice and Estimation of Daily Intake of Different Arsenic Species by Brazilians through Rice Consumption. *J. Hazard. Mater.* **2011**, *191*, 342–348. [CrossRef]
20. Santos, L.M.G.; Barata-Silva, C.; Neto, S.A.V.; Magalhães, C.D.; Moreira, J.C.; Jacob, S.C. Analysis and Risk Assessment of Arsenic in Rice from Different Regions of Brazil. *J. Food Compos. Anal.* **2021**, *99*, 103853. [CrossRef]
21. de Oliveira, V.F.; Busanello, C.; Viana, V.E.; Stafen, C.F.; Pedrolo, A.M.; Paniz, F.P.; Pedron, T.; Pereira, R.M.; Rosa, S.A.; de Magalhães Junior, A.M.; et al. Assessing Mineral and Toxic Elements Content in Rice Grains Grown in Southern Brazil. *J. Food Compos. Anal.* **2021**, *100*, 103914. [CrossRef]
22. Paulelli, A.C.C.; Martins, A.C.; Batista, B.L.; Barbosa, F. Evaluation of Uptake, Translocation, and Accumulation of Arsenic Species by Six Different Brazilian Rice (Oryza sativa L.) Cultivars. *Ecotoxicol. Environ. Saf.* **2019**, *169*, 376–382. [CrossRef]
23. Kato, L.S.; De Nadai Fernandes, E.A.; Raab, A.; Bacchi, M.A.; Feldmann, J. Arsenic and Cadmium Contents in Brazilian Rice from Different Origins Can Vary More than Two Orders of Magnitude. *Food Chem.* **2019**, *286*, 644–650. [CrossRef]
24. Segura, F.R.; de Oliveira Souza, J.M.; De Paula, E.S.; da Cunha Martins, A.; Paulelli, A.C.C.; Barbosa, F.; Batista, B.L. Arsenic Speciation in Brazilian Rice Grains Organically and Traditionally Cultivated: Is There Any Difference in Arsenic Content? *Food Res. Int.* **2016**, *89*, 169–176. [CrossRef] [PubMed]
25. U.S.EPA. *Chemical Assessment Summary: Arsenic (Inorganic)*; U.S.EPA: Washington, DC, USA, 1995.
26. U.S. EPA. *Risk Assessment Guidance for Superfund Volume I Human Health Evaluation Manual (Part A)*; U.S.EPA: Washington, DC, USA, 1989; Volume I.
27. U.S. EPA. *Guidance on Selecting Age Groups for Monitoring and Assessing Childhood Exposures to Environmental Contaminants*; U.S.EPA: Washington, DC, USA, 2005; p. 50.
28. Pelletier, B.G.; Box, P.O. YASAIw XIa—A Modified Version of an Open—Source Add—in for Excel to Provide Additional Functions for Monte Carlo Simulation; Installing YASAIw. *Wash. Dep. Ecol. Rep.* **2009**, *7710*, 1–17.
29. Batista, L.B. *Arsenic and Rice: Monitoring and (Bio)Remediation Studies for Food Safety*; FAPESP: Santo André, Brazil, 2015.
30. Paniz, F.P.; Pedron, T.; Freire, B.M.; Torres, D.P.; Silva, F.F.; Batista, B.L. Effective Procedures for the Determination of As, Cd, Cu, Fe, Hg, Mg, Mn, Ni, Pb, Se, Th, Zn, U and Rare Earth Elements in Plants and Foodstuffs. *Anal. Methods* **2018**, *10*, 4094–4103. [CrossRef]
31. *Manual de Orientação Para Centros de Educação Infantil—CEI. Esquema Alimentar e Porcionamentos*; SME: Sao Paulo, Brazil, 2011.
32. *Manual de Orientação Para EMEI e EMEF. Esquema Alimentar e Porcionamentos*; SME: Sao Paulo, Brazil, 2011.
33. Leroux, I.N.; da Silva Ferreira, A.P.S.; Paniz, F.P.; Pedron, T.; Salles, F.J.; da Silva, F.F.; Maltez, H.F.; Batista, B.L.; Olympio, K.P.K. Lead, Cadmium, and Arsenic Bioaccessibility of 24 h Duplicate Diet Ingested by Preschool Children Attending Day Care Centers in Brazil. *Int. J. Environ. Res. Public Health* **2018**, *15*, 1778. [CrossRef]
34. Bompem, K.C.M.; Canella, D.C.; Bandoni, D.H.; Jaime, P.C. *Manual de Medidas Caseiras e Receitas Para Cálculo Dietéticos*; M. Books do Brasil Ltd.: São Paulo, Brazil, 2012; ISBN 978-85-7680-137-5.

35. Tomita, L.Y.; Cardoso, M.A. *Relação de Medidas Caseiras, Composição Química e Receitas de Alimentos Nipo-Brasileiros*; Faculdade de Medicina de São José do Rio Preto: São José do Rio Preto, Brazil, 2000.
36. IBGE. Pesquisa de Orçamentos Familiares 2008–2009. In *Antropometria e Estado Nutricinal de Crianças, Adolescentes e Adultos No Brasil*; IBGE: Rio de Janeiro, Brazil, 2010; Volume 46.
37. U.S. EPA. Risk Assessment Guidance for Superfund (RAGS) Volume III—Part A: Process for Conducting Probabilistic Risk Assessment, Appendix B. *U.S. Environ. Prot. Agency* **2001**, *III*, B1–B51.
38. Ministry of Health. *RDC N° 42 de 29 de Agosto de 2013*; Ministry of Health: Chiyoda, Tokyo, 2013.
39. Joint FAO/WHO. *Report of the 12th Session of the Codex Committee on Contaminants in Foods*; Joint FAO/WHO: Geneva, Switzerland, 2018.
40. EC. *Amending Regulation (EC) No 1881/2006 as Regards Maximum Levels of Inorganic Arsenic in Foodstuffs*; EC: Brussels, Belgium, 2015; Volume 58.
41. Ministry of Health of China. *China's Maximum Levels for Contaminants in Foods China*; Ministry of Health of China: Beijing, China, 2014.
42. Joint FAO/WHO. *Joint FAO/WHO Codex Alimentarius Commission*; Joint FAO/WHO: Geneva, Switzerland, 2016.
43. Althobiti, R.A.; Sadiq, N.W.; Beauchemin, D. Realistic Risk Assessment of Arsenic in Rice. *Food Chem.* **2018**, *257*, 230–236. [CrossRef]
44. Conab. *A Cultura Do Arroz*; Conab: Brasília, Brazil, 2015.
45. Ministry of Agriculture. *Relatório de Gestão—Exercício 2018*; Ministry of Agriculture: New Delhi, India, 2019; Volume 53.
46. Batista, B.L.; Nigar, M.; Mestrot, A.; Rocha, B.A.; Júnior, F.B.; Price, A.H.; Raab, A.; Feldmann, J. Identification and Quantification of Phytochelatins in Roots of Rice to Long-Term Exposure: Evidence of Individual Role on Arsenic Accumulation and Translocation. *J. Exp. Bot.* **2014**, *65*, 1467–1479. [CrossRef]
47. Sharma, S.; Kumar, R.; Sahoo, P.K.; Mittal, S. Geochemical Relationship and Translocation Mechanism of Arsenic in Rice Plants: A Case Study from Health Prone South West Punjab, India. *Groundw. Sustain. Dev.* **2020**, *10*, 100333. [CrossRef]
48. Shibata, T.; Meng, C.; Umoren, J.; West, H. Risk Assessment of Arsenic in Rice Cereal and Other Dietary Sources for Infants and Toddlers in the U.S. *Int. J. Environ. Res. Public Health* **2016**, *13*, 361. [CrossRef] [PubMed]
49. Segura, F.R.; Franco, D.F.; da Silva, J.J.C.; Batista, B.L. Variations in Total As and As Species in Rice Indicate the Need for Crop-Tracking. *J. Food Compos. Anal.* **2020**, *86*, 103392. [CrossRef]
50. Senado Federal. *Constituição Da República Federativa Do Brasil*; Senado Federal, Centro Gráfico: Brasília, Brazil, 2016; Volume 6.
51. WHO. *Guideline: Protecting, Promoting and Supporting Breastfeeding in Facilities Providing Maternity and Newborn Services*; WHO: Geneva, Switzerland, 2017.
52. Senado Federal. *Lei n 11.770 de 9 de Setembro de 2008*; Senado Federal: Brasília, Brazil, 2008; Volume 2, p. 2008.
53. Brasil. *Trabalho e Família—Rumo a Novas Formas de Conciliação Com Co-Responsabilidade Social*; Brasil: Brasília, Brazil, 2009.
54. Chen, H.L.; Lee, C.C.; Huang, W.J.; Huang, H.T.; Wu, Y.C.; Hsu, Y.C.; Kao, Y.T. Arsenic Speciation in Rice and Risk Assessment of Inorganic Arsenic in Taiwan Population. *Environ. Sci. Pollut. Res.* **2016**, *23*, 4481–4488. [CrossRef] [PubMed]
55. Meharg, A.A.; Lawgali, Y.Y.; Deacon, C.M.; Williams, P.T. Levels of Arsenic in Rice—Literature Review. *Food Stand. Agency Contract CC101045* **2007**, *1*, 1–65.
56. Meharg, A.A.; Williams, P.N.; Adomako, E.; Lawgali, Y.Y.; Villada, A.; Cambell, R.C.J.; Sun, G.; Zhu, Y.; Raab, A.; Zhao, F.; et al. Geographical Variation in Total and Inorganic Arsenic Content of Polished (White) Rice. *Environ. Sci. Technol.* **2009**, *43*, 1612–1617. [CrossRef]
57. Lange, C.N.; Monteiro, L.R.; Freire, B.M.; Franco, D.F.; de Souza, R.O.; dos Reis Ferreira, C.S.; da Silva, J.J.C.; Batista, B.L. Mineral Profile Exploratory Analysis for Rice Grains Traceability. *Food Chem.* **2019**, *300*, 125145. [CrossRef]
58. Ministry of Health. *Guia Alimentar Para a População Brasileira. Ministério Da Saúde*; Ministry of Health: Chiyoda, Tokyo, 2014; ISBN 9788533421769.
59. Jo, G.; Todorov, T.I. Distribution of Nutrient and Toxic Elements in Brown and Polished Rice. *Food Chem.* **2019**, *289*, 299–307. [CrossRef]
60. Meharg, A.A.; Raab, A. Getting to the Bottom of Arsenic Standards and Guidelines. *Environ. Sci. Technol.* **2010**, *44*, 4395–4399. [CrossRef]
61. Yim, S.R.; Park, G.Y.; Lee, K.W.; Chung, M.S.; Shim, S.M. Determination of Total Arsenic Content and Arsenic Speciation in Different Types of Rice. *Food Sci. Biotechnol.* **2017**, *26*, 293–298. [CrossRef]
62. Upadhyay, M.K.; Majumdar, A.; Barla, A.; Bose, S.; Srivastava, S. An Assessment of Arsenic Hazard in Groundwater–Soil–Rice System in Two Villages of Nadia District, West Bengal, India. *Environ. Geochem. Health* **2019**, *41*, 2381–2395. [CrossRef] [PubMed]
63. Lin, K.; Lu, S.; Wang, J.; Yang, Y. The Arsenic Contamination of Rice in Guangdong Province, the Most Economically Dynamic Provinces of China: Arsenic Speciation and Its Potential Health Risk. *Environ. Geochem. Health* **2015**, *37*, 353–361. [CrossRef]
64. Cano-Lamadrid, M.; Munera-Picazo, S.; Burló, F.; Hojjati, M.; Carbonell-Barrachina, Á.A. Total and Inorganic Arsenic in Iranian Rice. *J. Food Sci.* **2015**, *80*, T1129–T1135. [CrossRef] [PubMed]
65. Cerveira, C.; Pozebon, D.; De Moraes, D.P.; Silva De Fraga, J.C. Speciation of Inorganic Arsenic in Rice Using Hydride Generation Atomic Absorption Spectrometry (HG-AAS). *Anal. Methods* **2015**, *7*, 4528–4534. [CrossRef]
66. Corguinha, A.P.B.; de Souza, G.A.; Gonçalves, V.C.; de Andrade Carvalho, C.; de Lima, W.E.A.; Martins, F.A.D.; Yamanaka, C.H.; Francisco, E.A.B.; Guilherme, L.R.G. Assessing Arsenic, Cadmium, and Lead Contents in Major Crops in Brazil for Food Safety Purposes. *J. Food Compos. Anal.* **2015**, *37*, 143–150. [CrossRef]

67. Fu, Y.; Chen, M.; Bi, X.; He, Y.; Ren, L.; Xiang, W.; Qiao, S.; Yan, S.; Li, Z.; Ma, Z. Occurrence of Arsenic in Brown Rice and Its Relationship to Soil Properties from Hainan Island, China. *Environ. Pollut.* **2011**, *159*, 1757–1762. [CrossRef]
68. Dittmar, J.; Voegelin, A.; Maurer, F.; Roberts, L.C.; Hug, S.J.; Saha, G.C.; Ali, M.A.; Badruzzaman, A.B.M.; Kretzschmar, R. Arsenic in Soil and Irrigation Water Affects Arsenic Uptake by Rice: Complementary Insights from Field and Pot Studies. *Environ. Sci. Technol.* **2010**, *44*, 8842–8848. [CrossRef]
69. Moreno-Jiménez, E.; Meharg, A.A.; Smolders, E.; Manzano, R.; Becerra, D.; Sánchez-Llerena, J.; Albarrán, Á.; López-Piñero, A. Sprinkler Irrigation of Rice Fields Reduces Grain Arsenic but Enhances Cadmium. *Sci. Total Environ.* **2014**, *485–486*, 468–473. [CrossRef] [PubMed]
70. Duan, G.; Shao, G.; Tang, Z.; Chen, H.; Wang, B.; Tang, Z.; Yang, Y.; Liu, Y.; Zhao, F.-J. Genotypic and Environmental Variations in Grain Cadmium and Arsenic Concentrations Among a Panel of High Yielding Rice Cultivars. *Rice* **2017**, *10*, 9. [CrossRef]
71. Sommella, A.; Deacon, C.; Norton, G.; Pigna, M.; Violante, A.; Meharg, A.A. Total Arsenic, Inorganic Arsenic, and Other Elements Concentrations in Italian Rice Grain Varies with Origin and Type. *Environ. Pollut.* **2013**, *181*, 38–43. [CrossRef]
72. Monteiro, L.R.; Lange, C.N.; Freire, B.M.; Pedron, T.; da Silva, J.J.C.; de Magalhães, A.M.; Pegoraro, C.; Busanello, C.; Batista, B.L. Inter- and Intra-Variability in the Mineral Content of Rice Varieties Grown in Various Microclimatic Regions of Southern Brazil. *J. Food Compos. Anal.* **2020**, *92*, 103535. [CrossRef]
73. Avelar, A.C.; Ferreira, W.M.; Pemberthy, D.; Abad, E.; Amaral, M.A. Dioxins, Furans, Biphenyls, Arsenic, Thorium and Uranium in Natural and Anthropogenic Sources of Phosphorus and Calcium Used in Agriculture. *Sci. Total Environ.* **2016**, *551–552*, 695–698. [CrossRef]
74. Ministry of Agriculture. *Adubação e Calagem Para o Arroz Irrigado No Rio Grande Do Sul*; Ministry of Agriculture: Pelotas, Brazil, 2007.
75. da Silva, F.B.V.; do Nascimento, C.W.A.; Araújo, P.R.M. Environmental Risk of Trace Elements in P-Containing Fertilizers Marketed in Brazil. *J. Soil Sci. Plant Nutr.* **2017**, *17*, 635–647. [CrossRef]
76. Campos, V. Arsenic in Groundwater Affected by Phosphate Fertilizers at São Paulo, Brazil. *Environ. Geol.* **2002**, *42*, 83–87. [CrossRef]
77. Mirlean, N.; Andrus, V.E.; Baisch, P.; Griep, G.; Casartelli, M.R. Arsenic Pollution in Patos Lagoon Estuarine Sediments, Brazil. *Mar. Pollut. Bull.* **2003**, *46*, 1480–1484. [CrossRef] [PubMed]
78. Alves, R.I.S.; Sampaio, C.F.; Nadal, M.; Schuhmacher, M.; Domingo, J.L.; Segura-Muñoz, S.I. Metal Concentrations in Surface Water and Sediments from Pardo River, Brazil: Human Health Risks. *Environ. Res.* **2014**, *133*, 149–155. [CrossRef] [PubMed]
79. Cagnin, R.C.; Quaresma, V.S.; Chaillou, G.; Franco, T.; Bastos, A.C. Arsenic Enrichment in Sediment on the Eastern Continental Shelf of Brazil. *Sci. Total Environ.* **2017**, *607–608*, 304–316. [CrossRef] [PubMed]
80. Espinoza-Quiñones, F.R.; Módenes, A.N.; De Pauli, A.R.; Palácio, S.M. Analysis of Trace Elements in Groundwater Using ICP-OES and TXRF Techniques and Its Compliance with Brazilian Protection Standards. *Water. Air. Soil Pollut.* **2015**, *226*, 1–12. [CrossRef]
81. Mirlean, N.; Baisch, P.; Diniz, D. Arsenic in Groundwater of the Paraiba Do Sul Delta, Brazil: An Atmospheric Source? *Sci. Total Environ.* **2014**, *482–483*, 148–156. [CrossRef]
82. Joint FAO/WHO. *Evaluation of Certain Contaminants in Food*; Joint FAO/WHO: Geneva, Switzerland, 2011.
83. Sengupta, M.K.; Hossain, M.A.; Mukherjee, A.; Ahamed, S.; Das, B.; Nayak, B.; Pal, A.; Chakraborti, D. Arsenic Burden of Cooked Rice: Traditional and Modern Methods. *Food Chem. Toxicol.* **2006**, *44*, 1823–1829. [CrossRef]
84. Naito, S.; Matsumoto, E.; Shindoh, K.; Nishimura, T. Effects of Polishing, Cooking, and Storing on Total Arsenic and Arsenic Species Concentrations in Rice Cultivated in Japan. *Food Chem.* **2015**, *168*, 294–301. [CrossRef] [PubMed]
85. Gray, P.J.; Conklin, S.D.; Todorov, T.I.; Kasko, S.M. Cooking Rice in Excess Water Reduces Both Arsenic and Enriched Vitamins in the Cooked Grain. *Food Addit. Contam. Part A-Chem. Anal. Control Expo. Risk Assess.* **2016**, *33*, 78–85. [CrossRef] [PubMed]
86. Nachman, K.E.; Punshon, T.; Rardin, L.; Signes-Pastor, A.J.; Murray, C.J.; Jackson, B.P.; Guerinot, M.L.; Burke, T.A.; Chen, C.Y.; Ahsan, H.; et al. Opportunities and Challenges for Dietary Arsenic Intervention. *Environ. Health Perspect.* **2018**, *126*, 6–11. [CrossRef] [PubMed]
87. United Nations. *Transforming Our World: The 2030 Agenda for Sustainable Development*; United Nations: San Francisco, CA, USA, 2015.
88. Pedron, T.; Segura, F.R.; Paniz, F.P.; de Moura Souza, F.; dos Santos, M.C.; de Magalhães Júnior, A.M.; Batista, B.L. Mitigation of Arsenic in Rice Grains by Polishing and Washing: Evidencing the Benefit and the Cost. *J. Cereal Sci.* **2019**, *87*, 52–58. [CrossRef]
89. Segura, F.R.; Paulelli, A.C.C.; Braga, G.Ú.L.; Dos Reis Pedreira Filho, W.; Silva, F.F.; Batista, B.L. Promising Filamentous Native Fungi Isolated from Paddy Soils for Arsenic Mitigation in Rice Grains Cultivated under Flooded Conditions. *J. Environ. Chem. Eng.* **2018**, *6*, 3926–3932. [CrossRef]
90. UNICEF-WHO-UNESCO. *Facts for Life*, 4th ed.; UNICEF-WHO-UNESCO: New York, NY, USA, 2010.

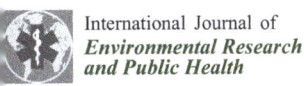

International Journal of
Environmental Research and Public Health

Article

A Low-Cost Method Shows Potentially Toxic Element Levels in Dust Correlated with Elevated Blood Levels of These Chemicals in Children Exposed to an Informal Home-Based Production Environment

Fairah Barrozo [1], Gilmar Alves de Almeida [2], Maciel Santos Luz [2] and Kelly Polido Kaneshiro Olympio [1,*]

1 Department of Environmental Health, School of Public Health, University of São Paulo, Sao Paulo 01246-904, Brazil
2 Advanced Materials, Laboratory of Metallurgical Processes, Institute for Technological Research of the State of São Paulo, Sao Paulo 05508-901, Brazil
* Correspondence: kellypko@usp.br

Abstract: Dust is recognized as a route of exposure to environmental pollutants. The city of Limeira, Sao Paulo state, Brazil, is a production center for jewelry and fashion jewelry, where part of this jewelry production is home-based, informal, and outsourced. The aim of this study was to evaluate exposure to Potentially Toxic Elements (PTE: Cr, Sn, Mn, Sb, Ni, Cu, Zn, Cd, Pb, and As) in dust among children from households of informal workers using electrostatic dust cloths (EDC). Dust samples were collected in 21 exposed and 23 control families using EDC from surfaces where dust deposits had accumulated for approximately 14 days. In exposed families, dust samples were also collected from welders' workstations. PTE concentrations were then determined using inductively coupled mass spectrometry (ICP-MS). The results raised concerns in relation to Cr, As, and Cd exposure among children within the informal home-based production environment. Blood PTE concentrations in children showed a moderate correlation with levels of Cr (Rho 0.40), Zn (Rho −0.43), and As (Rho 0.40), and a strong correlation with Cd (Rho 0.80) ($p < 0.05$), detected in dust. In conclusion, analyzing dust collected using EDC proved a potentially low-cost tool for determining PTE in dust. In addition, the results confirmed that informal home-based work poses a risk for children residing in these households. Public policies are needed to assist these families and promote better conditions of occupational health and safety for the whole family.

Keywords: blood; metals; child; environmental exposure; occupational exposure; dust; child health; worker health

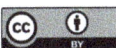

1. Introduction

Cottage industries are a subgroup of informal work characterized by artisan and craft production, usually with family participants and carried out within homes or backyards [1] as opposed to companies or purpose-built facilities [2]. This type of occupational activity is often outsourced and associated with the use of hazardous substances, such as lead, arsenic, and cadmium [3], with examples including cottage industries, subsistence fishing, artisanal pot making, battery dismantling, artisanal gold mining [2], and jewelry manufacturing.

A study of homes in Zuni Pueblo, New Mexico, a production center for this cottage industry, showed that residual metals from the jewelry-making process were a potential risk for chronic, low-level exposure to metals, such as silver, copper, lead, and cadmium [4]. However, it is difficult to convince workers who develop occupational diseases of the link between their exposure to hazardous materials and resultant illness. Furthermore, all members of the worker's family can be at risk, including young children and infants residing in the same environment [1]. Young children can be at particular risk because they spend more time at home, especially those engaging in hand-to-mouth behavior [3] and in the habit of eating non-nutritive substances (pica) [3,5].

A previous study investigated exposure to metals among people making cookware in informal foundries in South Africa [6]. The authors found a statistically significant difference in blood lead levels (BLL) between the group of artisanal pot makers and the non-exposed group on quantile regression (p = 0.0003). Moreover, the analysis of pot makers' handwipes pre- and post-work revealed variable exposure to Al, As, Ba, Bi, Cd, Ce, Co, Cr, Cu, Fe, Li, Mn, Mo, Ni, Pb, Sb, Sn, U, V, Zn, and Zr. Another study compared a small group of children with neurological complaints, such as convulsions and drowsiness, to a control group in Mumbai, a city which has a booming artificial jewelry cottage industry [7]. Mean BLL was 42.6 ± 22.5 µg/dL (range 16.6–85.4) in the exposed group versus 8.7 ± 1.2 µg/dL (range 7.0–10.2) in the control group, a statistically significant difference (p < 0.001) [7]. In addition, 80.0% of the exposed group had a history of lead smelting activities within the home to produce artificial jewelry, compared with only 35.7% of controls [7].

In Bangladesh, there are lead acid battery manufacturing industries, predominantly cottage industries with small, poorly ventilated environments [8]. A study involving these workers found high blood lead concentrations averaging 65.25 µg/dL, where 84% of the workers had blood Pb concentrations > 40 µg/dL [8]. Moreover, in Indonesia, 69.5% of the children living near a lead acid battery recycling site (deactivated but still working illegally) had high blood lead levels > 10 µg/dL [9]. Also, dust and blood samples of pottery artisans, in Brazil, showed an excessive exposure to Pb during the pottery-glazing process, which 2.3% of the artisans had blood lead levels above 40 µg/dL [10]. The city of Limeira, Brazil, is a large center of jewelry and fashion jewelry production [11] with a unique home-based outsourced informal production process. The exposure scenario is complex, with multiple sources of Potentially Toxic Elements (PTE), such as chrome (Cr), manganese (Mn), nickel (Ni), copper (Cu), zinc (Zn), arsenic (As), cadmium (Cd), antimony (Sn), and lead (Pb). Workers, and especially their children, are exposed to occupational exposure levels [12,13]. Moreover, most workers engaged in soldering and similar activities do not use personal protective equipment (PPE) [12], further increasing exposure levels.

Children breathe air faster as a function of their lower body weight, and their skin more readily absorbs some harmful substances [14]. Children's immune systems are also more vulnerable, as their organs have not fully matured, especially during the development of the central nervous system between the age of 6 months and 3 years [14,15]. Dust intake by infants and young children is proportionally higher than for other age groups [16]. Therefore, informal, outsourced, home-based jewelry production raises concern because of the potential presence of dust metals from welding processes. Thus, the aim of this study was to evaluate children's exposure to metals in house dust by determining PTE levels in household dust, through a low-cost method, and correlating them with blood PTE concentrations. Furthermore, the exposure scenario was evaluated, yielding recommendations of actions to protect the children's health.

2. Materials and Methods

2.1. Study Population

The present investigation is part of a larger research study, "The 'omics' era applied to society: the impact of formal and informal labor on the exposome of workers with an emphasis on metabolomics, transcriptomics and lipidomics" by the Human Exposome Research Group of the School of Public Health, University of São Paulo, which also involved collection of blood, urine, and whole saliva samples from informal workers of Limeira, and of blood and urine from the children who are members of the workers' families.

All of the families participating in this study were volunteers, comprising 21 exposed and 23 control families. The exposed group was made up of families who performed jewelry soldering in the domestic environment. In most cases, the same environment was used for both feeding and work activities, as shown in Figure 1 parts A and B. The families were selected with the assistance of the Health Secretariat of Limeira city. The control group consisted of families with no occupational chemical exposure, selected for invitation by counting the fourth household clockwise facing the street from the exposed households. In the event of refusal to accept the invitation, the neighboring house was invited [12].

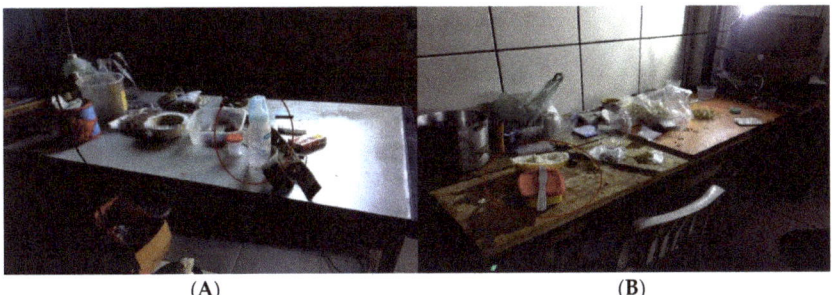

Figure 1. Welder's workstations with baby feeding bottle (**A**) and food items (**B**). Limeira, 2019.

2.2. Dust Sample Collection

Dust samples were collected with EDC (Procter and Gamble®) cloths. One EDC was placed inside an open pre-decontaminated plastic folder and affixed to the wall at a height of 1.5 m for 14 to 17 days before the collection of the biological samples (Figure 2). The folder was subsequently closed and transported to the laboratory at ambient temperature [17]. All of the samples were collected in duplicate, labeled for each household, and opened only at the time of analysis to avoid external contamination.

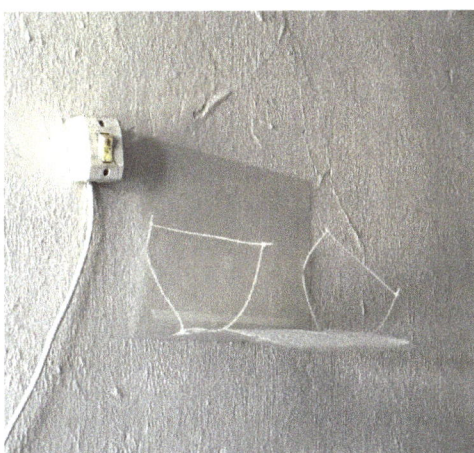

Figure 2. EDC. Limeira, 2019.

This method was adapted to simulate dust accumulation on furniture because prior visits showed that most families did not have furniture from which dust could be collected. In the workers' homes, the EDC was placed near the workstations, whereas in the control group, the EDC was placed in the room where the children spent most of their time (bedroom, living room, or kitchen), as informed by the children's parents or legal guardians.

In addition, surface dust samples were collected directly from welders' workstations. One EDC was used to clean part of the worktop, stored, and then transported in plastic vessels to the laboratory. All the areas cleaned were measured and recorded.

All of the materials used for sample collection and transport, such as the folders, were previously cleaned using nitric acid overnight and tested for PTE using XRF analyses.

2.3. Dust Sample Preparation and Chemical Analysis

All the EDCs were analyzed at the Institute for Technological Research of the State of São Paulo (IPT). For the chemical analysis, the tubes were decontaminated with the addition of 10 mL of 32.5% m/v nitric acid and heated to a high temperature in a microwave digester. After cooling, the tubes were rinsed with ultrapure water.

The sample preparation involved acid extraction with a microwave oven (Ethos UP model, Milestone). Each EDC sample was cut into four parts with stainless steel scissors previously cleaned with ethyl alcohol. Each part was then placed into a polytetrafluoroethylene tube with plastic forceps and 12 mL of 65% m/v nitric acid, 2 mL of 35% m/v hydrogen peroxide, and 0.4 mL of 48% m/v hydrofluoric acid were then added [18]. The tubes were sealed and placed in the microwave oven. The final solutions were transferred to conical tubes and bulked up with deionized water, and then analyzed by inductively coupled plasma mass spectrometry (ICP-MS) [19]. High purity deionized water was obtained using a Milli-Q water purification system (Millipore, Bedford, MA, USA) and used for the preparation of samples and solutions. The standard material NIST 1648A for Particulate Urban Material [20] was used as certified reference material.

The limits of detection (LOD) and quantification (LOQ), respectively, in µg/cloth, were: Cr (0.1667/0.5154), Mn (0.0049/0.0076), Ni (0.2954/0.3197), Cu (0.0050/0.0085), Zn (0.1124/0.1354), As (0.0032/0.0064), Cd (0.0004/0.0012), Sn (0.0035/0.0084), and Pb (0.0006/0.0011).

2.4. Exposure Questionnaires

As part of the exposure assessment, questionnaires were applied to the families regarding the chemicals used, exposure time, work shifts, working environment, ventilation conditions, use of personal protective equipment, and the presence and exposure time of children in the dwellings [21]. Additionally, a work diary was filled out by the workers engaged in soldering to quantify the hours worked during the dust sample collection periods (14 to 17 days), during which the EDC was placed in the homes. To this end, workers reported the time dedicated to soldering work and the place where they worked during the study period.

2.5. XRF Measurements

PTEs were determined in the solder powders and wires used for the jewelry and fashion jewelry production at the 17 exposed families' homes using a Thermo Fisher TM portable X-Ray Fluorescence Analyzer (NitonTM XL2®). Not all of the exposed families had solder powders and wires in the residence during the sample collection period.

All the measurements were performed in situ at workers' homes during the collection of dust samples in October and November 2019.

The analyzer was placed close to the material for 30 s with the trigger pulled [22] and readings were stored in the device until being downloaded to its program software, Standard Thermo Scientific™ Niton Data Transfer (NDT™). Additionally, for quality control, the device was calibrated, every time it was turned on, by standardization and measurement of a specific stainless-steel alloy (alloy 316) [13] and was previously calibrated by the manufacturer before commencement of the study.

2.6. Secondary Data Variables

As part of the larger research study by our group, the cited data on blood PTE concentrations of the children were obtained previously [23]. This dataset included concentrations from 29 children, comprising 14 exposed individuals (9 families) and 15 control individuals (14 families) aged 1–11 years. The blood samples were collected at the same time [23] as the dust samples at each house, between October and November 2019.

The blood collection methodology has been described elsewhere [23]. Briefly, the collections were performed by a trained nurse who collected six milliliters of whole blood in heparinized tubes free of trace elements (Vacutainer®). The biological samples were then stored at 80 °C before being transferred to the laboratory of the IPT, where determination of PTE was carried out using ICP-MS, in the same manner as for the dust samples.

2.7. Data Processing and Statistical Treatment

All statistical analyses were performed using the R and RStudio statistical package (version 1.3.1093). The concentrations of metals analyzed in the dust were expressed using descriptive statistics, including minimum and maximum, standard deviation, geometric mean (GM), and the 95th percentiles of each element. Participants were stratified by exposure group (exposed or control). In addition to comparison tests, Student's t-test and the Mann–Whitney test were performed, according to the distribution of the variables. Results were considered statistically significant for p-values < 0.05. Nonparametric Spearman correlations were computed to assess univariate correlations of PTE levels in house dust with concentrations in children's blood, number of workers and work time, and also for different dust sample collection methods.

Elemental concentrations in blood and dust samples below the limit of detection (LOD) were assigned a value of LOD/2 [24].

3. Results

The participants (n = 44) comprised 21 exposed and 23 control families. One of the exposed family used two rooms for working and three workstations. Correspondingly, two dust samples were collected from the rooms for approximately 14 days after installation of EDC (14 days before blood sample collection) and three dust samples were collected from the welders' workstations. Most of the welders were women (n = 41). Regarding the exposed group, the welders reported using chemical products during their work process, such as acid and soldering powder (23.8%), acid and soldering wire (23.8%), and soldering powder alone (47.6%). Furthermore, only 19.0% of the workers who engaged in soldering stated that they used PPE during the work, such as safety glasses, dust masks or respirators, face shields, gloves, and protective clothing. Overall, 42.9% of the welders stated that they used ventilation systems, while 80.9% worked with doors and windows open or in the open air. A total of 80.9% of welders stated that they worked in living rooms, bedrooms, laundry rooms, and backyards, as shown in Table 1. In 42.9% of households, welding activities were shared by spouses, siblings, and friends.

Table 1. Distribution of demographic characteristics and working conditions of study population by group. Limeira, Brazil, 2019.

Characteristics	N	%
Total number of participating families	44	100.0
Exposed	21	47.7
Control	23	52.3
Total number of participating children	29	100.0
Exposed	14	48.3
Control	15	51.7
Exposed group	21	
Chemicals used		
Acid and soldering powder	5	23.8
Acid and soldering wire	5	23.8
Soldering powder alone	10	47.6
None	1	4.8
Use of personal protective equipment		
Yes	4	19.0
No	17	80.9
Use of ventilation system		
Yes	9	42.9
No	12	57.1

Table 1. Cont.

Characteristics	N	%
Place of work		
Living room	3	14.3
Kitchen	1	4.8
Bedroom	2	9.5
Laundry	1	4.8
Work room	4	19.0
Open area (backyard)	10	47.6
Use of natural ventilation		
All doors and windows left open	17	80.9
Doors open and windows closed	2	9.5
Depends on temperature	1	4.8
Other	1	4.8

PTE concentrations in the house dust samples collected over approximately 14 days were significantly higher ($p < 0.05$) in the exposed group for all PTE included in this study, but levels of the elements detected in these accumulated dust samples (worktop cleaning) from homes in the exposed group were not correlated with concentrations found in welders' workstation dust, except for Sn ($p < 0.05$) (Table 2).

Table 2. PTE levels ($\mu g/cm^2$) in dust samples by group. Limeira, Brazil, 2019.

	Accumulated Dust [a]							Welders' Workstation Dust [b]		
	Exposed		Control		Total			Exposed		
	N = 21		N = 23		N = 44			N = 21		
	Mean	SD	Mean	SD	Mean	SD	p-Value [c]	Mean	SD	p-Value [d]
Cr	0.0061	0.0130	0.0004	0.0003	0.0032	0.0094	<0.05	0.11	0.53	>0.05
Mn	0.0052	0.0034	0.0014	0.0011	0.0033	0.0031	<0.05	0.01	0.03	>0.05
Ni	0.3979	0.2099	0.0005	0.0003	0.1948	0.2478	<0.05	0.02	0.11	>0.05
Cu	0.0044	0.0034	0.0004	0.0006	0.0024	0.0031	<0.05	0.26	0.73	>0.05
Zn	0.3483	1.3181	0.0002	0.0000	0.1704	0.9274	<0.05	0.46	0.91	>0.05
As	0.0002	0.0001	0.0000	0.0000	0.0001	0.0001	<0.05	0.00	0.00	>0.05
Cd	0.0017	0.0028	0.0000	0.0000	0.0009	0.0021	<0.05	0.03	0.09	>0.05
Sn	0.0529	0.2105	0.0001	0.0002	0.0259	0.1479	<0.05	0.07	0.17	<0.05
Pb	<LOD	<LOD	<LOD	<LOD	<LOD	<LOD	-	0.06	0.13	-

SD—Standard Deviation; <LOD—Below limit of detection. [a] Dust collected for approximately 14 days after installation of EDC. [b] Dust collected from welders' workstations. [c] Mann–Whitney test in exposed and control groups for dust deposits on EDC after approximately 14 days. [d] Spearman correlation between accumulated dust deposits on EDC after approximately 14 days and dust deposits on welders' workstations.

The PTE concentrations in Table 2 were calculated based on the area cleansed for the samples collected from welders' workstations and on the exposed EDC area for the accumulated dust samples.

The levels of Pb detected did not exceed the LOD in any of the dust samples collected for approximately 14 days. Additionally, PTEs in solder powders and wires were determined using a field-portable X-ray fluorescence analyzer, except for As. The following values for Cd (geometric mean (GM): 53,927.21 ppm; standard deviation (SD): 32,806.44 ppm; range: 5209.72–165,296.14 ppm), Cr (GM: 4115.78 ppm; SD: 2810.68 ppm; range: 465.31–14,550.51 ppm), Mn (GM: 1161.33 ppm; SD: 460.50 ppm; range: 1050.71–1471.06 ppm) and Ni (GM: 524.22 ppm; SD: 291.83 ppm; range: 102.03–1015.37 ppm) were found for solder powders only, while a value of Pb (GM: 249,973.13 ppm; SD: 165,157.41 ppm; range: 5840.90–522,785.34 ppm) was determined for solder wires only (Table 3), consistent with the results found in the dust exposure samples. Additionally, Cu and Zn were higher in solder powders and Sn was higher in solder wires.

Table 3. PTE levels (ppm) in soldering powders and wires. Limeira, Brazil, 2019.

	Soldering Powders N = 13			Soldering Wires N = 4		
	GM [a]	SD [b]	Min–Max	GM [a]	SD [b]	Min–Max
Cd	53,927	32,806	5209–165,296	<LOD	<LOD	<LOD
Mn	1161	460	1050–1471	<LOD	<LOD	<LOD
Ni	524	291	102–1015	<LOD	<LOD	<LOD
Cu	314,720	101,971	34,242–497,231	1800	8155	546–23,599
Zn	201,336	68,072	19,732–317,607	873	1159	202–2931
Cr	4115	2810	465–14,550	<LOD	<LOD	<LOD
Sn	1462	1244	635–5743	597,797	157,267	473,193–966,567
Pb	<LOD	<LOD	<LOD	249,973	165,157	5,840–522,785

<LOD—Below limit of detection. [a] GM—Geometric mean. [b] SD—Standard Deviation.

Spearman correlations between PTE concentrations in dust samples and the number of welders working in the same room and work time were not statistically significant ($p > 0.05$).

Moreover, Spearman correlations between PTE concentrations and the physical infrastructure of the workspaces (area, doors and windows areas, and ceiling height) were heterogeneous (Table 4). The correlation of PTE determined in dust deposits (cleaning worktop) (exposed group) with the area was statistically significant for Zn (Spearman correlation coefficient: Rho = 0.57) and Sn (Rho = 0.54), with door area for Mn (Rho = 0.71) and Sn (Rho = 0.45), and with ceiling height for Zn (Rho = 0.47), $p < 0.05$. Regarding the control group, correlations of PTE determined in dust deposits were statistically significant ($p < 0.05$) only with ceiling height for Cr (Rho = 0.48), Mn (Rho = 0.44), As (Rho = 0.65) and Sn (Rho = 0.46). Although PTE concentrations in welders' workstation dust proved statistically significant ($p < 0.05$) with area for Ni (Rho = 0.45) and Zn (Rho = 0.44) and with door area for Zn (Rho = 0.42), the correlation between window area and PTE dust deposits was not statistically significant ($p > 0.05$).

Socio-Demographic Data and Blood PTE Levels of Children

The subgroup of children, members of the families assessed, comprised 14 exposed and 15 control children aged 1–11 years. The mean age of the exposed group was 6 years (range: 1–11 years) comprising 4 females and 10 males, whereas the mean age of the control group was 6 years (range: 2–11 years) comprising 8 females and 7 males, showing the homogeneity of participants for the exposure groups. The mean time staying at home during the week for the children was approximately 7 h in both groups, ranging from 3–24 h for the exposed group and 10–24 h for the control group.

The blood samples of the exposed group had a mean and standard deviation (SD) of 1.62 µg/L (0.42), 9.9 µg/L (3.63), 3.35 µg/L (1.03), 1147.31 µg/L (278.13), 3698.25 µg/L (1155.84), 0.40 µg/L (0.19), 0.11 µg/L (0.11), 6.42 µg/L (20.99), and 3.31 µg/dL (2.29) for Cr, Mn, Ni, Co, Zn, As, Cd, Sn, and Pb, respectively. For the control group, the mean (SD) levels in blood were 1.49 µg/L (0.39), 10.43 µg/L (3.41), 3.23 µg/L (0.68), 1204.49 µg/L (205.56), 4227.96 µg/L (696.02), 0.34 µg/L (0.22), 0.01 µg/L (0.01), 0.80 µg/L (0.23), and 1.31 µg/dL (0.53) for Cr, Mn, Ni, Co, Zn, As, Cd, Sn, and Pb, respectively. The results showed a statistical difference for Cd and Pb ($p < 0.05$) between the control and exposed groups, as shown in Table 5.

Finally, the correlations between concentrations of PTEs in the blood samples and levels in dust deposits collected for approximately 14 days were moderate for Cr, Zn, and As, and strong for Cd. No statistically significant correlations were found between PTE levels in the blood and in dust collected from welders' workstations ($p > 0.05$) (Table 6).

Table 4. *p*-Values of Spearman correlations between PTE levels in dust samples and physical infrastructure by group. Limeira, Brazil, 2019.

	Accumulated Dust [a]																Welders' Workstation Dust [b]							
	Area				Window Area				Door Area				Ceiling Height				Area		Window Area		Door Area		Ceiling Height	
	Exposed N = 21		Control N = 23		Exposed N = 21		Control N = 23		Exposed N = 21		Control N = 23		Exposed N = 21		Control N = 23		Exposed N = 21							
	Rho	*p*-Value	Rho	*p*-Value	Rho	*p*-Value	Rho	*p*-Value	Rho	*p*-Value	Rho	*p*-Value	Rho	*p*-Value	Rho	*p*-Value	Rho	*p*-Value	Rho	*p*-Value	Rho	*p*-Value	Rho	*p*-Value
Cr	0.10	>0.05	−0.29	>0.05	−0.43	>0.05	0.08	>0.05	0.20	>0.05	−0.26	>0.05	−0.17	>0.05	0.48	<0.05	0.20	>0.05	−0.22	>0.05	0.29	>0.05	0.02	>0.05
Mn	0.40	>0.05	−0.34	>0.05	0.04	>0.05	−0.04	>0.05	0.71	<0.05	0.01	>0.05	−0.33	>0.05	0.44	<0.05	−0.08	>00.05	−0.15	>0.05	−0.10	>0.05	0.08	>0.05
Ni	0.30	>0.05	−0.11	>0.05	−0.33	>0.05	0.12	>0.05	0.03	>0.05	0.29	>0.05	0.12	>0.05	0.00	>0.05	0.45	<0.05	−0.04	>0.05	0.27	>0.05	0.29	>0.05
Cu	−0.09	>0.05	−0.08	>0.05	0.12	>0.05	0.08	>0.05	−0.06	>0.05	−0.05	>0.05	−0.37	>0.05	0.33	>0.05	0.13	>0.05	−0.11	>0.05	0.10	>0.05	0.05	>0.05
Zn	0.57	<0.05	0.22	>0.05	0.22	>0.05	0.00	>0.05	0.33	>0.05	−0.16	>0.05	0.47	<0.05	0.10	>0.05	0.44	<0.05	0.07	>0.05	0.42	<0.05	0.03	>0.05
As	0.39	>0.05	−0.01	>0.05	−0.45	>0.05	0.18	>0.05	0.38	>0.05	−0.09	>0.05	−0.19	>0.05	0.65	<0.05	0.06	>0.05	−0.39	>0.05	−0.10	>0.05	0.24	>0.05
Cd	−0.19	>0.05	−0.15	>0.05	0.05	>0.05	−0.36	>0.05	−0.22	>0.05	0.08	>0.05	−0.36	>0.05	−0.17	>0.05	0.04	>0.05	0.01	>0.05	0.06	>0.05	−0.26	>0.05
Sn	0.54	<0.05	−0.31	>0.05	0.14	>0.05	−0.13	>0.05	0.45	<0.05	0.05	>0.05	0.30	>0.05	0.46	<0.05	0.25	>0.05	−0.29	>0.05	0.32	>0.05	0.21	>0.05
Pb	<LOD	<LOD	<LOD	<LOD	<LOD	<LOD	<LOD	<LOD	<LOD	<LOD	<LOD	<LOD	<LOD	<LOD	<LOD	<LOD	0.30	>0.05	−0.19	>0.05	0.24	>0.05	0.26	>0.05

[a] Dust collected for approximately 14 days after installation of EDC. [b] Dust collected from welders' workstations. <LOD—Below limit of detection. **<0.05** represents the statistically significant correlations.

Table 5. Blood PTE levels determined in children. Limeira, Brazil, 2019.

	Exposed N = 14			Control N = 15			Total N = 29			
	Mean	SD	95th Percentile	Mean	SD	95th Percentile	Mean	SD	95th Percentile	p-Value *
Cr (µg/L)	1.62	0.42	2.30 (95)	1.49	0.39	2.05 (95)	1.55	0.40	2.27 (95)	>0.05
Mn (µg/L)	9.91	3.63	16.07 (95)	10.43	3.41	16.93 (95)	10.18	3.46	16.64 (95)	>0.05
Ni (µg/L)	3.35	1.03	5.05 (95)	3.23	0.68	4.13 (95)	3.28	0.85	4.81 (95)	>0.05
Cu (µg/L)	1147.31	278.13	1554.40 (95)	1204.49	205.56	1621.93 (95)	1176.90	240.60	1626.90 (95)	>0.05
Zn (µg/L)	3698.25	1155.84	6058.62 (95)	4227.96	696.02	5239.38 (95)	3972.00	966.98	5907.13 (95)	>0.05
As (µg/L)	0.40	0.19	0.78 (95)	0.34	0.22	0.62 (95)	0.37	0.21	0.83 (95)	>0.05
Cd (µg/L)	0.11	0.11	0.30 (95)	0.01	0.01	0.02 (95)	0.06	0.10	0.26 (95)	**<0.05**
Sn (µg/L)	6.42	20.99	28.51 (95)	0.80	0.23	1.08 (95)	3.61	14.85	1.12 (95)	>0.05
Pb (µg/dL)	3.31	2.29	7.14 (97.5)	1.31	0.53	2.17 (97.5)	2.28	1.90	6.66 (97.5)	**<0.05**

* Mann–Whitney tests in exposed and control groups, except Cr, Cu, and Zn, for which Student's t-test was applied. **<0.05** represents the statistically significant differences.

Table 6. Spearman correlations of PTE levels in children's blood (0–11 years) and in dust samples. Limeira, Brazil, 2019.

	Accumulated Dust [a] Total N = 29		Welders' Workstation Dust [b] Exposed N = 14	
	Rho	p-Value	Rho	p-Value
Cr	**0.40**	**<0.05**	−0.06	>0.05
Mn	−0.11	>0.05	0.05	>0.05
Ni	−0.04	>0.05	−0.46	>0.05
Cu	−0.22	>0.05	0.37	>0.05
Zn	**−0.43**	**<0.05**	−0.03	>0.05
As	**0.40**	**<0.05**	−0.05	>0.05
Cd	**0.80**	**<0.05**	0.08	>0.05
Sn	0.22	>0.05	−0.18	>0.05
Pb	-	-	−0.43	>0.05

[a] Dust collected for approximately 14 days after installation of EDC. [b] Dust collected from welders' workstations. Bold represents the statistically significant differences

4. Discussion

To the best of our knowledge, there are few studies [25] investigating the use of EDC in the assessment of PTE exposure, where most studies use EDC to investigate microbiological exposure. However, some studies have used the cloth method to analyze exposure to metals by surface cleaning [26,27]. During the soldering process, workers are often exposed to pollutants, ash and dust, fumes, and hazardous chemicals [28]. The present study found moderate (Cr Rho = **0.40**, As Rho = **0.40**) and strong (Cd Rho = **0.80**) positive correlations between levels of these PTEs in children's blood and in dust deposits collected for approximately 14 days (p-value < 0.05), confirming that PTE concentrations in blood can be influenced by dust concentrations. Oral contact is the most common route of exposure, but inhalation is also an important route [12]. The dust collected from welders' workstations proved to be a less relevant exposure route (p > 0.05) for all PTE except Sn. This finding can be explained by the complexity of the informal work scenario, with no fixed workstations or number of workers and the presence of unregistered cleaning routines or accidents related to handling soldering powder, such as dropping on floors and furniture, in the present study. Despite cleaning routines, the hazard of high PTE concentrations in dust from the floor or the air which can be inhaled or ingested by children remains.

In a previous study, 19 ash and dust samples were collected into glass beakers from jewelry workshops in Bangladesh and high concentrations of the compounds Cd, Cr, Pb, and As were found [28]. Other studies also showed that high metal concentrations in inexpensive jewelry [29,30] were a health concern. High metal concentrations can also pose a health risk after the production process during use of the items by children. High Pb concentrations in low-cost jewelry from Cambodia were detected using X-ray fluorescence (XRF) measurements [31]. These health risks can also be found in developed countries, where high Cd in inexpensive jewelry using XRF measurements was found [29]. Even in jewelry with high surface Cd levels, bioavailability to the wearer during dermal contact was low, although the same does not apply to manufacturing of the jewelry, since solder powder has a high Cd concentration [32].

The results of the present study showed statistically significant differences ($p < 0.05$) between exposed and control groups for blood levels of the metals Cd (mean: Control 0.001 µg/L; Exposed 0.011 µg/L) and Pb (mean: Control 1.31 µg/dL; Exposed 3.31 µg/dL). However, on the analysis of blood and dust PTE levels, Spearman correlations revealed statistically significant differences ($p < 0.05$) for Cr, Zn, As, and Cd in dust samples collected for approximately 14 days. A study analyzed associations for isotopic ratios in comparisons between lead concentrations in blood samples from 30 children and environmental samples (floor dust, soil, drinking water and paint) in Australia [33]. The authors concluded that floor dust collected using EDC showed the most significant correlation, as evidenced by regression analyses.

Surface dust samples were collected from the homes of Native American jewelry makers and from homes in which jewelry was not made in New Mexico [4]. The dust samples were collected by cleaning wall and floor areas near the workplace and the dining rooms of control participants, using Whatman® filter paper. The concentrations of Ag, Cu, Ni, Mg, and Sb were significantly higher in exposed homes than in control homes ($p \leq 0.02$). Moreover, Ag, Cu, Sn, B, Ni, Zn, Pb, and Cd concentrations were significantly higher in samples collected in work areas when compared with living areas in exposed homes ($p = 0.02$, paired t-test). These findings are corroborated by the results of the present study, revealing significantly higher concentrations in samples of accumulated dust in the exposed group for all PTEs assessed, except Pb ($p < 0.05$).

The Pb concentrations detected in accumulated dust were below the LOD. Although Pb was found only in soldering wires and not soldering powders, all of the materials (soldering powders and wires, jewelry, and acids) are employed informally and have no clear provenance and/or instructions on use and safety. Blood lead levels (BLL) of the children in the exposed group reached 7.5 µg/dL, and the US Centers for Disease Control and Prevention (CDC), based on results from the National Health and Nutrition Examination Survey (NHANES), has determined a Blood Lead Reference Value (BLRV) of 3.5 µg/dL [34]. The BLRV of the CDC serves as a guide to determine medical or environmental actions and prioritize communities for actions preventing exposure. No safe BLL in children exists, where even low levels can cause harm [35]. Children are especially sensitive to Pb damage, principally because their central nervous system is still developing and more vulnerable to toxic agents [5]. In Latin America, there is a dearth of legal instruments on exposure to lead [36]. In a study of 29 children (15 cases and 14 controls) from Mumbai exposed to a jewelry cottage industry, the authors described cases with neurological symptoms of seizures (n = 12) and drowsiness (n = 3), and mean blood lead level of cases was 42.6 ± 22.5 µg/dL (range 16.6–85.4 µg/dL) proving significantly higher in these exposed children than in controls (mean BLL 8.7 ± 1.2 µg/dL, range 7.0–10.2 µg/dL) ($p < 0.001$) [7].

A previous study of the same population of welders analyzed PTE concentrations in air of the breathing zone of the workers and in the blood of the workers and their relatives within the same household, raising concerns about the concentrations of Ni and Cd [12]. Moreover, PTEs are often intentionally added to jewelry items because they are good coating agents, can lower manufacturing costs, improve workability, produce shiny surfaces, and mimic famous jewelry items [30]. Blood PTE concentrations in adults from the same population were measured, showing higher blood levels in the exposure group for As (0.44 µg L^{-1}), Cd (0.21 µg L^{-1}) and Pb (1.88 µg L^{-1}) compared to the control group (0.35 µg L^{-1}, 0.01 µg L^{-1} and 1.04 µg L^{-1} for As, Cd, and Pb, respectively) [23].

Regarding physical infrastructure, correlations between physical infrastructure and dust PTE concentrations in the present investigation were heterogeneous. Another study measured the accumulation rate of ash and dust in jewelry workshops in Bangladesh by weighing the passive samples, the calculated accumulation rate of ash showed no strong correlation with workshop size or number of jewelry workers [28]. However, a slight difference was observed between the different types of manufacturing units, where smelting, polishing, cutting, and enameling units produced more ash and dust than soldering activities. It is important to note that a large number of households did not have appropriate workspaces, with rooms divided using cloth and cardboard, potentially impacting air circulation and results.

This study has some limitations. First, dust and children's blood sampled only once during the year, where the relationships observed between study variables and PTE concentrations may vary by season and work demand. Second, the number of participants was small, preventing different interactions from being further explored. The primary reason for parents or legal guardians refusing to participate was not wanting their child to have a venous blood draw. Third, only one exposure pathway was analyzed, namely, dust, but other pathways such as water, soil from the unpaved yard, and paint from the walls should be further analyzed. However, accessing home-based welders is difficult because most live in areas of high social vulnerability, change work constantly, and principally, the production of informal jewelry is not regulated by law and, therefore, most workers do not want to be exposed to authorities. Last, some studies have used different kinds of cloths to analyze metal exposure by cleaning surfaces [26,37], but Swiffer cloths were used in the present study as they are both accessible and low-cost and have proven effective for the proposed application.

5. Conclusions

The study results highlighted concerns regarding children's exposure to Cr, As, and Cd within the informal home-based environment. It is important to foster actions promoting safety, including preventing the involvement of children in this type of labor and restricting their access to workspaces and materials. In addition, EDC represents a potentially low-cost tool for evaluating PTE exposure, particularly in highly vulnerable areas and in studies with limited funding.

Author Contributions: Conceptualization, F.B. and K.P.K.O.; methodology, K.P.K.O., F.B., M.S.L. and G.A.d.A.; fieldwork, F.B.; software, F.B.; validation, K.P.K.O.; formal analysis, F.B., M.S.L. and G.A.d.A.; resources, K.P.K.O., M.S.L. and G.A.d.A.; data curation, F.B.; writing—original draft preparation, F.B.; writing—review and editing, K.P.K.O., M.S.L. and G.A.d.A.; supervision, K.P.K.O.; project administration, K.P.K.O.; funding acquisition, K.P.K.O., M.S.L. and G.A.d.A. All authors have read and agreed to the published version of the manuscript.

Funding: This study was supported by grants from the Fundação de Amparo à Pesquisa do Estado de São Paulo (2018/18391-0, 2017/20752-8, 2014/50887-4) and the Coordenação de Aperfeiçoamento de Pessoal de Nível Superior (CAPES). K.P.K.O. is the recipient of a scholarship from Conselho Nacional de Desenvolvimento Científico e Tecnológico (CNPq, #314637/2021-4).

Institutional Review Board Statement: The study was approved by the Ethics Committee of School of Public Health of University of São Paulo (CAAE 26665319.3.0000.5421).

Informed Consent Statement: Informed consent was obtained from all subjects involved in the study. Written informed consent has been obtained from the patient(s) to publish this paper.

Data Availability Statement: Not applicable.

Acknowledgments: The authors extend their thanks to the volunteers who agreed to participate in the study and acknowledge the support of the Health Secretariat of Limeira city, including all health agents and the coordinator of Limeira's primary healthcare units.

Conflicts of Interest: The authors declare no conflict of interest.

References

1. McCann, M. Hazards in Cottage Industries in Developing Countries. *Am. J. Ind. Med.* **1996**, *30*, 125–129. [CrossRef]
2. Mathee, A.; Street, R.; Teare, J.; Naicker, N. Lead exposure in the home environment: An overview of risks from cottage industries in Africa. *Neurotoxicology* **2020**, *81*, 34–39. [CrossRef] [PubMed]
3. Teare, J.; Kootbodien, T.; Naicker, N.; Mathee, A. The Extent, Nature and Environmental Health Implications of Cottage Industries in Johannesburg, South Africa. *Int. J. Environ. Res. Public Health* **2015**, *12*, 1894–1901. [CrossRef] [PubMed]
4. Gonzales, M.; Shah, V.; Bobelu, A.; Qualls, C.; Natachu, K.; Bobelu, J.; Jamon, E.; Neha, D.; Paine, S.; Zager, P. Concentrations of Surface-Dust Metals in Native American Jewelry-Making Homes in Zuni Pueblo, New Mexico. *Arch. Environ. Health* **2004**, *59*, 245–249. [CrossRef] [PubMed]
5. Olympio, K.P.K.; Gonçalves, C.; Günther, W.M.R.; Bechara, E.J.H. Neurotoxicity and aggressiveness triggered by low-level lead in children: A review. *Rev. Panam. Salud. Publica* **2009**, *26*, 266–275. [CrossRef] [PubMed]
6. Street, R.A.; Goessler, W.; Naidoo, S.; Shezi, B.; Cele, N.; Rieger, J.; Ettinger, K.; Reddy, T.; Mathee, A. Exposure to lead and other toxic metals from informal foundries producing cookware from scrap metal. *Environ. Res.* **2020**, *191*, 109860. [CrossRef]
7. Goel, A.D.; Chowgule, R.V. Outbreak investigation of lead neurotoxicity in children from artificial jewelry cottage industry. *Environ. Health Prev. Med.* **2019**, *24*, 30. [CrossRef]
8. Ahmad, S.A.; Khan, M.H.; Khandker, S.; Sarwar, A.F.M.; Yasmin, N.; Faruquee, M.H.; Yasmin, R. Blood Lead Levels and Health Problems of Lead Acid Battery Workers in Bangladesh. *Sci. World J.* **2014**, *2014*, 974104. [CrossRef]
9. Irawati, Y.; Kusnoputranto, H.; Achmadi, U.F.; Safrudin, A.; Sitorus, A.; Risandi, R.; Wangsamuda, S.; Asih, P.B.S.; Syafruddin, D. Blood lead levels and lead toxicity in children aged 1-5 years of Cinangka Village, Bogor Regency. *PLoS ONE* **2022**, *17*, e0264209. [CrossRef]
10. Bandeira, M.J.; Santos, M.R.; Cardoso, M.S.; Hlavinicka, N.; Anjos, A.L.S.; Wândega, E.L.; Bah, H.A.F.; Oliva, S.T.; Rocha, A.R.; Souza-Júnior, J.A.; et al. Assessment of potters' occupational exposure to lead and associated risk factors in Maragogipinho, Brazil: Preliminary results. *Int. Arch. Occup. Environ. Health* **2021**, *94*, 1061–1071. [CrossRef]
11. Lacorte, L.E.C.; Vilela, R.A.G.; Silva, R.C.; Chiesa, A.M.; Tulio, E.S.; Franco, R.R.; Bravo, E.S. The knots in the network for eradicating child labor in the production of jewelry and costume jewelry in Limeira-SP. (in Portuguese). *Rev. Bras. Saúde Ocup.* **2013**, *38*, 199–215. [CrossRef]
12. Ferreira, A.P.S.S.; Pereira, E.C.; Salles, F.J.; Silva, F.F.; Batista, B.L.; Handakas, E.; Olympio, K.P.K. Home-based and informal work exposes the families to high levels of potentially toxic elements. *Chemosphere* **2019**, *218*, 319–327. [CrossRef] [PubMed]
13. Salles, F.J.; Tavares, D.J.B.; Freire, B.M.; Ferreira, A.P.S.S.; Handakas, E.; Batista, B.L.; Olympio, K.P.K. Home-based informal jewelry production increases exposure of working families to cadmium. *Sci. Total Environ.* **2021**, *785*, 147297. [CrossRef]
14. USEPA. United States Environmental Protection Agency. *Guide to Considering Children's Health When Developing EPA Actions: Implementing Executive Order 13045 and EPA's Policy on Evaluating Health Risks to Children*; EPA: Washington, DC, USA, 2006.
15. Tong, S.T.Y.; Lam, K.C. Home sweet home? A case study of household dust contamination in Hong Kong. *Sci. Total Environ.* **2000**, *256*, 115–123. [CrossRef] [PubMed]
16. Schultz, I.R.; Cade, S.; Kuo, L.J. The Dust Exposome. In *Unraveling the Exposome*; Dagnino, S., Macherone, A., Eds.; Springer: Berlin/Heidelberg, Germany, 2019; pp. 247–254. [CrossRef]
17. Noss, I.; Wouters, I.M.; Visser, M.; Heederik, D.J.J.; Thorne, P.S.; Brunekreef, B.; Doekes, G. Evaluation of a Low-Cost Electrostatic Dust Fall Collector for Indoor Air Endotoxin Exposure Assessment. *Appl. Environ. Microbiol.* **2008**, *74*, 5621–5627. [CrossRef] [PubMed]
18. Wang, C.F.; Huang, M.F.; Chang, E.E.; Chiang, P.C. Assessment of closed vessel digestion methods for elemental determination of airborne particulate matter by ICP-AES. *Anal. Sci.* **1996**, *12*, 201–207. [CrossRef]
19. Karthikeyan, S.; Joshi, U.M.; Balasubramanian, R. Microwave assisted sample preparation for determining water-solubre fraction of trace elements in urban airbone particulate matter: Evaluation of bioavailability. *Anal. Chim. Acta* **2006**, *576*, 23–30. [CrossRef]
20. Lum, K.R.; Betteridge, J.S.; Macdonald, R.R. The potential availability of P, Al, Cd, Co, Cr, Cu, Fe, Mn, Ni, Pb and Zn in urban particulate matter. *Environ. Technol. Lett.* **1982**, *3*, 57–62. [CrossRef]
21. American Industrial Hygiene Association. *A Strategy for Assessing and Managing Occupational Exposures*, 4th ed.; American Industrial Hygiene Association: Washington, DC, USA, 2015.
22. Silva, J.P.R.; Salles, F.J.; Leroux, I.N.; Ferreira, A.P.S.S.; Silva, A.S.; Assunção, N.A.; Nardocci, A.C.; Sato, A.P.S.; Barbosa, F., Jr.; Cardoso, M.R.A.; et al. High blood lead levels are associated with lead concentrations in households and day care centers attended by Brazilian preschool children. *Environ. Pollut.* **2018**, *239*, 681–688. [CrossRef]
23. Salles, F.J.; Luz, M.S.; Olympio, K.P.K. Occupational exposure to potentially toxic elements in home-based and informal workers. In Proceedings of the Abstract, 33rd Annual Conference of the International Society for Environmental Epidemiology, New York, NY, USA, 23–26 August 2021; Environmental Health Perspectives: Durham, UK, 2021.
24. Croghan, C.; Egeghy, P.P. Methods of Dealing With Values Below the Limit Of Detection Using SAS. In Proceedings of the Southeastern SAS User Group, St. Petersburg, FL, USA, 22–24 September 2003.
25. Lewis, R.D.; Ong, K.H.; Emo, B.; Kennedy, J.; Brown, C.A.; Condoor, S.; Thummalakunta, L. Do new wipe materials outperform traditional lead dust cleaning methods? *J. Occup. Environ. Hyg.* **2012**, *9*, 524–533. [CrossRef]
26. Harper, M.; Hallmarka, T.S.; Bartolu, A.A. A comparison of methods and materials for the analysis of leaded wipes. *J. Environ. Monit.* **2002**, *4*, 1025–1033. [CrossRef] [PubMed]

27. Cox, J.; Indugula, R.; Vesper, S.; Zhu, Z.; Jandarov, R.; Reponen, T. Comparison of indoor air sampling and dust collection methods for fungal exposure assessment using quantitative PCR. *Environ. Sci. Process Impacts* **2017**, *19*, 1312–1319. [CrossRef] [PubMed]
28. Sikder, A.M.; Hossain, T.; Khan, M.H.; Hasan, M.A.; Fakhruzzaman, M.; Turner, J.B.; Pestov, D.; McCallister, L.S.; Elahi, K.M. Toxicity assessment of ash and dust from handmade gold jewelry manufacturing workshops in Bangladesh. *Environ. Monit. Assess* **2017**, *189*, 279. [CrossRef]
29. Kern, M.S.; Boron, M.L.; Weidenhamer, J.D. Buyer beware: Inexpensive, high cadmium jewelry can pose severe health risks. *Sci. Total Environ.* **2021**, *764*, 142926. [CrossRef]
30. Adie, G.U.; Oyebade, E.O.; Atanda, B.M. Preliminary Study of Heavy Metals in Low-Cost Jewelry Items Available in Nigerian Markets. *J. Health Pollut.* **2020**, *10*, 201202. [CrossRef] [PubMed]
31. Murphy, T.; Lim, S.; Kim, S.; Irvine, K.; Chaiwat, W.; Wilson, K. Metal Contamination in Low-Cost Jewelry and Toys in Cambodia. *J. Health Pollut.* **2016**, *6*, 47–57. [CrossRef]
32. Pouzar, M.; Zvolská, M.; Jarolím, O.; Vavrušová, L.A. The Health Risk of Cd Released from Low-Cost Jewelry. *Int. J. Environ.* **2017**, *14*, 520. [CrossRef]
33. Gulson, B.; Anderson, P.; Taylor, A. Surface dust EDC are the best predictors of blood leads in young children with elevated blood lead levels. *Environ. Res.* **2013**, *126*, 171–178. [CrossRef]
34. Centers for Disease Control and Prevention. USA. 2022. Available online: https://www.cdc.gov/nceh/lead/data/blood-lead-reference-value.htm (accessed on 25 March 2022).
35. Ruckart, P.Z.; Jones, R.L.; Courtney, J.G.; LeBlanc, T.T.; Jackson, W.; Karwowski, M.P.; Cheng, P.; Allwood, P.; Svendsen, E.R.; Breysse, P.N. Update of the Blood Lead Reference Value-United States, 2021. *MMWR Morb. Mortal. Wkly. Rep.* **2021**, *70*, 1509–1512. [CrossRef]
36. Olympio, K.P.K.; Gonçalves, C.G.; Salles, F.J.; Ferreira, A.P.S.S.; Soares, A.S.; Buzalaf, M.A.R.; Cardoso, M.R.A.; Bechara, E.J.H. What are the blood lead levels of children living in Latin America and the Caribbean? *Environ. Int.* **2017**, *101*, 46–58. [CrossRef]
37. Beaucham, C.; Ceballos, D.; King, B. Lessons learned from surface wipe sampling for lead in three workplaces. *J. Occup. Environ. Hyg.* **2017**, *14*, 611–619. [CrossRef] [PubMed]

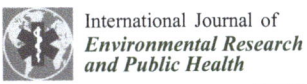

Article

Agrochemical Residues in Fish and Bivalves from Sepetiba Bay and Parnaiba River Delta, Brazil

Joyce Aparecida Tavares Miranda [1,*], Fabíola Helena S. Fogaça [2], Sara C. Cunha [3], Mariana Batha Alonso [1], João Paulo M. Torres [1] and José Oliveira Fernandes [3]

1. Biophysics Institute Carlos Chagas Filho, Universidade Federal do Rio de Janeiro (IBCCF-UFRJ), Av. Carlos Chagas Filho, 373, Rio de Janeiro 21941-902, RJ, Brazil
2. Brazilian Agricultural Research Company, Agroindústria de Alimentos (EMBRAPA), Av. das Américas, nº 29.501, Guaratiba, Rio de Janeiro 23020-470, RJ, Brazil
3. Laboratory of Bromatology and Hydrology (LAQV-REQUIMTE), Faculty of Pharmacy, University of Porto, Rua Jorge de Viterbo Ferreira 228, 4050-313 Porto, Portugal
* Correspondence: joycetmiranda@gmail.com

Abstract: Accumulation of pesticides has a harmful impact on the environment and human health. The main goal of this work was to develop a method to determine and quantify the residues of thirteen pesticides in edible fish and bivalves such as parati (*Mugil curema*), seabass (*Centropomus* ssp.), mullet (*Mugil brasiliensis*), clams (*Anomalocardia brasiliana*) and mussel (*Mytilus galloprovincialis*) collected from Sepetiba Bay and Parnaiba River Delta (Brazil) between 2019 and 2020. Matrix solid-phase dispersion (MSPD) was used for extraction and quantification through gas chromatography coupled to tandem mass spectrometry (GC-MS/MS). The method was validated (linearity, accuracy and precision) for fatty fish (*Salmo salar*), lean fish (*Mugil curema*) and bivalves (*Mytilus edulis*). The survey found linear correlation coefficients (r) equal to or greater than 0.9 for almost all analytes. The relative standard deviations (RSD) of five replicates were less than 20% for almost all analytes at different concentrations in lean fish, fatty fish and bivalves. Most analytes showed satisfactory accuracy. Alachlor herbicide was found in samples of seabass, mussels, clams and parati with levels ranging between 0.55 to 420.39 $\mu g\ kg^{-1}$ dw. Ethion was found in parati (maximum 211.22 $\mu g\ kg^{-1}$ dw), mussels (15.1 $\mu g\ kg^{-1}$ dw) and clams (maximum 44.50 $\mu g\ kg^{-1}$ dw). Alachlor was found in clams (maximum 93.1 $\mu g\ kg^{-1}$ dw), and bifenthrin was found in parati (maximum 43.4 $\mu g\ kg^{-1}$ dw) and clams (maximum 42.21 $\mu g\ kg^{-1}$ dw). The validated method was satisfactory for the determination of eleven pesticides in the fatty fish matrix, and thirteen pesticides in the samples of lean fish and bivalves. The presence of alachlor, ethion and bifenthrin stands out.

Keywords: organochlorine; organophosphorus; pyrethroids; seafood; MSPD; GC-MS/MS

1. Introduction

Pollution by industrial, domestic and agricultural waste severely affects the aquatic ecosystem. Endocrine disruptors (EDs) are exogenous substances or mixtures that alter functions of the endocrine system and consequently cause adverse health effects in an intact organism, or its progeny, or (sub)populations [1]. ED substances have the ability to alter the functions of the endocrine system and cause adverse effects on human and animal health [2–8]. Moreover, the EDs may be persistent organic pollutants (POPs). POPs are classes of environmental micropollutants—compounds that are present in the environment in approximate concentrations of $\mu g\ L^{-1}$ and $ng\ L^{-1}$—and the main concerns related to these classes of substances are that they can produce adverse effects in organisms exposed to very low concentrations, remain for decades in the environment, under mechanisms of bioaccumulation and biomagnification, passing through the food chain of the species [3]. The impacts of pesticides on the environment and ecosystems can vary from contamination of groundwater and imbalances in soil microbial populations to the emergence of new pathogens, or imbalance of some existing ones.

Some studies suggest that contamination with chlorinated pesticides can be related to neurodegenerative diseases and cancers and contribute to the development of type 2 diabetes mellitus (T2D), due to the interference in glucose uptake and adiposity function, resulting in proinflammatory responses and disrupted energy metabolism [9–11]. These substances can follow the transplacental route, and be transferred through lactation; therefore, individuals can be exposed to these compounds before birth and in early childhood [10,12,13]. Despite the ban on certain organochlorine pesticides (OCPs) in some parts of the world in the early 1970s, these compounds still contaminate the environment because they are POPs [9–11,14–16]. Exposure to organophosphorus pesticides (OPs) is related to acute neurotoxicity, possibly due to the inhibition of acetylcholinesterase (AChE). Exposure to this agrochemical is also related to attention deficit disorders (ADHD) and autism in children [8,17]. Pyrethroids are highly efficient against a large range of insect pests, with relatively low toxicity for mammalian species [18]. Despite their low human toxicity, there have been several reports of poisoning related to occupational exposure and deliberate ingestion. Pyrethroids act on several channels and proteins, and interfere with the excitatory neurons, inducing cholinergic syndrome (CS), hyperexcitability, choreoathetosis, and profuse salivation; these pesticides are also related to T-syndrome, characterized by tremors [18,19].

Surveys concerning the anthropic impacts caused by POPs, such as pesticides, on aquatic food chains depend on the use of bioindicator species. Bivalves are intensively employed as sentinel bioindicators in various ecological studies, and spatial–temporal assessments of marine and freshwater contaminants [20–23]. Morphological malformation in the embryos of fish was detected in response to OPs exposure, [24] and there is evidence of tuna hepatic alteration under OCPs exposure [11]. Transplacental transfer of pyrethroid pesticides and OCPs was also observed in aquatic mammals [25,26].

The choice of the analysis method for pesticide residues determination requires consideration of a huge number of factors, such as: chemical class of the analyte and metabolites, and their chemical properties such as boiling point or polarity; appropriate solvent and mobile phases; pesticides' stability in injector ports, on-column, or in-mass ion sources; chromatographic behavior; interferences in detection; detection method and limit or regulatory requirements. In mass spectrometry methods, one of the most important parameters to consider, particularly when selectivity or sensitivity criteria are required, is the ionization mode. In gas chromatography (GC), the electron ionization (EI) method clearly has an advantage due to the availability of extensive libraries in full scan mode for confirmation of compound identity through library search matching, when sufficient sample concentration is available. GC-MS/MS can provide additional selectivity when compared with the GC/MS method [27]. Regarding extraction techniques, matrix solid-phase dispersion (MSPD) has been successfully used in the extraction of multiple trace pesticide residues analysis in several foods [28]. MSPD is based on thorough mechanical homogenization of the sample with a sorbent, after which the analytes are eluted with an appropriate solvent. MSPD has advantages such as speed, inexpensiveness, simplicity, adaptability, and ease of handling in comparison to traditional techniques such as liquid–liquid extraction [8,21,22,29–33].

As for the environmental concern, aquatic contamination by pesticides can compromise the marine ecosystem. Regarding human nutrition and food security, the exposure of seafood to these compounds in their natural habitats leads to the loss of their quality and compromises their safety for consumption, directly affecting fishing activity. Thus, the objective of the present work was to develop a method for the quantification of 13 pesticide residues belonging to the organochlorine, organophosphorus and pyrethroid classes, in 84 samples of Brazilian seafood from Sepetiba Bay, including parati (*Mugil curema*), seabass (*Centropomus* spp.) and mussel (*Mytilus galloprovincialis*), and from Parnaiba River Delta, including mullet (*Mugil brasiliensis*) and clam (*Anomalocardia brasiliana*) species. Additionally, to demonstrate the presence of pesticides in marine animals for human consumption and the potential deleterious impact on human health and how much it impacts the decisions of control agencies.

2. Materials and Methods

2.1. Sampling Area

The fish and bivalve samples studied in the present work—seabass, parati, mullet, clams and mussels—were caught by fishermen between 2019 and 2020 in estuaries and adjacent coastal areas of Brazil, a country bathed by the Atlantic Ocean. The collected samples were desiccated, and the edible and nonedible parts were separated. The edible part (muscle) was then stored at approximately $-20\,°C$ for 90 days; afterward, the 84 samples were lyophilized and stored in Petri dishes covered with aluminum foil in order to avoid contamination before being transported to Portugal for analysis.

The Parnaiba River Delta is located in the northeast of Brazil, in the state of Piauí. It is considered one of the three largest sedimentary basins in Brazilian territory with an extent of about 2750 km^2 [34]. The biome is divided between caatinga and tropical forest, housing important plant and animal communities. The tropical climate of the region is characterized by a rainy summer and a dry winter, with 1200 mm annual average rainfall [34–36]. The Sepetiba Bay is located on the southeastern coast of Brazil, in the state of Rio de Janeiro, with ~447 km^2 of extension area at high tide [37]. It is a body of saline and brackish water, which communicates with the Atlantic Ocean through two passages, one on the west and another on the east, as well as having great influence on rivers and tidal channels in its innermost part. The region is highly urbanized with intense industrial activity, such as metallurgical, petrochemical and pyrometallurgical foundries. In this way, the aquatic environment is severely impacted, which in turn contributes to the social impact on the lives of fishing communities, which depend on this activity for subsistence and income [36,38]. Brazil is one of the countries in the world that most uses a wide variety of agrochemicals, so it is expected to find the presence of many classes of these compounds in different Brazilian aquatic biomes.

2.2. Reagents and Standards

The compounds analyzed were organophosphorus: lindane, chlorpyrifos-methyl, chlorpyrifos, fipronil, ethion; organochlorines: aldrin, chlordene, hexachlorobenzene, mirex; organochlorine: alachloro; pyrethroids: bifenthrin, permethrin; and the dicarboximide vincozoline. We used a standard compound with purity >98%, supplied by Sigma Aldrich (Saint Louis, MO, USA). Triphenyl phosphate (TPP, purity 99%), purchased from Sigma Aldrich (Saint Louis, MO, USA), was used as an internal standard.

Acetonitrile and methanol (HPLC grade) were purchased from Honeywell/Riedel-de-Haën TM (Muskegon, MI, USA); acetone, toluene, and carbon tetrachloride from Panreac Quimica SA (Barcelona, Spain). Anhydrous magnesium sulphate and sodium chloride, all reagent grades, were obtained from Honeywell/Fluka (Muskegon, MI, USA), and anhydrous potassium carbonate from Fluka Chemie GmbH (Buchs, France). Ultrapure water (18.2 mΩ cm^{-1}) was purified using a Milli-Q gradient system from Millipore (Milford, MA, USA).

Individual standard solutions were prepared at a concentration of 1000 µg mL^{-1} in acetonitrile, acetone, methanol or toluene, according to the analyte solubility. Then, the solutions were stored in amber screw-capped glass flasks in the dark at $-20\,°C$. Working standard solutions at a concentration of 100 µg mL^{-1} were obtained by diluting the stock solutions in acetonitrile and storing them at $-20\,°C$. Mixing solutions of 1.0, 0.5 and 0.25 µg mL^{-1} were prepared in acetonitrile and used to spike the samples in order to obtain matching calibration curves.

2.3. Sample Preparation

To extract the analytes, ~500 mg of each sample (dry weight basis, dw) was weighed in amber glass vials (15 mL bottles). One hundred mg of magnesium sulphate, 100 mg of acidified silica [39] and 20 µL of TPP (5 mg L^{-1}) were added to the flasks and shaken for 1 min. Then, after mixing overnight (~12 h) at 420 rpm and ~21 °C (D-72379 Hechingen, Edmund Bühler GmbH, Germany), 3.0 mL of acetonitrile: toluene (4:1, v/v, pH 3.0) was added and mixed for 15 min at 420 rpm at ~21 °C. After centrifugation (3 min at 1500× g) 1 mL of supernatant was added to a small aluminum oxide column (100 mg, preactivated with 500 µL of the extracting solvent), and eluted with 500 µL of acetonitrile: toluene (4:1, v/v, pH 3.0). Finally, the eluted was evaporated under a gentle stream of nitrogen at 40 °C, then reconstitute to a total volume of 70 µL in toluene, and transferred to a 2 mL amber bottle containing a 100 µL insert.

2.4. Instrumental Analysis and Optimization of the Analytical Method

The sample extracts (1 µL) were analyzed using a gas chromatograph Agilent 7890B (Agilent Technologies, Santa Clara, CA, USA) coupled to an Agilent 7000C triple quadrupole mass spectrometer (Agilent Technologies, USA), in electron ionization mode (EI), using a 5MS capillary column (30 m × 0.25 mm × 0.25 mm, Agilent J&W USA). The oven was programmed to start at 95 °C, hold for 1.5 min, ramp at 20 °C min^{-1} to 130 °C, ramp again at 5 °C min^{-1} to 230 °C, then ramp at 25 °C min^{-1} to 290 °C, with a total run time of 30 min. The flow rate was 1.3 mL min^{-1} using helium gas as a carrier. The temperatures of the transfer line, ion source, 1st and 2nd quadrupole were 250, 320 and 150 °C, respectively. The collision cell gases were nitrogen (1.5 mL min^{-1}) and helium (2.25 mL min^{-1}). The triple quadrupole MS was operated in multiple reaction monitoring (MRM) mode detecting two transitions per analyte (Table 1).

Table 1. GC-MS/MS parameters for determination of target analytes by MRM.

Target Compounds	Log K$_{ow}$	Transition m/z		Collision Energy (KV)
Lindane	3.72	218.8> 181> 180.9>	183 109 145	5 30 12
Chlorpyriphos-methyl	4.31	288> 286>	93 271 270.0	15 26 16
Chlorpyriphos	4.96	318.8> 314> 313.8> 28.8>	286 258 272.9	5 14 15
Fipronil	4.00	367>	228 225 224 213	30 25 20 30
Ethion	5.07	231>	175 129	5 25
Aldrin	6.50	298> 263> 257>	263 191 193 222	8 30 12

Table 1. Cont.

Target Compounds	Log K_{ow}	Transition m/z		Collision Energy (KV)
Chlordene	5.57	230>	195	25
			160	40
HCB	5.73	283.9>	248.8	25
		284>	213.9	35
			142	50
Mirex	6.89	272>	237	20
		271.9>	167	40
			235	15
Bifenthrin	6.00	166>	116.9	25
		181>	165	16
		182>	166	25
			167	12
Permethrin	6.50	183.1>	168.1	15
		183>	153.1	25
		163>	115.2	38
			77.1	5
			127	
Alachlor	3.52	270>	161.5	20
		238>		
Vinclozolin	3.10	187	145.0	15
			172.2	

2.5. Analytical Method Validation

The defined method was validated by studies of linearity, recovery, repeatability, limit of detection (LOD) and of quantification (LOQ) applied to a fish species with low lipid content (parati, *Mugil curema*), a species of fatty fish (*Salmon salar*), and a species of bivalve (mussels). Linearity was evaluated by calibration-matched curves. For this purpose, an analytical curve was obtained with spiked matrices (free of analytes), with levels ranging from 10 to 840 µg kg^{-1} dw of the analytes (between 5 and 8 different concentrations depending to the analyte). The limit of detection (LOD) and limit of quantification (LOQ) were calculated, by adopting the signal/noise ratio of 3:1 and 10:1, respectively, using the relative standard deviation (RSD) of ten injections from the low calibration level. Microsoft Excel 2016™ software was applied in the validation methods.

2.6. Determination of Analytes in Samples

Samples of seabass (*Centropomus* spp., $n = 16$), parati (*Mugil curema*, $n = 17$), and blue mussel (*Mytilus edulis*, $n = 6$ pools of 12 units each) from Sepetiba Bay; and mullet (*Mugil* spp., $n = 39$) and clams (*Anomalocardia brasiliana*, $n = 19$ pools of 60 units each) from Parnaiba River Delta were analyzed by GC-MS/MS, according to the description in Sections 2.3 and 2.4. The differences between the concentrations of compounds present in the samples were compared using Tukey's *t*-test, with 5% error probability, using Graphpad Prism™ software.

3. Results and Discussion

3.1. Optimization of Extraction Method

Linearity, represented by linear correlation coefficients (r), was equal to or greater than 0.99 for almost all pesticides found in the three different matrices, except for fipronil in fatty fish (salmon). However, in lean fish species, vinclozolin, alachlor, chlorpyrifos, mirex and bifenthrin had coefficients lower than 0.9. Concerning the precision interlay for the lean fish matrix, the relative standard deviations (RSD) of five replicates were less than 20% for almost all analytes at different levels, except fipronil at 320 µg kg^{-1} dw, showing satisfactory repeatability of the method. In fatty fish, RSD was higher than 20% for all pesticides in at least some of the dilutions analyzed, and for lindane and mirex in all dilutions. In bivalves, RSD was higher than 20% for chlorpyrifos-methyl, chlorpyrifos, alachlor, mirex and atrazine in at least some of the dilutions analyzed (Table 2).

Table 2. RSD, referring to repeatability of the analysis method in three concentrations for the lean fish, fatty fish and bivalve matrices.

	Lean Fish ($\mu g\ kg^{-1}$ dw)			Fatty Fish ($\mu g\ kg^{-1}$ dw)			Mussel ($\mu g\ kg^{-1}$ dw)		
	10	80	320	20	120	270	20	120	400
Lindane	1.7	1.0	5.4	43.8	22.3	27.3	6.5	12.8	4.3
Chlorpyrifos-methyl	0.8	2.3	3.2	15.8	40.6	32.3	26.6	12.6	7.5
Chlorpyrifos	0.4	1.5	5.8	40.0	16.0	20.4	33.0	13.4	2.4
Fipronil	5.8	5.4	41.0	33.5	8.8	18.7	20.12	7.4	6.0
Ethion	0.7	2.6	15.4	36.9	20.5	14.5	18.16	80.0	7.5
Aldrin	1.2	2.2	5.7	29.4	14.6	14.9	16.9	10.9	9.3
Chlordene	3.4	2.5	4.0	25.5	14.3	23.8	9.4	10.4	9.0
HCB	1.9	2.5	4.2	41.3	7.2	14.3	16.6	15.8	3.6
Mirex	2.6	1.2	3.0	22.7	24.2	30.4	23.4	26.4	44.7
Bifenthrin	1.1	1.3	2.4	21.6	26.4	19.1	8.4	6.8	3.6
Permethrin	10.1	3.1	2.2	16.8	26.9	32.9	11.1	20.5	30.6
Alachlor	0.9	2.3	2.1	-	-	-	25.0	105.3	31.9
Vinclozolin	3.3	3.8	4.0	7.2	9.3	20.1	17.8	16.0	6.6

The method verified using mackerel fillet by Wongmaneepratip, Leong and Yanga [40] for pyrethroids achieved standard deviations (SD) of 4.91 to 13.69%. The majority of agrochemicals analyzed by Petrarca et al. [41] and Kaczyński et al. [42] achieved a repeatability RSD $\leq$ 20% in the analysis of agrochemicals in seafood.

Regarding accuracy studies, by standard recovery, at a concentration of 10 $\mu g\ kg^{-1}$ for lean fish, most analytes showed an extractive yield (%) greater or less than the accepted margin (70 to 120%) [43], indicating that in this concentration the analytes do not present reliable values. For this reason, the recovery of the other matrices was analyzed from 20 $\mu g\ kg^{-1}$ dw. In the other concentrations, the vast majority of the compounds that could be analyzed showed a yield between 70 and 120%, except chlorpyrifos-methyl at 80 $\mu g\ kg^{-1}$ dw, and atrazine at 320 $\mu g\ kg^{-1}$ dw, as shown in Table 3.

Table 3. Interval (minimum–maximum) of mean extractive recoveries (%) and RSD for the analytes at three concentrations for the lean fish matrix.

	10 $\mu g\ kg^{-1}$ dw		80 $\mu g\ kg^{-1}$ dw		320 $\mu g\ kg^{-1}$ dw	
	Recovery (%)	RSD (%)	Recovery (%)	RSD (%)	Recovery (%)	RSD (%)
Lindane	81.0	1.2	81.9	2.6	102.5	5.5
Chlorpyrifos-me	85.7	0.2	44.3	58.1	101.7	1.9
Chlorpyrifos	55.3	8.0	89.6	2.5	103.1	1.6
Fipronil	45.3	18.4	77.9	14.2	81.8	18.9
Ethion	103.4	4.9	84.9	7.2	94.5	4.9
Aldrin	46.3	2.2	96.9	3.8	104.6	10.5
Chlordene	50.3	14.5	100.8	4.6	99.4	1.5
HCB	98.1	4.8	92.1	4.0	99.9	4.6
Mirex	7.3	7.8	101.9	0.8	103.9	1.3
Bifenthrin	35.1	10.3	98.3	3.3	99.1	1.4
Permethrin	89.6	12.2	120.8	21.9	113.6	9.7
Alachlor	59.3	0.1	88.9	1.8	98.6	1.5
Vinclozolin	44.4	10.1	102.0	3.5	111.9	4.4

Concerning the fatty fish matrix, most analytes showed extractive yields (%) within the accepted range (70 to 120%) [43], except for ethion, mirex and bifenthrin at 270 $\mu g\ kg^{-1}$ and permethrin at all analyzed concentrations. Table 4 presents these values.

Table 4. Interval (minimum–maximum) of mean extractive recoveries (%) and RSD for the analytes at three concentrations for the fatty fish matrix.

	20 µg kg^{-1} dw		120 µg kg^{-1} dw		270 µg kg^{-1} dw	
	Recovery (%)	RSD (%)	Recovery (%)	RSD (%)	Recovery (%)	RSD (%)
Lindane	69.6	12.3	84.9	10.5	79.6	12.0
Chlorpyrifos-me	88.5	14.6	74.2	10.2	71.7	25.0
Chlorpyrifos	97.2	7.3	109.1	11.1	86.3	24.4
Fipronil	105.3	0.9	87.3	3.7	92.4	8.9
Ethion	85.5	2.3	79.4	38.2	68.5	64.2
Aldrin	89.3	2.4	87.9	1.9	82.7	39.8
Chlordene	74.7	1.3	90.5	37.2	71.3	48.9
HCB	85.4	11.2	103.5	10.4	89.3	5.6
Mirex	65.9	0.3	71.5	64.4	57.8	79.3
Bifenthrin	79.8	1.0	88.1	47.1	62.8	66.2
Permethrin	64.7	0.6	55.1	70.4	39.4	121.2
Vinclozolin	95.7	0.4	82.5	6.6	75.6	21.7

Regarding the bivalve samples, many pesticides showed an extractive yield (%) above the accepted margin by 20 µg kg^{-1} dw [43]. At 120 µg kg^{-1} dw the findings were satisfactory, except for atrazine. At 400 µg kg^{-1} dw only aldrin, mirex and permethrin had unsatisfactory yields (Table 5).

Table 5. Interval (minimum–maximum) of mean extractive recoveries (%) and RSD for the analytes at three concentrations for the bivalve matrix.

	20 µg kg^{-1} dw		120 µg kg^{-1} dw		400 µg kg^{-1} dw	
	Recovery (%)	RSD (%)	Recovery (%)	RSD (%)	Recovery (%)	RSD (%)
Lindane	106.3	2.7	97.0	4.3	99.5	5.5
Chlorpyrifos-me	115.5	12.5	105.9	7.5	99.0	14.9
Chlorpyrifos	114.2	5.4	100.4	2.3	102.8	20.0
Fipronil	107.4	3.2	74.5	6.0	77.1	28.8
Ethion	91.8	9.1	88.5	7.5	96.6	4.2
Aldrin	102.7	10.0	111.5	9.3	10.0	7.0
Chlordene	108.7	18.3	64.8	9.0	86.3	14.7
HCB	170.3	9.2	93.0	3.6	97.2	10.7
Mirex	105.7	40.3	63.4	44.8	51.3	92.2
Bifenthrin	99.1	5.7	98.0	3.6	101.4	10.6
Permethrin	370.8	35.6	106.1	30.6	50.5	165.7
Alachlor	99.3	2.6	95.4	31.9	70.6	3.9
Vinclozolin	131.3	34.8	83.3	6.6	109.9	10.5

The mean concentration of organochlorine recoveries in spiked fish samples was 91% with RSD < 20% in the Cho, Lee and Jung [44] study. The majority of agrochemicals presented mean recoveries within the range of 70–120% and repeatability RSD ≤ 20% in bivalves, lean and fatty fishes [41]. The method proposed by Wongmaneepratip, Leong and Yanga [40] applied to pyrethroid analysis in salmon, seabass, threadfin fish, tiger prawn, vannamei prawn, shrimp, squid, grand jackknife clam, and oyster provided recoveries of 75.95–96.81%. Table 6 presents LOD and LOQ values for the three matrices.

Table 6. LOD and LOQ for the three matrices.

	Lean Fish ($\mu g\ kg^{-1}$ dw)		Fatty Fish ($\mu g\ kg^{-1}$ dw)		Mussel ($\mu g\ kg^{-1}$ dw)	
	LOD	LOQ	LOD	LOQ	LOD	LOQ
Lindane	1.5	4.5	8.2	24.9	0.1	0.4
Chlorpyrifos-me	0.5	1.5	12.5	37.9	7.0	21.2
Chlorpyrifos	4.3	13.2	10.4	31.4	6.9	20.8
Fipronil	1.9	5.7	20.3	61.4	15.9	48.3
Ethion	21.2	64.4	12.8	38.5	1.5	4.6
Aldrin	6.3	18.9	13.3	40.2	6.0	18.3
Chlordene	9.5	28.7	10.4	31.5	9.0	27.2
HCB	0.4	1.3	10.6	32.0	21.0	63.2
Mirex	12.1	36.6	11.9	36.1	0.1	0.4
Bifenthrin	12.3	37.2	12.9	30.1	37.2	39.1
Permethrin	17.2	52.3	11.54	35.0	280.1	484.7
Alachlor	5.2	15.7	-	-	0.5	1.4
Vinclozolin	8.4	25.3	16.3	49.4	0.5	1.4

In the trace analysis of organic pollutants in seafood, it is very important to remove some compounds, such as lipids, in order to decrease interference with the analysis, to achieve a low detection limit and to protect the analytical instruments [44]. In the present work, the values of LOD and LOQ found in each analyte of lean fish were between 0.4 $\mu g\ kg^{-1}$ (HCB) and 21.2 $\mu g\ kg^{-1}$ (ethion) and from 1.3 $\mu g\ kg^{-1}$ (HCB) to 64.4 $\mu g\ kg^{-1}$ (ethion), respectively. The values found for LOD and LOQ in each analyte of fatty fish were from 8.2 $\mu g\ kg^{-1}$ (lindane) to 20.3 $\mu g\ kg^{-1}$ (fipronil) and 24.9 $\mu g\ kg^{-1}$ (lindane) to 61.4 $\mu g\ kg^{-1}$ (fipronil), respectively. In the bivalve matrix, the values of LOD and LOQ found in each analyte varied from 0.1 $\mu g\ kg^{-1}$ to 0.4 $\mu g\ kg^{-1}$ (lindane and mirex), respectively. However, for permethrin in the bivalve matrix, the values found for LOD and LOQ were 280.1 $\mu g\ kg^{-1}$ and 484.7 $\mu g\ kg^{-1}$, respectively, suggesting that the extraction method was not effective for this compound determination and quantification from bivalve matrices.

Kaczyński et al. [42] obtained LOD values ranging from 0.05 to 1.2 $\mu g\ kg^{-1}$ for fishes' muscles and liver. Wongmaneepratip, Leong and Yanga [40] achieved LOQs of 0.54–0.85 $ng\ g^{-1}$ for pyrethroids in seafood. The method's detection limits ranged from 0.05 to 1.2 $\mu g\ kg^{-1}$ in the Petrarca et al. [41] study.

3.2. Determination of Analytes in Samples

The presence of alachlor, ethion, bifenthrin and permethrin was determined by analyzing some samples. The herbicide alachlor was found in four seabass samples (levels from 6.77 to 32.36 $\mu g\ kg^{-1}$ dw), in five mussel samples (levels from 0.66 to 33.41 $\mu g\ kg^{-1}$ dw), eighteen clam samples (levels from 0.55 and 93.17 $\mu g\ kg^{-1}$ dw), and in three parati samples (levels from 8.90, 9.01 and 420.39 $\mu g\ kg^{-1}$ dw). The parati samples that were more contaminated with alachlor was also found to contain ethion with a level of 211.22 $\mu g\ kg^{-1}$ dw. The presence of ethion was also observed in three samples of mussels, with levels ranging from LOQ to 15.13 $\mu g\ kg^{-1}$ dw, and in 13 samples of clams, with levels ranging from LOQ to 44.50 $\mu g\ kg^{-1}$ dw. Regarding the pyrethroid class, permethrin and bifenthrin were the pesticide residues analyzed. Permethrin was observed in two samples of mullet with levels below the LOQ. Bifenthrin was found in four samples of parati, two of them with levels above the LOQ, in concentrations of 41.01 and 43.41 $\mu g\ kg^{-1}$ dw. Bifenthrin was also found in 23 samples of mullet, but only two with levels above the LOQ, in concentrations of 32.14 and 36.06 $\mu g\ kg^{-1}$ dw, and in two samples of clams, only one of which had a value above the LOQ, in a concentration of 42.20 $\mu g\ kg^{-1}$ dw. There are no differences between the concentrations of compounds present in the samples, compared using Tukey's t-test, with 5% error probability. Table 7 shows the levels of the analytes found in the samples (in $\mu g\ kg^{-1}$ dw).

Table 7. Concentrations of analytes found in the analyzed samples (µg kg^{-1} dw).

Found Analyte	Class	Seafood Species	Concentrations
Alachlor	Herbicide	seabass (n = 4)	6.8 to 32.4 µg kg^{-1}
		mussels (n = 5)	0.7 to 33.4 µg kg^{-1}
		clams (n = 18)	0.5 to 93.1 µg kg^{-1}
		parati (n = 3)	8.9; 9.0 and 420.4 µg kg^{-1}
Ethion	organophosphorus	parati (n = 1)	211.2 µg kg^{-1}
		mussels (n = 3)	<LOQ (4.6 µg kg^{-1}), 12.9 and 15.1 µg kg^{-1}
Permethrin	Pyrethroid	clams (n = 13)	<LOQ to 44.5 µg kg^{-1}
		clams (n = 2)	<LOQ
Bifenthrin		parati (n = 4)	<LOQ to 43.4 µg kg^{-1}
		mullet (n = 23)	<LOQ
		clams (n = 2)	<LOQ and 42.2 µg kg^{-1}

The European Union (EU) recommends an MLR of 0.01 mg kg^{-1} for tall oil repellents in fish, fish products and any other marine and freshwater food products [43], which is the case of bifenthrin in parati and clams. There is literature on the lethal and sublethal effects of these agrochemical classes on fish, including alteration of behavior (sensation, locomotion, feeding, learning, etc.), physiology (respiration, metabolism, reproduction, etc.), alteration of biochemistry of enzymes, blood and hormones, carcinogenicity and mutagenicity [45,46].

A mutagenic response has been observed for alachlor metabolites as ethanesulfonic and oxanilic acid, which are more persistent in soil than alachlor itself [47]. The ethion metabolite monoxon may be hazardous to human health [48]. Regarding the pyrethroid bifenthrin, its metabolites, such as benzene 1,1(methylthio)ethylidene, may be less toxic than bifenthrin for some organisms [49].

Pesticides have caused serious health problems as they accumulate in fat-rich foods such as meat and milk and affect the food chain. Human exposure to these pesticides could occur through diet, including food items such as meat, fish, poultry, and dairy products [50]. Fishermen and coastal populations are especially exposed to the chronic effects of dietary pesticide ingestion, such as hypertension, cardiovascular disorders, endocrine system disorders and other health-related problems in humans.

The basic characteristics of organochlorine pesticides are high persistence, low polarity, low aqueous solubility, and high lipid solubility. Their toxicity is mainly due to stimulation of the central nervous system, as cyclodines, such as the GABA antagonists endosulphan and lindane, inhibit the calcium ion influx and Ca- and Mg-ATPase causing the release of neurotransmitters. Epidemiological studies have exposed the etiological relationship between Parkinson's disease and organochlorine pollutants [51].

Pyrethroid insecticides are also reported to be found in seafood. Rocha et al. [52] identified transfluthrin, cyhalothrin, permethrin, cyfluthrin, cypermethrin, fenvalerate, bifenthrin, phenothrin, fluvalinate, deltamethrin, and flumethrin in the roe or gonads of sea urchins (*Paracentrotus lividus*) from the northwest (NW) Portuguese coast, and Gadelha et al. [53] reported five pyrethroid (tetramethrin, bifenthrin, cyhalothrin, fenvalerate and permethrin) insecticides in farmed oysters from Aveiro (Portugal, north coast). Riaz et al. [54] determined the concentrations of cypermethrin, deltamethrin, permethrin, and bifenthrin in the samples of water, sediments, and fish collected from various locations of the Chenab River, Pakistan, during summer and winter seasons. In their study, the highest mean concentrations of pyrethroid (1248 µg g^{-1} dw) were detected in fish collected in winter, as compared with summer (0.087 µg L^{-1} dw).

Traces of organophosphorus pesticides (OPs) present in fish fed in aquaculture can affect the organisms [24,55,56]. Fenthion (0.0026–0.0037 mg kg^{-1}) exhibited values above the limit of quantification in tilapia from Aracoiaba, Castanhão, and Ilha Solteira [57]. Martins, Costa & Bianchini [58] found a maximum concentration 4.93 ng g^{-1} of chlorpyriphos in the muscle of Brazilian guitarfish (*Pseudobatos horkelli*). Zhang et al. [13] found Fipronil sulfone in 16 seafood samples (ten shrimp and six fish) with concentrations ranging from 17.2 µg kg^{-1} to 181.5 µg kg^{-1}, and in two shrimp samples, above 50.3 µg kg^{-1}.

Several authors around the world reported the presence of pesticides in seafood [8]. The OCPs class of pesticides, especially DDE, a DDT metabolite, is commonly found in muscle samples of fish such as tuna (*Thunnus* spp.), swordfish (*Xiphias gladius*), king mackerel (*Scomberomorus cavalla*), sardines (*Sardinella* spp.), corvina (*Argyrosomus regius*), mullet, mackerel (*Trachurus* spp.), mussels, blue crabs (*Callinectes sapidus*), clams, tilapia (*Oreochromis niloticus*), bigeye barracuda (*Sphyraena forsteri*), and cod fish (*Gadus morhua*). Despite the fact that some OCP compounds have been restricted and banned, isomers of DDT are frequently detected in top predators, due to bioaccumulation and biomagnification along with the food web [59–69].

Moraes [70] described a scientific trend of studies on the effect of pesticides on the fish endocrine system. Data were compiled through the Web of Science, Scopus and Scielo databases, through a diagnosis that identified studies from 1970 to 2017. The author identified a significant increase in publications for this period ($r = 0.83$; $p < 0.0001$). It was observed that most of the studies took place ex situ, and pesticides such as endosulfan, dichlorodiphenyltrichloroethane (DDT), together with its metabolic dichlorodiphenyldichloroethylene (DDE), atrazine, and chlorpyrifos were the most investigated. On the other hand, the groups of contaminants most studied in situ were organochlorines, organophosphates and alkylphenols. Countries like the United States, China and India dominated the polls. The most used species in the research were zebrafish (*Danio rerio*), rainbow trout (*Oncorhynchus mykiss*) and medaka (*Oryzias latipes*). Effects such as hormonal and histological changes, genetic expressions and gonadal damage were significant in fish in the presence of these chemicals. According to the author, this area is still a little lacking in research for endocrine analysis.

4. Conclusions

Considering that the indiscriminate use of pesticides can contaminate groundwater, and that the inappropriate discharge of effluents results in rivers, seas and oceans being the final destinations of these residues, studies on the contamination of aquatic biota are necessary, especially concerning biomagnification among species. Through the application of this validated method, it was possible to determine 11 pesticides in the fatty fish matrix, and 13 in the lean fish and bivalve matrices by GC-MS/MS. Hence, in this study the presence of three concerning classes of pesticides, organochlorine, organophosphorus and pyrethroids, was found in seafood samples. The solid-phase matrix dispersion method for analyte extraction, associated with mass spectrometry for detection and quantification of agrochemicals, provided a 95% reduction in analysis time and in the amount of solvent used compared with conventional methods. In addition, quick and multianalyte techniques for the detection and prevention of chemical and biological contaminants in fresh and industrialized foods can contribute to government programs and the productive sector, in the control and mitigation of food contamination, strengthening safety and zoosanitary defense.

Author Contributions: Conceptualization, F.H.S.F., S.C.C., J.O.F., M.B.A. and J.P.M.T.; Writing—review & editing, J.A.T.M., S.C.C., F.H.S.F. and J.O.F.; Validation, formal analysis and investigation, J.A.T.M.; Data curation and supervision, S.C.C. and J.O.F.; Resources, J.O.F.; Project administration and funding acquisition, F.H.S.F., M.B.A. and J.P.M.T. All authors have read and agreed to the published version of the manuscript.

Funding: This work was supported by UIDB/50006/2020 and Program Capes-FCT (project 88887.309193/2018-00).

Institutional Review Board Statement: Not applicable.

Informed Consent Statement: Not applicable.

Data Availability Statement: Not applicable.

Acknowledgments: The authors would like to thank the Brazilian Coordenação de Aperfeiçoamento de Pessoal de Nível Superior (Capes); Portuguese national funding agency Fundação para a Ciência e a Tecnologia (FCT/MCTES) (Grant 34/2018), Program Capes-FCT (project 88887.309193/2018-00) and EMBRAPA. This work was supported by FEDER (Programa Operacional Competitividade e Internacionalização—COMPETE 2020), from PIDDAC through FCT/MCTES project POCI-01-0145-FEDER-028708-PTDC/ASP-PES/28708/2017, and AgriFood XXI R&D&I project, operation No. NORTE-01-0145-FEDER-000041, co-financed by the European Regional Development Fund (ERDF) through NORTH 2020 (Northern Regional Operational Program 2014/2020). Sara C. Cunha acknowledges FCT for IF/01616/2015 contract. The authors also thank Renata S. Nunes for the english review.

Conflicts of Interest: The authors declare that they have no known competing financial interest or personal relationships that could have appeared to influence the work reported in this paper.

References

1. IPCS, W. *Global Assessment of the State-of-the-Science of Endocrine Disruptors*; World Health Organization: Geneva, Switzerland, 2002; Available online: https://apps.who.int/iris/handle/10665/67357 (accessed on 25 November 2022).
2. Bila, D.M.; Dezotti, M. Endocrine disruptors in the environment: Effects and consequences. *New Chem.* **2007**, *30*, 651–666.
3. Cunha, D.L.; Silva, S.M.C.; Bila, D.M. *Regulation of Synthetic Estrogen 17α-Ethinylestradiol in Aquatic Matrices in Europe, United States and Brazil. Public Health Notebooks*; 2016; Volume 32, pp. 1–13. Available online: https://www.scielo.br/j/csp/a/sMfbYgmKM9yMTFpNVzPFStf/?format=pdf&lang=en (accessed on 25 November 2022).
4. Brasil, 2002. Decreto No. 4074, 4 January 2002. Brasília: Federal Official Gazette. Available online: http://www.planalto.gov.br/ccivil_03/decreto/2002/d4074.htm (accessed on 25 November 2022).
5. EFSA 2014. Conclusion on the peer review of the pesticide human health risk assessment of the active substance chlorpyrifos. *EFSA J.* **2014**, *12*, 3640. Available online: https://www.efsa.europa.eu/en/efsajournal/pub/3640 (accessed on 18 March 2022).
6. Tornero, V.; Hanke, G. Chemical contaminants entering the marine environment from sea-based sources: A review with a focus on European seas. *Mar. Pollut. Bull.* **2016**, *112*, 17–38. [CrossRef] [PubMed]
7. EC, European Comission 2020. European Commission Pesticide Residue Database. Available online: https://ec.europa.eu/food/plant/pesticides/eu-pesticides-db_en (accessed on 13 February 2022).
8. Cunha, S.C.; Menezes-Sousa, D.; Mello, F.V.; Miranda. J., A.T.; Fogaça, F.H.; Alonso, M.B.; Torres, J.P.; Fernandes, J.O. Survey on endocrine-disrupting chemicals in seafood: Occurrence and distribution. *Environ. Res.* **2022**, *210*, 112886. [CrossRef] [PubMed]
9. Govett, G.; Genuis, S.J.; Govett, H.E.; Beesoon, S. Chlorinated pesticides and cancer of the head and neck: A retrospective case series. *Eur. J. Cancer Prev.* **2011**, *20*, 320–325. [CrossRef] [PubMed]
10. Burns, J.S.; Williams, P.L.; Korrick, S.A.; Hauser, R.; Sergeyev, O.; Revich, B.; Lam, T.; Lee, M.M. Association between chlorinated pesticides in the serum of prepubertal Russian boys and longitudinal biomarkers of metabolic function. *Am. J. Epidemiol.* **2014**, *180*, 909–919. [CrossRef] [PubMed]
11. Maisano, M.; Cappello, T.; Oliva, S.; Natalotto, A.; Giannetto, A.; Parrino, V.; Battaglia, P.; Romeo, T.; Salvo, A.; Spanò, N.; et al. PCB and OCP accumulation and evidence of hepatic alteration in the Atlantic bluefin tuna, *T. thynnus*, from the Mediterranean Sea. *Mar. Environ. Res.* **2016**, *121*, 40–48. [CrossRef] [PubMed]
12. Lam, T.; Williams, P.L.; Burns, J.S.; Sergeyev, O.; Korrick, S.A.; Lee, M.M.; Birnbaum, L.S.; Revich, B.; Altshul, L.M.; Patterson, D.G., Jr.; et al. Predictors of serum chlorinated pesticide concentrations among prepubertal Russian boys. *Environ. Health Perspect.* **2013**, *121*, 1372–1377. [CrossRef] [PubMed]
13. Zhang, Y.; Zhao, Y.G.; Cheng, H.L.; Muhammad, N.; Chen, W.S.; Zeng, X.Q.; Zhu, Y. Fast determination of fipronil and its metabolites in seafood using PRiME pass-through cleanup followed by isotope dilution UHPLC-MS/MS. *Anal. Methods* **2018**, *10*, 1673–1679. [CrossRef]
14. Bettinetti, R.; Quadroni, S.; Boggio, E.; Galassi, S. Recent DDT and PCB contamination in the sediment and biota of the Como Bay (Lake Como, Italy). *Sci. Total Environ.* **2016**, *542*, 404–410. [CrossRef] [PubMed]
15. Ferreira, V.B.; Estrella, L.F.; Alves, M.G.R.; Gallistl, C.; Vetter, W.; Silva, T.T.C.; Malm, O.; Torres, J.P.M.; Abadio-Finco, F.D.B. Residues of legacy organochlorine pesticides and DDT metabolites in highly consumed fish from the polluted Guanabara Bay, Brazil: Distribution and assessment of human health risk. *J. Environ. Sci. Health* **2020**, *55*, 30–41. [CrossRef]
16. Li, Y.; Lohmann, R.; Zou, X.; Wang, C.; Zhang, L. Air-water exchange and distribution pattern of organochlorine pesticides in the atmosphere and surface water of the open Pacific ocean. *Environ. Pollut.* **2020**, *265*, 114956. [CrossRef] [PubMed]
17. Lim, L.; Bolstad, H.M. Organophosphate insecticides: Neurodevelopmental effects. *Encycl. Environ. Health* **2019**, *2*, 785–791.
18. Matsuo, N. Discovery and development of pyrethroid insecticides. *Proc. Jpn. Acad.* **2019**, *95*, 378–400. [CrossRef] [PubMed]
19. Ramchandra, A.M.; Chacko, B.; Victor, P.J. Pyrethroid poisoning. *Indian J. Crit. Care Med. Peer-Rev. Off. Publ. Indian Soc. Crit. Care Med.* **2019**, *23* (Suppl. 4), S267. [CrossRef]

20. Ulusoy, S.; Özden, Ö.; Päpke, O. Organochlorine pesticide and polychlorinated biphenyl levels of horse mackerel (*Trachurus* sp.) caught from Marmara Sea coastal sites. Marine Biological Association of the United Kingdom. *J. Mar. Biol. Assoc. UK* **2017**, *97*, 401. [CrossRef]
21. Beyer, J.; Green, N.W.; Brooks, S.; Allan, I.J.; Ruus, A.; Gomes, T.; Brate, I.L.N.; Schøyen, M. Blue mussels (*Mytilus edulis* spp.) as sentinel organisms in coastal pollution monitoring: A review. *Mar. Environ. Res.* **2017**, *130*, 338–365. [CrossRef]
22. Campillo, J.A.; Fernández, B.; García, V.; Benedicto, J.; León, V.M. Levels and temporal trends of organochlorine contaminants in mussels from Spanish Mediterranean waters. *Chemosphere* **2017**, *182*, 584–594. [CrossRef] [PubMed]
23. Milun, V.; Grgas, D.; Radman, S.; Štefanac, T.; Ibrahimpašić, J.; Landeka Dragičević, T. Organochlorines Accumulation in Caged Mussels *Mytilus galloprovincialis*—Possible Influence of Biological Parameters. *Appl. Sci.* **2020**, *10*, 3830. [CrossRef]
24. Jeon, H.J.; Lee, Y.H.; Kim, M.J.; Choi, S.D.; Park, B.J.; Lee, S.E. Integrated biomarkers induced by chlorpyrifos in two different life stages of zebrafish (*Danio rerio*) for environmental risk assessment. *Environ. Toxicol. Pharm.* **2016**, *43*, 166–174. [CrossRef] [PubMed]
25. Alonso, M.B.; Feo, M.L.; Corcellas, C.; Gago-Ferrero, P.; Bertozzi, C.P.; Marigo, J.; Flach, L.; Meirelles, A.C.O.; Carvalho, V.L.; Azevedo, A.F.; et al. Toxic heritage: Maternal transfer of pyrethroid insecticides and sunscreen agents in dolphins from Brazil. *Environ. Pollut.* **2015**, *207*, 391–402. [CrossRef] [PubMed]
26. Barbosa, A.P.M.; Méndez-Fernandez, P.; Dias, P.S.; Santos, M.C.O.; Taniguchi, S.; Montone, R.C. Transplacental transfer of persistent organic pollutants in La Plata dolphins (Pontoporia blainvillei; Cetartiodactyla, Pontoporiidae). *Sci. Total Environ.* **2018**, *631*, 239–245. [CrossRef] [PubMed]
27. Raina, R. Chemical Analysis of Pesticides Using GC/MS, GC/MS/MS, and LC/MS/MS. In *Pesticides—Strategies for Pesticides Analysis*; InTech: Rijeka, Croatia, 2011; p. 105.
28. Cunha, S.C.; Fernandes, J.O.; Oliveira, M.B.P. Comparison of matrix solid-phase dispersion and liquid–liquid extraction for the chromatographic determination of fenthion and its metabolites in olives and olive oils. *Food Addit. Contam.* **2007**, *24*, 156–164. [CrossRef] [PubMed]
29. Viñas, L.; Pérez-Fernández, B.; Soriano, J.A.; López, M.; Bargiela, J.; Alves, I. Limpet (*Patella* sp.) as a biomonitor for organic pollutants. A proxy for mussel? *Mar. Pollut. Bull.* **2018**, *133*, 271–280. [CrossRef] [PubMed]
30. Cunha, S.C.; Trabalón, L.; Jacobs, S.; Castro, M.; Fernandez-Tejedor, M.; Granby, K.; Verbeke, W.; Kwadijk, C.; Ferrari, F.; Robbens, J.; et al. UV-filters and musk fragrances in seafood commercialized in Europe Union: Occurrence, risk and exposure assessment. *Environ. Res.* **2018**, *161*, 399–408. [CrossRef] [PubMed]
31. Chang, H.Y.; Yang, W.C.; Xue, Y.J.; Tsai, M.Y.; Wang, J.H.; Chang, G.R. Phthalates and organophosphorus insecticide residues in shrimp determined by liquid/gas chromatography–tandem mass spectrometry and a health risk assessment. *Mar. Pollut. Bull.* **2019**, *144*, 140–145. [CrossRef] [PubMed]
32. Mijangos, L.; Ziarrusta, H.; Zabaleta, I.; Usobiaga, A.; Olivares, M.; Zuloaga, O.; Etxebarria, N.; Prieto, A. Multiresidue analytical method for the determination of 41 multiclass organic pollutants in mussel and fish tissues and biofluids by liquid chromatography coupled to tandem mass spectrometry. *Anal. Bioanal. Chem.* **2019**, *411*, 493–506. [CrossRef] [PubMed]
33. Preedy, V.R.; Watson, R. (Eds.) *Olives and Olive Oil in Health and Disease Prevention*; Academic Press: Cambridge, MA, USA, 2020.
34. De Paula Filho, F.J.; Marins, R.V.; de Lacerda, L.D.; Aguiar, J.E.; Peres, T.F. Background values for evaluation of heavy metal contamination in sediments in the Parnaíba River Delta estuary, NE/Brazil. *Mar. Pollut. Bull.* **2015**, *2*, 424–428. [CrossRef] [PubMed]
35. Santos, T.A.; Gonçalves, T.S.; Nascimento, P.S.D.; Fernandes, C.A.F.; Cunha, F.E.D.A. Seasonal variation on diet of juvenile Elops saurus Linnaeus, 1766 (Ladyfish) in the Parnaiba River Delta. *Acta Limnol. Bras.* **2020**, *32*, e11. [CrossRef]
36. Mello, F.V.; Cunha, S.C.; Fogaça, F.H.; Alonso, M.B.; Torres, J.P.M.; Fernandes, J.O. Occurrence of pharmaceuticals in seafood from two Brazilian coastal areas: Implication for human risk assessment. *Sci. Total Environ.* **2022**, *803*, 149744. [CrossRef]
37. Da Silva, L.C.; Martins, M.V.A.; Castelo, W.F.L.; Saibro, M.B.; Rangel, D.; Pereira, E.; Bergamaschi, S.; Mello-Sousa, S.H.; Varela, J.; Laut, L.; et al. Trace metals enrichment and potential ecological risk in sediments of the Sepetiba Bay (Rio de Janeiro, SE Brazil). *Mar. Pollut. Bull.* **2022**, *177*, 113485. [CrossRef] [PubMed]
38. Molisani, M.M.; Marins, R.V.; Machado, W.; Paraquetti, H.H.M.; Bidone, E.D.; Lacerda, L.D. Environmental changes in Sepetiba bay, SE Brazil. *Reg. Environ. Chang.* **2004**, *4*, 17–27.
39. Mello, F.V.; Roscales, J.L.; Guida, Y.S.; Menezes, J.F.; Vicente, A.; Costa, E.S.; Jiménez, B.; Torres, J.P.M. Relationship between legacy and emerging organic pollutants in Antarctic seabirds and their foraging ecology as shown by δ13C and δ15N. *Sci. Total Environ.* **2016**, *573*, 1380–1389. [CrossRef] [PubMed]
40. Wongmaneepratip, W.; Leong, M.; Yang, H. Quantification and risk assessment of pyrethroid residues in seafood based on nanoparticle-extraction approach. *Food Control* **2022**, *133*, 108612. [CrossRef]
41. Petrarca, M.H.; Fernandes, J.O.; Marmelo, I.; Marques, A.; Cunha, S.C. Multi-analyte gas chromatography-mass spectrometry method to monitor bisphenols, musk fragrances, ultraviolet filters, and pesticide residues in seafood. *J. Chromatogr. A* **2022**, *1663*, 462755. [CrossRef] [PubMed]
42. Kaczyński, P.; Łozowicka, B.; Perkowski, M.; Szabuńko, J. Multiclass pesticide residue analysis in fish muscle and liver on one-step extraction-cleanup strategy coupled with liquid chromatography tandem mass spectrometry. *Ecotoxicol. Environ. Saf.* **2017**, *138*, 179–189. [CrossRef]

43. European Commission, Document N0. SANTE/12682/2019, Analytical Quality Control and Method Validation Procedures for Pesticide Residues Analysis in Food and Feed, 2020. Available online: https://www.eurl-pesticides.eu/userfiles/file/EurlALL/AqcGuidance_SANTE_2019_12682.pdf (accessed on 25 November 2022).
44. Choi, M.; Lee, I.S.; Jung, R.H. Rapid determination of organochlorine pesticides in fish using selective pressurized liquid extraction and gas chromatography–mass spectrometry. *Food Chem.* **2016**, *205*, 1–8. [CrossRef] [PubMed]
45. Stanley, J.; Preetha, G. Pesticide Toxicity to Fishes: Exposure, Toxicity and Risk Assessment Methodologies. In *Pesticide Toxicity to Non-Target Organisms*; Springer: Dordrecht, The Netherlands, 2016.
46. Al-Ghanim, K.A.; Mahboob, S.; Vijayaraghavan, P.; Al-Misned, F.A.; Kim, Y.O.; Kim, H.J. Sub-lethal effect of synthetic pyrethroid pesticide on metabolic enzymes and protein profile of non-target Zebra fish, Danio rerio. *Saudi J. Biol. Sci.* **2020**, *27*, 441–447. [CrossRef]
47. USEPA. *Reregistration Eligibility Decision: Alachlor*; United States Environmental Protection Agency: Washington, DC, USA, 1998. Available online: http://www3.epa.gov/pesticides/chem_search/reg_actions/reregistration/red_PC-090501_1-Dec-98.pdf (accessed on 19 November 2022).
48. Rusiecki, J.A.; Baccarelli, A.; Bollati, V.; Tarantini, L.; Moore, L.E.; Bonefeld-Jorgensen, E.C. Global. DNA hypomethylation is associated with high serum-persistent organic pollutants in Greenlandic Inuit. *Environ. Health Perspect.* **2008**, *116*, 1547–1552. [CrossRef] [PubMed]
49. Jan, I.; Dar, A.A.; Mubashir, S.; Alam Wani, A.; Mukhtar, M.; Sofi, K.A.; Dar, I.H.; Sofi, J.A. Quantification, dissipation behavior and risk assessment of ethion in green pea by gas chromatography-electron capture detector. *J. Sep. Sci.* **2018**, *41*, 1990–1994. [CrossRef] [PubMed]
50. Mali, G.V. Toxicological study of bifenthrin and its metabolites on earthworm (Eisenia fetida). *Nat. Environ. Pollut. Technol.* **2019**, *18*, 1387–1391.
51. Jayaraj, R.; Megha, P.; Sreedev, P. Organochlorine pesticides, their toxic effects on living organisms and their fate in the environment. *Interdiscip. Toxicol.* **2016**, *9*, 90–100. [CrossRef] [PubMed]
52. Rocha, A.C.; Camacho, C.; Eljarrat, E.; Peris, A.; Aminot, Y.; Readman, J.W.; Boti, V.; Nannou, C.; Marques, A.; Nunes, M.L.; et al. Bioaccumulation of persistent and emerging pollutants in wild sea urchin Paracentrotus lividus. *Environ. Res.* **2018**, *161*, 354–363. [CrossRef] [PubMed]
53. Gadelha, J.R.; Rocha, A.C.; Camacho, C.; Eljarrat, E.; Peris, A.; Aminot, Y.; Readman, J.W.; Boti, V.; Nannou, C.; Kapsi, M.; et al. Persistent and emerging pollutants assessment on aquaculture oysters (Crassostrea gigas) from NW Portuguese coast (Ria De Aveiro). *Sci. Total Environ.* **2019**, *666*, 731–742. [CrossRef]
54. Riaz, G.; Tabinda, A.B.; Kashif, M.; Yasar, A.; Mahmood, A.; Rasheed, R.; Khan, M.I.; Iqbal, J.; Siddique, S.; Mahfooz, Y. Monitoring and spatiotemporal variations of pyrethroid insecticides in surface water, sediment, and fish of the river Chenab Pakistan. *Environ. Sci. Pollut. Res.* **2018**, *25*, 22584–22597. [CrossRef]
55. Ismail, M.; Ali, R.; Shahid, M.; Khan, M.A.; Zubair, M.; Ali, T.; Mahmood Khan, Q. Genotoxic and hematological effects of chlorpyrifos exposure on freshwater fish Labeo rohita. *Drug Chem. Toxicol.* **2018**, *41*, 22–26. [CrossRef]
56. Olsvik, P.A.; Larsen, A.K.; Berntssen, M.H.; Goksøyr, A.; Karlsen, O.A.; Yadetie, F.; Sanden, M.; Kristensen, T. Effects of agricultural pesticides in aquafeeds on wild fish feeding on leftover pellets near fish farms. *Front. Genet.* **2019**, *10*, 794. [CrossRef] [PubMed]
57. Lopes, T.O.M.; Passos, L.S.; Vieira, L.V.; Pinto, E.; Dorr, F.; Scherer, R.; Salustriano, N.A.; Carneiro, M.T.W.D.; Postay, L.F.; Gomes, L.C. Metals, arsenic, pesticides, and microcystins in tilapia (Oreochromis niloticus) from aquaculture parks in Brazil. *Environ. Sci. Pollut. Res.* **2020**, *27*, 20187–20200. [CrossRef] [PubMed]
58. Martins, M.F.; Costa, P.G.; Bianchini, A. Contaminant screening and tissue distribution in the critically endangered Brazilian guitarfish Pseudobatos horkelii. *Environ. Pollut.* **2020**, *265*, 114923. [CrossRef] [PubMed]
59. Nicklisch, S.C.; Bonito, L.T.; Sandin, S.; Hamdoun, A. Geographic differences in persistent organic pollutant levels of yellowfin tuna. *Environ. Health Perspect.* **2017**, *125*, 067014. [CrossRef]
60. Klinčić, D.; Romanić, S.H.; Katalinić, M.; Zandona, A.; Čadež, T.; Sarić, M.M.; Sarić, T.; Aćimov, D. Persistent organic pollutants in tissues of farmed tuna from the Adriatic Sea. *Mar. Pollut. Bull.* **2020**, *158*, 111413. [CrossRef] [PubMed]
61. Klinčić, D.; Romanić, S.H.; Kljaković-Gašpić, Z.; Tičina, V. Legacy persistent organic pollutants (POPs) in archive samples of wild Bluefin tuna from the Mediterranean Sea. *Mar. Pollut. Bull.* **2020**, *155*, 111086. [CrossRef] [PubMed]
62. Munschy, C.; Bely, N.; Héas-Moisan, K.; Olivier, N.; Pollono, C.; Hollanda, S.; Bodin, N. Tissue-specific bioaccumulation of a wide range of legacy and emerging persistent organic contaminants in swordfish (Xiphias gladius) from Seychelles, Western Indian Ocean. *Mar. Pollut. Bull.* **2020**, *158*, 111436. [CrossRef] [PubMed]
63. Miranda, D.A.; Yogui, G.T. Polychlorinated biphenyls and chlorinated pesticides in king mackerel caught off the coast of Pernambuco, northeastern Brazil: Occurrence, contaminant profile, biological parameters and human intake. *Sci. Total Environ.* **2016**, *569*, 1510–1516. [CrossRef]
64. Kilercioglu, B.G.; Cengizler, I.; Daglioglu, N.; Kilercioglu, S. Organochlorine Pesticides and Polychlorinated Biphenyls in Blue Crabs Callinectes sapidus (Rathbun, 1896) from Akyatan Lagoon in the Eastern Mediterranean Region of Turkey. *Mediterr. Mar. Sci.* **2018**, *19*, 376–382. [CrossRef]
65. Saber, T.M.; Khedr, M.H.; Darwish, W.S. Residual levels of organochlorine pesticides and heavy metals in shellfish from Egypt with assessment of health risks. *Slov. Vet. Res.* **2018**, *55*, 101–113. [CrossRef]

66. Khallaf, E.A.; Authman, M.M.; Alne-na-ei, A.A. Evaluation of organochlorine and organophosphorus pesticides residues in the sediment and muscles of Nile tilapia *Oreochromis niloticus* (Linnaeus, 1758) fish from a River Nile Canal, Egypt. *Int. J. Environ. Stud.* **2018**, *75*, 443–465. [CrossRef]
67. Qian, Z.; Luo, F.; Wu, C.; Zhao, R.; Cheng, X.; Qin, W. Indicator polychlorinated biphenyls (PCBs) and organochlorine pesticides (OCPs) in seafood from Xiamen (China): Levels, distributions, and risk assessment. *Environ. Sci. Pollut. Res.* **2017**, *24*, 10443–10453. [CrossRef]
68. Chang, G.R. Persistent organochlorine pesticides in aquatic environments and fishes in Taiwan and their risk assessment. *Environ. Sci. Pollut. Res.* **2018**, *25*, 7699–7708. [CrossRef]
69. Zhang, X.; Wu, X.; Lei, B.; Jing, Y.; Zhang, X.; Fang, X.; Yu, Y. Transplacental transfer characteristics of organochlorine pesticides in paired maternal and cord sera, and placentas and possible influencing factors. *Environ. Pollut.* **2018**, *233*, 446–454. [CrossRef]
70. Moraes, B. Global Scenario with Research Involving Agricultural Contaminants in Fish Endocrine System. Thesis. IFGoiano. 2019. Available online: https://repositorio.ifgoiano.edu.br/handle/prefix/588 (accessed on 13 February 2022).

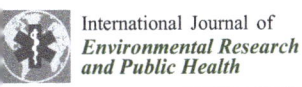

Article

Potential Transformation of Contaminated Areas into Public Parks: Evidence from São Paulo, Brazil

Camila Vitorino dos Santos and Helena Ribeiro *

Faculdade de Saúde Pública, Universidade de São Paulo, Sao Paulo 01246-904, Brazil
* Correspondence: lena@usp.br

Abstract: Waste-contaminated areas have been reused and requalified environmentally across the globe, aiming to reintegrate them into urban dynamics with new functions such as public parks. This practice has attracted the attention of public health and environmental control agencies due to the scarcity of free areas and vacant spaces for creation of green areas, and d the need for more sustainable planning guidelines in large cities. The present work aimed to study processes of requalification of waste-contaminated areas for transformation in parks, using as study two cases located in the city of São Paulo, Brazil. Method: Documentary research in environmental agencies, literature review and field visit. Results: In the two cases the process of requalification was unequal, with emphasis on three aspects: the actors involved in the case, the role of civil society and the action of the Public Prosecutor's Office of the State of São Paulo. Thus, it becomes evident that successful cases of waste-contaminated areas in the city of São Paulo are linked to the direct support of these aspects complemented with the private sector. Furthermore, a consensus is necessary among the public authorities regarding the laws of contaminated areas versus environmental damage full repair in the process of requalification.

Keywords: contaminated areas; urban residues; urban areas; environmental health

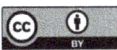

1. Introduction

In the last thirty years, as ecological awareness grows around the world, there has been a need for the implementation of more sustainable planning guidelines in large cities. With the disordered urban expansion in the territory, there is a notable scarcity of free land and vacant spaces for the creation of new vegetated areas in cities.

The insertion of a green area in urban space depends on urban and economic factors, which sometimes are unfeasible. The reuse of waste-contaminated areas, transforming them into public parks is a particularly well-executed solution performed in many countries.

A contaminated area is one in which there is evidence of contaminants on the ground or site, in quantities or concentrations above the environmentally acceptable reference values and may cause harm to human or ecological health or other goods to be protected [1].

Contaminated areas degrade the urban landscape and interfere in the quality of life of the population, since they alter the natural characteristics of the compartments and go unnoticed by the population. In addition, they are considered polluting sources of great magnitude and importance for public health, due to the risks to human health and public safety, and their complexity of management [2].

The measures of rehabilitation are based on the use of the area that may still be contaminated, with the guarantee that there are no transport routes of contaminants or receptors exposed to them. Remediation measures refer to those aimed at containing and/or isolating and/or treating contaminated environments, seeking to eliminate or reduce contaminant levels to acceptable concentrations according to legislation, allowing the area to be rehabilitated later [1].

Worldwide, there are several accidents, leaks, disposals and improper handling of materials and waste that have resulted in tens of thousands of contaminated sites. In the United States, it is estimated that there are more than 450,000 contaminated areas that require environmental intervention [3] and more than 340,000 contaminated sites in the European Union, posing risks to health and the environment and preventing the revitalization of urban neighborhoods [4].

In Brazil, despite the advance of technology and the constant search for compliance with environmental legislation, only three Brazilian states (São Paulo, Rio de Janeiro, and Minas Gerais) have data and information provided by environmental agencies on contaminated areas and their main characteristics.

According to the survey by the Environmental Company of the State of São Paulo—CETESB, on 6 December 2020, 571 contaminated areas were recorded in the state of São Paulo, Brazil. In the city of São Paulo, the largest Brazilian metropolis, there were 1103 areas that had undergone the rehabilitation process and were able to be declared rehabilitated, indicating a tendency to change land use and occupation [5].

Solid waste was the fourth source of contamination, with 208 contaminated areas registered in the state of São Paulo. For the safe reuse of these areas, remediation measures should be carried out to recover them, or to make current use compatible with the future [5].

In the State of Minas Gerais, Brazil, an inventory carried out by the State Environmental Foundation (FEAM), in December 2021, indicated 687 contaminated and rehabilitated areas, 20 of which were managed by the City Hall of Belo Horizonte. As in the state of São Paulo, the largest number of enterprises with contaminated sites corresponds to the activity of fuel stations, including the retail trade in fuels and dealers of gasoline, alcohol, and diesel [6].

Geographically, the metropolitan region of Belo Horizonte is the one with the highest number of areas in the list of contaminated and rehabilitated areas. Regarding areas rehabilitated for declared use, there was an increase in compliance with legal requirements, from 224 areas in 2020 to 251 areas in 2021, indicating an improvement in the management of contaminated areas [6]. Municipal solid waste was the second polluting source, due to irregular disposal points on public roads and many clandestine dumps [6].

In the state of Rio de Janeiro, according to the Institute of the Environment (INEA), the Register of Contaminated and Rehabilitated Areas identified, in 2019, 327 contaminated areas in 48 municipalities. Sites were contaminated by gas stations, industries, and waste landfill. In that year, only nine areas were rehabilitated for declared use, i.e., for new uses and functions [7].

The dumping of solid waste in the open varies significantly between different regions of the world since it is related to income and standard of living of cities [8].

In the richest countries that generate larger amounts of waste, there is more capacity to equate management, by a sum of factors that include economic resources, environmental concern of the population and technological development.

Globally, in cities of low- and middle-income countries, due to the very accelerated urbanization, there are deficits in the financial and administrative capacity for providing essential infrastructure and services such as water, sanitation, collection and proper disposal of garbage, housing, and in ensuring safety and control of environmental quality for the population. Thus, dumps continue to be the main method of disposal of municipal solid waste, significantly impacting the environment and public health [8,9].

A rehabilitated area for declared use is one that, after being submitted to intervention measures, presents a level of tolerable risk for future use, considering human health. Reusing a contaminated area means reinserting it back into the urban fabric, making it an instrument of urban requalification [10].

The city of São Paulo has many areas subject to the management of contaminated sites compared to others, especially due to the environmental licensing program conducted by CETESB, required by the federal government since 2000 [11].

The creation of green areas and the requalification of public spaces are relevant to public health and the environment. They are considered as one of the essential items for the well-being of the population living in large cities and a great tool to plan and develop a more sustainable urban environment [12].

Among these benefits are the conservation and reintroduction of species of native fauna and flora, the improvement of air and water quality, the climate balance and consequently thermal comfort. Due to this, they are used as indicators of quality of life and collective satisfaction, being directly linked to leisure and recreation activities through social interaction [12–14].

In addition, green spaces are associated with psychological well-being, decreased symptoms of depression, anxiety, and stress, providing a higher quality of life to the population [15,16]. With this, to alleviate urban problems stemming from urban expansion and the difficulty of creating public parks, managers have been rethinking the potential for reuse of contaminated areas as a sustainable tool for land use and occupation.

Considering this scenario, the present study aimed to analyze two case studies of requalification of urban solid waste-contaminated areas for transformation into parks, in the city of São Paulo, Brazil.

2. Materials and Methods

For the present study, the methods adopted were case studies, using documentary and bibliographic research and field visit. A case study of two parks located in rehabilitated areas in the city of São Paulo, Brazil was carried out. The municipality of São Paulo has 11,811,516 inhabitants residing in its territory of 1521 km^2 and a population density of 7765 inhabitants/km^2, being the main one in the metropolitan São Paulo area. It concentrates all the activities of economic, cultural, and social interests of the city [17].

Two areas contaminated by solid waste located within the municipality were selected, with declared use for the implementation of a public park.

The selection criteria were based on the following aspects: area insufficiently studied and explored; time in the scheduling of environmental studies at the Municipal Bureau of Green and the Environment (Secretaria Municipal do Verde e do Meio Ambiente de São Paulo—SVMA); time for the implementation and completion of the park's construction; the potential for reuse of the area for new uses, and the benefits that the park might bring to the surrounding community and future users.

The first case selected was the contaminated area of the Jardim Primavera Municipal Park (Figure 1), inserted at the eastern part of the municipality, in the district of Vila Jacuí, in São Miguel Paulista.

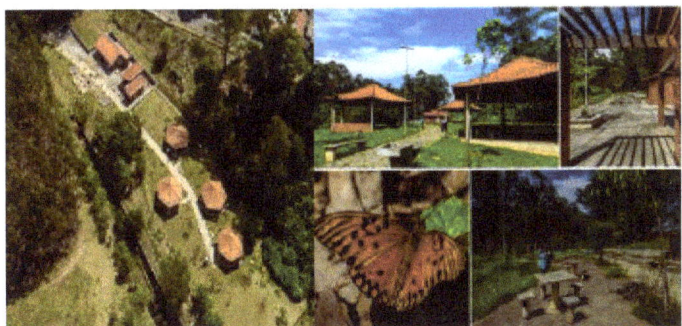

Figure 1. Municipal Park Jardim Primavera [18].

The second case was the contaminated area of the Villa-Lobos State Park (Figure 2) already fully implemented in the city of São Paulo. The Villa-Lobos State Park is in the neighborhood of Alto de Pinheiros, in the west, in Pinheiros district.

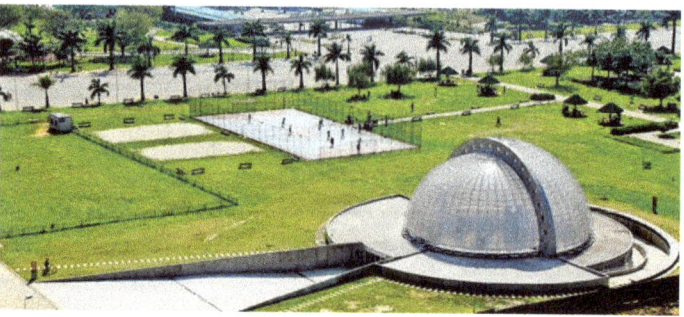

Figure 2. Villa-Lobos State Park [19].

The selection criteria were similar characteristics such as land use and occupation and source of pollution; operation period and deactivation of the polluting source; contaminated compartments (soil, surface, and groundwater); and considered as a successful case of requalification of waste-contaminated area and the current or future use of the area.

The documentary research was carried out after telephone appointments at the public institutions Municipal Bureau of Green and the Environment (Secretaria Municipal do Verde e do Meio Ambiente de São Paulo—SVMA) and the Environmental Company of the State of São Paulo (Companhia Ambiental do Estado de São Paulo—CETESB) to consult the administrative processes and environmental studies on the sites of the parks.

The survey of secondary data on the contaminated area of Jardim Primavera municipal park was carried out from February to December 2018. This survey included data on the background of land use and occupation; type of contamination; impacted means; contaminants; environmental management steps performed; actors involved; intervention measures taken; implementation of the park and current environmental situation of the area.

Subsequently, from May to June 2019, an appointment was made at the Department of Infrastructure and Environment of the State of São Paulo (Secretaria de Infraestrutura e Meio Ambiente do Estado de São Paulo—SIMA), Urban Park Coordination (Coordenadoria de Parque Urbanos—CPU) to carry out consultations with environmental and technical documents about the Villa-Lobos State Park. This consultation aimed to obtain the same detailed information as for the Jardim Primavera Municipal Park. The visits and photographic records were carried out concomitantly with the documentary research.

2.1. Background: Soil Use and Occupation

2.1.1. Jardim Primavera Municipal Park

The area occupied by the Jardim Primavera Municipal Park until the 1950s presented a small earthmoving operation, but around 1968 the exploration of sand by a private company began, a common activity in various regions of the city. This activity resulted in the formation of two pits, one larger and the other smaller, practically occupying the entire property, representing great environmental damage (Figure 3). Due to the interception of the groundwater, ponds were formed in these pits [20].

The mining pits had an average depth of 25 m in relation to the natural level of the terrain, reaching up to 40 m. The larger pit had an area of 60,784 m^2 and the smaller one measured 11,750 m^2, and due to this depth and rainfall at the site, the area began to present risks of drowning for the population living in the surroundings, Figure 3 [18,20].

Around 1979, the city of São Paulo was pressured by the local population to ground the pits that began to receive urban solid waste at the site. In an immediate response to the population, the smaller pit was grounded with soil from the leveling of the land, and the larger pit continued to receive construction residues (rubble), but there was no control for its disposal. The site also received other types of waste from 1979 to 1988 [18,21]. Urban solid waste was arranged randomly on the larger mining pit in precarious operating conditions and without technical measures for soil and groundwater protection, turning it into a dump [22].

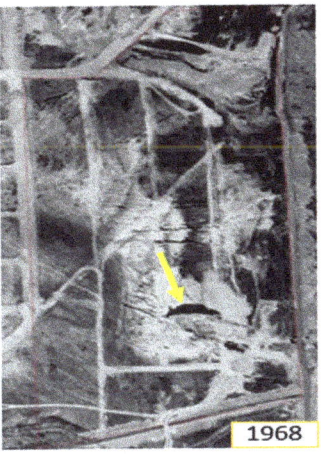 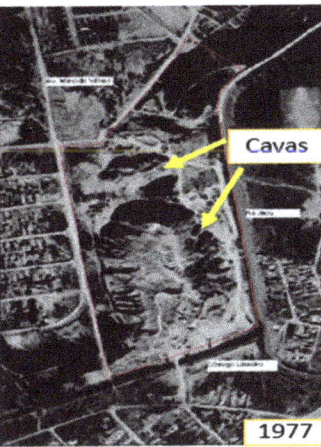

Figure 3. Pit formation in 1968 and 1977. Municipal Park Jardim Primavera [18].

In mid-1981, with the complaint of the population to the government (Regional Administration of São Miguel Paulista, currently the subprefecture) because of the precarious conditions of the area and the need for another place for the disposal of garbage in the east, the City Hall of São Paulo proposed to build a landfill site. Thus, the Jacuí landfill project was elaborated in October 1983, which had a favorable technical report by CETESB [23].

The Jacuí landfill was designed in such a way that it would consist of two smaller landfills, to take advantage of the two pits. However, due to the urgency of a place for the disposal of waste, gas drains were installed in the pit area, which collected and burned the gases generated by the 2.5 tons of waste deposited, until operation ended in 1988 [20].

Also in 1988, near the end of the landfill's useful life, CETESB was triggered by the residents of the neighborhood to verify the migration of gases from the landfill to some surrounding residences. This migration caused an explosion accident in a surrounding house, with two people injured, due to the presence of biogas in a nearby well [23].

From then on, between 1988 and 1994, in successive technical inspections of CETESB, it was verified by means of measures with explosimeters the presence of biogas in several places of neighboring residences, such as at the exit point of the conduit of installation of a doorbell, on the sidewalk, in a water well, in stormwater drainage drains, in existing cracks in the ground and in the paving of the streets. As a result, CETESB determined the closure of all water supply wells in the region, retaining only one for monitoring, and requested the construction of deeper drains in the area [23].

In parallel, in 1990, the municipality developed the pilot project of the park called Primavera. The project was elaborated through the Department of Parks and Green Areas (Departamento de Parques e Áreas Verdes—DEPAVE) linked at the time to the Municipal Bureau of Services and Works (Secretaria Municipal de Serviços e Obras—SSO), without previous studies to evaluate soil and groundwater contamination [22].

However, the project already raised concerns about the possible risks to human health that the area presented. Few buildings and sports courts with lawns were planned to be built outside the area grounded with solid waste, avoiding direct contact with soil and confinement of gases. In addition, afforestation should consider planting species of surface roots in the grounded area, and deeper roots in places that maintained natural soil [22,23].

Without previous studies, the execution of the project began, which was then paralyzed due to the detection of gases during the implantation, making it impossible to use the land for the intended purpose. Among the identified problems there were strong odor of gas, bubbles caused by fumes, bubbles in the puddles of water including external to the landfill massif and the difficulty for planting the lawns. These problems caused the work to stop in 1991, with the suggestion of waiting for the stabilization of the terrain and elimination of gases [23].

2.1.2. Villa—Lobos State Park

Villa-Lobos State Park is already finished and in use. It belongs to the government of the state of São Paulo. In the area of the park, located in an old floodplain of the Pinheiros River, the occupation began in 1958, where it presented grassy vegetation, some paths of earthmoving and the Boaçava stream (Figure 4).

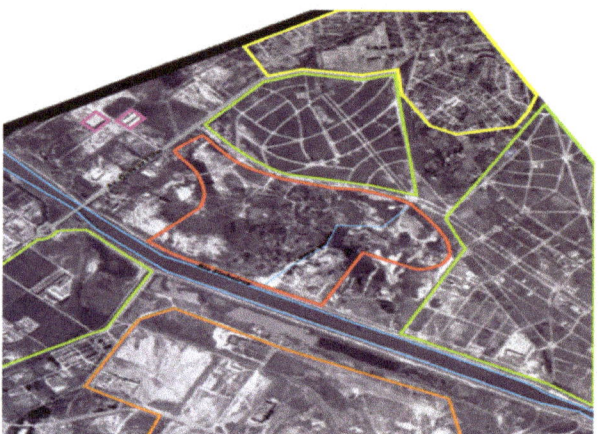

Figure 4. Villa-Lobos site. Occupation of the area and neighborhood in 1958. Colors: Red: Villa-Lobos Park Area; Brown: Earth movement; Green: green area/allotment; Blue: Body of water; Yellow: residences; Purple: industries; Orange: University of São Paulo [19].

In its surroundings, there were allotments and residential occupation, in addition to some developments in the process of construction, such as the Olympic Rowing Lane of the University of São Paulo—USP, empty land and two industrial sheds. In 1968, the area had more dense stretches of vegetation, and in its southern portion, near the Pinheiros River, a great earthmoving with ditches and roads used for the extraction of sand [19].

The tailings formed in the area ranged from 5 to 11 m high, in the form of piles in the northern part. There were also small ponds in the western part (Figure 5). Its surroundings, to the north, had denser residential occupation and allotments, to the west the expansion of industrial occupation, and to the south, bordering the Pinheiros River, the implementation of CPTM Railway Road-CPTM, the current Esmeralda line [19].

Later, in 1974, in the southern stretch of the area, vegetation was recomposed in a pit, and in the northeast portion, a new area of earthmoving was made. In 1977, the pit was completely grounded, in which it was also possible to notice two sediment dredging ferries of the Pinheiros River in front of the park area, and signs of dredged material released in a lagoon formed in the central part, next to the old sand extraction pit.

As for its surroundings, the north and east were completely occupied by residences, the University City of the University of São Paulo was installed to the south, as well as its Olympic Rowing Lane, and to the west there was the increase in industrial activity. It was possible to observe the Avenida Marginal of Pinheiros river already implanted. In 1986, new paths and decanting dikes of dredged material from the river were formed within the area. In the central area, a soil landfill of high proportions, apparently without construction debris, is identified and in the northwest a stretch with residential occupation and a soccer field [19].

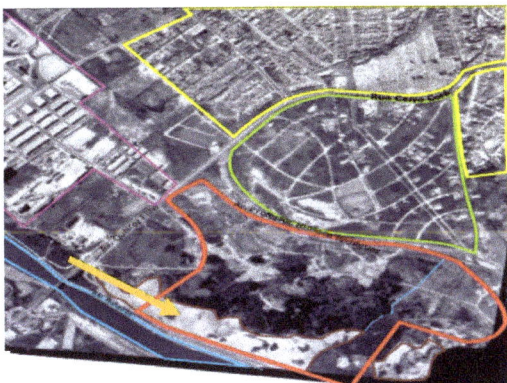

Figure 5. Villa-Lobos site. Earth movement in the south part of the area in 1968 [19].

During this period, near the site where the administration of the park operates nowadays, an area was identified that received metal materials for recycling, apparently scrap from underground storage tanks. The surroundings at that time had the same characteristics as in 1968, but with increased occupation (Figure 6).

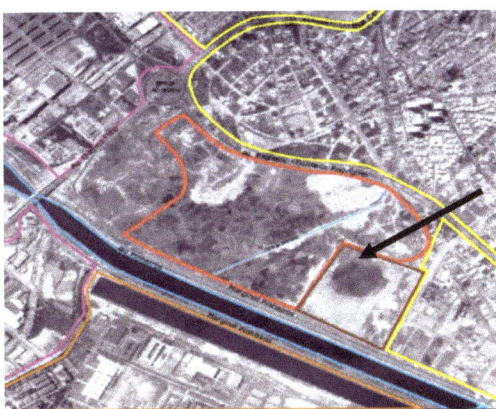

Figure 6. Villa-Lobos. Disposal of dredged material next to the old sand mine in 1977 [19].

Still in 1986, the area was used in its westernmost portion as a garbage dump of the Entrepots and General Warehouses Company of the State of São Paulo (Companhia Entrepostos e Armazéns Gerais do Estado de São Paulo—CEAGESP), from where about eighty families collected food and packaging. In the eastern part, adjacent to the current Villa-Lobos Shopping Mall, dredged material from the Pinheiros River was deposited and in the central portion, the former owner allowed the deposit of rubble, derived from construction sites.

In the early 1980s, the architect Decio Tozzi, on his way back and forth from FAU-USP, passed daily through this immense and degraded area, which was one of the last urban voids of the expanded center of São Paulo. The architect had the idea of recovering the area, transforming this open-air dump into a park, for which he elaborated a project. A contemporary park was designed, with large and dense biodiverse forest, composed of 50,000 trees divided into 300 species and 12 grassy clearings intended for free use of the population [24].

In the center, an area was designed by rows of imperial palm trees where an urban landscaping was developed, composed of a succession of small squares with shade trees, aiming to represent the landscaping of the squares and urban gardens of Brazilian cities. Continuing, the architect presented the project to three councilors who liked the idea. Later, for two and a half years, he sought to arouse the interest of the population, disseminating the project in neighborhood associations, community chambers, schools, clubs and even in communities. Once popular support was gained, the idea was brought to the state government, which took charge of expropriating the land.

In 1987, the year of commemoration of the centenary of the birth of composer and musician Heitor Villa-Lobos, the first studies were presented, aiming at the implementation of the contemporary park, which had music as the main theme [24]. The executive project was completed by the architect and the construction was put in charge of the Camargo Correa construction company, the winner of the bid. Existing buildings in the park area were removed in 1988.

In 1989, the Villa-Lobos State Park began to be deployed, starting with earthworks, Figure 7.

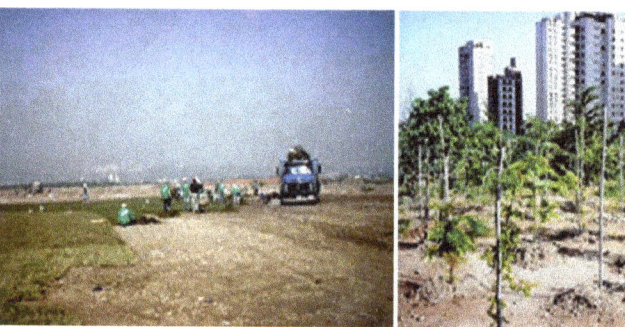
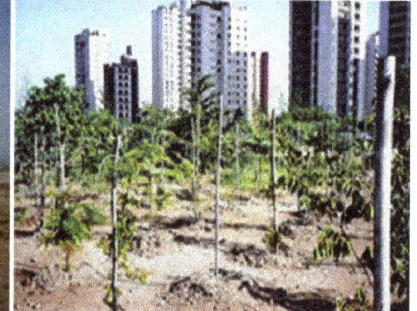

Figure 7. Building of Villa-Lobos State Park in 1989 [24].

The entire area of the park received a clean soil cover with known origin, in variable layers to level the existing elevations, preventing direct contact with the deposited material and the flow of rainwater (Figure 7). The Boaçava stream, which passed through the area, was channeled. All the residue was kept in the ground. After earthmoving, the park was 6 m taller than the avenue next to it. In this period, families living on the site were removed, 500,000 m^3 of rubble more than 1 m in diameter was removed, and 2 million m^3 of rubble was moved.

The next step was to convert the degraded and poorly permeable surface into fertile soil. To this end, a rigorous program of organic fertilization was developed using mainly vermicompost. In the space between the pits of the trees the green fertilization—the planting of legumes of annual cycle to incorporate nitrogen and organic matter into the soil—was also made. However, before the fruits and seeds appear, the green mass was cut. Finally, the soil underwent correction with application of limestone and chemical fertilizers based on NPK.

In the early 1990s, the trees began to be planted and organize the formation of the forests, the land was divided into modules of 10 m × 10 m and each of them received 25 seedlings with an interval of 2 m. The planted species are distinct among native pioneers (Angico, Candeia, Embaúba), non-pioneer natives (Cedar, Fig tree, Jatobá), species of marked flowering (Ipê-amarelo, Ipê-branco, Ipê-roxo) and species that attract birds (Mulberry, Guava, Jerivá palm tree), totaling 50,000 trees and 300 different species [24].

In 1994, the park was inaugurated unfinished, not in the original size proposed, with several sound installations, exhibition buildings and schools of ballet and music. The eastern area was incorporated after ten years. In 2006, the park was delivered completed with approximately 24,000 trees planted in pits of 1000 L of substrate and soil exchange.

Two-sport and tennis courts, Cooper track, skater track, amphitheater, bike lanes, soccer grounds and parking with 730 spaces [19] were made.

In that same year of 2006, civil society composed of environmental entities opened a Public Civil Action against the state, with the participation of the Public Prosecutor's Office, which ended in the form of an agreement. The action questioned many points of the park as: the delay of the opening of the entire area of the Villa-Lobos State Park to the population; the priority in the implementation of forests, lawn spaces, pedestrian paths; the interest of the population in expanding the spaces of culture, leisure, sport and green areas available; the need to meet and have equipment for people with locomotion disabilities; the restriction for the practice of large sporting or musical events; among others [25]. Faced with these issues, an agreement was established between civil society and state stakeholders with the participation of the Public Prosecutor's Office, clearly stating the attributions and responsibilities of each one regarding the operation and conservation of the Villa-Lobos State Park.

In 2008, 800 more seedlings were planted for Autoban's Environmental Recovery Commitment Term (TCRA) for forest enrichment. In 2009, the Villa Ambiental space was inaugurated, the new headquarters of the park's administration and a headquarters of the 1st Company of the 23rd Battalion of the Military Police were also opened in the park. In 2010, the Ouvillas space and the Ruth Cardoso Orchid Greenhouse were inaugurated, and in 2013, the environmental education center [19].

3. Results

The results found in the contaminated areas of the respective parks are presented. In both cases, contamination was derived from the irregular disposal of urban waste directly in the soil, which was submitted to the management of contaminated areas established by CETESB for the process of reuse and rehabilitation, in the form of a public park.

The practices adopted in the requalification process presented common and different aspects, although both areas are located within the city of São Paulo.

The main common aspects identified areas related to legislation, sources of contamination, environmental, and restriction measures for the implementation of parks.

3.1. Environmental Research—Contamination

3.1.1. Jardim Primavera Municipal Park

In 2004, CETESB signaled to the Municipal Bureau of Green and Environment (SVMA) that only after a detailed investigation on site the environmental problems in the area could be identified and, from then on, determine recovery and mitigation measures to be adopted.

The SVMA, still in 2004, conducted an on-site inspection, verifying the existence of drains without maintenance, which would allow clogging and accumulation of gases. Furthermore, in view of the suspicion of contamination, the bureau considered it essential to carry out full studies to ascertain the necessary intervention measures [18].

The environmental study in Jardim Primavera municipal park area was executed in two phases. The first lasted from 29 March 2007 to 16 May 2007, and involved services and the geotechnical situation assessment studies, gas emanation investigations and confirmatory investigation (laboratory analyses of soil and groundwater). And the second phase was performed from 20 August 2007 to 1 April 2008, in which detailed research was undertaken, as well as preparation of the risk assessment and remediation proposals [20].

The inspections made did not detect conditions of instability, erosion, and leakage of surface percolates from the landfill, as well as exposed waste. It was also identified that the drainage and slurry treatment facilities were disabled.

Local geology was identified by a sequence of alluvial and floodplain deposition, resulting in stacking by sand packets, interspersed with the presence of thinner sediments such as silts and clay with varying colors [26].

The results obtained in step I indicated contamination in groundwater: metals (aluminum, barium, boron, total chromium, iron, manganese, nitrate); fecal coliforms resulting from the former effluent treatment plant (TEE) and total coliforms. And in the soil: methane gas present also in the drains and visiting boxes of SABESP arranged in the vicinity of the property. There were indications of the impact on the aquifer under study, especially in the downstream to the landfill in the direction of the Jacu stream by slurry [20].

In step II, aiming to expand the sampling and laboratory analyses, 36 investigative surveys were carried out, which required the installation of multilevel wells and monitoring wells. Soil contamination by metals (vanadium, iron, and aluminum) and groundwater by metals (aluminum, barium, cadmium, lead, cobalt, total chromium, iron, manganese, nickel), fecal coliforms and total coliforms were identified.

In phase II, the presence of methane gas in the soil was also confirmed, concluding that there was an imminent risk resulting from concentrations higher than 2000 ppm. The exception was a grounded shallow well, with concentrations above 10,000 ppm in explosive conditions [20,22,26].

The results obtained from the analysis in stages I and II in 2008 indicated risks in the three different scenarios, their exposure routes and the receivers, Table 1.

In view of the results and the damage caused to the environment, the Public Ministry of the State of São Paulo (Ministério Público do Estado de São Paulo—MPSP), in 2012, filed a Public Civil Action in defense of the Environment under the terms of Law N.7347/1985 (regulates the Public Civil Action of Liability for Damage Caused to the Environment and provides other measures) against the City of São Paulo, requiring the total suspension of any work aimed at the implementation of the park [25].

The MPSP granted this injunction with the obligation of exhausting the gases present in the soil, if CETESB or GTAC did not find the absence of environmental risk, under penalty of a daily fine of ten thousand reais [27].

Table 1. Results of Human Health Risk Assessment [28].

Scenarios	Receptors	Exposure Routes	Toxicological Risk
Current (Deactivated Landfill)	Commercial workers, security guards and construction workers	Accidental ingestion, inhalation of particles and dermal contact with soil.	Aluminum
Future (Park)	Children	Accidental soil ingestion	Aluminum and iron
Hypothetical (Park)	Children, youth, adults, and the elderly	Ingestion and dermal contact with groundwater	Aluminum, Iron and Manganese

In 2013, a monitoring of possible gases existing in the area for a period of 2 years was proposed by SVMA. This monitoring served as an initial measure to update the current scenario, and to establish the procedures to be applied in the area, aiming at the health risks for employees and regulars of Parque Primavera [28].

Aiming at environmental compensation for damage, in the period from 29 January 2014 to 5 February 2014, phase I services were started, which included a soil *gas survey* and the installation of 40 gas monitoring wells.

Measurements of concentrations of volatile organic compounds and methane were performed in the underground facilities located around the study area (sewage, water, gas, drainage, and telephony networks), in addition to the inlet and outlet of pipes from existing buildings [21].

The results of the analyses obtained from volatile organic compounds in the soil showed concentrations above the standards adopted for benzene, tetrachloroethene, chlorobenzene, ethylbenzene, n-propylbenzene, 1,3,5-trimethylbenzene and 1,2,4-trimethylbenzene. Methane measurements performed in the three campaigns indicated concentrations above the Lower Explosive Limit (LEL), being: 22.5%, 20% and 7.5% above the LEL with explosive potential [29].

On February 2014, a soil sample was collected for the characterization and proper disposal of the residues, as established by ABNT NBR 10004/2004. The residue was characterized in excavated soil and classified as Inert IIB [21].

In phase II, gas levels were measured for a period of 2 years (2014 to 2016) with quarterly reports of their results, in addition to the intervention plan and the updated risk assessment [21] (Supplementary Material).

3.1.2. Villa-Lobos State Park

Given the size of the area and the diversity of places and types of materials arranged in Villa-Lobos State Park, environmental investigations began to be carried out in two campaigns (7 May 2007 to 15 May 2007 and 24 July 2008 to 1 August 2008), considering the type of current occupation and the routes of exposure. Between 7 January 2008 and 18 January 2008, new samples were collected to confirm results for phthalates.

According to the surveys (from 0 to 15 m deep) carried out throughout the park, the presence of several materials at different depth levels was confirmed, as well as thickness and varied sizes, highlighting civil construction debris and dredging sediments of the Pinheiros River. However, the presence of plastic bags, pieces of dishes and glasses was also verified, indicating that the area may have received waste of domestic origin, but not on a regular basis. The presence of residues of industrial origin was not detected [19].

The analytical data of the collected samples indicated the existence of contamination in the subsurface soil (phenanthrene, PCBs, Bis (2-ethyl) phthalate and methane gas) and in groundwater (Indene (1,2,3-cd) pyrene, lead, and arsenic).

During the vapor surveys in the soil, an upward flow of gas under pressure was observed in one of the points investigated close to the administration buildings, with concentrations higher than 10,000 ppm or 100% UEL. The monitoring only indicated the presence of methane gas, generated from the degradation of organic matter. In view of this confirmation, the presence of gases in all underground utilities (rainwater galleries, passage boxes, drainage gallery) was monitored, which, according to CETESB emergency technical team, did not show significant explosiveness risk.

The exposure of the intake of free aquifer groundwater was not characterized in the area and its surroundings, due to installation of the wells in deeper parts. However, the existence of cisterns and other rainwater accumulation points used for irrigation was observed, characterizing the routes of dermal contact exposure and inhalation of water vapors for users and park employees, in open and closed environments.

With the need for more detailed research for soil vapors, the results of the 2009 analyses of groundwater samples showed that only zinc exceeded the intervention value (IV) established by CETESB (2005). It was found that although the zinc contaminant exceeded the IV, according to the risk assessment, the value found at the time was below the concentration that represents risk to the residential intake scenario for workers and users of the future park (consumption of 2 L/day).

Thus, it was recommended not to use local groundwater and monitoring every six-months, at least until the end of the investigation of the area. Continuing environmental management in the area, in November 2012, thirty areas were defined for surface soil sampling, twenty-nine monitoring wells for groundwater and for gas monitoring, fifty-nine for open environments and twenty areas for indoor environments, since it has few confined environments.

In view of the results obtained from the surveys, the identified residues were classified as non-hazardous and inert waste, and its use is allowed by the park itself. It was also verified the extensive presence of dredged material of the Pinheiros River, characterized by sandy clay, light gray to dark with odor and debris, deposited in several parts of the park [19].

In groundwater, contamination by metals (barium, boron, lead, manganese, nickel, and selenium) and volatile organic compounds (bromodichloromethane) and in the soil several points with phthalate and PAHS (polycyclic aromatic hydrocarbons) were identified: dietilexil phthalate, benzo(b)fluoranthene and benzo(k)fluoranthene, in addition to dissolved and total metals (cobalt and nickel).

For methane gas, residential use was considered, considering the use of the park by employees and users. Concentrations ranging from 52,300 ppm (5.23%) to 983,000 ppm (98.3%) were detected in the sampled monitoring wells, with a number above the flammability range of the compound, which is 5% to 15%. In the monitored indoor environments, no concentrations higher than 217 ppm (0.21%) were found [10]. However, considering the risk assessment, concentrations above the IV were detected for benzene and ethylbenzene in the wells located next to the buildings, which have underground environments, being the Orchid greenhouse and Reference Center in Environmental Education of the park.

In view of this situation, it was recommended to immediately install monitoring systems for volatile organic compounds—VOC—and methane in other constructions, in addition to ventilation, exhaust and/or inflation systems; continuous monitoring of indoor environments for the evaluation of intrusion; use of personal protective equipment (PPE) for any intervention made in the park and the maintenance of quarterly gas monitoring campaigns, evaluating VOC and methane (Supplementary Material).

3.2. Common Aspects—Case Studies

Considering that there is no specific Brazilian legislation addressing the subject, the legislation adopted as a reference for the process of requalification and the implementation of parks were those established by the environmental agency of the state: CETESB, according to similar ruling from the Environmental Protection Agency EPA of the United States of America, starting from 2005.

It is pointed out that the areas of those properties belong to the government, and that, in the mid-1960s, they were initially used for the activity of sand mining, followed later by the irregular disposal of urban solid waste and dredged materials, characterizing the two sites as dumps. Both sites were contaminated by PAHS, and methane in soil and water. It was evidenced that the main aspect considered for the requalification of the areas was the acceptable risk of exposure to human health, aiming at the safety of future users and the correct principle of operation of the parks.

In addition, in both cases there were similarities as to the measures required for the park area, such as the restriction of the use of groundwater for any purpose within the property; the final cover with clean soil preferably of clay origin; the restriction on the planting of fruit trees in the entire property; the construction of buildings in confined spaces and the monitoring of gases and groundwater.

3.3. Different Aspects—Case Studies

According to the contaminated area management procedure and CONAMA Resolution N. 420/2009, it was possible to identify that the objectives of the requalification of contaminated areas in São Paulo are not always achieved successfully and guaranteed by the Brazilian legislation.

There was unequal treatment in the requalification process, with emphasis on three specific aspects: the actors involved in the case, the role of civil society, and the action of the Public Prosecutor's Office.

Regarding the actors involved, one can perceive the importance of private participation in projects of contaminated areas. In the area of the Villa-Lobos State Park, with the presence of the private sector, it was possible for its construction to begin quickly and with no major interruption during the environmental investigation, being fully completed as projected in 2013, demanding twenty-four years. As for the Jardim Primavera Municipal Park, it was observed that the municipal administration, as much as it has been committed to meeting all the requirements for safety and requalification of the area, was unable to have an active and swift participation in the process.

Another aspect observed in the Villa-Lobos State Park was the participation of the neighborhood and resident population of the surrounding area. This participation of the population occurred from the deactivation of the area until its total conversion into a park. Civil society, through non-governmental organizations (NGOs), actively participated in the entire process of requalification of the area, given its benefits from future land use and occupation.

On the other hand, regarding Jardim Primavera Municipal Park, the participation of the community occurred mainly through complaints and claims made to the environmental agency, denouncing the risks that the former controlled landfill represented, and the problems encountered in the attempt to build the park.

Another issue of great relevance identified in the requalification process was the participation of the Public Prosecutor's Office of the State of São Paulo.

In Brazil, according to the Constitution of the Federative Republic of Brazil (art. 225, §3) and Law 6.938/1981 (art. 4, item VII) of the National Environmental Policy, it was established that once the environmental damage has been caused, it must always be fully repaired [22]. This total repair is considered a determining economic aspect in the sphere of sustainability because it adheres to the Polluter-Pays Principle, which emerged in principle 16 of the Declaration of the United Nations Conference of RIO 92, defined as: "the one who infects must, in principle, bear the costs of contamination" [23].

However, when analyzing this idea in a contaminated area such as the studied parks, there are divergences between the current norms related to the recovery of contaminated areas versus repair of environmental damage. These divergences, although they are still under debate in major technical events, often lead to legal conflicts between the actors involved, which can directly compromise the urban requalification and sustainable development of land use in important regions of the city of São Paulo.

As in the areas of the parks there is buried waste, it is recorded that it is not feasible to fully recover the environmental damage caused, that is, it is impossible to have an ecologically balanced environment as recommended by the entire legislative framework focused on environmental damage, and its recovery.

Another point that is worth mentioning is that the Villa-Lobos State Park, because it was able to quickly start the first environmental studies to investigate contamination in the area, was able to avoid the legal process and the deviation from the planned purposes for the area, such as that identified by the Jardim Primavera municipal park area. In a way, it is pointed out that the lawsuit promoted by the population in this site ended up contributing to the State, showing the importance of the principle of participation in the decision-making process.

In general, the importance of effective efforts and investments in the institutions and individuals involved can be highlighted. One solution that could be applied in these cases is knowledge management or 3D creativity management.

This management is based on a conceptual structure in three large blocks to obtain something innovative, being: 1-block: of absorption and filtering of information; 2-block: processing of creativity and the 3-block: results of innovation [30]. In the case of Jardim Primavera Park, it is evident that the government has failed to absorb and filter the information to monitor, control and manage the entire process of requalification of the area to develop appropriate responses and strategies [31]. In the Villa-Lobos State Park, with civil society commitment and investments, in a public–private partnership, it was possible to process and collect all information effectively and efficiently throughout the requalification process. Later, it was possible to evaluate, compare and monitor the entire system to develop viable strategies and to complete the park, achieving an innovative result for the city of São Paulo.

4. Discussion

In the city of São Paulo, enactment and care of green areas and public parks may be the responsibility of the municipal or state administration, which is the responsibility of SVMA through DEPAVE, or SIMA.

In the contaminated areas of the case studies, it was evidenced that the practice of sand extraction was very common at the time and many areas that were converted into green areas, previously housed extraction pits. These pits, for the most part, were used for disposal of urban solid waste without adequate engineering recommendations and resulted in soil contamination and risks to human health. The current situation has no relation to the original uses. As examples, other parks, such as the Embu Das Artes Ecological Park, the Olympic Rowing Lane of USP, Ibirapuera Park and Toronto City Park, have been transformed into public areas, taking advantage of the mining pits [32].

Urban parks worldwide are considered places of integration and exercise of citizenship for all social classes and ages, as well as ideal for the development of permanent programs and campaigns of environmental education. Once inserted in urban areas, they promote various benefits to the population, the environment, and the conservation of biodiversity [33,34].

Studies confirm the benefits and importance of parks in the socioeconomic, public health and environmental spheres. These include improving air quality, soil permeabilization and environmental comfort; increasing physical, social, and psychological health; promoting well-being and health; preventing chronic diseases such as depression; social inclusion; and improving mood and self-esteem, evidencing that contact with nature leads to positive results for health in the short and long term [14,35,36].

Studies found that just five minutes of walking in green areas brings improvements in people's mental health, such as mood and self-esteem. Such evidence suggests that sedentary people and/or people with mental problems would have mental health benefits by committing to short-term exercises in accessible green areas [35]. Thus, parks are places that promote the feeling of well-being of users, sports practices, greater socialization, and stimulation of the identity of the community with the place, playing a motivator and social inclusion role.

Additionally, a reduction of 20–25% of diseases is estimated among children who do not live near contaminated places; the increase in the value of residential property between 19–24%; the creation of jobs and the increase in local taxes for new uses and functions, evidencing the importance of a healthy, clean, and accessible environment for the population [36].

Considering that in both areas there was soil and groundwater contamination, it might be stated that environmental investigations were managed adequately, following the technical protocol of the environmental agency CETESB.

As for the different aspects identified, the importance of the participation of investors and construction companies is emphasized, as they assume two roles, that of financial-economic viability and the execution of the revitalization itself. In addition, they seek and involve other actors concerned, and together they promote the necessary synergy for the requalification of the area [37]. In this scenario, the difficulty of the municipal administration of the Jardim Primavera Municipal Park of having to exercise the role of the government and that of investor at the same time can be justified, making it difficult to complete the project, which lasts inconclusive until now.

Thus, a possible solution would be that of reviewing the planned project for the area and verifying whether it is possible to implement another use for the benefit of the community, such as the project carried out at the municipal landfill in Brick Township, New Jersey, USA. That landfill received materials from contaminated sewage and liquids, which led to groundwater contamination and was added in 1983 to the EPA's list of national priorities for its cleanup [38]. Due to the extent of the contamination, the EPA required Brick Township to install a waterproof cover in the landfill to prevent rainwater from infiltrating the landfill floor. In addition, it required that the municipality conduct a long-term monitoring groundwater and use of drinking water for human consumption.

Therefore, Brick Township decided to turn this former landfill into a solar power facility, providing electricity to the surrounding government buildings, residences and community parks, Figure 8.

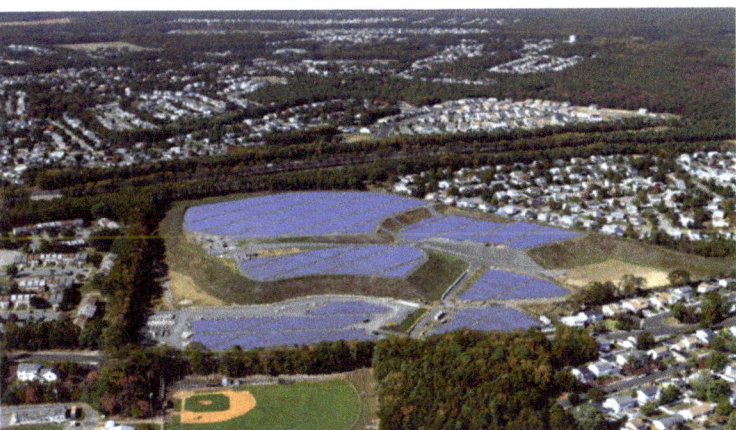

Figure 8. Brick Town landfill. Solar panel view [38].

Another important situation is the direct insertion of the population even before the elaboration of the project, as in the case of Villa-Lobos Park, where it ended up stimulating environmental education, not only to inform about the problem, but to provide sufficient and adequate knowledge for better understanding, transparency, and decision-making regarding the problem [38]. In addition, with the creation of the Orientation Council of the Villa-Lobos State Park, the State was able to arouse community interest, later counting on its support, dialogue and dissemination of all actions concerning the requalification process of the area, in a receptive and transparent way.

Social participation is one of the main ways to stimulate the population in identifying, planning, and implementing actions that help create healthier environments and improve quality of life. However, in the decision-making process regarding Jardim Primavera Municipal Park there was not a participatory moment of direct and conscious exchange through education, but only meetings and consultation spaces without participatory instance between representatives and represented.

In other words, the right to information is the one that establishes a duty-power, that is, the whole of the public power and the community (State and Society) in a participatory and active way of the different groups and segments interested in the formulation and execution of the decision-making circumstances [28].

The public authorities must assume and present a more educational, effective, and qualified function in the implementation of the Jardim Primavera Municipal Park regarding the real problems that affect the area. It is also necessary to objectively provide access to information, and better disseminate and explain it to the population, showing how this requalification will be made for the region, clearly addressing all their interfaces.

A successful case that highlights the importance of civil society in environmental requalification participation and direct government participation is Chambers Gully Park in Australia. Chambers Gully Park, located in the suburbs of Adelaide, Australia, was a local landfill.

The recovery of the area was carried out through the joint action of volunteers and residents of the area and with the help of government funds. The area today is a sanctuary for wildlife, including mainly kangaroos and koalas that are often seen perched on the park's eucalyptus trees (Figure 9), as well as a 9.6 km trail with a 3-h duration. The circuit cannot be accessed directly by road, but it is an easy 1.2 km walk to reach an access point, from Chambers Gully parking lot [39].

As far as environmental liabilities are concerned, it was evident that the Public Prosecutor's Office needs to reach consensus with the public authorities so that it can admit, at first, another form of environmental repair other than integral.

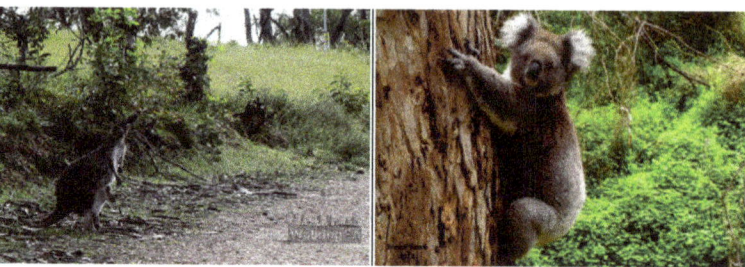

Figure 9. Chambers Gully Park, Adelaide, Australia [39].

According to CONAMA Resolution No. 420/2009, the process of recovery of contaminated areas does not guarantee the promotion of environmental quality prior to contamination, as it aims to adopt corrective measures based on the set of actions aimed at isolating, containing, minimizing, or eliminating contamination, enabling them to be recovered for a use compatible with the established goals, thus adopting the principle of declared use. With this rehabilitation of the area, a new occupation is possible, whether residential, commercial, or agricultural, a procedure adopted worldwide.

A solution would be public policies aimed at environmental management and recovery based on mechanisms of tax incentives and specific laws that stimulate the requalification of contaminated areas. Among the options we can mention the national funds for orphan contaminated areas, list of priority contaminated areas, creation of taxes, partnership between agencies of different spheres, participation of civil society in the process of requalification, decentralization and flexibilization of soil protection legislation and financial support and partnership with the private sector, of great importance to achieve a successful requalification case.

The present work directly contributes to a more sustainable planning for cities since it considers a viable alternative for the use and occupation of soil in urban space.

Although one of the case studies—Parque Jardim Primavera—has not been successfully completed, Villa-Lobos Park has evidenced that this practice can be carried out safely, as well as in the international context. This sustainable tool aims at government efforts, funding, public policies, and public–private partnership, thereby promoting the environmental quality of life of cities and population, reducing crime, irregular occupation, degraded places and preserving biodiversity.

5. Conclusions

The studied cases allowed us to know that the areas contaminated by solid waste, considered as successful cases in the city of São Paulo, had the direct support of civil society and the public authorities complemented with the private sector. Another issue is that for these urban projects to be completed with greater depth and ease, it is necessary to reformulate and/or modify the Brazilian legislation, especially in the thesis of Integral Repair advocated by the Public Ministry versus Management of Contaminated Areas.

It was evident that before sanctioning a law creating a park, the government needs to stimulate/insert direct private participation in the projects of contaminated areas, because they are essential for unfinished cases such as the Jardim Primavera Municipal Park. It should also actively and directly insert civil society support in the requalification process, enabling practical, in loco, knowledge. In addition, it needs to seek the support of other competent bodies such as urban policy, public health, tourism, aiming to create better solutions and projects for the requalification of waste-contaminated areas as a tool for sustainable urban development of land use and promotion of quality of life.

For future actions in other areas contaminated by municipal solid waste, not only for the city of São Paulo but for the world, it is first recommended to study the contaminated area/site in a thorough manner, so that it is possible to identify its interaction with the environment and its surroundings. In addition, in requalification planning it should be identified whether the ideal is really a park project for the area, and whether there is another utility option.

Another important factor is to respect the natural conditions of the place, changing only what is necessary, and when altered, seek projects that require low maintenance costs, thus avoiding new degraded spaces, abandoned and/or idle by the city. It is necessary to consider the gains and impacts for the region with the new requalification of the area, as well as its attributions/responsibilities, whether social, environmental, economic, or cultural.

The research's positive points include the scope and interdisciplinary view on the subject. Finally, it is recommended to further explore the theme discussed in the research and the evaluation of the actions of the public authorities in relation to areas contaminated by waste. Although actions aimed at the creation of parks in these areas have been proposed, it is important that there is a strengthening of legislation, planning, supervision and monitoring so that success cases are obtained as a result.

Supplementary Materials: The following supporting information can be downloaded at: https://www.mdpi.com/article/10.3390/ijerph191911933/s1, Table S1. History and Actions carried out in the areas of case studies.

Author Contributions: Formal analysis, C.V.d.S.; Funding acquisition, H.R.; Investigation, C.V.d.S.; Methodology, C.V.d.S. and H.R.; Supervision, H.R.; Writing—original draft, C.V.d.S.; Writing—review & editing, H.R. All authors have read and agreed to the published version of the manuscript.

Funding: C.V.d.S.: Graduate Program in Public Health of the School of Public Health of the University of São Paulo and the Coordination for the Improvement of Personnel Higher Education—Brazil (CAPES)—Funding Code—001. H.R.: CNPq productivity grant.

Institutional Review Board Statement: Not applicable.

Informed Consent Statement: Not applicable.

Data Availability Statement: Not applicable.

Conflicts of Interest: The authors declare no conflict of interest.

References

1. Companhia Ambiental Do Estado de São Paulo. *Manual de Gerenciamento de áreas Contaminadas*, 2nd ed.; Cetesb/Gtz: São Paulo, Brazil, 2001. Available online: https://cetesb.sp.gov.br/manual-de-gerenciamento-de-areas-contaminadas (accessed on 18 March 2018).
2. Günther, W.M.R. Áreas Contaminadas no contexto da Gestão Urbana. *Revista São Paulo em Perspectiva* **2006**, *20*, 105–117.
3. USEPA—United States Environmental Protection Agency. Brownfields-Basic Information: Overview. USA. May 2022. Available online: https://www.epa.gov/brownfields/overview-epas-brownfields-program (accessed on 6 February 2019).
4. van Liedekerke, M.; Sabine Rabl-Berger, G.P.; Kibblewhite, M.; Louwagie, G. JRC Reference Reports. In *Progress in the Management of Contaminated Sites in Europe*; Publications Office of the European Union: Luxembourg, 2014. [CrossRef]
5. Companhia Ambiental Do Estado de São Paulo-Cetesb. *Relatório de Áreas Contaminadas e Reabilitadas de São Paulo 2002 a 2020*; Companhia Ambiental Do Estado de São Paulo-Cetesb: São Paulo, Brazil, 2020. Available online: https://mapas.infraestruturameioambiente.sp.gov.br/portal/apps/MapJournal/index.html?appid=28e7bb2238a443819447a8ec3ae4abe5 (accessed on 2 September 2022).
6. Fundação Estadual de Meio Ambiente-Feam. *Inventário de Áreas Contaminadas, 2021*; Minas Gerais: Belo Horizonte, Brasil, 2021; 31p.
7. Ministério do Meio Ambiente (MMA). *Programa de Recuperação de Áreas Contaminadas*; Ministério do Meio Ambiente: Brasília, Brasil, 2020; 40p. Available online: https://www.gov.br/mma/pt-br/agendaambientalurbana/recuperacao-de-areas-contaminadas (accessed on 3 September 2022).
8. Jacobi, P.R.; Besen, G.R. Gestão de resíduos sólidos em São Paulo: Desafios da sustentabilidade. *Estudos Avançados* **2011**, *25*, 135–158. [CrossRef]
9. World Bank Group. *What a Waste 2.0: A Global Snapshot of Solid Waste Management to 2050*; World Bank Group: Washington, DC, USA, 2018; 272p, Available online: https://www.worldbank.org/en/news/immersive-story/2018/09/20/what-a-waste (accessed on 2 September 2022).
10. Habermann, M.; Gouveia, N. Requalificação Urbana em Áreas Contaminadas na Cidade de São Paulo. *Estudos Avançados* **2014**, *28*, 129–137. [CrossRef]

11. BRASIL. Resolução Conama. N. 273, de 29 de Novembro de 2000. In *Estabelece Diretrizes para o Licenciamento Ambiental de Postos de Combustíveis e Serviços e Dispõe Sobre a Prevenção e Controle da Poluição. Diário Oficial da União. de 29 de Novembro de 2000. Poder Executivo, Brasília, DF, Brazil, 8 de Janeiro de 2001*; SP: Brasília, Brazil, 2000; Section 1; pp. 20–23.
12. Santos, T.B.; Nascimento, A.P.N.; Regis, M.M. Áreas verdes e qualidade de vida: Uso e percepção ambiental de um parque urbano na cidade de São Paulo, Brasil. *Rev. Gest. Ambient. Sustentabilidade-GeAS* **2019**, *8*, 363–388. [CrossRef]
13. Maia, B.S.; Ferreira, D.G.; Paula, G.F.; Santana, H.C. Influência das áreas verdes a qualidade de vida nos centros urbanos: Estudo em Governador Valadares/MG. In *Anais do XV Congresso Nacional do Meio Ambiente-Poços de Caldas*; Espaço Cultura da Urca: Poços de Caldas, Brazil, 2018; pp. 440–445.
14. Mensah, C.A.; Andres, L.; Perera, U.; Roji, A. Enhancing quality of life through the lens of green spaces: A systematic review approach. *Int. J. Wellbeing* **2016**, *6*, 142–163. [CrossRef]
15. Locatelli, M.M.; Arantes, B.L.; Polizel, J.L.; Filho, D.F.S.; Franco, M.A.R.O. panorama atual da cobertura arbórea da cidade de São Paulo. *Rev. Labverde* **2018**, *9*, 29–48. [CrossRef]
16. Kim, D.; Jin, J. Does happiness data say urban parks are worth it? *Landsc. Urban Plan.* **2018**, *178*, 1–11. [CrossRef]
17. Fundação Seade. *Perfil dos Municípios Paulistas*; Fundação Seade: São Paulo, Brasil, 2019. Available online: https://perfil.seade.gov.br/# (accessed on 11 April 2020).
18. Weber Ambiental Ltda. *Relatório de Avaliação Ambiental e Análise de Risco- Tier 2- Fase 2*; Projeto n° 01.257.07; Antigo Aterro Municipal Jacuí: São Paulo, Brazil, November 2007; 59fls.
19. Weber Ambiental Ltda. *Relatório Técnico: Investigação Complementar de Contaminação do Solo e Água Subterrânea do Parque Villa-Lobos*; Processo N° 6.204/2011; Junho: São Paulo, Brasil, 2013; 2179fls.
20. SVMA-Secretaria Municipal do Verde e do Meio Ambiente. *Aterro Sanitário de Vila Jacuí*; Informação Técnica N° 26/GTAC/2012. Ofício 031/12/CLE; SVMA: São Paulo, Brasil, 2012; 2fls.
21. Geointegra Engenharia Ambiental Ltda. *Serviços Ambientais na área do Aterro Jacuí*; Geointegra Engenharia Ambiental Ltda: Vila Jacuí, Brazil, 2013; Fase I; Volume 2, 347fls.
22. Ramires, J.Z.S.; Vitor, J.D.S. O impacto ambiental oriundo do descarte irregular de resíduos: A contaminação do solo e das águas subterrâneas no município de São Paulo. In *Anais do XVI Congresso Brasileiro de Águas Subterrâneas*; Encontro Nacional de Perfuradores de Poços: São Luís, Brasil, 2010; pp. 1–17.
23. CETESB—Companhia Ambiental do Estado de São Paulo. *Inspeção Técnica ao Aterro Sanitário Jacuí*; SI/30.0002/98; Mai: São Paulo, Brazil, 1998; 5fls.
24. Jornal Da USP. *Urbanismo: Arquitetura, Luz, Espaço, Matéria*; N. 748, Ano XXI. 12 a 18 de Dezembro; Jornal Da USP: São Paulo, Brasil, 2005; pp. 1–5.
25. MPSP-Ministério Público do Estado de São Paulo. *Estado de São Paulo: Ação Civil Pública*; Autos n°1177/053.00.018822-6; MPSP: São Paulo, Brazil, 2006; 4fls.
26. Weber Ambiental Ltda. *Relatório de Avaliação Ambiental e Análise de Risco- Tier 2- Fase 2*; Projeto n° 01.257.07; Antigo Aterro Municipal Jacuí: São Paulo, Brazil, April 2008; 102f.
27. MPSP—Ministério Público do Estado de São Paulo. *Prefeitura do Município de São Paulo: Ação Civil Pública N°0004793-03.2012.8.26.0053. Poder Judiciário*; 2ª Vara da Fazenda Pública: São Paulo, Brasil, 2012; 11fls.
28. SVMA—Secretaria do Verde e do Meio Ambiente. *Aterro Jacuí Parque Municipal Jardim Primavera*; Informação Técnica N° 20/GTAC/2017. Processo n° 30.104915; SVMA—Secretaria do Verde e do Meio Ambiente: São Paulo, Brasil, 2017; 4fls.
29. Geointegra Engenharia Ambiental Ltda. *Serviços Ambientais na área do Aterro Jacuí*; Informações Complementares da Fase I. Atendimento ao PT n° 068/GTAC/2014; Geointegra Engenharia Ambiental Ltda: São Paulo, Brasil, 2014.
30. Vuong, Q.H.; Le, T.T.; La, V.P.; Nguyen, H.T.T.; Ho, M.T.; Khuc, Q.V.; Nguyen, M.H. COVID-19 vaccines production and societal immunization under the serendipity-mindsponge-3D knowledge management theory and conceptual framework. *Humanit. Soc. Sci. Commun.* **2022**, *9*, 1–12. [CrossRef]
31. MPSP—Ministério Público do Estado de São Paulo. *Cria Grupo de Trabalho para Análise e Fixação de Premissas Relativas à Valoração de dano Ambiental. Ato N°036/2011-PG, 06 de Maio de 2011. Diário Oficial da Cidade de São Paulo, de Maio de 2011*; Poder Executivo: São Paulo, Brasil, 2011; p. 50.
32. Bononi, V.L.R. Controle Ambiental de Áreas Verdes. In *Curso de Gestão Ambiental*, 2nd ed.; Philippi, J.R.A., Romero, M.A., Bruna, G.C., Eds.; Manole: São Paulo, Brasil, 2014; pp. 257–305.
33. Sanches, P.M. Potencialidades de paisagens degradadas e residuais: O caso de São Bernardo do Campo. In *Estratégias Para uma Infraestrutura Verde*; Pellegrino, P., Moura, N.B., Eds.; Manole: São Paulo, Brasil, 2017; pp. 147–181.
34. Barton, J.; Pretty, J.N. What is the Best Dose of Nature and Green Exercise for Improving Mental Health? A Multi-Study Analysis. *Environ. Sci. Technol.* **2010**, *44*, 3947–3955. [PubMed]
35. el Khateeb, S.; Shawket, I.M. A new perception; generating well-being urban public spaces after the era of pandemics. *Dev. Built Environ.* **2022**, *9*, 100065. [CrossRef]
36. *Superfund Remedial Annual Accomplishments Fiscal Year 2021 Report*; USEPA—United States Environmental Protection Agency: Washington, DC, USA, 2021; 38p. Available online: https://semspub.epa.gov/work/HQ/100003048.pdf (accessed on 2 September 2022).
37. Marker, A. *Manual: Revitalização de Áreas Degradadas e Contaminadas (Brownfields) na América Latina*; Iclei-Brasil; Departamento de Proteção Ambiental da Cidade de Stuttgart, Alemanha: São Paulo, Brasil, 2013.

38. Superfund Success Stories. *EPA Region 2-Brick Township Landfill*; USEPA—United States Environmental Protection Agency: Washington, DC, USA, 2018. Available online: https://www.epa.gov/superfund/superfund-success-stories-epa-region-2 (accessed on 6 February 2019).
39. Walking, S.A. Chambers Hike. Adelaide, Australia. 2019. Available online: https://www.walkingsa.org.au/walk/find-a-place-to-walk/chambers-hike/ (accessed on 25 February 2019).

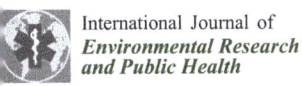

Article

Acute Kidney Failure among Brazilian Agricultural Workers: A Death-Certificate Case-Control Study

Armando Meyer [1,*], Aline Souza Espindola Santos [1], Carmen Ildes Rodrigues Froes Asmus [2], Volney Magalhaes Camara [1], Antônio José Leal Costa [3], Dale P. Sandler [4] and Christine Gibson Parks [4]

[1] Occupational and Environmental Health Branch, Public Health Institute, Federal University of Rio de Janeiro, Rio de Janeiro 21941-598, Brazil; esp.aline@gmail.com (A.S.E.S.); camaravolney@gmail.com (V.M.C.)
[2] Maternity-School, School of Medicine, Federal University of Rio de Janeiro, Rio de Janeiro 22240-000, Brazil; carmenfroes@iesc.ufrj.br
[3] Epidemiology and Biostatistics Branch, Public Health Institute, Federal University of Rio de Janeiro, Rio de Janeiro 21941-598, Brazil; ajcosta@iesc.ufrj.br
[4] Epidemiology Branch, National Institute of Environmental Health Sciences, National Institutes of Health, Research Triangle Park, NC 27709, USA; sandler@niehs.nih.gov (D.P.S.); parks1@niehs.nih.gov (C.G.P.)
* Correspondence: armando@iesc.ufrj.br; Tel.: +55-21973732000

Abstract: Recent evidence suggests that pesticides may play a role in chronic kidney disease. However, little is known about associations with acute kidney failure (AKF). We investigated trends in AKF and pesticide expenditures and associations with agricultural work in two Brazilian regions with intense use of pesticides, in the south and midwest. Using death certificate data, we investigated trends in AKF mortality (1980–2014). We used joinpoint regression to calculate annual percent changes in AKF mortality rates by urban/rural status and, in rural municipalities, by tertiles of per capita pesticide expenditures. We then compared AKF mortality in farmers and population controls from 2006 to 2014 using logistic regression to estimate odds ratios and 95% confidence intervals adjusted by age, sex, region, education, and race. AKF mortality increased in both regions regardless of urban/rural status; trends were steeper from the mid-1990s to 2000s, and in rural municipalities, they were higher by tertiles of pesticide expenditures. Agricultural workers were more likely to die from AKF than from other causes, especially at younger ages, among females, and in the southern municipalities. We observed increasing AKF mortality in rural areas with greater pesticide expenditures and an association of AKF mortality with agricultural work, especially among younger workers.

Keywords: acute renal failure; agricultural occupation; death certificates; kidney diseases; mortality; pesticides

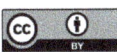

1. Introduction

Acute kidney failure (AKF; ICD-10: N17) is characterized by an abrupt decrease in renal function that increases toxins and nitrogenous metabolites concentration in the blood [1]. According to the Kidney Disease Improving Global Outcomes organization (KDIGO), AKF is defined by changes in serum creatinine of ≥ 0.3 mg/dL or ≥ 26.5 mmol/L within 48 h or increases of ≥ 1.5 times the baseline within the previous 7 days, or urine volume <0.5 mL/kg/h for 6 h [2]. Biochemical abnormalities in patients with AKF require intensive therapy until metabolic alterations can be reversed, but delayed diagnosis and treatment are some of the factors that make AKF a syndrome with high mortality [3].

A meta-analysis reported geographic differences in the incidence of AKF in hospitalized patients, with the highest rates in southern Europe (31.5%; 95% CI: 23.1–41.3) and South America (29.6%; 95% CI:19.1–42.7), followed by North America 24.5% (95% CI: 21.7–27.5), south Asia 23.7% (95% CI: 7.5–54.4), and eastern Europe 22.0% (95% CI: 9.5–43.3) [4]. Overall, AKF incidence is higher in low-to-middle-income countries than in high-income ones [5,6]. In the United States, racial disparities in AKF incidence rates appear associated with socioeconomic factors [7], and the incidence is higher in the elderly [8,9], consistent with what is seen in other high-income countries where the disease is more common among the elderly. By contrast, low-to-middle-income countries show a higher incidence of AKF among younger adults and children [8,10,11].

Known risk factors for AKF include chronic kidney disease (CKD), nephrotoxic drug ingestion, iodinated contrast, heart failure, liver diseases, sepsis, and diabetes [12,13]. Few environmental or occupational risk factors have been identified. Agricultural pesticides have been associated with CKD [14,15], and growing evidence suggests a positive association of AKF with pesticides and farming activities [16]. Clinical reports have described AKF cases related to accidental or intentional organophosphate (OP) poisonings [17,18]. In a retrospective cohort study, Lee and coworkers [19] observed a higher risk of AKF (hazard ratios (HR) = 6.17, 3.28–11.6 adjusted for age, sex, and comorbidities) among patients with OP poisoning than in controls, especially at younger ages (age 34 years or less HR: 9.65; 95% CI: 4.75–19.6).

Nephrotoxic effects of pesticides have been documented, along with their underlying pathomechanisms, in animal studies. For example, organophosphates insecticides seem to induce changes in epithelial cell and intratubular edema, focal hemorrhage, and inflammatory infiltration in the rat's kidney (Georgiadis et al. 2018; Kaya et al. 2018). Herbicides' effects on rat kidneys include marked proximal and distal tubular lesions showing coagulation necrosis with tubular cell loss [20–22]. Fungicides have also been related to degeneration of some tubular epithelial cells and hemorrhage in rat kidneys [23,24].

Brazil is one of the top consumers of pesticides in the world. Between 1999 and 2014, pesticide use increased in Brazil from 3.06 to 5.71 Kg/ha (86.6%; average annual increase 4.62%), compared with a global increase from 2.37 to 2.74 Kg/ha (15.6%; average 1.83% annual increase) [25]. Soybean, corn, and sugar cane crops account for about 70% of commercial pesticide use, and the south and midwest regions are the primary users of these substances [26]. Despite the relevance of pesticide use in both areas, the midwest is a region with the highest number of large farms. In contrast, the south region comprises small farms over the total agricultural area [27]. Although there is evidence of acute and chronic adverse health effects of pesticide exposure in Brazilian farmers [28–32], to our knowledge, no studies have examined the association between farming, pesticide exposure, and AKF in Brazil. Our study evaluated time trends in AKF mortality rates in Brazilian south and midwest regions, where most agricultural production is located, for the period 1980–2014. We also compared the AKF mortality risk among southern and midwestern Brazilian agricultural workers with that experienced by the general population in the period 2006–2014.

2. Materials and Methods

2.1. Studied Area

Agriculture in the midwest is mainly dedicated to the plantation of soybean and other grains on very large farms. Although in the south there are also large farms dedicated to soybean and other grains, in this region there is also a more significant number of medium and small farms, operated by family farmers, which produce many other agricultural commodities. These differences in crop diversity observed in the two regions may result in pesticide use and possible exposure differences in these regions [27,33].

2.2. Data Collection

Mortality data were retrieved from the Brazilian Mortality Information System, which uses the International Classification of Diseases' 10th edition (ICD-10) to organize and codify the main and auxiliary causes of death. Occupations were classified according to the Brazilian Standard Classification of Occupations, which follows the International Classification of Occupations (ISCO). Data on pesticide expenditure on each Brazilian farm in southern and midwestern municipalities were obtained from the Agricultural Census of

1996. National data on pesticide expenditure at the municipality level from the Brazilian agricultural censuses are electronically available for 1985, 1996, 2006, and 2017. We used the 1996 pesticide data to allow time for the exposure to induce biological alterations that could lead to the development and AKF deaths between 2006 and 2014. Mortality data used in the current study are publicly available through the Brazilian Public Health System's Informatics Department (http://datasus.saude.gov.br/; accessed on 6 April 2022), which does not allow the identification of the cases and therefore does not require Institutional Review Board-IRB review.

2.3. Trends in AKF Mortality Sample

We evaluated deaths due to AKF (ICD-10: N17) occurring between 1980 and 2014 in individuals of both sexes aged 20 years or older who lived in a Brazilian south and midwest municipality. Mortality rates were calculated using the number of deaths from AKF in each year of the study period divided by the population of the same year and multiplied by 100,000.

Per capita use of pesticides was calculated by dividing the total pesticide expenditure, in the Brazilian currency of 1996, in each municipality of the south and midwest regions, by its population in the same year.

2.4. Death-Certificate-Based Case-Control Sample

We also compared the odds of being an agricultural worker among those who died from AKF against the odds of being an agricultural worker among those who died from other causes. To do so, we retrieved data on all deaths due to AKF (ICD-10: N17) between 2006 and 2014 in individuals 20 years of age or older, of both sexes, who lived in a Brazilian southern and midwestern municipality. Cases (n = 6041) were individuals whose primary (underlying) cause of death was AKF, and controls (n = 2,010,829) were those who died from any other disease but AKF.

2.5. Statistical Analyses

2.5.1. AKF Mortality Time Trend Analysis

AKF mortality rates were calculated for each Brazilian southern and midwestern municipality. They were then grouped into urban and rural status according to the Brazilian Institute of Geography and Statistics' classification, and for rural states, grouped into low, medium, and high use of pesticides based on the tertiles (T1, T2, and T3) of per capita pesticide expenditure. For each of these groups, we calculated annual AKF mortality rates from 1980 to 2014. We used a joinpoint regression model (Joinpoint version 4.5.0.1; National Cancer Institute, Bethesda, MD, USA; 2017) to identify the years of significant inflection in AKF mortality rates' linear trends. We also estimated the annual percentage change (APC) and the average annual percent change (AAPC) in AKF mortality rates over the last 15 years of the studied period, stratified by urban/rural status and, within rural municipalities, by tertiles of pesticide use, using Poisson regression that allows for adjusting a data series from the smallest possible number of inflection points [34]. We calculated the AAPC between 2000 and 2014 because mortality data quality in Brazil has been considered better since then [35].

2.5.2. Case-Control Analysis

Logistic regression models were used to calculate odds ratios (OR) and 95% confidence intervals (95% CI) for AKF mortality risk associated with agricultural work, stratified, and adjusted (all other variables) for sex, age (20–50, 51–70, ≥71 years), the region of residence (south and midwest), ethnicity (non-white and white), and education (more than high school and high school or less). Stratified analyses were performed to explore the magnitude of the association between AKF mortality risk and agricultural work within the covariate categories for descriptive purposes but not analytical comparisons. The association of

AKF mortality and agricultural occupation was also assessed across 10-year birth cohorts (Supplemental Table S1) and 10-year age strata.

3. Results

3.1. Mortality Trends

In the south, the average annual percent change (AAPC) in AKF mortality for 2000–2014 was 3.41 (95% CI: 1.70, 5.15) (Figure 1a), which was significant in the rural (AAPC: 3.72; 95% CI: 2.14, 5.33) but not in the urban (AAPC: 3.05; 95% CI: 0.82, 5.33) municipalities. Using joinpoint software, we also calculated annual percent changes (APC) for specific periods. Overall AKF mortality rates showed a significant decrease between 1980 and 2006 (APC: −0.88; 95% CI: −1.48, −0.27) but an increasing trend between 2006 and 2014 (APC: 6.75; 95% CI: 3.59, 10.01). In rural municipalities, we observed only a small, non-significant decreasing trend in AKF mortality rates (APC: −0.42; 95% CI: −1.13, 0.30) from 1980 to 2006 compared to a steeper decline for urban areas (−1.82; 95% CI: −2.59, −1.04) for the same period. Subsequently, the parallel rise in both regions maintained higher mortality from AKI in rural compared to urban areas between 2006 and 2014.

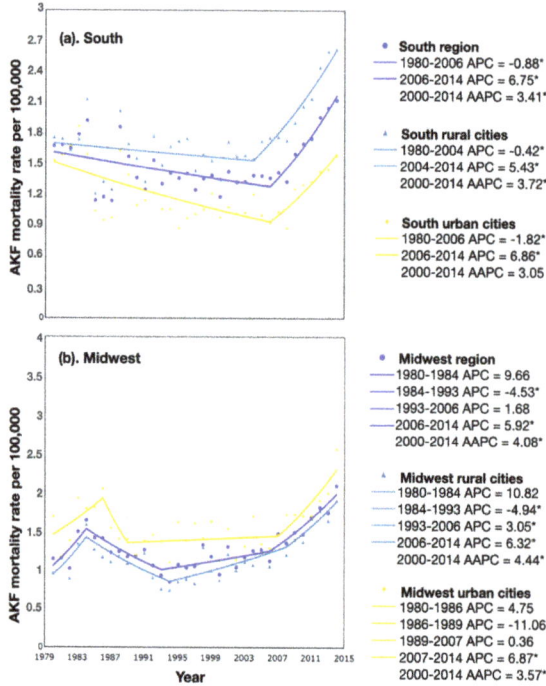

Figure 1. Mortality trends for acute kidney failure, 1980–2014. (**a**) Acute kidney failure mortality crude rates for the south region and its rural and urban municipalities. (**b**) Acute kidney failure mortality crude rates for the midwest region and its rural and urban municipalities. * Significant at $p < 0.05$.

In the midwest, the overall AAPC in AKF mortality rates was 4.08 (95% CI: 2.61, 5.58) between 2000 and 2014 (Figure 1b), with a significant increase in both urban and rural municipalities, slightly higher in the latter (Urban: AAPC: 3.57; 95% CI: 1.55, 5.62 and Rural: AAPC: 4.44; 95% CI: 2.22, 6.71). AKF mortality significantly decreased between 1984 and 1993 (APC: −4.53; 95% CI: −7.69, −1.26) and increased between 2006 and 2014 (APC: 5.92; 95% CI: 3.52, 8.37) (Figure 1b). In rural municipalities of midwest Brazil, a significant decrease in AKF mortality (from 1.4 to 0.8 deaths per 100,000 population) between 1984 and 1993 (APC: −4.94; 95% CI: −8.60, −1.14) was followed by two periods of a significant increase in AKF mortality between 1993 and 2006 (APC: 3.05; 95% CI: 1.08, 5.07) and between 2006 and 2014 with APC of 6.32 (95% CI: 1.54, 11.32). Rates were somewhat higher in urban municipalities, but changes in 1984 to 1993 and 1993 to 2006 were less pronounced than in the rural areas.

We then looked at AKF mortality rate trends, across tertiles of per capita pesticide expenditures. In the south (Figure 2a), AKF mortality rates were stable for the first 20 years; joinpoint regression detected an earlier, significant shift in the highest (third) tertile starting in 2000–2014 (APC 5.43; 95% CI: 2.19, 8.79) compared to the second (in 2004) and first (in 2005) tertiles. In the subsequent 9–14 years of follow-up, we observed a significant increase in AKF mortality rates in all three groups. The 2000–2014 AAPC reinforces the more recent increasing trends of AKF mortality rates in the southern municipalities, especially in the higher two tertiles of per capita pesticide expenditure (AAPC 4.56 and 4.13, respectively). In the midwest, AKF mortality rates by pesticide expenditures were more variable (Figure 2b). In the lowest (first) tertile, there was a significant decrease in AKF mortality from 1980 to 1995 (APC: −4.82; 95% CI: −7.93, −1.61), followed by a significant increase (APC:3.98; 95% CI: 2.19, 5.79), while in the third tertile (high), AKF mortality rates showed a slight decrease between 1980 and 2004, followed by a period of significant increase (2004–2014; APC: 5.11; 95% CI: 1.72, 8.61). The average annual percent change (AAPC) for the last 15 years of the studied period showed an increasing trend regardless of per capita pesticide expenditure.

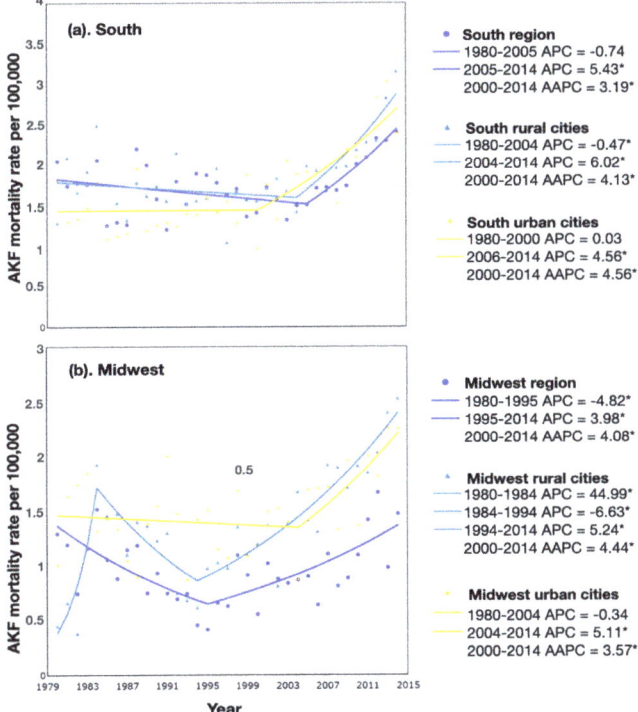

Figure 2. Mortality trends for acute kidney failure by tertiles of pesticide consumption, 1980–2014. (a) Acute kidney failure mortality rates for south rural municipalities. (b) Acute kidney failure mortality crude rates for midwest rural municipalities. * Significant at $p < 0.05$.

3.2. Agricultural Work and AKF

The characteristics of AKF cases and controls are shown in Table 1. Persons who died from AKF (cases) were older and more often from the midwest compared to cases who died from other causes. They were also more likely to be white, lower educated, and agricultural workers.

Table 1. Characteristics of AKF cases and controls, based on death certificates for southern and midwestern Brazilian states from 2006 to 2014.

	Cases	Controls	OR * (95% CI)	OR ** (95% CI)
	N (%)	N (%)		
Sex				
Male	3215 (53.2)	1,155,237 (57.5)	1.00	1.00
Female	2826 (46.8)	855,142 (42.5)	1.19 (1.13–1.25)	1.05 (0.99–1.11)
Age at death				
≤50	539 (8.9)	409,646 (20.4)	1.00	1.00
51–70	1656 (27.4)	660,093 (32.8)	1.91 (1.73–2.10)	1.90 (1.70–2.13)
>70	3846 (63.7)	941,090 (46.8)	3.11 (2.84–3.40)	3.07 (2.76–3.42)
Region of residence				
South	4236 (70.1)	1,509,866 (75.1)	1.00	1.00
Midwest	1805 (29.9)	500,963 (24.9)	1.28 (1.22–1.36)	1.37 (1.28–1.47)
Race/Ethnicity				
Non-white	1416 (23.4)	502,380 (25.0)	1.00	1.00
White	4625 (76.6)	1,508,449 (75.0)	1.09 (1.03–1.16)	1.21 (1.11–1.30)
Education				
More than high school	166 (3.6)	81,147 (5.3)	1.00	1.00
High school or less	4413 (96.4)	1,438,597 (94.7)	1.50 (1.28–1.75)	1.30 (1.11–1.52)
Occupation *				
Non-agricultural workers	4030 (79.2)	1,436,019 (83.9)	1.00	1.00
Agricultural workers	1057 (20.8)	274,834 (16.1)	1.37 (1.28–1.47)	1.32 (1.22–1.42)

* Crude odds ratio; ** Odds ratio adjusted by sex, age at death, region of residence, race/ethnicity, education; *** Missing occupation data on 15.8% of cases and 14.9% of controls.

After adjusting for sex, age at death, region of residence, race/ethnicity, and level of education, persons who died from AKF were more likely to have been agricultural workers than persons who died from other causes (OR (95% CI) 1.23 (1.22–1.42) (Table 2). Agricultural work was associated with AKF mortality in both women (OR: 1.40; 95% CI: 1.23–1.59) and men (OR: 1.27; 95% CI: 1.15–1.39). The odds of being an agricultural worker among those who died from AKF was greatest among younger workers (50 years or less; OR: 1.56; 95% CI: 1.16–2.11) but increased at every age group. The association between agricultural work and AKF mortality was most evident among those from Brazilian southern states (OR: 1.40; 95% CI: 1.29–1.53 versus OR: 1.06; 95% CI: 0.90–1.25 in the midwest states) and appeared stronger among whites (OR: 1.37; 95% CI: 1.26–1.49) than among non-whites (OR: 1.12; 95% CI: 0.94–1.34). The association between agricultural work and death due to AKF did not differ meaningfully by level of education.

Because of the differences observed in the age-stratified analysis, we conducted a further exploratory analysis across the 10-year age strata (Table 3). The association between dying from AKF and agricultural work was highest among the youngest (20–29 years old) agricultural workers (OR: 3.07; 95%: 1.71, 6.26) and lowest among those aged 50–59 years (OR: 0.95; 95% CI: 0.71, 1.26). According to the birth cohort, the odds of being an agricultural worker born in past periods (until 1940–1949) among those who died from AKF were higher than those born after 1950–1959 (Supplementary Table S1).

Table 2. Overall, adjusted, and stratified AKF mortality among Brazilian southern and midwestern agricultural workers, 2006–2014.

	Cases	Controls	OR * (95% CI)	OR ** (95% CI)
	N (%)	N (%)		
Sex				
Male				
Non-agricultural workers	1909 (72.1)	758,357 (78.9)	1.00	1.00
Agricultural workers	739 (27.9)	202,515 (21.1)	1.45 (1.33–1.58)	1.27 (1.15–1.39)
Female				
Non-agricultural workers	2121 (87.0)	677,551 (90.4)	1.00	1.00
Agricultural workers	318 (13.0)	72,307 (9.6)	1.41 (1.25–1.58)	1.40 (1.23–1.59)
Age at death				
≤50				
Non-agricultural workers	369 (86.4)	296,921 (89.2)	1.00	1.00
Agricultural workers	58 (13.6)	35,774 (10.8)	1.31 (0.99–1.72)	1.56 (1.16–2.11)
51–70				
Non-agricultural workers	1147 (83.4)	474,278 (84.7)	1.00	1.00
Agricultural workers	229 (16.6)	85,743 (15.3)	1.10 (0.96–1.27)	1.13 (0.97–1.32)
>70				
Non-agricultural workers	2514 (76.6)	664,820 (81.3)	1.00	1.00
Agricultural workers	770 (23.4)	153,317 (18.7)	1.33 (1.23–1.44)	1.36 (1.25–1.49)
Region of residence				
South				
Non-agricultural workers	2851 (77.4)	1,098,465 (83.7)	1.00	1.00
Agricultural workers	831 (22.6)	214,252 (16.3)	1.49 (1.38–1.62)	1.40 (1.29–1.53)
Midwest				
Non-agricultural workers	1179 (83.9)	337,554 (84.8)	1.00	1.00
Agricultural workers	226 (16.1)	60,582 (15.2)	1.07 (0.93–1.23)	1.06 (0.90–1.25)
Race/Ethnicity				
Non-white				
Non-agricultural workers	908 (82.7)	342,478 (84.4)	1.00	1.00
Agricultural workers	190 (17.3)	63,539 (15.6)	1.13 (0.96–1.32)	1.12 (0.94–1.34)
White				
Non-agricultural workers	3122 (78.3)	1,093,541 (83.8)	1.00	1.00
Agricultural workers	867 (21.7)	211,295 (16.2)	1.44 (1.33–1.55)	1.37 (1.26–1.49)
Education ***				
More than high school				
Non-agricultural workers	146 (96.7)	71,879 (98.1)	1.00	1.00
Agricultural workers	5 (3.3)	1390 (1.9)	1.77 (0.73–4.33)	1.82 (0.74–4.46)
High school or less				
Non-agricultural workers	3036 (76.3)	1,051,486 (81.6)	1.00	1.00
Agricultural workers	941 (23.7)	237,012 (18.4)	1.38 (1.28–1.48)	1.32 (1.22–1.42)

* Crude odds ratio; ** Odds ratio adjusted by sex, age at death, region of residence, race/ethnicity, education; *** Missing data: 31.67% for cases and 32.28% for controls.

Table 3. AKF mortality among Brazilian southern and midwestern agricultural workers, according to 10-year age strata, 2006–2014.

	Cases	Controls	OR * (95% CI)	OR ** (95% CI)
	N (%)	N (%)		
Age				
20–29				
Non-agricultural workers	50 (83.3)	72,588 (92.3)	1.00	1.00
Agricultural workers	10 (16.7)	6024 (7.7)	2.41 (1.22–4.75)	3.07 (1.71–6.26)

Table 3. Cont.

	Cases	Controls	OR * (95% CI)	OR ** (95% CI)
	N (%)	N (%)		
Age				
30–39				
Non-agricultural workers	92 (82.5)	81,309 (89.7)	1.00	1.00
Agricultural workers	16 (14.8)	9349 (10.3)	1.51 (0.89–2.57)	1.57 (0.84–2.91)
40–49				
Non-agricultural workers	196 (87.9)	126,365 (87.6)	1.00	1.00
Agricultural workers	27 (12.1)	17,886 (12.4)	0.97 (0.65–1.46)	1.25 (0.81–1.93)
50–59				
Non-agricultural workers	430 (86.7)	196,179 (85.9)		
Agricultural workers	66 (13.3)	32,237 (14.1)	0.93 (0.72–1.21)	0.95 (0.71–1.26)
60–69				
Non-agricultural workers	671 (82.4)	264,325 (84.2)	1.00	1.00
Agricultural workers	143 (17.6)	49,687 (15.8)	1.13 (0.95–1.36)	1.16 (0.95–1.41)
70–79				
Non-agricultural workers	1049 (76.1)	326,149 (81.7)	1.00	1.00
Agricultural workers	329 (23.9)	72,913 (18.3)	1.40 (1.24–1.59)	1.42 (1.24–1.63)
80+				
Non-agricultural workers	1542 (76.8)	369,104 (81.0)	1.00	1.00
Agricultural workers	466 (23.2)	86,738 (19.0)	1.29 (1.16–1.43)	1.31 (1.17–1.47)

* Crude odds ratio; ** Odds ratio adjusted by sex, age at death, region of residence, race/ethnicity, education.

4. Discussion

The current study was designed to explore the role of agricultural work and pesticide exposure in the development of acute kidney failure in regions of Brazil with the greatest concentration of agricultural production. In this population-based study in the Brazilian south and midwest, AKF mortality rates showed increasing trends, especially in the last 10–15 years, but regardless of their urban/rural status or level of pesticide expenditure. Although evidence from case reports suggests an association of AKF with pesticides [36,37], few occupational studies have evaluated this relationship. In addition, we observed an association between AKF mortality and agricultural occupation.

CKD is a risk factor for AKF, and the relationship between pesticide exposure and CKD has been evaluated in epidemiological studies. In a prospective analysis of the Agricultural Health Study (AHS) cohort, an increased rate of end-stage renal disease (ESRD) was associated with several specific herbicides in licensed male pesticide applicators [15], while increased risk (HR: 4.22; 95% CI: 1.26, 14.2) was also seen in their female spouses who reported high cumulative overall pesticide use when compared with low pesticide use [14]. CKD of unknown etiology (CKDu) has occurred in Latin America and Sri Lanka, primarily affecting young agricultural workers without known CKD risk factors [38–40]. CKDu has been considered multifactorial, with pesticide and metal exposure along with long working hours, intense heat, low fluid intake, and dehydration having been associated with its development [40,41]. A case–control study conducted by Jayasumana et al. [42] found an elevated risk of CKDu (OR 5.12, 95% CI 2.33–11.26) among farmers exposed to the herbicide glyphosate compared with controls. Although there is no evidence of CKDu-induced AKF in rural areas, this hypothesis cannot be ruled out, especially in tropical countries, due to the presence of physical, chemical, and social risk factors. In our study, the youngest agricultural workers (ages 20–29 years) had a higher risk of dying of AKF than from other causes, with a stronger association than in older workers who had higher rates of AKF likely due to other risk factors.

As far as we know, no previous study has assessed trends in AKF mortality in rural areas or areas with pesticide use in Brazil. In our study, rural and urban municipalities and municipalities with low, medium, and high pesticide-per-capita expenditure in the Brazilian south and midwest experienced an increase in AKF mortality in recent years compared to the whole studied period. These results reinforce the hypothesis that different and "traditional" risk factors can contribute to the development of AKF in urban and rural areas. In Brazilian midwestern municipalities, excess mortality from AKF began in the mid-1990s, the same period when there was an increase in pesticide use and planted areas with grains [43]. In the following decades, the midwestern region became the highest pesticide user in terms of liters in Brazil [26], and the progressive and gradual use of these substances was accompanied by a gradual increase in AKF. By contrast, in the south, the increase did not begin until the mid-2000s. The southern region's long-standing agricultural tradition includes many smallholder farms and diversified crops.

It's been shown that pesticides have nephrotoxic effects in animal studies. Rats exposed orally to acute and sub-acute levels of the insecticide chlorpyrifos showed tubular dilation, glomerular hypercellularity, and degeneration of renal tubules [44]. Urea nitrogen and creatinine levels were increased in rats treated by oral gavage with the herbicide atrazine [45]. Low oral doses of methyl parathion were related to structural and functional damage to the proximal tubules of male rat kidneys [46]. The herbicide 2,4-D has been related to tubular damage, glomerular alterations, vascular congestion, and an increased number of pyknotic nuclei in the kidneys of rats [21]. In addition, azoxystrobin fungicide administration in rats showed degeneration of tubular epithelial cells and hemorrhage in the intratubular spaces [24].

This study has several limitations. The data on risk factors, such as drug/medication ingestion, iodinated contrast, heart failure, liver disease, infections, and diabetes, were not available. Underreporting and misclassification can introduce biases when comparisons are made of mortality rates among areas or time periods with differences in information quality. In this study, CKD and unspecified kidney failure (UKD; ICD-10: N19) frequency reported as contributory causes of death among AKF cases were 0.54% (33) and 1.27% (77), respectively. Among controls, these numbers were 38,553 (1.92%) for CKD and 39,164 (1.95%) for UKD. However, AKF mortality might include cases of undiagnosed CKD in areas with limited access to healthcare. While the community healthcare system in Brazil has provided basic services to citizens since the mid-1990s, it does not routinely obtain data on pre-clinical laboratory markers of kidney disease. Farmers are exposed to several factors in addition to pesticides that may increase the risk of kidney diseases, and AKF specifically, such as heat and dehydration, metals, infections, and snake bites. In the current study, it was not possible to evaluate which agricultural-related risk factors could be specifically associated with AKF deaths.

A growing number of studies have focused on the acute renal effects of heat stress in agriculture. Moyce and coworkers [47] observed an increased cumulative incidence of AKF (OR: 4.52, 95% CI: 1.61–12.70) after a single day of summer agricultural work, with urine osmolality and creatinine increased among agricultural workers. Another study with the same design found renal alteration, including increased serum creatinine, uric acid, and urea nitrogen, and reduced glomerular filtration rate in sugarcane workers [48]. In rural settings, other common exposures may include leptospirosis, gastroenteritis, and hemolytic-uremic syndrome [5], but these and other individual-level risk factors were not included in our analysis. Overall trends suggest that AKF mortality rates are increasing in rural areas of the southern region, which may similarly be reflected in the stratified regression models showing increased odds of AKF in agricultural workers in this region. In addition to climatic differences (the midwest tends to be dryer) and, therefore, types of crops, specific pesticides and farming practices may also vary. Finally, in rural areas, prior episodes of AKF or pre-existing conditions, such as glomerulonephritis, may go unrecognized, increasing the potential severity of subsequent AKF episodes and associated mortality risk. Complications of pregnancy, such as sepsis and gestational hypertension/preeclampsia, are the other important pre-existing conditions. Excluding deaths prior to age 35 (i.e., most women of reproductive age) did not alter the odds of AKF mortality in females, suggesting pregnancy-related renal failure did not explain the elevated mortality odds in women. Indeed, most AKF mortality in agricultural workers under age 35 occurred in males. The association with agricultural occupation was seen in both males and females, though it appeared somewhat stronger among females. Moreover, we observed an increased chance of AKI mortality in women compared to men in models adjusting for occupation and the other health covariates. Given the possibility of gender-related differences in pathophysiological mechanisms, more research is needed specifically among males and females separately.

The main strength of our study was that we were able to examine AKF mortality related to the farming occupation in a large national database in Brazil, which also allowed us to look at contemporary time trends in AKF mortality across recent decades, a time of increasing pesticide use in Brazil. To evaluate the potential associations of pesticides with AKF mortality, we focused our analyses on the Brazilian south and midwest regions, where pesticide use is very high (mainly used in soybeans, corn, and cotton crops) [26]. Studies that evaluated the risk of renal outcomes in farmers suggest a synergism between environmental factors and increased risk of AKI mortality [49,50]. Our findings reinforce the need for more robust epidemiological studies that account for co-exposures and conditions of agricultural work in the relationship between pesticide exposure and kidney health in Brazil.

5. Conclusions

Our results suggest that mortality rates by AKF are increasing in both rural and urban Brazilian municipalities. In the south, AKF mortality rates increased faster in rural municipalities. In addition, in more recent periods (2004–2014), rural municipalities with medium and high pesticide-per-capita expenses showed, in general, higher and faster increases (higher AAPC) in AKF mortality rates. Our study also provides novel and robust evidence of the association between AKF mortality and agricultural work in Brazil, especially among younger workers.

Supplementary Materials: The following supporting information can be downloaded at: https://www.mdpi.com/article/10.3390/ijerph19116519/s1, Table S1: AKF mortality among agricultural workers according to the 10-year birth cohort.

Author Contributions: Conceptualization, A.M., A.S.E.S., A.J.L.C. and C.G.P.; methodology, A.M., A.S.E.S., A.J.L.C. and C.G.P.; data analysis, A.M. and A.S.E.S.; writing—original draft preparation, A.M.; writing—review and editing, A.M., A.S.E.S., A.J.L.C., C.I.R.F.A., V.M.C., D.P.S. and C.G.P. All authors have read and agreed to the published version of the manuscript.

Funding: This work was supported in part by the Intramural Research Program of the NIH, National Institute of Environmental Health Sciences (Z01-ES049028). A.M. was funded by the Brazilian Coordination for the Improvement of Higher Education Personnel (CAPES; grant No. 2478/2015-03), and National Council for Scientific and Technological Development (CNPq; grant No. 309152/2018-6).

Institutional Review Board Statement: Mortality data used in the current study are publicly available through the Brazilian Public Health System's Informatics Department (http://datasus.saude.gov.br/; accessed on 6 April 2022), which does not allow the identification of the cases and, therefore, does not require IRB review.

Informed Consent Statement: Not applicable.

Data Availability Statement: The data presented in this study are openly available in the DATASUS database at https://datasus.saude.gov.br/transferencia-de-arquivos/, accessed on 6 April 2022.

Conflicts of Interest: The authors declare no conflict of interest.

References

1. Bellomo, R.; Kellum, J.A.; Ronco, C. Acute Kidney Injury. *Lancet* **2012**, *380*, 756–766. [CrossRef]
2. Khwaja, A. KDIGO Clinical Practice Guidelines for Acute Kidney Injury. *Nephron. Clin. Pract.* **2012**, *120*, c179–c184. [CrossRef] [PubMed]
3. Soares, D.M.; Pessanha, J.F.; Sharma, A.; Brocca, A.; Ronco, C. Delayed Nephrology Consultation and High Mortality on Acute Kidney Injury: A Meta-Analysis. *Blood Purif.* **2017**, *43*, 57–67. [CrossRef] [PubMed]
4. Susantitaphong, P.; Cruz, D.N.; Cerda, J.; Abulfaraj, M.; Alqahtani, F.; Koulouridis, I.; Jaber, B.L. Acute Kidney Injury Advisory Group of the American Society of Nephrology World Incidence of AKI: A Meta-Analysis. *Clin. J. Am. Soc. Nephrol.* **2013**, *8*, 1482–1493. [CrossRef]
5. Cerdá, J.; Bagga, A.; Kher, V.; Chakravarthi, R.M. The Contrasting Characteristics of Acute Kidney Injury in Developed and Developing Countries. *Nat. Clin. Pract. Nephrol.* **2008**, *4*, 138–153. [CrossRef]
6. Hoste, E.A.; Kellum, J.A.; Selby, N.M.; Zarbock, A.; Palevsky, P.M.; Bagshaw, S.M.; Goldstein, S.L.; Cerdá, J.; Chawla, L.S. Global Epidemiology and Outcomes of Acute Kidney Injury. *Nat. Rev. Nephrol.* **2018**, *14*, 607–625. [CrossRef]
7. Grams, M.E.; Matsushita, K.; Sang, Y.; Estrella, M.M.; Foster, M.C.; Tin, A.; Kao, W.L.; Coresh, J. Explaining the Racial Difference in AKI Incidence. *J. Am. Soc. Nephrol.* **2014**, *25*, 1834–1841. [CrossRef]
8. Xue, J.L.; Daniels, F.; Star, R.A.; Kimmel, P.L.; Eggers, P.W.; Molitoris, B.A.; Himmelfarb, J.; Collins, A.J. Incidence and Mortality of Acute Renal Failure in Medicare Beneficiaries, 1992 to 2001. *J. Am. Soc. Nephrol.* **2006**, *17*, 1135–1142. [CrossRef]
9. Hsu, C.-Y.; McCulloch, C.; Fan, D.; Ordonez, J.; Chertow, G.; Go, A. Community-Based Incidence of Acute Renal Failure. *Kidney Int.* **2007**, *72*, 208–212. [CrossRef]
10. Cerdá, J.; Lameire, N.; Eggers, P.; Pannu, N.; Uchino, S.; Wang, H.; Bagga, A.; Levin, A. Epidemiology of Acute Kidney Injury. *Clin. J. Am. Soc. Nephrol.* **2008**, *3*, 881–886. [CrossRef]
11. Ponce, D.; Balbi, A. Acute Kidney Injury: Risk Factors and Management Challenges in Developing Countries. *Int. J. Nephrol. Renov. Dis.* **2016**, *9*, 193–200. [CrossRef] [PubMed]
12. Rewa, O.; Bagshaw, S.M. Acute Kidney Injury-Epidemiology, Outcomes and Economics. *Nat. Rev. Nephrol.* **2014**, *10*, 193–207. [CrossRef] [PubMed]
13. Rossaint, J.; Zarbock, A. Acute Kidney Injury: Definition, Diagnosis and Epidemiology. *Minerva Urol. Nefrol.* **2016**, *68*, 49–57. [PubMed]
14. Lebov, J.F.; Engel, L.S.; Richardson, D.; Hogan, S.L.; Sandler, D.P.; Hoppin, J.A. Pesticide Exposure and End-Stage Renal Disease Risk among Wives of Pesticide Applicators in the Agricultural Health Study. *Environ. Res.* **2015**, *143*, 198–210. [CrossRef] [PubMed]
15. Lebov, J.F.; Engel, L.S.; Richardson, D.; Hogan, S.L.; Hoppin, J.A.; Sandler, D.P. Pesticide Use and Risk of End-Stage Renal Disease among Licensed Pesticide Applicators in the Agricultural Health Study. *Occup. Environ. Med.* **2016**, *73*, 3–12. [CrossRef]
16. Petejova, N.; Martinek, A.; Zadrazil, J.; Teplan, V. Acute Toxic Kidney Injury. *Renal. Fail.* **2019**, *41*, 576–594. [CrossRef]
17. Agostini, M.; Bianchin, A. Acute Renal Failure from Organophospate Poisoning: A Case of Success with Haemofiltration. *Hum. Exp. Toxicol.* **2003**, *22*, 165–167. [CrossRef]
18. Rubio, C.R.; Felipe Fernández, C.; Manzanedo Bueno, R.; Del Pozo, B.A.; García, J.M. Acute Renal Failure Due to the Inhalation of Organophosphates: Successful Treatment with Haemodialysis. *Clin. Kidney J.* **2012**, *5*, 582–583. [CrossRef]
19. Lee, F.-Y.; Chen, W.-K.; Lin, C.-L.; Lai, C.-Y.; Wu, Y.-S.; Lin, I.-C.; Kao, C.-H. Organophosphate Poisoning and Subsequent Acute Kidney Injury Risk: A Nationwide Population-Based Cohort Study. *Medicine* **2015**, *94*, e2107. [CrossRef]
20. Dinis-Oliveira, R.J.; Duarte, J.A.; Remiao, F.; Sanchez-Navarro, A.; Bastos, M.L.; Carvalho, F. Single high dose dexamethasone treatment decreases the pathological score and increases the survival rate of paraquat-intoxicated rats. *Toxicology* **2006**, *227*, 73–85. [CrossRef]
21. Tayeb, W.; Nakbi, A.; Trabelsi, M.; Miled, A.; Hammami, M. Biochemical and histological evaluation of kidney damage after sub-acute exposure to 2,4-dichlorophenoxyacetic herbicide in rats: Involvement of oxidative stress. *Toxicol. Mech. Methods* **2012**, *22*, 696–704. [CrossRef] [PubMed]
22. Wunnapuk, K.; Liu, X.; Peake, P.; Gobe, G.; Endre, Z.; Grice, J.E.; Roberts, M.S.; Buckley, N.A. Renal biomarkers predict nephrotoxicity after paraquat. *Toxicol. Lett.* **2013**, *222*, 280–288. [CrossRef] [PubMed]
23. Parsons, P.P. Mammalian Toxicokinetics and Toxicity of Chlorothalonil. In *Hayes' Handbook of Pesticide Toxicology*; Academic Press: Cambridge, MA, USA, 2010; pp. 1951–1966. [CrossRef]
24. Ziada, R.M.; Abdulrhman, S.M.; Nahas, A.A. Hepato-nephro-toxicity Induced by Premium Fungicide and Protective Effect of Sesame Oil. *Egypt. J. Hosp. Med.* **2020**, *81*, 2445–2450. [CrossRef]
25. Zhang, W. Global Pesticide Use: Profile, Trend, Cost/Benefit and More. *Proc. Int. Acad. Ecol. Environ. Sci.* **2018**, *8*, 1–27.
26. Pignati, W.A.; Lima, F.A.; Correa, M.L.M.; Barbosa, J.R.; Leão, L.H.; Pignatti, M.G. Spatial distribution of pesticide use in Brazil: A strategy for Health Surveillance. *Cienc. Saude Colet.* **2017**, *22*, 3281–3293. [CrossRef]
27. De Castro, C.N. *Agriculture in Brazil's Midwest Region: Limitations and Future Challenges to Development*; Texto Para Discussão: Brasília, Brazil, 2014.
28. Meyer, A.; Chrisman, J.; Moreira, J.C.; Koifman, S. Cancer Mortality among Agricultural Workers from Serrana Region, State of Rio de Janeiro, Brazil. *Environ. Res.* **2003**, *93*, 264–271. [CrossRef]

29. Meyer, A.; Koifman, S.; Koifman, R.J.; Moreira, J.C.; de Rezende Chrisman, J.; Abreu-Villaca, Y. Mood Disorders Hospitalizations, Suicide Attempts, and Suicide Mortality among Agricultural Workers and Residents in an Area with Intensive Use of Pesticides in Brazil. *J. Toxicol. Environ. Health A* **2010**, *73*, 866–877. [CrossRef]
30. Santana, V.S.; Moura, M.C.P.; Ferreira e Nogueira, F. Occupational pesticide poisoning mortality, 2000-2009, Brazil. *Rev. Saude Publica* **2013**, *47*, 598–606. [CrossRef]
31. Krawczyk, N.; de Souza Espíndola Santos, A.; Lima, J.; Meyer, A. Revisiting Cancer 15 Years Later: Exploring Mortality among Agricultural and Non-agricultural Workers in the Serrana Region of Rio de Janeiro. *Am. J. Ind. Med.* **2017**, *60*, 77–86. [CrossRef]
32. de Boccolini, P.M.M.; Boccolini, C.S.; de Chrisman, J.R.; Koifman, R.J.; Meyer, A. Non-Hodgkin Lymphoma among Brazilian Agricultural Workers: A Death Certificate Case-Control Study. *Arch. Environ. Occup. Health* **2017**, *72*, 139–144. [CrossRef]
33. Nunes, E.P.; da Costa Côrtes, S.; Bivar, W.S.B.; Fortes, L.P.S.; Simões, P.C.M.; Tai, D.W.; Quintslr, M.M.M.; Lima, U.T.; Gadelha, P.; Instituto Brasileiro de Geografia e Estatística-IBGE. *Atlas do Espaço Rural Brasileiro*, 2nd ed.; IBGE: Rio de Janeiro, Brazil, 2020. Available online: https://biblioteca.ibge.gov.br/visualizacao/livros/liv101773_pre_textual.pdf (accessed on 6 April 2022).
34. Kim, H.J.; Fay, M.P.; Feuer, E.J.; Midthune, D.N. Permutation Tests for Joinpoint Regression with Applications to Cancer Rates. *Stat. Med.* **2000**, *19*, 335–351. [CrossRef]
35. De Lima, E.E.C.; Queiroz, B.L. Evolution of the Deaths Registry System in Brazil: Associations with Changes in the Mortality Profile, under-Registration of Death Counts, and Ill-Defined Causes of Death. *Cad. Saude Publica* **2014**, *30*, 1721–1730. [CrossRef] [PubMed]
36. Bashir, B.; Sharma, S.G.; Stein, H.D.; Sirota, R.A.; D'Agati, V.D. Acute Kidney Injury Secondary to Exposure to Insecticides Used for Bedbug (Cimex Lectularis) Control. *Am. J. Kidney Dis.* **2013**, *62*, 974–977. [CrossRef]
37. Mohamed, F.; Endre, Z.H.; Buckley, N.A. Role of Biomarkers of Nephrotoxic Acute Kidney Injury in Deliberate Poisoning and Envenomation in Less Developed Countries. *Br. J. Clin. Pharmacol.* **2015**, *80*, 3–19. [CrossRef] [PubMed]
38. Cerdas, M. Chronic Kidney Disease in Costa Rica. *Kidney Int.* **2005**, *68*, S31–S33. [CrossRef] [PubMed]
39. Orantes Navarro, C.M.; Herrera Valdés, R.; López, M.A.; Calero, D.J.; Fuentes de Morales, J.; Alvarado Ascencio, N.P.; Vela Parada, X.F.; Zelaya Quezada, S.M.; Granados Castro, D.V.; Orellana de Figueroa, P. Epidemiological Characteristics of Chronic Kidney Disease of Non-Traditional Causes in Women of Agricultural Communities of El Salvador. *Clin. Nephrol.* **2015**, *83*, 24–31. [CrossRef] [PubMed]
40. Pearce, N.; Caplin, B. Let's Take the Heat out of the CKDu Debate: More Evidence Is Needed. *Occup. Environ. Med.* **2019**, *76*, 357–359. [CrossRef]
41. Jayatilake, N.; Mendis, S.; Maheepala, P.; Mehta, F.R. Chronic Kidney Disease of Uncertain Aetiology: Prevalence and Causative Factors in a Developing Country. *BMC Nephrol.* **2013**, *14*, 180. [CrossRef]
42. Jayasumana, C.; Paranagama, P.; Agampodi, S.; Wijewardane, C.; Gunatilake, S.; Siribaddana, S. Drinking Well Water and Occupational Exposure to Herbicides Is Associated with Chronic Kidney Disease, in Padavi-Sripura, Sri Lanka. *Environ. Health* **2015**, *14*, 6. [CrossRef]
43. Brandão, A.S.P.; de Rezende, G.C.; da Marques, R.W.C. Crescimento Agrícola No Período 1999/2004: A Explosão Da Soja e Da Pecuária Bovina e Seu Impacto Sobre o Meio Ambiente. *Econ. Apl.* **2006**, *10*, 249–266. [CrossRef]
44. Raina, S.; Hamid, S. Histopathological Effects of Pesticide-Cholopyrifos on Kidney in Albino Rats. *Int. J. Res. Med. Sci.* **2013**, *1*, 465–475.
45. Liu, W.; Du, Y.; Liu, J.; Wang, H.; Sun, D.; Liang, D.; Zhao, L.; Shang, J. Effects of Atrazine on the Oxidative Damage of Kidney in Wister Rats. *Int. J. Clin. Exp. Med.* **2014**, *7*, 3235–3243. [PubMed]
46. Fuentes-Delgado, V.H.; Martínez-Saldaña, M.C.; Rodríguez-Vázquez, M.L.; Reyes-Romero, M.A.; Reyes-Sánchez, J.L.; Jaramillo-Juárez, F. Renal Damage Induced by the Pesticide Methyl Parathion in Male Wistar Rats. *J. Toxicol. Environ. Health Part A* **2018**, *81*, 130–141. [CrossRef] [PubMed]
47. Moyce, S.; Joseph, J.; Tancredi, D.; Mitchell, D.; Schenker, M. Cumulative Incidence of Acute Kidney Injury in California's Agricultural Workers. *J. Occup. Environ. Med.* **2016**, *58*, 391–397. [CrossRef] [PubMed]
48. García-Trabanino, R.; Jarquín, E.; Wesseling, C.; Johnson, R.J.; González-Quiroz, M.; Weiss, I.; Glaser, J.; Vindell, J.J.; Stockfelt, L.; Roncal, C. Heat Stress, Dehydration, and Kidney Function in Sugarcane Cutters in El Salvador–a Cross-Shift Study of Workers at Risk of Mesoamerican Nephropathy. *Environ. Res.* **2015**, *142*, 746–755. [CrossRef] [PubMed]
49. Correa-Rotter, R.; Wesseling, C.; Johnson, R.J. CKD of Unknown Origin in Central America: The Case for a Mesoamerican Nephropathy. *Am. J. Kidney Dis.* **2014**, *63*, 506–520. [CrossRef]
50. Gunatilake, S.; Seneff, S.; Orlando, L. Glyphosate's Synergistic Toxicity in Combination with Other Factors as a Cause of Chronic Kidney Disease of Unknown Origin. *Int. J. Environ. Res. Public Health* **2019**, *16*, 2734. [CrossRef]

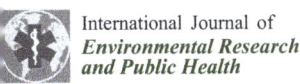

Article

Neurological Impacts of Chronic Methylmercury Exposure in Munduruku Indigenous Adults: Somatosensory, Motor, and Cognitive Abnormalities

Rogério Adas Ayres de Oliveira [1], Bruna Duarte Pinto [1], Bruno Hojo Rebouças [1], Daniel Ciampi de Andrade [1], Ana Claudia Santiago de Vasconcellos [2] and Paulo Cesar Basta [3],*

[1] Centro de Dor, Departamento de Neurologia, Hospital das Clínicas, Faculdade de Medicina, Universidade de São Paulo (USP), São Paulo 05403-000, Brazil; roger.adas.doc@gmail.com (R.A.A.d.O.); brunaduartencl@gmail.com (B.D.P.); bruhojo@hotmail.com (B.H.R.); ciampi@usp.br (D.C.d.A.)
[2] Laboratório de Educação Profissional em Vigilância em Saúde, Escola Politécnica de Saúde Joaquim Venâncio, Fundação Oswaldo Cruz (EPSJV/Fiocruz), Rio de Janeiro 21040-900, Brazil; anacsvasconcellos@gmail.com
[3] Departamento de Endemias Samuel Pessoa, Escola Nacional de Saúde Pública, Fundação Oswaldo Cruz (ENSP/Fiocruz), Rio de Janeiro 21041-210, Brazil
* Correspondence: paulobasta@gmail.com; Tel.: +55-21-2598-2503

Abstract: There has been increasing evidence about mercury (Hg) contamination in traditional populations from the Amazon Basin due to illegal gold mining. The most concerning health impact is neurotoxicity caused by Hg in its organic form: methylmercury (MeHg). However, the severity and extent of the neurotoxic effects resulting from chronic environmental exposure to MeHg are still unclear. We conducted a clinical-epidemiological study to evaluate the neurological impacts of chronic MeHg exposure in Munduruku indigenous people, focusing on somatosensory, motor, and cognitive abnormalities. All participants were subjected to a systemized neurological exam protocol, including Brief Cognitive Screening Battery (BCSB), verbal fluency test, and Stick Design Test. After the examination, hair samples were collected to determine MeHg levels. Data collection took place between 29 October and 9 November 2019, in three villages (*Sawré Muybu*, *Poxo Muybu*, and *Sawré Aboy*) from *Sawré Muybu* Indigenous Land, Southwest of Pará state. One hundred and ten individuals >12 years old were included, 58 of which were men (52.7%), with an average age of 27.6 years (range from 12 to 72). Participants' median MeHg level was 7.4 µg/g (average: 8.7; S.D: 4.5; range: 2.0–22.8). In *Sawré Aboy* village, the median MeHg level was higher (12.5 µg/g) than in the others, showing a significant statistical exposure gradient (Kruskal–Wallis test with p-value < 0.001). Cerebellar ataxia was observed in two participants with MeHg levels of 11.68 and 15.68 µg/g. Individuals with MeHg exposure level ≥10 µg/g presented around two-fold higher chances of cognitive deficits (RP: 2.2; CI 95%: 1.13–4.26) in BCSB, and in the verbal fluency test (RP: 2.0; CI 95%: 1.18–3.35). Furthermore, adolescents of 12 to 19 years presented three-fold higher chances of verbal development deficits, according to the fluency test (RP: 3.2; CI 95%: 1.06–9.42), than individuals of 20 to 24 years. The worsened motor and cognitive functions are suggestive of neurotoxicity due to chronic MeHg exposure. In conclusion, we believe monitoring and follow-up measures are necessary for chronic mercury exposed vulnerable people, and a basic care protocol should be established for contaminated people in the Brazilian Unified Health System.

Keywords: mercury exposure; neurological abnormalities; indigenous people; Amazon; environmental impacts; illegal mining

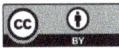

1. Introduction

Methylmercury (MeHg) is a toxic organo-mercurial compound which acts systemically in the human body [1,2]. The intake dose, exposure duration, and frequency, in addition to the exposure route and age of the individual (or stage of development), are factors that determine the extent of damage caused by MeHg and which organs or systems are worst affected [3].

After the Minamata and Niigata disasters in Japan in the 1950s and 1960s, the international scientific community agreed that methylmercury's main target is the Central Nervous System (CNS) [4]. During that time, it was observed that adult individuals who regularly consumed contaminated fish presented neurological abnormalities such as paresthesia, ataxia, dysarthria, visual field alterations, and hearing impairments. In addition, these events showed that the prenatal period is the most vulnerable stage to the deleterious effects of MeHg. Many women who were exposed during pregnancy gave birth to children with severe congenital malformations and significant cognitive impairments [5–7]. Years later, the clinical manifestation caused by the exposure to high MeHg levels during adult life or pregnancy became known as Minamata Disease [8,9].

The MeHg intoxication episode in Iraq, in the early 1970s, was even more devastating than Japan's tragedy. Because it was an acute exposure episode, there were more than 6000 hospitalizations due to intoxication and hundreds of deaths in a short period of time [10,11]. In that time, the refinement of the spectrometry of atomic absorption technique for analyzing Hg in human tissue made laboratory measurements more precise. Consequently, it was possible to establish a consistent relationship between the signs and symptoms presented by the exposed individuals and mercury concentration in exposure biomarkers (e.g., hair and blood) [6]. Based on scientific evidence, the World Health Organization established [4] that the neurological effects of MeHg exposure can be found in 5% of adult individuals who ingest 3 to 7 µg daily of MeHg per kilogram of body weight (kg bw). This daily intake dose corresponds to levels of 200 µg/L in blood or 50 µg/g in hair. However, these indexes are constantly revised, and some are updated as a result of new technologies and current research carried out in different parts of the world.

Since the 1990s, research conducted in the Amazon region identified adult individuals with neurological abnormalities probably associated with the consumption of contaminated fish. In those individuals, levels of methylmercury in hair samples varied between 10 and 20 µg/g [12–17]. Similar findings were reported in riparian populations in Bolivia and Suriname [18,19].

It is worth noting that the peculiar characteristics of the Amazon's ecosystem and the social dynamics of its traditional populations may be responsible for the different thresholds for the onset of neurological effects. In that region, the majority of the mercury human exposure is due to artisanal small-scale gold mining (ASGM) [20]. ASGM causes the liberation of large quantities of Hg in the ecosystem and, at the same time, mobilizes natural Hg present in the soil. In addition to ASGM, the construction of hydroelectric plants and dams, deforestation, and fires also alter the Hg cycle in the region, increasing the risk of human contamination [20–24]. Moreover, the traditional people living there are considered to be among the largest consumers of fish in the world [25–27].

In the aquatic environment, the Hg released by the ASGM suffers methylation, mediated by microorganisms, transforming it into methylmercury (MeHg). Most of the toxicity attributed to MeHg is due to its biomagnification capacity in aquatic trophic chains and to the ability to overcome blood–brain and placenta barriers. Because fish consumption is the main protein source in many traditional populations in the Amazon, chronic exposure to high levels of mercury can cause various negative consequences and create health problems in local populations [20,28–32]. After intake of contaminated fish, almost all MeHg is quickly absorbed by the gastrointestinal tract. The absorbed MeHg forms a conjugate with the cysteine molecules present in the blood and, afterward, is distributed to virtually all human body tissue. When the MeHg reaches the CNS, it undergoes oxidation and tends to accumulate, leading to potentially irreversible cerebral tissue damage [33].

Experimental evidence shows that MeHg neurotoxicity is marked by an increase in oxidative stress, by the presence of mitochondrial lesions, by the release of excitatory amino acids, and by proteomic expression alterations, which can lead to cellular dysfunction and death [34–36]. Furthermore, the chronic exposure to high levels of MeHg has been associated with memory and learning deficits, motor function abnormalities, hearing loss, and a reduced visual field [3,20,37–42].

In the Amazon region, few clinical studies have correlated MeHg exposure levels with neurological symptoms [12–14,16,17]. Nevertheless, none of these studies included indigenous populations. Therefore, there is insufficient evidence about neurotoxicity concerning indigenous populations chronically exposed to MeHg in the Amazon Basin.

With the lack of evidence on this topic in mind, this study aimed to describe neurological clinical manifestations, focusing on somatosensory, motor, and cognitive abnormalities, in adults indigenous from three Munduruku villages in the Amazon Basin. The ultimate goal was to explore possible associations between neurological abnormalities with chronic methylmercury exposure.

2. Materials and Methods
2.1. Study Design and Field Work

We conducted a cross-sectional clinical-epidemiological study including indigenous people older than 12 years old living in three villages: *Sawré Muybu* (SM), *Poxo Muybu* (PM), and *Sawré Aboy* (SA), in the *Sawré Muybu* Indigenous Land (IL), located at Middle-Tapajós River, in the southwest region of Pará state, Brazilian Amazon.

Data collection occurred between 29 October and 9 November 2019, according to a multidisciplinary and inter-institutional study developed to clarify the consequences and assess the impacts of illegal mining in the *Sawré Muybu* IL. For additional information, see Basta et al. [43].

2.2. Evaluated Population

We performed a census in the three villages mentioned above, and all indigenous individuals aged 12 or older were invited to participate in the study. Therefore, probabilistic sampling methods were not used to select participants. A 15-year-old man from *Sawré Muybu* village, who had cerebral palsy, was excluded from the study.

Fish Consumption Estimates

Like the majority of the traditional groups living in the Amazon Basin, Munduruku people consume large quantities of fish. Recently, Vasconcellos et al. [44] carried out an investigation to estimate the fish consumption of the Munduruku indigenous people living in the study area and compared their findings with the acceptable levels proposed by the FAO/WHO [45] and by the U.S.EPA [46].

During one week, the authors collected 88 fish specimens representing 17 species and four trophic levels to analyze the total mercury (THg) concentration in muscle tissue. They also developed an empirical method to estimate fish consumption from catch effort. The average daily fish consumption estimated for adult men was 216.75 g, and for women of childbearing age was 168.58 g. Considering that about 90–95% of total mercury species detected in fish samples is in the form of MeHg [47–49], we assume that all of the Hg detected in the fish samples is compounded by MeHg.

The average MeHg levels in samples of non-piscivorous fish (n = 57) was 0.10 µg/g (SD = 0.09) and the average for piscivorous fish (n = 31) was 0.44 µg/g (SD = 0.34). The highest level of methylmercury in muscle tissue (1.95 µg/g) was observed in the *Serrasalmus rhombeus* (also known as *piranha preta* in Portuguese), a fish not only located at the top of the food chain, but also highly appreciated and regularly consumed by the Munduruku [44].

Moreover, the authors devised four scenarios to estimate the MeHg exposure, considering the fish consumption from catch effort: (i) in the rainy season; (ii) in the dry season; (iii) based on the weighted average of medium mercury levels detected in piscivorous and non-piscivorous species; and (iv) based on the 95th percentile of mercury concentrations in piscivorous and non-piscivorous species (1.42 and 0.29 µg/g, respectively).

According to the authors, scenario (iii) most closely matches the local reality, in which the estimates of MeHg ingestion for Munduruku adult men ranged from 1.84- to

8.28-fold above the safe daily methylmercury intake recommended by FAO/WHO [45] and U.S.EPA [46], respectively. The estimates ranged from 3.17- to 7.29-fold above the FAO/WHO [45] and U.S.EPA [46], respectively, for women of childbearing age.

Summarizing, the studied Munduruku villages are at severe risk of harm due to the ingestion of MeHg-contaminated fish.

2.3. Neurological Examination

All participants were submitted to a systemized neurological examination protocol, specifically developed for this research, to make the evaluation feasible in the adverse conditions of the fieldwork in the villages. The evaluations were conducted by neurologists (BDP, BHR, and RAAO) familiar with clinical neurological semiology and duly trained to apply the protocol and use the examining instruments.

The explanations about the clinical procedures for the neurological exam were verbally presented to the participants in Brazilian Portuguese. When necessary, for indigenous individuals that had difficulties with Portuguese, an indigenous translator (indigenous health agents, teachers, or chiefs) from the village would assist.

2.3.1. Static Balance and Walking Evaluation

The evaluation of static balance and walking was performed by visual inspection. Participants were asked to remain in an orthostatic position to perform the Romberg test, with eyes open and closed, sequentially. Then, participants were asked to walk towards the examiner.

2.3.2. Cranial Nerve Examination

The following parameters were evaluated: visual campimetry by confrontation, pupil reflex and external ocular motricity, facial motricity and symmetry, facial sensibility, palate elevation, gag reflex and tongue motricity.

2.3.3. Sensory Testing

The following instruments were used to evaluate the respective somatosensory modalities:

(a) Sharp nickel-plated pin (Bacchi® number 29): mechanical nociceptive perception.
(b) Sorri Bauru esthesiometer/Von Frey 10g monofilament: tactile sensitivity.
(c) Dry cotton wad: dynamic tactile sensitivity.
(d) 128 Hz diapason: tactile vibration sensitivity and thermic sensitivity to cold [50].

The sensitivity was tested in upper and lower limbs at three distinct points for each sensory modality, in the proximal and distal segments. The sensitivity was classified as normal (0) or abnormal (1) depending on the abnormality occurrence in at least one parameter.

For the clinical diagnosis of distal symmetric polyneuropathy, criteria from the American Academy of Neurology were used, which consider the occurrence of distal sensory deficits, in addition to the clinical signs of neuropathy, defined as the presence of abnormalities in at least one somatic sensory domain and/or alterations in the ankle jerk reflex [51].

2.3.4. Motor Function

Muscular strength was evaluated through maneuvers against resistance in all four limbs, on proximal and distal segments. Muscular hypertonia and bradykinesia were evaluated through passive mobilization of the four members, through finger tapping maneuvers, facial expression mimicking, and spontaneous mobilization. Coordination was evaluated through finger to nose, heel to knee, and diadochokinesis (ability to make alternating quick movements) tests. The deep osteotendinous ankle jerk reflex was tested with the Babinski hammer, according to the Hallett [52] myotatic reflex score. Toe amyotrophy was investigated through inspection.

2.3.5. Cognitive Evaluation

All individuals were submitted to a cognitive evaluation by the authors (BDP, BHR and RAAO), immediately after the neurological exam, as part of the evaluation protocol.

An indigenous translator from the village was present in the interviews to help with the communication with indigenous individuals who had difficulties with Portuguese.

The Brief Cognitive Screening Battery (BCSB) [53], the verbal fluency test in the animal category [54], and the stick design test [55] were used as instruments of cognitive evaluation. These instruments were selected given their appropriateness for populations with low levels of education and for the easy application in adverse conditions in the field.

Brief Cognitive Screening Battery (BCSB)

The BCSB is an instrument developed by the Cognitive and Behavior Neurology Group of the *Hospital das Clínicas* of the Medical School of the *Universidade de São Paulo* [53], which entails naming and remembering 10 drawings of simple and known objects in black and white presented in a single picture. This instrument evaluates, in sequence, the following domains: (a) visual perception and naming, (b) incidental memory, (c) immediate memory, (d) learning, (e) verbal fluency test (described below), (f) 5 min belated memory, and g) recognition.

The following cutoffs were used in the tests to evaluate the domains' normality: immediate memory (≥ 5), learning (≥ 7), verbal fluency (≥ 9), and delayed recall (≥ 6). Alteration in at least one of these domains was considered a criterion for abnormality for the BCSB, finally classified as: (0) normal or (1) abnormal.

Verbal Fluency Test in the Animal Category

To evaluate verbal fluency, participants were asked to name as many animals as they could in one minute. The individuals received the following instructions: *"you must say the animal names you remember, as quickly as possible. Any animal will do, four-legged, fish, birds, the more you say, the better"*. The cutoff for verbal fluency test normality was ≥ 9. This test was applied as part of the BCSB, as an interference factor.

Stick Design Test

To evaluate logical thinking, participants were asked to reproduce geometric shapes, presented on a sheet of paper one after the other, with matches. The number of sides, the image and stick orientation in each of the four images were criteria considered for the test score, which varies from zero to 12. Scores ≥ 10 were considered the cutoff for normality and classified as normal (0) or abnormal (1).

2.4. MeHg Exposure Biomarker

According to the guidance published by the World Health Organization [56], and described by other authors [57,58], hair samples are considered the best biomarker of the MeHg human exposure, because almost all Hg detected in this kind of biological matrix is in the MeHg form. In addition, because the main Hg exposure route observed in the studied population is the consumption of Hg-contaminated fish, and almost all Hg present in the fish muscle is in the MeHg form, hair samples were used as its exposure biomarker [47–49]. Therefore, we assume for this study that all Hg present in hair samples is MeHg.

The hair's samples were collected from the occipital region, with the aid of stainless-steel dissection scissors, from all participants. The samples were stored in individually identified paper envelopes and sent for total mercury concentration (THg) analysis in the Toxicology Laboratory in the Environmental Section of the *Instituto Evandro Chagas* (IEC).

In the laboratory, before starting the analyses, hair samples were repeatedly washed with Extran detergent (Merck KGaA, Darmstadt, Germany) to remove any exogenous contamination. After drying, the samples were finely homogenized in glass flasks before weighing. This methodology comprises chemical opening, wet digestion, and subsequent reduction with SnCl$_2$ to quantify total Hg in a Cold Vapor Atomic Absorption Spectrometer (CVAAS).

The protocols for Quality Assurance (QA)/Quality Control (QC) included the following parameters: (i) a method blank; (ii) a 6-point calibration curve (concentration ranging from 0.4 to 4 ng/g); (iii) the Human Hair Certified Reference Material (IAEA-86), whose average recovery rate was 101% (n = 8, recovery ranging from 83.4 to 106.6%) from the International Atomic Energy Agency; and (iv) the relative standard deviation (RSD) of 8.32%. Sample replicates (n = 10), whose RSD was 2.49%, were also randomly selected. The detection and quantification limits (LOD/LOQ) obtained were 0.0083 ng/mg and 0.027 ng/mg, respectively.

For further detail on hair sample analysis, see Basta et al. [43].

2.5. Statistical Analysis

A descriptive analysis of the participants was undertaken according to sociodemographic variables: sex (female / male), age (12 to 19; 20 to 24, 25 to 29, and $\geq$30 years old) and village of residence (*Sawré Muybu*, *Poxo Muybu*, and *Sawré Aboy*), in contrast to the evaluated neurological parameters.

To estimate the prevalence of exposure, in the numerator we included participants older than 12 who presented with methylmercury levels $\geq$10.0 μg/g. In the denominator, the population sampled for the study in the same age group was considered. The prevalence was presented for the three villages under study: *Sawré Muybu*, *Poxo Muybu*, and *Sawré Aboy*.

The main neurological abnormalities detected in the clinical exam were compared between two groups, according to the participants' level of methylmercury exposure: $\geq$10.0 vs. <10.0 μg/g.

Because mercury levels do not show a normal distribution, the Kruskal–Wallis non-parametric test was used to evaluate differences in methylmercury levels in all comparisons that showed measures of central tendency (medians). The difference in proportion between variables was evaluated using Pearson's chi-squared test.

We used a Poisson regression model with robust variance to estimate the association between alterations observed in the BCSB and the verbal fluency test in the animal category with independent variables: (i) methylmercury exposure level (<10.0 vs. $\geq$10.0 μg/g); age (12 to 19; 20 to 24, 25 to 29, and $\geq$30 years old); and (ii) sex (female vs. male). Prevalence Ratio (PR), with the respective confidence interval of 95%, was used as an association measure.

Variables with a *p*-value < 0.20 in the simple analysis were selected and included in the multiple model. Variables that presented significance levels of 5% ($p < 0.05$) remained in the final model. The data was analyzed with the statistical software SPSS version 9.0 (Chicago, IL, USA).

3. Results

During the field work, 110 indigenous individuals were evaluated, 50 of whom were from the *Sawré Muybu* (SM) village, 37 from the *Poxo Muybu* (PM) village, and 23 from the *Sawré Aboy* (SA) village. Fifty-eight were men (52.7%) and 52 were women (47.3%). The participants age ranged from 12 to 72 years (average: 27.6 years; standard deviation: 13.7). The participants' distribution, according to age group, was heterogenous in the studied villages. There was a predominance of adolescents (12 to 19 years) in PM and SA villages, with 16 (43.2%) and 11 (47.8%) participants, respectively, compared to nine (18.0%) participants in the SM village. In contrast, in *Sawré Muybu* there was the highest concentration of young adults between 25 and 29 years of age (26.0%) ($p = 0.032$) (Table 1).

Table 1. Sociodemographic variables, hair-methylmercury level groups, somatosensory and motor functions, and cognitive alterations, according to the village of residence. *Sawré Muybu* Indigenous Land, Pará state, Brazilian Amazon, 2019.

Sociodemographic Variables	Villages						Total		p-Value
	Sawré Muybu		*Poxo Muybu*		*Sawré Aboy*				
	n	%	n	%	n	%	n	%	
Sex									0.857
Female	25	50.0	17	45.9	10	43.5	52	47.3	
Male	25	50.0	20	54.1	13	56.5	58	52.7	
Total	50		37		23		110		
Age range (years)									0.032
12 to 19	9	18.0	16	43.2	11	47.8	36	32.7	
20 to 24	11	22.0	6	16.2	3	13.0	20	18.2	
25 to 29	13	26.0	2	5.4	2	8.7	17	15.5	
≥30	17	34.0	13	35.1	7	30.4	37	33.6	
Total	50		37		23		110		
Hair-methylmercury levels									
≥10 µg/g	11	22.4	4	10.8	18	78.3	33	30.3	0.001
<10 µg/g	38	77.6	33	89.2	5	21.7	76	69.7	
Total	49		37		23		109		
Somatosensory signs									
Distal pinprick perception									0.012
Normal	40	80.0	37	100.0	18	78.3	95	86.4	
Abnormal	10	20.0	0	0.0	5	21.7	15	13.6	
Total	50		37		23		110		
Distal Thermal Sensitivity									0.004
Normal	38	76.0	37	100.0	17	73.0	92	83.6	
Abnormal	12	24.0	0	0.0	6	26.1	18	16.4	
Total	50		37		23		110		
Hallux or Thumb Vibration Sensitivity									0.042
Normal	46	92.0	36	97.3	18	78.3	100	90.9	
Abnormal	4	8.0	1	2.7	5	21.7	10	9.1	
Total	50		37		23		110		
Feet mechanical detection threshold									0.001
Normal	33	66.0	37	100.0	15	65.2	85	77.3	
Abnormal	17	34.0	0	0.0	8	34.8	25	22.7	
Total	50		37		23		110		
Clinical signs of polyneuropathy (Neuropathy burden)									0.003
No	29	58.0	33	89.2	13	56.4	75	68.2	
Yes	21	42.0	4	10.8	10	43.5	35	31.8	
Total	50		37		23		110		
Motor functions									
Toe amyotrophy									0.331
Absent	48	96.0	34	91.9	23	100.0	105	95.5	
Present	2	4.0	3	8.1	0	0.0	5	4.5	
Total	50		37		23		110		
Ankle jerk reflex									0.025
Normal	40	80.0	36	97.3	17	73.9	92	83.6	
Abnormal	10	20.0	1	2.7	6	26.1	17	16.4	
Total	50		37		23		110		
Bradykinesia									0.121
Absent	49	98.0	37	100.0	21	91.3	107	97.3	
Present	1	2.0	0	0.0	2	8.7	3	2.7	
Total	50		37		23		110		
Cerebellar Ataxia									0.468
Absent	49	98.0	37	100.0	21	95.5	108	98.2	
Present	1	2.0	0	0.0	1	4.5	2	1.8	
Total	50		37		22		110		
Cognition									
Brief Cognitive Screening Battery (BCSB)									0.124
Normal	42	82.4	29	78.4	14	60.9	85	76.6	
Abnormal	9	17.6	8	21.6	9	39.1	26	23.4	
Total	51		37		23		111		
Stick design test									0.466
Normal	50	98.0	37	100.0	22	95.7	109	98.2	
Abnormal	1	2.0	0	0.0	1	4.3	2	1.8	
Total	51		37		23		111		
Verbal Fluency test									0.046
Normal	47	94.0	33	89.2	17	73.9	97	88.2	
Abnormal	3	6.0	4	10.8	6	26.1	13	11.8	
Total	50		37		23		110		

3.1. Overall Data by Village

No participant showed static balance, walking, or cranial nerve function alterations. There were significant somatosensory alterations in the SM and SA villages in contrast to PM, represented here by the distal pinprick perception ($p = 0.012$), distal thermal sensitivity ($p = 0.004$), hallux or thumb vibration sensitivity (pallesthesia) ($p = 0.042$), and feet mechanical detection threshold ($p = -0.001$). Clinical signs of polyneuropathy were detected in 21 (42.0%) participants from *Sawré Muybu* village and 10 (43.5%) participants from *Sawré Aboy* village, revealing a significant superior prevalence compared to *Poxo Muybu* village, where only 4 (10.8%) participants were affected ($p = 0.003$) (Table 1).

Two (1.9%) indigenous people presented with alterations in cerebellar motor alterations ataxy, one from SM and one from SA villages, and three (2.8%) presented with bradykinesia, two of which were from SA and one from SM village, with no significant differences in the distribution between the villages. No signs of hypertonia or rigidity were detected in participants (Table 1).

Five (4.5%) participants were diagnosed with toe amyotrophy, three of which were from PM village and two from SM village (p-value = 0.331). There were no recorded cases of amyotrophy in SA.

The absence of ankle jerk reflex was detected in 10 (20%) and six (26.1%) participants from SM and SA village, respectively, and was more prevalent than in PM village, where it was observed in only one (2.7%) individual ($p = 0.025$) (Table 1).

Regarding cognitive manifestations, there were BCSB abnormalities in 39.1% (n = 9) of participants from SA village, whereas in SM and PM the alterations affected 17.6% (n = 9) and 21.6% (n = 8) of participants, respectively ($p = 0.089$) (Table 1).

Impairments in the verbal fluency test were detected in 21.6% (n = 6) of participants from SA village. In contrast, in PM and SM, the verbal fluency affected 10.8% (n = 4) and 6.0% (n = 3) of participants, respectively ($p = 0.046$) (Table 1).

Alterations in the stick design test were observed in only one (2.0%) individual from SM village and in one (4.3%) individual from SA ($p = 0.466$).

3.2. Neurological Abnormalities According to MeHg Exposure Levels

In general, the median MeHg level in participants was 7.4 µg/g (average: 8.7; standard deviation: 4.5; range from 2.0 to 22.8). In *Poxo Muybu* village, the median MeHg level in participants was 7.3 µg/g (average: 7.3; standard deviation: 2.3; range from 2.3 to 12.9). In *Sawré Muybu* village, the median MeHg level in participants was 6.5 µg/g (average: 7.4; standard deviation: 4.2; range from 2.0 to 22.1). Finally, in *Sawré Aboy* village, the median MeHg level in participants was 12.5 µg/g (average: 13.5; standard deviation: 4.6; range from 4.8 to 22.8), showing a significant statistical exposure gradient (Kruskal–Wallis Test with p-value < 0.001).

The MeHg exposure prevalence over 10 µg/g also varied according to the studied villages, 78.3% of which from SA, 22.4% from SM, and 10.8% from PM (p-value = 0.001) (Table 1). However, there were no significant differences in MeHg exposure considering age group and sex (Table 2).

3.2.1. Somatic Sensitivity (Somatosensory)

Alterations in distal pinprick perception were found in 14.5 and 12.1% of participants in the exposure groups of <10 and ≥10 µg/g MeHg, respectively (p-value = 0.743) (Table 2).

Distal thermal sensitivity alterations were observed in 14.5% of participants of exposure group of <10 µg/g, in comparison to 21.2% in the group of ≥10 µg/g MeHg (p-value = 0.384) (Table 2).

Hallux or thumb vibration sensitivity alterations were seen in 6.6% of participants in the exposure group of <10 µg/g, in contrast to 15.2% in the exposure group of ≥10 µg/g MeHg ($p = 0.154$) (Table 2).

Table 2. Sociodemographic variables, somatosensory and motor functions, and cognition signs, according to hair-MeHg levels (<10 vs. ≥10 µg/g), *Sawré Muybu* Indigenous Land, Pará state, Brazilian Amazon, 2019.

Sociodemographic Variables	Hair-MeHg Levels						p-value
	<10.0 µg/g		≥10.0 µg/g		Total		
	n	%	n	%	n	%	
Sex							0.915
Female	36	47.4	16	48.5	52	47.7	
Male	40	52.6	17	51.5	57	52.3	
Total	76		33		109		
Age range (years)							0.774
12 to 19	26	34.2	10	30.3	36	33.0	
20 to 24	12	15.8	8	24.2	20	18.3	
25 to 29	12	15.8	5	15.2	17	15.6	
≥30	26	34.2	10	30.3	36	33.0	
Total	76		33		109		
Somatosensory signs							
Distal pinprick perception							0.743
Normal	65	85.5	29	87.9	94	86.2	
Abnormal	11	14.5	4	12.1	15	13.8	
Total	76		33		109		
Distal Thermal Sensitivity							0.384
Normal	65	85.5	26	78.8	91	83.5	
Abnormal	11	14.5	7	21.2	18	16.5	
Total	76		33		109		
Hallux or Thumb Vibration Sensitivity							0.154
Normal	71	93.4	28	84.8	99	90.8	
Abnormal	5	6.6	5	15.2	10	9.2	
Total	76		33		109		
Feet mechanical detection threshold							0.089
Normal	62	81.6	22	66.7	84	77.1	
Abnormal	14	18.4	11	33.3	25	22.9	
Total	76		33		109		
Clinical signs of polyneuropathy (neuropathy burden)							0.531
No	53	69.7	21	63.6	74	67.9	
Yes	23	30.3	12	36.4	35	32.1	
Total	76		33		109		
Motor function							
Toe amyotrophy							0.131
Absent	71	93.4	33	100.0	104	95.4	
Present	5	6.6	0	0.0	5	4.6	
Total	76		33		109		
Ankle jerk reflex							0.287
Normal	66	86.8	26	78.8	92	84.4	
Abnormal	10	13.2	7	21.2	17	15.6	
Total	76		33		109		
Bradykinesia							0.164
Absent	75	98.7	31	93.9	106	97.2	
Present	1	1.3	2	6.1	3	2.8	
Total	76		33		109		
Cerebellar incoordination (ataxia)							0.030
Absent	76	100.0	31	93.9	107	98.2	
Present	0	0.0	2	6.1	2	1.8	
Total	76		33		109		
Cognition							
Brief Cognitive Screening Battery (BCSB)							0.028
Normal	63	82.9	21	63.6	84	77.1	
Abnormal	13	17.1	12	36.4	25	22.9	
Total	76		33		109		
Stick design test							0.540
Normal	75	98.7	32	97.0	107	98.2	
Abnormal	1	1.3	1	3.0	2	1.8	
Total	76		33		109		
Verbal Fluency test							0.049
Normal	70	92.1	26	78.8	96	88.1	
Abnormal	6	7.9	7	21.2	13	11.9	
Total	76		33		109		

Feet mechanical detection threshold (hypoesthesia) alterations were detected in 18.4% of participants in the exposure group of <10 µg/g, in contrast to 33.3% in the exposure group of ≥10 µg/g MeHg ($p = 0.089$) (Table 2).

Finally, the clinical signs of polyneuropathy, indicative of distal symmetric polyneuropathy, were similar in the groups, and were reported in 30.3% of indigenous individuals with the exposure <10 µg/g and in 36.4% of those with exposure ≥10 µg/g MeHg ($p = 0.531$) (Table 2).

3.2.2. Motor Function

Toe amyotrophy was recorded in five individuals (6.6%) in SM village. The ankle jerk reflex absence appeared in 13.2 and 21.2% of indigenous individuals exposed to levels of MeHg <10 µg/g and ≥10.0 µg/g ($p = 0.287$), respectively (Table 2).

The occurrence of bradykinesia was detected in three indigenous individuals: an individual with a methylmercury exposure level of 9.08 µg/g, and in two other participants with exposure levels of 11.68 and 20.18 µg/g ($p = 0.164$) (Table 2).

Cerebellar motor incoordination (ataxia) was observed in two participants with exposure levels of 11.68 and 15.86 µg/g MeHg ($p = 0.030$).

3.2.3. Cognitive Alterations

According to the BCSB, cognitive alterations were observed in 17.1% of indigenous individuals with MeHg exposure levels of <10 µg/g, in contrast with 36.4% of those with an exposure of ≥10 µg/g ($p = 0.028$) (Table 2).

Moreover, the participants with MeHg exposure levels of <10 µg/g showed 7.9% of alteration in the verbal fluency test in the animal category, whereas 21.2% of participants with MeHg exposure levels of ≥10 µg/g presented alterations ($p = 0.049$) (Table 2).

Two individuals (1.8% of the total) presented with alterations in the stick design test, one with a MeHg exposure level of 9.67 µg/g, and the other with 22.75 µg/g (Table 2). It is worth noting that the recorded exposure level in the latter was the highest in the studied population.

3.2.4. Main Findings Considering the Neurological Abnormalities, According to MeHg Exposure Levels

Table 3 summarizes the main results, highlighting neurological clinical variables that presented an association with hair-MeHg levels (≥10 µg/g). Considering the presence of somatosensory signs, abnormalities in the feet mechanical detection threshold affected 33.3% of the participants with MeHg levels above 10 µg/g, in contrast to 18.4% of the participants with MeHg levels below 10 µg/g. Regarding motor function, only two cases of ataxia were detected. However, both were observed in participants with MeHg levels above 10 µg/g.

Regarding the cognition abilities, 36.4% of the participants with MeHg levels above 10 µg/g presented abnormalities in the Brief Cognitive Screening Battery (BCSB). In contrast, 17.1% of the participants with MeHg levels below 10 µg/g showed abnormalities in the BCSB. Finally, concerning the verbal fluency test, 21.2% of the participants with MeHg levels above 10 µg/g presented abnormalities, in contrast to 7.9% of the participants with MeHg levels below 10 µg/g (Table 3).

3.2.5. Poisson's Regression Model Findings, Considering Cognition Abilities of the Participants

Poisson's regression modeling revealed that participants with MeHg exposure levels ≥10 µg/g showed approximately two-fold higher chances of suffering from cognitive deficits in the BCSB (PR: 2.2; CI 95%: 1.13–4.26) and the verbal fluency test (PR: 2.0; CI 95%: 1.18–3.35). Furthermore, the final model showed that 12 to 19 year old adolescents presented with around a three-fold chance of developing deficits in the verbal fluency test (PR: 3.2; CI 95%: 1.06–9.42), compared to 20 to 24 year old young adults, even controlling for the effect of mercury exposure level and sex (Table 4).

Table 3. Summary of the main results highlighting clinical variables that presented an association (p-value < 0.10) with hair-MeHg levels (≥10 μg/g), *Sawré Muybu* Indigenous Land, Pará state, Brazilian Amazon, 2019.

Clinical Variables	Hair-MeHg Levels						
	<10.0 μg/g		≥10.0 μg/g		Total		
Somatosensory Signs	N	%	n	%	n	%	p-Value
Feet mechanical detection threshold							
Normal	62	81.6	22	66.7	84	77.1	0.089
Abnormal	14	18.4	11	33.3	25	22.9	
Total	76		33		109		
Motor function							
Cerebellar incoordination (ataxia)							
Absent	76	100.0	31	93.9	107	98.2	0.030
Present	0	0.0	2	6.1	2	1.8	
Total	76		33		109		
Cognition							
Brief Cognitive Screening Battery (BCSB)							
Normal	63	82.9	21	63.6	84	77.1	0.028
Abnormal	13	17.1	12	36.4	25	22.9	
Total	76		33		109		
Verbal Fluency test							
Normal	70	92.1	26	78.8	96	88.1	0.049
Abnormal	6	7.9	7	21.2	13	11.9	
Total	76		33		109		

Table 4. Logistic regression model (crude and adjusted) of prevalence ratios (PR) in the Brief Cognitive Screening Battery (BCSB) and verbal fluency test, *Sawré Muybu* Indigenous Land, Pará state, Brazilian Amazon, 2019.

Cognitive Screening Brief Battery				
Variables	PR Crude (CI 95%)	p-Value	PR Adjusted (CI 95%)	p-Value
Hair-MeHg level				
<10 μg/g	1.0		1.0	
≥10 μg/g	2.1 (1.08–4.15)	0.027	2.2 (1.13–4.26)	0.028
Age range (years)				
20 to 24	1.0		1.0	
12 to 19	1.3 (0.38–4.47)	0.681	1.5 (0.44–4.80)	0.424
25 to 29	1.7 (0.51–5.46)	0.399	1.9 (0.60–6.05)	0.280
≥30	2.2 (0.65–7.61)	0.204	2.4 (0.74–7.82)	0.144
Sex				
Female	1.0		1.0	
Male	1.1 (0.57–2.29)	0.71	1.2 (0.61–2.32)	0.492
Verbal Fluency Test				
Variables	PR Crude (CI 95%)	p-Value	PR Adjusted (CI 95%)	p-Value
Hair-MeHg level				
<10 μg/g	1.0		1.0	
≥10 μg/g	1.9 (1.07–3.38)	0.03	2.0 (1.18–3.35)	0.010
Age range (years)				
20 to 24	1.0		1.0	
12 to 19	3.0 (0.98–8.95)	0.054	3.2 (1.06–9.42)	0.039
25 to 29	0.8 (0.15–4.16)	0.775	0.9 (0.16–4.64)	0.871
≥30	1.8 (0.56–5.81)	0.324	2.0 (0.63–6.46)	0.239
Sex				
Female	1.0		1.0	
Male	0.6 (0.31–1.05)	0.071	0.6 (0.34–1.11)	0.109

4. Discussion

This exploratory clinical-epidemiological study was the first to produce evidence about the neurotoxic effects of consuming contaminated fish by MeHg in adults from the Munduruku indigenous population. The findings were produced with a comparative analysis of systemized neurological evaluation data in contrast to hair-MeHg concentration, used as a biomarker of chronic mercury exposure.

There is strong evidence substantiating MeHg neurotoxicity in experimental models and humans [33–35,42]. The neurological manifestations, classically described after the acute intoxication by MeHg, in Minamata Bay, Japan, in 1953, are characterized by somatosensory dysfunctions, ataxia, incoordination, tremors, and visual and neuropsychiatric symptoms [8,9]. A study conducted by Yorifuji et al. [59] also confirms that the neurological manifestations are due to the methylmercury contamination and are irrefutable evidence that the toxicity produced by this chemical element lasts for decades.

However, in the context of chronic environmental exposure, there is still no solid causal connection between the neurological dysfunction and toxicity due to methylmercury, as highlighted by Puty et al. [60], who conducted a systematic review of this theme. Despite the relevance of this systematic review in consolidating the scientific knowledge, it is essential to emphasize that this study included only six papers, and most of these (i.e., four) do not provide data on mercury concentration in exposure biomarkers. Consequently, we can conclude that almost all selected research in that review presumptively reported human mercury exposure.

Nonetheless, when we focus only on research conducted in the Amazon region, we observe that most of these studies indicate that exposure to MeHg may be responsible for neurological alterations in adult individuals [13–19]. In this region, the mercury levels detected in exposure biomarkers can be up to 10-fold higher than the limits recommended by health agencies [45,46]. The main neurological alterations include cognitive, visual, motor, somatosensory, and behavioral changes [13–19,61–68].

The impact of gold mining on human mercury exposure has been described by some studies that compared exposed populations to control groups (for example, populations living in areas with no previous history of mining activities) [16,69–72]. These studies indicate that hair mercury levels detected in areas impacted by mining activities are considerably higher than those observed in control groups. Even considering the natural mercury available in the Amazon soil, these findings reinforce the hypothesis that the region's primary source of human mercury contamination is mining activities.

In the present study, somatosensory, motor, and cognitive abnormalities were researched in indigenous adults from the Munduruku people who live in three villages, located in the region of Middle-Tapajos River. The participants with higher mercury exposure levels ($\geq$10 µg/g MeHg) presented the highest prevalence of cognitive impairment, according to the BCSB and the verbal fluency test results, and cerebellar incoordination, both indicating CNS dysfunctions. Distal somatosensory deficits and verbal fluency reduction were also reported. These alterations were more frequent in *Sawré Aboy* village, where there was the highest mercury exposure, compared to *Sawré Muybu* and *Poxo Muybu* villages. Again, this finding strengthens the hypothesis that the primary source of mercury exposure in the studied villages is mining activities.

4.1. Somatosensory Abnormalities

In the group with the highest MeHg exposure ($\geq$10 µg/g), there was also a higher prevalence of abnormalities in the feet mechanical detection threshold, in comparison to the group with lower exposure (33.3% vs. 18.4%, $p = 0.089$). There was a slim predominance of temperature and vibrant hypoesthesia in participants with methylmercury exposure higher than 10 µg/g (Table 2), however, there was no statistical significance. Even considering different methodological approaches, our findings revealed the highest somatosensory abnormalities in comparison to the study conducted by Khoury et al. [63,64], in which there was a decrease in hypoesthesia, tactile sensitivity, and pain, in 11.5% (n = 9) of riparian residents in Barreiras and 13.3% (n = 4) of residents in São Luiz do Tapajós, areas in the Pará State, in the Amazon Basin, equally affected by mining activities. In turn, the somatosensory alterations reported here were higher than those observed in a region known as *Furo do Maracujá* (n = 1; 2.0%), an area considered free of mercury exposure, and therefore classified as a control area by the authors [63,64]. However, due to the small number of participants, the differences highlighted in the study were not statistically significant.

The comparison by village revealed a significantly lower prevalence of somatosensory abnormalities in *Poxo Muybu* village, in contrast to *Sawré Aboy* and *Sawré Muybu* villages (Table 1). The difference in occurrence of alterations was revealed in all sensory modalities investigated, either in the tactile superficial sensory ($p = 0.001$), temperature sensitivity ($p = 0.004$) and pain sensitivity (nociceptive) ($p = 0.012$), and hallux and thumb deep sensitivity (vibration) ($p = 0.042$). In the same manner, *Poxo Muybu* was the village where lower frequencies were reported of ankle jerk reflex alterations ($p = 0.025$) and clinical signs of polyneuropathy ($p = 0.003$).

These findings provide evidence of the toxic effects of methylmercury, because *Poxo Muybu* village recorded the lowest proportion of participants with exposure levels above 10 µg/g MeHg (10.8%), whereas in *Sawré Muybu* and *Sawré Aboy* villages the exposure prevalence was approximately two to eight times higher, reaching 22.4% and 78.3% of participants, respectively.

However, although there is a tendency of major abnormalities in distal thermal sensory, deep vibration, and tactile superficial sensitivity, the magnitude of the somatosensory alterations observed in the comparative analysis by village was not confirmed, according to the methylmercury exposure groups. In part, this contradiction can be explained by the reduced size of our sample. However, it is important to note that the average methylmercury levels in all participants were high (average: 8.7 µg/g; range from 2.0 to 22.8), which makes it difficult for more robust analysis, because we did not have a control group, without mercury exposure, for comparison.

It is important to note that distal somatosensory alterations and clinical signs of polyneuropathy are indicative of peripheral nervous system (PNS) dysfunctions that can be induced by several clinical conditions in addition to mercury contamination. The presence of chronic alcoholism, diabetes mellitus, and sexually transmittable diseases was actively researched in our study population, via interview, blood glucose level testing, or rapid HIV, syphilis, and viral hepatitis testing, with no positive cases identified (for further detail see Basta et al. [43]). Nutritional deficits, especially B12 deficiency, are also potential causes of polyneuropathy and somatosensory abnormalities. However, these nutritional deficiencies were not researched and may add a degree of bias to our findings. It must also be noted that the use of a hair sample as a biomarker for mercury exposure may not be adequate, especially in the adult population, for detecting the neuropathy cases [33]. It is possible that the clinical signs of neuropathy detected here may have begun prior to our research for reasons not evaluated.

However, it cannot by overlooked that the clinical signs of polyneuropathy, diagnosed in approximately one-third of all participants, were more frequent in *Sawré Muybu* and *Sawré Aboy* villages, where the highest levels of MeHg exposure were detected.

Similar to the results reported in this study, Takaoka et al. [73] compared an indigenous population in Canada who lived in a region affected by chloralkali industrial waste, with two populations in Japan, one exposed to mercury in Minamata Bay and the other in a non-affected area (control). The authors reported complaints and neurological abnormalities as more prevalent. In addition, somatosensory signs were more evident in the Canadian indigenous group and in the Japanese group exposed to mercury compared to the control group.

In another study conducted in Japan, Takaoka et al. [38] presented a detailed description of somatosensory symptoms that included perioral numbness, hands and feet numbness, cramps, difficulty in hearing, smelling, and tasting, difficulty in buttoning shirts, and difficulty executing fine tasks with fingers. The authors reported that the symptoms were more frequently observed in individuals who ate fish with Hg concentrations higher than levels considered to be safe. They concluded that their findings indicated that the effects of Minamata disease were observed almost 50 years after Chisso Corporation stopped polluting water with methylmercury, in 1968.

In our study, the presence of distal hypoesthesia and clinical signs of polyneuropathy were respectively observed in 33.3% and 36.4% in the group with the highest mercury exposure (≥ 10 µg/g). These findings were similar to those reported by Yorifuri et al. [59], who showed somatosensory abnormalities in 25 and 58% of participants with mercury exposure higher than 10 µg/g in the contaminated areas of Minamata and Goshonoura, Japan, respectively.

In the Amazon region, Khoury et al. [63,64] described somatosensory complaints of numbness of the extremities in 11.5 and 13.3% of participants of riparian communities in two areas of the state of Pará, which are under the influence of mining and, therefore, exposed to mercury.

Due to communication difficulties arising because Munduruku people express themselves in their native language and do not speak fluent Portuguese, in this study, we exclusively evaluated clinical signs through a patterned neurological exam. In contrast to other authors [8,63,64,73], we opted not to include any complaints or symptoms reported by participants in the collected data.

4.2. Motor Functions Abnormalities

Cerebellar signs were only detected in two indigenous individuals, who presented with methylmercury exposure higher than 10 µg/g. Similarly, Takaoka et al. [39] described alterations in the finger to nose test, which indicates cerebellar dysfunction, in 21 and 47% of two groups with high mercury exposure, in Japan. Cerebellar symptomatology was also described in other empirical studies [15,39,59] and in revision papers [8,60,74]. In turn, Khoury et al. [63,64] described altered walking in participants with high mercury exposure levels compared to the control group. However, there was no mention of cerebellar signs.

Bradykinesia or slowness of movement were identified in three indigenous individuals in our study. They did not present rigidity or tremors. Bradykinesia, usually found in rigid-hypokinetic or parkinsonian syndromes, is not part of the classical manifestation of acute mercury intoxication, as described in Japan [8,59].

Nonetheless, experimental evidence associates mercury toxicity with dopaminergic depletion in the CNS [40] and establishes a possible correlation with parkinsonian and neurodegenerative diseases [75], even considering the latency period after mercury exposure [76]. In this sense, we propose two possibilities: (i) bradykinesia is an isolated symptom, or (ii) it may be a part of an incomplete parkinsonian syndrome falling within the spectrum of neurological manifestations of mercury contamination in this indigenous population from the Amazon. To clarify this question, we suggest a longitudinal evaluation in those populations at risk of chronic methylmercury exposure, with a priority for those cases with bradykinesia and other neurological signs and symptoms. In this manner, we believe that it will be possible to broaden the knowledge on this subject, which is surrounded by controversy and uncertainty.

4.3. Cognitive Abnormalities

Cognitive evaluation in individuals with a low education level is a challenging task, especially in indigenous populations who live in diverse sociocultural and environmental contexts. Language and communication barriers, in addition to the lack of appropriate evaluation instruments, were some of the difficulties experienced by our team. When choosing the evaluation instruments, we selected those that allowed us to overcome communication barriers, had references to the local population's everyday elements, and were easily applicable in the context of the fieldwork in the villages. The BCSB domains used in this study allowed the evaluation of immediate memory, verbal fluency, and belated memory. It is essential to consider years of schooling, a factor significantly related to some cognitive tests [77] but not related to the ability to solve everyday problems, as highlighted in our evaluation.

Despite the limitations, the proportion of higher impairment rates in the BCSB in participants with high methylmercury exposure levels (≥ 10 µg/g) was more than two-fold (36.4%) those observed (17.1%) in participants with lower exposure levels (<10 µg/g) ($p = 0.028$). Similarly, Yorifuji et al. [59], in an enquiry that analyzed the Minamata population in the early 1970s, revealed significantly more frequent intelligence limitations (RP 5.2, 95% CI 3.7–7.3) and behavior alterations (RP 4.4, 95% CI 2.9–6.7) in the group exposed to methylmercury, in contrast to the control group.

It is worth noting that the neuropsychiatric manifestations, including irritability, depression, social isolation, aggressiveness, or even psychotic cases (*"mad hatter disease"*) were described in association with acute mercury intoxication [74]. In a bibliography review, Jackson [74] concluded that methylmercury poisoning causes chronic neurological illness, mainly due to direct neural lesions in the brain, particularly involving the cerebral cortex and granular cells, and reinforces the importance of detailed clinical evaluation to assess the extent of neurological deficits in chronically exposed populations.

In the Amazon scenario, the neuropsychiatric manifestations are more frequently associated with occupational exposure and are reported in miners who burn amalgam to separate mercury from gold and inhale mercury's toxic vapors. Considering environmental exposure through the consumption of contaminated fish, which is manifested chronically and insidiously, there are few studies that report cognitive deficiencies and neuropsychiatric manifestations. Khoury et al. [63,64] analyzed depression complaints and symptoms such as fear, sadness, and insomnia in the riparian population in two areas in the Amazon with different mercury exposure levels. Despite the effort made in the analysis, the authors found that there were no statistical differences between the exposed and control groups.

In our study, the detected memory and verbal fluency impairments indicate cognitive deficits are more frequent in the indigenous people with the highest methylmercury levels (≥ 10 µg/g). Moreover, cognitive impairment was more frequent in 12- to 19-year-old adolescents. Because chronic methylmercury exposure may cause cognitive, motor, and somatosensory losses, this finding requires caution in interpretation and warrants deeper analysis. The investigated communities, who live in a highly contaminated environment, at present, in addition to the future generations (women of childbearing age and babies), are under permanent threat. Our findings emphasize the need for new studies that deepen cognitive and psychiatric evaluation to generate even more robust evidence about the MeHg toxicity in vulnerable populations, and demand interventions from the authorities and social leadership.

4.4. Limitations

Bradykinesia, temperature sensitivity, tactile and deep distal alterations, and clinical signs of polyneuropathy were more prevalent in the group with methylmercury exposure higher than 10 µg/g. However, due to the limited size of our sample, the differences were not statistically significant. The broadening of the study to other areas with the inclusion of a greater number of participants may result in more conclusive data.

In this study, we prioritized the evaluation of somatosensory abnormalities aimed at detecting PNS lesions. Somatosensory alterations from CNS lesions were described in anatomo-clinical studies [39] and clinical trials [8]. The two-point discrimination test, graphesthesia, and stereognosis have the potential to evaluate central somatosensory dysfunctions and should also be considered in future studies.

The absence of a control group with low environmental MeHg exposure, which would allow comparisons, was also a limiting factor in our approach. In the preparatory phase of the study, we expected that *Poxo Muybu* village, which is farther from the mining zones, would be a control group for comparison. However, like the other villages, *Poxo Muybu* also presented high average levels of MeHg exposure (average: 7.3 µg/g; range from 2.3 to 12.9), above the safe levels according to international health agencies [45,46]. Therefore, it was not possible to have a control group.

It is also important to consider that the reference levels of mercury exposure vary between international health agencies, and do not necessarily reflect biological security parameters. The safety limits recommended are based on daily or weekly maximum intake parameters of MeHg. The intake criteria have a strong relationship with MeHg levels detected in blood and hair. Therefore, FAO/WHO [45] recommends maximum intake doses of 1.6 µg/kg (body weight)/week for more sensitive groups such as women of childbearing age and pregnant women, and 3.2 µg/kg bw/week for the general population. Thus, the reference intake limit doses considered to be safe, for those still not reported to have poisonous effects in human beings, correspond to mercury levels of 2.3 and 4.5 µg/g in hair samples, respectively [45].

Although our results may show promise in revealing higher cognitive deficits in participants with the highest methylmercury exposure levels, the BCSB has not yet been validated for use in traditional Amazonian populations. The use of simplified and validated instruments for evaluation of cognition in populations chronically exposed to mercury and ethnically differentiated can produce new evidence to consolidate the knowledge on this topic. Tools such as the mini-mental state examination [78], previously used in Amazonian populations [77], appear to be equally promising, and mainly associated with the BCSB.

5. Conclusions

The present study produced evidence concerning the association between motor and cognitive impairments in the CNS with chronic MeHg exposure among the Munduruku indigenous adults. The majority of people who suffered from neurological abnormalities presented MeHg exposure levels above 10 µg/g.

Somatosensory abnormalities reported in the villages where the highest methylmercury exposures were registered also indicate toxicity signs in the PNS. However, the differences reported between the two exposure groups were not statistically significant. Due to the limited sample size, we believe it is necessary to conduct broader studies to deepen the knowledge about the neurotoxic effects of methylmercury in the traditional populations living in the Amazon Basin, and particularly indigenous populations.

In conclusion, despite its limitations, this study indicates that neurotoxicity due to chronic environmental methylmercury exposure in the Munduruku indigenous population provides evidence of the long-lasting persistent environmental impacts in the Amazon [20–24]. The context revealed here highlights the risk looming over the present and future generations, who represent a substantial social, ethnic, and culturally diverse community, and should be considered and treated as the country's most significant wealth.

Finally, we believe monitoring and follow-up measures are necessary for the vulnerable populations chronically exposed to methylmercury who live in the Amazon basin. Moreover, we consider it essential to establish a basic care protocol for contaminated people in the Brazilian Unified Health System (SUS) with the support of specialists.

Author Contributions: Proposal design, study design and methodology, R.A.A.d.O., D.C.d.A. and P.C.B. Fieldwork data collection, R.A.A.d.O., B.D.P. and B.H.R.; writing—original draft preparation, R.A.A.d.O. and P.C.B.; writing—review and editing, R.A.A.d.O., D.C.d.A., B.D.P., B.H.R., A.C.S.d.V. and P.C.B.; supervision, obtaining resources and project management, P.C.B. All authors have read and agreed to the published version of the manuscript.

Funding: This research was funded by the Vice-Presidency of Environment, Care and Health Promotion (VPAAPS) of Fundação Oswaldo Cruz (Fiocruz) through Decentralized Execution of Resources Document No. 175/2018, Process: 25000.209221/2018-18, signed between the Fiocruz and the Special Secretariat for Indigenous Health, both under the Ministry of Health. The non-governmental organization WWF-Brazil offered financial support to disseminate the results of the research.

Institutional Review Board Statement: The study was conducted in accordance with the guidelines of the Declaration of Helsinki and was approved by the Research Ethics Committee of the National School of Public Health at Fiocruz (REC/ENSP) and the Brazilian National Research Ethics Commission of the National Health Council (CONEP/CNS), CAAE: 65671517.1.0000.5240, with Opinion No. 2.262.686 favorable to its performance. In compliance with Convention No. 169 of the International Labor

Organization (ILO), the study began with a pre-study consultation, carried out in August 2019, during a visit to the villages, in which the author PCB, and local indigenous leaders participated. At the time, the study objectives were presented and discussed (https://www.youtube.com/watch?v=oFEYEGxNmns&t=704s, accessed on 20 September 2019). After answering questions and approval of the proposal by the communities, we received support from the coordination of the Special Indigenous Sanitary District of the Tapajós River through the multidisciplinary indigenous health team to carry out the study. In addition, the interviews and data collection started only after the participants had their questions answered and formal consent was given via the Informed Consent Form (ICF) by the children's guardians.

Informed Consent Statement: Informed consent was obtained from all subjects involved in the study. Written informed consent was obtained from the patients to publish this paper.

Data Availability Statement: Data sharing not applicable.

Acknowledgments: On behalf of chiefs Juarez Saw, Jairo Saw, and Valdemar Poxo, and the leader Alessandra Korap, we thank the Munduruku people for the trust placed in our team and the support in carrying out the research. On behalf of Rio Tapajós Indigenous Special Sanitary District, we thank the coordination Cleidiane C.R. Santos and the nurses Alan Marcelo Simon and Lygia Catarina de Oliveira. We also thank to Marcelo de Oliveira Lima, Iracina Maura de Jesus and João Paulo Goes Pereira who performed the mercury laboratory analysis. We also thank Marcelo Oliveira-da-Costa from World-Wide Fund for Nature (WWF-Brazil) for technical and financial support for this scientific communication.

Conflicts of Interest: The authors declare no conflict of interest. The funders had no role in the design of the study; in the collection, analyses, or interpretation of data; in the writing of the manuscript, or in the decision to publish the results.

References

1. Hong, Y.S.; Kim, Y.M.; Lee, K.E. Methylmercury exposure and health effects. *J. Prev. Med. Public Health* **2012**, *45*, 353. [CrossRef]
2. Mergler, D.; Anderson, H.A.; Chan, L.H.M.; Mahaffey, K.R.; Murray, M.; Sakamoto, M.; Stern, A.H. Methylmercury exposure and health effects in humans: A worldwide concern. *AMBIO J. Hum. Environ.* **2007**, *36*, 3–11. [CrossRef]
3. Díez, S. Human health effects of methylmercury exposure. *Rev. Environ. Cont. Toxicol.* **2008**, *198*, 111–132.
4. World Health Organization. *Environmental Health Criteria 1. Mercury*; World Health Organization: Geneva, Switzerland, 1976.
5. World Health Organization. *Mercury: Environmental Aspects-Environmental Health Criteria 86*; World Health Organization: Geneva, Switzerland, 1989.
6. World Health Organization. *IPCS Environmental Health Criteria 101: Methylmercury. International Programme of Chemical Safety*; World Health Organization: Geneva, Switzerland, 1990.
7. National Research Council (US). *Committee on the Toxicological Effects of Methylmercury. Toxicological Effects of Methylmercury*; National Academies Press: Washington, DC, USA, 2000.
8. Ekino, S.; Susa, M.; Ninomiya, T.; Imamura, K.; Kitamura, T. Minamata disease revisited: An update on the acute and chronic manifestations of methyl mercury poisoning. *J. Neurol. Sci.* **2007**, *262*, 131–144. [CrossRef] [PubMed]
9. Sakamoto, M.; Tatsuta, N.; Izumo, K.; Phan, P.T.; Vu, L.D.; Yamamoto, M.; Nakamura, M.; Nakai, K.; Murata, K. Health impacts and biomarkers of prenatal exposure to methylmercury: Lessons from Minamata, Japan. *Toxics* **2018**, *6*, 45. [CrossRef]
10. Bakir, F.; Damluji, S.F.; Amin-Zaki, L.; Murtadha, M.; Khalidi, A.; Al-Rawi, N.Y.; Tikriti, S.; Dhahir, H.I.; Clarkson, T.W.; Smith, J.C.; et al. Methylmercury poisoning in Iraq. *Science* **1973**, *181*, 230–241. [CrossRef]
11. Bakir, F.; Rustam, H.; Tikriti, S.; Al-Damluji, S.F.; Shihristani, H. Clinical and epidemiological aspects of methylmercury poisoning. *Postgrad. Med. J.* **1980**, *56*, 1–10. [CrossRef] [PubMed]
12. Lebel, J.; Mergler, D.; Lucotte, M.; Amorim, M.; Dolbec, J.; Miranda, D.; Arantes, G.; Rheault, I.; Pichet, P. Evidence of early nervous system dysfunction in Amazonian populations exposed to low-levels of methylmercury. *Neurotoxicology* **1996**, *17*, 157–167. [PubMed]
13. Lebel, J.; Mergler, D.; Branches, F.; Lucotte, M.; Amorim, M.; Larribe, F.; Dolbec, J. Neurotoxic effects of low-level methylmercury contamination in the Amazonian Basin. *Environ. Res.* **1998**, *79*, 20–32. [CrossRef] [PubMed]
14. Dolbec, J.; Mergler, D.; Passos, C.J.S.; De Morais, S.S.; Lebel, J. Methylmercury exposure affects motor performance of a riverine population of the Tapajos river, Brazilian Amazon. *Int. Arch. Occup. Environ. Health* **2000**, *73*, 195–203. [CrossRef] [PubMed]
15. Harada, M.; Nakanishi, J.; Yasoda, E.; Maria da Conceicâo, N.P.; Oikawa, T.; de Assis Guimarâes, G.; da silva Cardoso, B.; Kizaki, T.; Ohno, H. Mercury pollution in the Tapajos River basin, Amazon: Mercury level of head hair and health effects. *Environ. Int.* **2001**, *27*, 285–290. [CrossRef]
16. Khoury, E.D.T.; Souza, G.D.S.; da Costa, C.A.; de Araújo, A.A.K.; de Oliveira, C.S.B.; Silveira, L.C.D.L.; Pinheiro, M.D.C.N. Somatosensory psychophysical losses in inhabitants of riverside communities of the Tapajós River Basin, Amazon, Brazil: Exposure to methylmercury is possibly involved. *PLoS ONE* **2015**, *10*, e0144625. [CrossRef] [PubMed]

17. Lacerda, E.M.D.C.B.; Souza, G.D.S.; Cortes, M.I.T.; Rodrigues, A.R.; Pinheiro, M.C.N.; Silveira, L.C.D.L.; Ventura, D.F. Comparison of Visual Functions of Two Amazonian Populations: Possible Consequences of Different Mercury Exposure. *Front. Neurosci.* **2020**, *13*, 1428. [CrossRef] [PubMed]
18. Benefice, E.; Luna-Monrroy, S.; Lopez-Rodriguez, R. Fishing activity, health characteristics and mercury exposure of Amerindian women living alongside the Beni River (Amazonian Bolivia). *Int. J. Hyg. Environ. Health* **2010**, *213*, 458–464. [CrossRef] [PubMed]
19. Peplow, D.; Augustine, S. Neurological abnormalities in a mercury exposed population among indigenous Wayana in Southeast Suriname. *Environ. Sci. Process. Impacts* **2014**, *16*, 2415–2422. [CrossRef] [PubMed]
20. Crespo-López, M.E.; Augusto-Oliveira, M.; Lopes-Araújo, A.; Santos-Sacramento, L.; Takeda, P.Y.; Macchi, B.M.; do Nascimento, J.L.M.; Maia, C.S.F.; Lima, R.R.; Arrifano, G.P. Mercury: What can be learn from the Amazon? *Environ. Int.* **2021**, *146*, 106223. [CrossRef] [PubMed]
21. Azevedo, L.S.; Pestana, I.A.; Almeida, M.G.; da Costa Nery, A.F.; Bastos, W.R.; Souza, C.M.M. Mercury biomagnification in an ichthyic food chain of an amazon floodplain lake (Puruzinho Lake): Influence of seasonality and food chain modeling. *Ecotoxicol. Environ. Saf.* **2021**, *207*, 111249. [CrossRef] [PubMed]
22. Siqueira-Gay, J.; Soares-Filho, B.; Sanchez, L.E.; Oviedo, A.; Sonter, L.J. Proposed Legislation to Mine Brazil's Indigenous Lands Will Threaten Amazon Forests and Their Valuable Ecosystem Services. *One Earth* **2020**, *3*, 356–362. [CrossRef] [PubMed]
23. Lino, A.S.; Kasper, D.; Guida, Y.S.; Thomaz, J.R.; Malm, O. Total and methyl mercury distribution in water, sediment, plankton and fish along the Tapajós River basin in the Brazilian Amazon. *Chemosphere* **2019**, *235*, 690–700. [CrossRef] [PubMed]
24. Arrifano, G.P.; Martín-Doimeadios, R.C.; Jiménez-Moreno, M.; Ramírez-Mateos, V.; da Silva, N.F.; Souza-Monteiro, J.R.; Augusto-Oliveira, M.; Paraense, R.S.; Macchi, B.M.; do Nascimento, J.L.; et al. Large-scale projects in the amazon and human exposure to mercury: The case-study of the Tucuruí Dam. *Ecotoxicol. Environ. Saf.* **2018**, *147*, 299–305. [CrossRef]
25. Cerdeira, R.G.P.; Ruffino, M.L.; Isaac, V.J. Consumo de Pescado e Outros Alimentos Pela População Ribeirinha do Lago Grande de Monte Alegre, PA-Brasil. *Acta Amaz.* **1997**, *27*, 213–227. [CrossRef]
26. Santos, G.M.D.; Santos, A.C.M.D. Sustentabilidade da pesca na Amazônia. *Estud. Av.* **2005**, *19*, 165–182. [CrossRef]
27. Arruda, M.C.F.D. Avaliação dos Indicadores da Política de Pesca do Programa Zona Franca Verde: Perspectivas Econômicas e Ambientais. Master's Thesis, Programa de Pós-Graduação em Engenharia de Produção, Universidade Federal do Amazonas (UFAM), Manaus, Brasil, 2017. Available online: https://tede.ufam.edu.br/handle/tede/6068 (accessed on 19 June 2021).
28. Santos-Lima, C.D.; Mourão, D.S.; Carvalho, C.F.; Souza-Marques, B.; Vega, C.M.; Gonçalves, R.A.; Argollo, N.; Menezes-Filho, J.A.; Abreu, N.; Hacon, S.S. Neuropsychological Effects of Mercury Exposure in Children and Adolescents of the Amazon Region, Brazil. *Neurotoxicology* **2020**, *79*, 48–57. [CrossRef]
29. Basu, N.; Horvat, M.; Evers, D.C.; Zastenskaya, I.; Weihe, P.; Tempowski, J. A State-of-the-Science Review of Mercury Biomarkers in Human Populations Worldwide between 2000 and 2018. *Environ. Health Perspect.* **2018**, *126*, 106001. [CrossRef] [PubMed]
30. Sharma, S.; Baligar, R.S.; Singh, H.B.; Butcher, R.J. Reaction of a metallamacrocycle leading to a mercury(II)...palladium(II)...mercury (II) interaction. *Angew. Chem. Int. Ed. Engl.* **2009**, *48*, 1987–1990. [CrossRef] [PubMed]
31. Bauch, S.C.; Birkenbach, A.M.; Pattanayak, S.K.; Sills, E.O. Public health impacts of ecosystem change in the Brazilian Amazon. *Proc. Natl. Acad. Sci. USA* **2015**, *112*, 7414–7419. [CrossRef] [PubMed]
32. Berzas Nevado, J.J.; Rodríguez Martín-Doimeadios, R.C.; Guzmán Bernardo, F.J.; Jiménez Moreno, M.; Herculano, A.M.; do Nascimento, J.L.; Crespo-López, M.E. Mercury in the Tapajós River basin, Brazilian Amazon: A review. *Environ. Int.* **2010**, *36*, 593–608. [CrossRef] [PubMed]
33. Karri, V.; Schuhmacher, M.; Kumar, V. Heavy metals (Pb, Cd, As and MeHg) as risk factors for cognitive dysfunction: A general review of metal mixture mechanism in brain. *Environ. Toxicol. Pharmacol.* **2016**, *48*, 203–213. [CrossRef] [PubMed]
34. Oliveira, C.S.; Segatto, A.L.A.; Nogara, P.A.; Piccoli, B.C.; Loreto, É.L.S.; Aschner, M.; Rocha, J.B.T. Transcriptomic and Proteomic Tools in the Study of Hg Toxicity: What Is Missing? *Front. Genet.* **2020**, *11*, 425. [CrossRef] [PubMed]
35. Birdsall, R.E.; Kiley, M.P.; Segu, Z.M.; Palmer, C.D.; Madera, M.; Gump, B.B.; MacKenzie, J.A.; Parsons, P.J.; Mechref, Y.; Novotny, M.V.; et al. Effects of lead and mercury on the blood proteome of children. *J. Proteome Res.* **2010**, *9*, 4443–4453. [CrossRef]
36. Santos-Sacramento, L.; Arrifano, G.P.; Lopes-Araújo, A.; Augusto-Oliveira, M.; Albuquerque-Santos, R.; Takeda, P.Y.; Souza-Monteiro, J.R.; Macchi, B.M.; do Nascimento, J.L.M.; Lima, R.R.; et al. Human neurotoxicity of mercury in the Amazon: A scoping review with insights and critical considerations. *Ecotoxicol. Environ. Saf.* **2021**, *208*, 111686. [CrossRef]
37. Day, J.J.; Reed, M.N.; Newland, M.C. Neuromotor deficits and mercury concentrations in rats exposed to methyl mercury and fish oil. *Neurotoxicol. Teratol.* **2005**, *27*, 629–641. [CrossRef] [PubMed]
38. Takaoka, S.; Fujino, T.; Kawakami, Y.; Shigeoka, S.I.; Yorifuji, T. Survey of the Extent of the Persisting Effects of Methylmercury Pollution on the Inhabitants around the Shiranui Sea, Japan. *Toxics* **2019**, *6*, 39. [CrossRef] [PubMed]
39. Takaoka, S.; Kawakami, Y.; Fujino, T.; Oh-ishi, F.; Motokura, F.; Kumagai, Y.; Miyaoka, T. Somatosensory disturbance by methylmercury exposure. *Environ. Res.* **2008**, *107*, 6–19. [CrossRef]
40. Shao, Y.; Chan, H.M. Effects of methylmercury on dopamine release in MN9D neuronal cells. *Toxicol. Mech. Methods* **2015**, *25*, 637–644. [CrossRef] [PubMed]
41. Farias, L.A.; Fávaro, D.I.T.; Pessoa, A.; Aguiar, J.P.L.; Yuyama, L.K.O. Mercury and methylmercury concentration assessment in children's hair from Manaus, Amazonas state, Brazil. *Acta Amaz.* **2012**, *42*, 279–286. [CrossRef]
42. Crespo-López, M.E.; Herculano, A.M.; Corvelo, T.C.; Do Nascimento, J.L. Mercurio y neurotoxicidad [Mercury and neurotoxicity]. *Rev. Neurol.* **2005**, *40*, 441–447. [PubMed]

43. Basta, P.C.; Viana, P.V.S.; Vasconcellos, A.C.S.; Périssé, A.R.S.; Hofer, C.B.; Paiva, N.S.; Kempton, J.W.; Ciampi de Andrade, D.; Oliveira, R.A.A.; Achatz, R.W.; et al. Mercury exposure in Munduruku indigenous communities from Brazilian Amazon: Methodological background and an overview of the principal results. *Int. J. Environ. Res. Public Health* **2021**, *18*, 9222. [CrossRef] [PubMed]
44. Vasconcellos, A.C.S.; Hallwass, G.; Bezerra, J.G.; Aciole, A.N.S.; Meneses, H.N.M.; Lima, M.O.; Jesus, I.M.; Hacon, S.S.; Basta, P.C. Health Risk Assessment of Mercury Exposure from Fish Consumption in Munduruku Indigenous Communities in the Brazilian Amazon. *Int. J. Environ. Res. Public Health* **2021**, *18*, 7940. [CrossRef] [PubMed]
45. FAO/WHO. Evaluation of certain food additives and contaminants: Sixty-first report of the Joint FAO/WHO Expert Committee on Food Additives. In Proceedings of the Joint FAO/WHO Expert Committee on Food Additives (JECFA), Rome, Italy, 10–19 June 2003.
46. U.S. EPA. *Reference Dose for Methylmercury*; U.S. Environmental Protection Agency: Washington, DC, USA, 2000.
47. Marrugo-Negrete, J.; Verbel, J.O.; Ceballos, E.L.; Benitez, L.N. Total mercury and methylmercury concentrations in fish from the Mojana region of Colombia. *Environ. Geochem. Health* **2008**, *30*, 21–30. [CrossRef] [PubMed]
48. Kehrig, H.; Malm, O.; Akagi, H.; Guimarães, J.R.; Torres, J.P.M. Methylmercury in fish and hair samples from the Balbina Reservoir, Brazilian Amazon. *Environ. Res.* **1998**, *77*, 84–90. [CrossRef] [PubMed]
49. Souza-Araujo, J.; Giarrizzo, T.; Lima, M.O.; Souza, M.B.G. Mercury and methyl mercury in fishes from Bacaja River (Brazilian Amazon): Evidence for bioaccumulation and biomagnification. *J. Fish Biol.* **2016**, *89*, 249–263. [CrossRef] [PubMed]
50. Campbell, W.W. *DeJong's the Neurological Examination*, 6th ed.; Lippincott Williams $ Wilkins: Philadelphia, PA, USA, 2005.
51. England, J.D.; Gronseth, G.S.; Franklin, G.; Miller, R.G.; Asbury, A.K.; Carter, G.T.; Cohen, J.A.; Fisher, M.A.; Howard, J.F.; Kinsella, L.J.; et al. Distal symmetric polyneuropathy: A definition for clinical research: Report of the American Academy of Neurology, the American Association of Electrodiagnostic Medicine, and the American Academy of Physical Medicine and Rehabilitation. *Neurology* **2005**, *64*, 199–207. [CrossRef] [PubMed]
52. Hallett, M. NINDS Myotactic reflex scale. *Neurology* **1993**, *43*, 2723. [CrossRef] [PubMed]
53. Brucki, S.M.; Nitrini, R. Subjective memory impairment in a rural population with low education in the Amazon rainforest: An exploratory study. *Int. Psychogeriatr.* **2009**, *21*, 164–171. [CrossRef]
54. Brucki, S.M.; Malheiros, S.M.; Okamoto, I.H.; Bertolucci, P.H. Dados normativos para o teste de fluência verbal categoria animais em nosso meio [Normative data on the verbal fluency test in the animal category in our milieu]. *Arq. Neuropsiquiatr.* **1997**, *55*, 56–61. [CrossRef]
55. Baiyewu, O.; Unverzagt, F.W.; Lane, K.A.; Gureje, O.; Ogunniyi, A.; Musick, B.; Gao, S.; Hall, K.S.; Hendrie, H.C. The Stick Design test: A new measure of visuoconstructional ability. *J. Int. Neuropsychol. Soc.* **2005**, *11*, 598–605. [CrossRef] [PubMed]
56. World Health Organization (WHO). *Guidance for Identifying Populations at Risk from Mercury Exposure*; Mercury Publications: Geneva, Switzerzeland, 2008; Available online: https://wedocs.unep.org/.../IdentifyingPopnatRiskExposuretoMercury_2008 (accessed on 22 June 2021).
57. Berglund, M.; Lind, B.; Björnberg, K.A.; Palm, B.; Einarsson, O.; Vahter, M. Inter-individual variations of human mercury exposure biomarkers: A cross-sectional assessment. *Environ. Health* **2005**, *4*, 20. [CrossRef]
58. Clarkson, T.W.; Magos, L. The toxicology of mercury and its chemical compounds. *Crit. Rev. Toxicol.* **2006**, *36*, 609–662. [CrossRef] [PubMed]
59. Yorifuji, T.; Tsuda, T.; Takao, S.; Suzuki, E.; Harada, M. Total mercury content in hair and neurologic signs: Historic data from Minamata. *Epidemiology* **2009**, *20*, 188–193. [CrossRef]
60. Puty, B.; Leão, L.K.R.; Crespo-Lopez, M.E.; Almeida, A.P.C.P.S.C.; Fagundes, N.C.F.; Maia, L.C.; Lima, R.R. Association between methylmercury environmental exposure and neurological disorders: A systematic review. *J. Trace Elem. Med. Biol.* **2019**, *52*, 100–110. [CrossRef]
61. Fillion, M.; Lemire, M.; Philibert, A.; Frenette, B.; Weiler, H.A.; Deguire, J.R.; Guimaraes, J.R.; Larribe, F.; Barbosa, F.; Mergler, D. Visual acuity in fish consumers of the Brazilian Amazon: Risks and benefits from local diet. *Public Health Nutr.* **2011**, *14*, 2236–2244. [CrossRef] [PubMed]
62. Fillion, M.; Philibert, A.; Mertens, F.; Lemire, M.; Passos, C.J.; Frenette, B.; Guimaraes, J.R.; Mergler, D. Neurotoxic sequelae of mercury exposure: An intervention and follow-up study in the Brazilian Amazon. *EcoHealth* **2011**, *8*, 210–222. [CrossRef] [PubMed]
63. Khoury, E.D.T.; Souza, G.D.S.; Silveira, L.C.D.L.; Costa, C.A.D.; Araújo, A.A.D.; Pinheiro, M.D.C.N. Neurological manifestations in riverine populations from areas exposed to mercury in the Brazilian Amazon. *Cad. Saude Publica* **2013**, *29*, 2307–2318. [CrossRef] [PubMed]
64. Khoury, E.D.T.; Souza, G.S.; Silveira, L.C.L.; Costa, C.A.; Araújo, A.A.; Pinheiro, M.C.N. Manifestações neurológicas em ribeirinhos de áreas expostas ao mercúrio na Amazônia brasileira. *Cad. Saude Publica* **2013**, *29*, 2307–2318. [CrossRef] [PubMed]
65. Cardoso, N.A.; Hoshino, A.C.H.; Perez, M.A.; Bastos, W.R.; Carvalho, D.P.D.; Câmara, V.D.M. Zumbido em uma população ribeirinha exposta ao metilmercúrio. *Audiol. Commun. Res.* **2014**, *19*, 40–44. [CrossRef]
66. Hoshino, A.; Pacheco-Ferreira, H.; Sanches, S.G.G.; Carvallo, R.; Cardoso, N.; Perez, M.; Câmara, V.D.M. Mercury exposure in a riverside Amazon population, Brazil: A study of the ototoxicity of methylmercury. *Int. Arch. Otorhinolaryngol.* **2015**, *19*, 135–140. [CrossRef] [PubMed]

67. Costa Junior, J.M.F.; Lima, A.A.D.S.; Rodrigues Junior, D.; Khoury, E.D.T.; Souza, G.D.S.; Silveira, L.C.D.L.; Pinheiro, M.D.C.N. Emotional and motor symptoms in riverside dwellers exposed to mercury in the Amazon. *Rev. Bras. de Epidemiol.* **2017**, *20*, 212–224. [CrossRef] [PubMed]
68. Arrifano, G.P.; Martín-Doimeadios, R.C.; Jiménez-Moreno, M.; Fernández-Trujillo, S.; Augusto-Oliveira, M.; Souza-Monteiro, J.R.; Macchi, B.M.; Alvarez-Leite, J.I.; do Nascimento, J.L.; Amador, M.T.; et al. Genetic susceptibility to neurodegeneration in amazon: Apolipoprotein e genotyping in vulnerable populations exposed to mercury. *Front. Genet.* **2018**, *9*, 285. [CrossRef]
69. Dos Santos Freitas, J.; Lacerda, E.M.; da Silva Martins, I.C.; Rodrigues, D., Jr.; Bonci, D.M.; Cortes, M.I.; Corvelo, T.C.; Ventura, D.F.; de Lima Silveira, L.C.; Pinheiro, M.D.; et al. Cross-sectional study to assess the association of color vision with mercury hair concentration in children from Brazilian Amazonian riverine communities. *Neurotoxicology* **2018**, *65*, 60–67. [CrossRef] [PubMed]
70. Domingues, M.M.; Cury, E.D.; de Araújo, A.A.; Junior, J.M.; Pinheiro, M.D. Somatosensory psychophysic losses in inhabitants of riverside communities of the Tapajós river basin, Amazonas, Brazil: The possible involvement of exposure to methylmercury. *J. Neurol. Sci.* **2019**, *405*, 255–256. [CrossRef]
71. Pinheiro, M.D.; Oikawa, T.; Vieira, J.L.; Gomes, M.S.; Guimarães, G.D.; Crespo-López, M.E.; Müller, R.C.; Amoras, W.W.; Ribeiro, D.R.; Rodrigues, A.R.; et al. Comparative study of human exposure to mercury in riverside communities in the Amazon region. *Braz. J. Med. Biol. Res.* **2006**, *39*, 411–414. [CrossRef] [PubMed]
72. Marinho, J.S.; Lima, M.O.; Santos, E.C.; de Jesus, I.M.; Pinheiro, M.D.; Alves, C.N.; Muller, R.C. Mercury speciation in hair of children in three communities of the Amazon, Brazil. *BioMed Res. Int.* **2014**, *2014*, 945963. [CrossRef]
73. Takaoka, S.; Fujino, T.; Hotta, N.; Ueda, K.; Hanada, M.; Tajiri, M.; Inoue, Y. Signs and symptoms of methylmercury contamination in a First Nations community in Northwestern Ontario, Canada. *Sci. Total Environ.* **2014**, *468–469*, 950–957. [CrossRef]
74. Jackson, A.C. Chronic Neurological Disease Due to Methylmercury Poisoning. *Can. J. Neurol. Sci.* **2018**, *45*, 620–623. [CrossRef]
75. Cariccio, V.L.; Samà, A.; Bramanti, P.; Mazzon, E. Mercury Involvement in Neuronal Damage and in Neurodegenerative Diseases. *Biol. Trace Elem. Res.* **2019**, *187*, 341–356. [CrossRef] [PubMed]
76. Weiss, B.; Clarkson, T.W.; Simon, W. Silent latency periods in methylmercury poisoning and in neurodegenerative disease. *Environ. Health Perspect.* **2002**, *110* (Suppl. 5), 851–854. [CrossRef] [PubMed]
77. Souza-Talarico, J.N.; de Carvalho, A.P.; Brucki, S.M.; Nitrini, R.; Ferretti-Rebustini, R.E. Dementia and Cognitive Impairment Prevalence and Associated Factors in Indigenous Populations: A Systematic Review. *Alzheimer Dis. Assoc. Disord.* **2016**, *30*, 281–287. [CrossRef] [PubMed]
78. Folstein, M.F.; Folstein, S.E.; McHugh, P.R. Mini-mental state. A practical method for grading the cognitive state of patients for the clinician. *J. Psychiatr. Res.* **1975**, *12*, 189–198. [CrossRef]

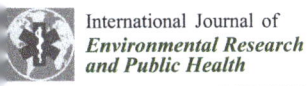

Article

An Assessment of Health Outcomes and Methylmercury Exposure in Munduruku Indigenous Women of Childbearing Age and Their Children under 2 Years Old

Joeseph William Kempton [1], André Reynaldo Santos Périssé [2], Cristina Barroso Hofer [3], Ana Claudia Santiago de Vasconcellos [4], Paulo Victor de Sousa Viana [5], Marcelo de Oliveira Lima [6], Iracina Maura de Jesus [6], Sandra de Souza Hacon [2] and Paulo Cesar Basta [2,*]

[1] Faculty of Medicine, St Mary's Hospital, Imperial College London, London W2 1PG, UK; joe.kempton@nhs.net
[2] Departamento de Endemias Samuel Pessoa, Escola Nacional de Saúde Pública, Fundação Oswaldo Cruz (ENSP/Fiocruz), Rua Leopoldo Bulhões, 1480, Manguinhos, Rio de Janeiro 21041-210, Brazil; aperisse41@gmail.com (A.R.S.P.); sandrahacon@gmail.com (S.d.S.H.)
[3] Instituto de Pediatria e Puericultura Martagão Gesteira, Faculdade de Medicina, Universidade Federal do Rio de Janeiro (UFRJ), Rua Bruno Lobo, 50, Cidade Universitária, Rio de Janeiro 21941-912, Brazil; cbhofer@hucff.ufrj.br
[4] Laboratório de Educação Profissional em Vigilância em Saúde, Escola Politécnica de Saúde Joaquim Venân-cio, Fundação Oswaldo Cruz (EPSJV/Fiocruz), Av. Brasil, 4365, Manguinhos, Rio de Janeiro 21040-900, Brazil; anacsvasconcellos@gmail.com
[5] Centro de Referência Professor Hélio Fraga, Escola Nacional de Saúde Pública, Fundação Oswaldo Cruz (CRPHF/ENSP/Fiocruz), Estrada de Curicica, 2000, Curicica, Rio de Janeiro 22780-195, Brazil; paulovictorsviana@gmail.com
[6] Seção de Meio Ambiente, Instituto Evandro Chagas, Secretaria de Vigilância em Saúde, Ministério da Saúde (SEAMB/IEC/SVS/MS), Rodovia BR-316 km 7 s/n, Levilândia 67030-000, Brazil; marcelolima@iec.gov.br (M.d.O.L.); iracinajesus@iec.gov.br (I.M.d.J.)
* Correspondence: paulobasta@gmail.com; Tel.: +55-21-2598-2503

Abstract: In line with the 1000-day initiative and the Sustainable Development Goals (SDG) 2 and 3, we present a cross-sectional analysis of maternal health, infant nutrition, and methylmercury exposure within hard-to-reach indigenous communities in the state of Pará, Brazilian Amazon. We collected data from all women of childbearing age (i.e., 12–49) and their infants under two years old in three Munduruku communities (*Sawré Muybu*, *Sawré Aboy*, and *Poxo Muybu*) along the Tapajos River. We explored health outcomes through interviews, vaccine coverage and clinical assessment, and determined baseline hair methylmercury (H-Hg) levels. Hemoglobin, infant growth (Anthropometric Z scores) and neurodevelopment tests results were collected. We found that 62% of women of childbearing age exceeded the reference limit of 6.0 µg/g H-Hg (median = 7.115, IQR = 4.678), with the worst affected community (*Sawré Aboy*) registering an average H-Hg concentration of 12.67 µg/g. Half of infants aged under 24 months presented with anemia. Three of 16 (18.8%) infants presented H-Hg levels above 6.0 µg/g (median: 3.88; IQR = 3.05). Four of the 16 infants were found to be stunted and 38% of women overweight, evidencing possible nutritional transition. No infant presented with appropriate vaccination coverage for their age. These communities presented with an estimated Infant Mortality Rate (IMR) of 86.7/1000 live births. The highest H-Hg level (19.6 µg/g) was recorded in an 11-month-old girl who was found to have gross motor delay and anemia. This already vulnerable indigenous Munduruku community presents with undernutrition and a high prevalence of chronic methylmercury exposure in women of childbearing age. This dual public health crisis in the context of wider health inequalities has the potential to compromise the development, health and survival of the developing fetus and infant in the first two critical years of life. We encourage culturally sensitive intervention and further research to focus efforts.

Keywords: environmental health; indigenous people; Amazon; 1000 days; childbearing women; nutrition; vaccine coverage; mercury exposure

Citation: Kempton, J.W.; Périssé, A.R.S.; Hofer, C.B.; de Vasconcellos, A.C.S.; de Sousa Viana, P.V.; de Oliveira Lima, M.; de Jesus, I.M.; de Souza Hacon, S.; Basta, P.C. An Assessment of Health Outcomes and Methylmercury Exposure in Munduruku Indigenous Women of Childbearing Age and Their Children under 2 Years Old. *Int. J. Environ. Res. Public Health* **2021**, *18*, 10091. https://doi.org/10.3390/ijerph181910091

Academic Editors: José Garrofe Dórea, Rejane C. Marques and Rafael Junqueira Buralli

Received: 17 June 2021
Accepted: 16 September 2021
Published: 25 September 2021

Publisher's Note: MDPI stays neutral with regard to jurisdictional claims in published maps and institutional affiliations.

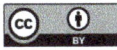

Copyright: © 2021 by the authors. Licensee MDPI, Basel, Switzerland. This article is an open access article distributed under the terms and conditions of the Creative Commons Attribution (CC BY) license (https://creativecommons.org/licenses/by/4.0/).

1. Introduction

Nutrition during the first 1000 days from a woman's pregnancy to the child's second birthday is a critical stage in determining the child's prospects of both growth and learning [1]. This period represents a stage of life with great potential for human development, but equally, of enormous vulnerability to the harm associated with factors such as a lack of essential elements (e.g., vitamins, minerals, fatty acids), infections caused by microorganisms (e.g., diarrhea, pneumonia), and exposure to toxic substances such as medicines (e.g., antibiotics) and environmental pollutants (e.g., pesticides, lead, mercury) [2–4]. An understanding of the importance of this period drives government policy and intervention worldwide with the 1000 Day Initiative outlining how poor nutrition during this period can keep families and communities trapped in poverty [5–7]. In the same vein, the United Nations adopted the Sustainable Development Goals (SGDs) in 2015 as a planetary alert to end poverty by 2030. Goals 2 and 3 set out to ensure access to safe and nutritious food all year round and reduce illness from hazardous chemicals and water contamination [8,9].

Indigenous communities living in remote areas of the Brazilian Amazon have limited access to varied food sources, relying heavily on fish from nearby rivers for their supply of protein [10–15]. Besides this food insecurity, these communities also face risk factors such as gastrointestinal infections, respiratory diseases, poor sanitation, and alarming rates of anemia [16–18]. This condition of vulnerability imposed on the indigenous people in Brazil is known to negatively impact children's cognitive development, physical growth and immunity [16,19–21]. In fact, indigenous children are twice as likely to be affected than other children of the same age [17]. Similarly, studies have also found deficits in height-for-age, weight-for-age, and weight-for-height [18,19,22], as well as increased rates of infant mortality [23,24].

Another important health risk factor faced by indigenous populations living in the Amazon is mercury exposure, which has been described in several scientific papers [11–15]. Mercury is an extremely toxic heavy metal widely used in artisanal gold mines, installed in practically the entire Amazon region [10,25–27]. Mercury used in mines is methylated by bacteria at the bottom of rivers and transformed into its most dangerous form to health, methylmercury (MeHg) [28]. This organomercurial form is a potent neurotoxin and biomagnifies along the entire aquatic trophic chain, contaminating fish, which are often the main source of protein in the diet of many indigenous and riverine communities in the Amazon [29,30]. Factors such as deforestation, burning and the construction of dams for hydroelectric plants intensify the formation of methylmercury and increase human exposure to this toxic substance [10]. The toxicological effects of chronic human exposure to methylmercury through the consumption of fish are pernicious with symptoms including cognitive, visual, motor, somatosensory, attention and emotional deficits as well as immunotoxic or immunomodulatory effects [29–37].

It is important to emphasize that neurotoxic effects related to methylmercury exposure are most serious during the prenatal period, since the fetal brain is particularly sensitive to the action of any neurotoxic substances [38–41]. When methylmercury contaminated fish is consumed, this mercurial form is almost completely absorbed by the gastrointestinal tract and rapidly circulates throughout the body, ultimately reaching its principal target, the central nervous system. In pregnant women, this toxicokinetic pattern is repeated, with methylmercury then crossing the placental barrier and entering the fetal circulatory system [38–40]. Some studies indicate that cord blood corresponds to maternal blood at a ratio of 1.7, leaving the developing nervous system exposed to amplified neurotoxic effects [40–42]. Exposure to a neurotoxin at such a critical period of development has been shown to lead to physical and mental developmental delay, altered muscle tone and reduced neurological test scores, even after exposure to levels of methylmercury that had little effect on the mother [38–42]. Mercury exposed infants specifically have been found to have reduced cognitive abilities [43].

There is little (or no) consensus amongst agencies in their recommendations for the safe ingestion of methylmercury. In 1972, the Joint Food and Additive Organization/World Health Organization (FAO/WHO) Expert Committee on Food Additives (JECFA) established a provisional tolerable weekly intake (PTWI) for methylmercury equal to 3.3 μg/kg bw/week, drawing on health endpoints from poisoning episodes in Minamata and Niigata in the 1950s [44]. Years later, in 1997, the United States Environmental Protection Agency (U.S.EPA) proposed a Reference Dose (RfD) for methylmercury of 0.1 μg/kg bw/day based on the intoxication tragedy in Iraq, which was revised and maintained after the Faroes Island cohort study [45]. More recently, in 2003, the JEFCA established PTWI for most vulnerable groups, as women of childbearing age and children, of 1.6 μg/kg bw/week, and for adults in general of 3.2 μg/kg bw/week [46].

These safe intake doses proposed by different agencies correlate with mercury exposure biomarkers, such as blood and hair, and the levels detected in these matrices can be used as a risk exposure indicator. For example, in 1989, the JEFCA proposed a PTWI of 0.3 mg of total mercury per person of which cannot surpass 0.2 mg of methylmercury [47]. This PTWI was converted to hair mercury levels of 6.0 μg/g for identifying individuals with high mercury exposure in the New Zealand cohort [48]. Many studies developed in the Amazon region used this mercury level as a reference for the appearance of health effects [49–51], including research with indigenous peoples with a history of or suspected exposure to mercury used in illegal gold mining [13,52].

The Munduruku indigenous people living in the Middle Tapajós Region have been subjected to invasions of their territories by gold miners for decades. However, in recent years, the process of invasion has intensified and caused enormous concern for local communities. With this in mind, the *Pariri* Indigenous Association, representing the Munduruku living in the Middle Tapajós, asked the Oswaldo Cruz Foundation to carry out a survey to investigate the extent of mercury contamination amongst the Munduruku indigenous people.

In a recent study, Vasconcellos et al. [12] found that the fish consumed by three Munduruku villages in the Middle Tapajós region showed mercury levels above the limits for commercialization established by FAO/WHO [53] and showed the methylmercury intake in these communities to be several times higher than the safety doses proposed by U.S.EPA [45] and FAO/WHO [46], including the most vulnerable groups of women of childbearing age and children. This study indicates that these communities ingest methylmercury daily at levels that can cause illness and highlights the importance of further research into mercury exposure and its health effects amongst indigenous people.

Thus, in line with the *Pariri* Indigenous Association's request, the 1000 Day initiative and UN Development Goals 2 and 3, the objective of this study was to explore the nutritional status, health outcomes and baseline methylmercury levels of all Munduruku indigenous infants and women of childbearing age in these communities with a focus on mothers who had given birth within the last two years.

2. Materials and Methods

2.1. Study Area and Population

The study was conducted in three Munduruku communities located in the *Sawré Muybu* Indigenous Land (IL) in the Tapajós River Basin, located in the municipalities of Itaituba and Trairão, in the state of Pará, Brazilian Amazon. In total, *Sawré Muybu* IL covers 178,173 hectares, with a population of approximately 800 indigenous people divided between eight villages. The people of these villages are largely subsistence farmers and fisherman, with a small number of teachers and miners [52]. The *Sawré Muybu* IL is of particular historical significance to the Munduruku community, adding further significance to the survival of Munduruku communities in this area [54].

2.2. Study Design

Over 10 days from 29 October to 9 November 2019, a cross-sectional study was carried out in three villages selected from *Sawré Muybu* IL (*Sawré Muybu*, *Poxo Muybu*, and *Sawré Aboy*), following the direct request from the *Pariri* Indigenous Association to the Oswaldo Cruz Foundation (Fiocruz). In the designated villages, we conducted a population census, and all residents were invited to participate in the study. There was no refusal and, therefore, no probabilistic sampling methods were used to include participants.

2.3. Data Collection

2.3.1. Interviews

Interviews exploring mothers' obstetric history and household information were conducted based on a data collection instrument prepared especially for this study. The questions were broadened to explore dietary patterns, information on breastfeeding practices, and pre- and post-natal complications (including miscarriages or infant deaths). In order to analyze vaccination coverage, we revised the health booklets of all indigenous infants enrolled in the study. Based on the data recorded in the child's health booklet, it was possible to check the vaccine records, with dates and corresponding doses, and compare the records with the current national immunization program schedule for the population studied [55].

Each participant was given a unique code for identification and the questionnaire was delivered with the support of Indigenous Health Agents who work in the communities and/or with the support of the local Indigenous leaders, such as chiefs and teachers.

Responses were recorded on electronic forms with the aid of portable electronic devices (tablets), and there was no use of paper forms. After conducting home visits and interviews, families were invited to participate in a standardized clinical (i.e., neurological, and nutritional status) and laboratory evaluation (i.e., mercury analysis and hemoglobin dosage), described in the next section.

Within indigenous communities, there is a younger observational age for commencing sexual initiation and for starting families; with many already married, recent studies exploring maternal health among indigenous groups have used 10 and 14 years of age as their initial starting age [56,57]. However, for this investigation we included women between 12 and 49 years of age.

2.3.2. Mercury Analysis

Hair samples were collected from all participants, removed close to the scalp in the occipital region with the aid of stainless-steel dissection scissors. The samples were stored in paper envelopes, individually identified, and sent for analysis of total mercury levels (THg) in the Toxicology Laboratory, in the Environment Section of the Evandro Chagas Institute (IEC), in Belém (Pará), Brazil. The entire methodology for determining total mercury levels can be found in Basta et al. [52], including the quality control protocol used.

We chose hair samples as methylmercury exposure biomarkers because the principal source of mercury exposure in the studied population is the intake of mercury contaminated fish and from 90% to 95% of mercury forms observed in the fish muscle samples is methylmercury [58–60]. Besides that, almost all mercury present in hair samples is in the methylmercury form, allowing us to assume that all mercury detected in the hair is compounded by methylmercury [61–63].

In addition, we also assume that the methylmercury concentration found in the mother's hair postnatally (i.e., at the time of collection) can be used as an estimate of pre-natal exposure, during pregnancy. This assumption is because, in these communities, diet and environmental exposure patterns are consistent and relatively stable [12].

2.3.3. Nutritional Status

All participants had their weight and height/length measured during the field visit using a vertical anthropometer or stadiometer from Alturexata® (with adapter for infantometer and precision of 0.1 cm—length measurement) (Alturexata®, Belo Horizonte, Minas Gerais, Brazil) and portable digital scale from Seca® (SECA®, model 770, Vogel & Halke, Hamburg, Germany), with a maximum capacity of 150 kg and accuracy of 0.1 kg. The measures of weight and height/length of children under 2 years old were transformed into Z-scores (adjusted for sex and age), according to the reference population of the World Health Organization (WHO), with those scoring below -2 classed as stunted [64].

Given the isolated circumstances of the fieldwork, a measurement of capillary hemoglobin was assessed using the HemoCue® device (HemoCue®, model HB 301-System, Angelholm, Sweden) to give a point of care result, without the need to collect and store venous blood samples. Anemia was diagnosed using the WHO guidance on Anemia with those aged

6–24 months and measuring <11.0 g/dL being classed as anemic. Women of childbearing age were classed as anemic at <12.0 g/dL, however this does not signify anemia during pregnancy, which is of a lower threshold and takes dilutional activity into account.

2.3.4. Neurological Status

An assessment of neurodevelopment was carried out using the Denver II developmental screening test in children aged 0 to 2 years [65]. The Denver II test assesses and identifies children at risk for developmental delay, but it is not intended to measure the intelligence quotient (IQ) and is not designed to diagnose learning or emotional disorders. The test consists of 125 items divided into 4 areas: (i) personal-social (25 items): socialization inside and outside the family environment; (ii) fine motor skills (29 items): hand-eye coordination, manipulation of small objects; (iii) language (39 items): sound production, ability to recognize, understand and use language; iv) gross motor skills (32 items): body motor control, sitting, walking, jumping and the other movements performed by the wide musculature.

2.4. Statistical Analysis

To commence the analyses, we performed a detailed description of the studied population, including children under two years of age and women of childbearing age, according to health parameters and hair mercury levels. The methylmercury concentration used as a reference level in women of childbearing age and their infants was 6.0 µg/g in hair samples (H-Hg) to identify individuals with high mercury exposure.

In the first stage of analysis, given the small sample size, we used the Wilcoxon signed-rank test to compare infants and women of child-bearing age to the reference limit. We then wished to examine whether levels of methylmercury in the hair of the groups of individuals we had tested differed depending on the village. Due to the small sample size and unequal variances between the groups, the Kruskal Wallis test was selected as a robust method of establishing whether any observed differences in the levels between groups were statistically relevant, with post-hoc analyses using the Mann-Whitney U test.

The next phase of the analysis focused on the relationship between maternal H-Hg and infant H-Hg levels, which was assessed using a Spearman correlation. Further descriptive analyses are given to review infant's Denver II developmental screening test scores and the relationship between H-Hg level. Prevalence of infant stunting and infant anemia is explored in relation to Z-scores of −2 and below and <11.0g/dL, respectively.

As a proxy of the Infant Mortality Rate (IMR), we used data extracted from the household interviews where the number of infant deaths was recorded (in the numerator) in contrast to the number of live births (in the denominator), considering each mother's response. The obtained value was multiplied by 1000.

The data were analyzed using the SciPy Open-Source library in Python, and figures were produced using the Seaborn visualization library. Throughout all statistical analyses, we set $\alpha < 0.05$.

3. Results

3.1. Description of the Studied Population

In total, we examined 15 women and their 16 infants under two years old. The average age of the women was 22 years old (S.D. = 7.8; range from 16 to 45), while for children the average age was 10.4 months of age (S.D. = 5.3; range from 4.7 to 21.0) (Table 1). In the *Poxo Muybu* village, we examined five women and five children (three boys and two girls), between 5 to 21 months. In the *Sawré Aboy*, we evaluated four women and five children (one boy and four girls), between 5 to 23 months. Finally, in the *Sawré Aboy*, we assessed six women and six children (two boys and four girls), between 5 to 11 months. Only one woman from *Sawré Aboy* had two children: one girl was 5 months, and one boy was 21 months of age (Table 1).

Table 1. Demographic (sex and age) and clinical (methylmercury and hemoglobin levels, as well nutritional status) characteristics of mothers and their children under 2 years, Sawré Muybu Indigenous Land, Brazilian Amazon, 2019.

Mothers to Infants ID	H-Hg (µg/g)	Age (Years)	Mother's Hb (g/dL)	Mother's BMI (kg/m²)	Infant ID	Sex	Age (months)	H-Hg (µg/g)	Hb (g/dL)	Height for Age (Z-Score)	Weight for Age (Z-Score)	Denver II Passed (Y/N)?
Poxo Muybu												
PM-01-03-01	6.02	16	12.1	19.6	PM-01-03-01-01	M	9	2.25	12.2	−1.43	−0.22	Y
PM-03-01-02	6.08	45	11.9	26.3	PM-03-01-02-05	F	20	2.97	12.1	−2.02	−1.68	Y
PM-05-03-01	5.91	22	14.6	24.0	PM-05-03-01-02	M	8	2.35	10.3	0.68	1.75	Y
PM-06-01-02	7.12	31	12.5	29.2	PM-06-01-02-03	M	21	2.22	11.1	−3.28	−2.71	Y
PM-13-02-02	9.20	19	12.4	19.0	PM-13-02-02-02	F	5	3.88	-	−0.41	0.38	Y
Sawré Aboy												
SA-01-01-02	10.1	19	11.4	19.6	SA-01-01-02-02	F	5	5.36	-	−0.62	−0.63	Y
SA-04-01-02	12.0	17	12.6	19.9	SA-04-01-02-01	F	19	7.85	11.3	−2.03	−0.87	Y
SA-06-01-02	13.8	19	14.4	24.4	SA-06-01-02-01	M	21	6.12	11.3	−1.23	−0.91	Y
					SA-06-01-02-02	F	5	4.84	-	0.57	−0.41	Y
SA-07-02-02	7.25	19	11.9	20.4	SA-07-02-02-02	F	21	2.59	10.7	−0.95	−0.18	N
Sawré Muybu												
SM-01-02-02	12.1	23	13.8	21.4	SM-01-02-02-04	M	9	3.28	10.4	−1.10	−1.85	Y
SM-04-03-02	4.10	18	13.4	26.3	SM-04-03-02-03	F	7	-	9.80	−2.81	−1.95	Y
SM-12-01-02	6.18	16	11.1	25.6	SM-12-01-02-01	F	11	19.6	10.7	−1.37	−0.45	N
SM-14-01-02	2.44	24	13.4	25.8	SM-14-01-02-04	M	7	5.78	9.40	−0.18	−0.18	Y
SM-15-01-02	4.31	16	12.8	24.2	SM-15-01-02-02	F	9	2.44	12.0	0.15	0.91	N
SM-20-01-02	3.34	29	15.3	23.6	SM-20-01-02-05	F	5	3.98	-	−1.16	−1.23	Y

No infant presented with appropriate vaccination coverage for their age with health booklets of all 16 infants showing missing routine vaccines.

Three boys (7, 9, and 10 months) were missing the pentavalent vaccine that includes protection against Diphtheria, Tetanus, Pertussis, Hepatitis B, and *Haemophilus influenza* B. One girl (9 months) was missing the pentavalent and Polio vaccines. One girl (11 months) was missing the Influenza (second dose) and Meningitis vaccines. One girl (5 months) was missing the pentavalent, Meningitis, and Pneumococcus vaccines. One boy (21 months) was missing the pentavalent, Meningitis, and Influenza (second dose) vaccines. One girl (18 months) was missing the Meningitis, Hepatitis B, and Pneumococcus vaccines. One girl (7 months) was missing the pentavalent, Pneumococcus, Meningitis, Polio, and Rotavirus vaccines. One girl (4 months) missed the pentavalent, Pneumococcus and Meningitis vaccines as well as all routine vaccines that should be offered at 2, 3, and 4 months. One girl (5 months) was missing the pentavalent, Pneumococcus, Meningitis, and Rotavirus vaccines. One girl (11 months) was missing the pentavalent, Pneumococcus, Meningitis, and yellow fever vaccines, as well as all routine vaccines that should be offered from 4 months. One girl (5 months) was missing the pentavalent, Pneumococcus, Meningitis, Hepatitis B and BCG vaccines, as well as all routine vaccines that should be offered at 3 and 4 months. One boy (8 months) was missing the pentavalent, Pneumococcus, Meningitis, Rotavirus, Polio, and BCG vaccines. One girl (20 months) was missing the pentavalent, Pneumococcus, yellow fever, Influenza (second dose), and triple viral (measles, mumps, and rubella) vaccines. Finally, a boy (9 months) missed all vaccines indicated at his age.

3.2. Interviews

Most women described their main occupation as supporting the home, with 14 women also working in agriculture alongside domestic activities. Two women were teachers. No women described themselves as miners (also called *garimpeiros* in Portuguese). Male partners described themselves as fisherman and farmers, with five involved in mining activities.

All women described eating a variety of herbivorous and piscivorous fish frequently with *Aracu* (Herbivorous), *Barbado* (Piscivorous), *Curimata* (Detritivorous) and *Piranha* (Piscivorous) being the most common, a median frequency of three times per week was established. Nuts were eaten in varied amounts during the rainy season by all families. Hunted meat was eaten in all communities with the most common being tapir and tortoise. Fruits were eaten with banana, pineapple, and *açaí* most mentioned, access to these fruits and frequency of consumption was not established. Average income gave a monthly figure of US$242 with a range (US$0–US$1250), median US$175.

All infants aged six months and under were exclusively breastfed. Following this, a weaning process began with most infants starting to consume alternative foods, including small amounts of hunted meat and fish in the form of fish soup. Fish soup consumption varied from once per week to three times per day, with the majority of infants consuming fish soup alongside breastfeeding three times per week.

There were 53 women of childbearing age within our cohort with 35 women having given birth at least once. Five women were pregnant at the time of analysis. The number of completed pregnancies ranged from 1 to 14, with an average parity of four. Five women (9%) described a history of spontaneous abortion whilst 11 women (21%) described having at least one infant that had passed away, with a total of 13 infant deaths (Table 2). Considering the 150 live births accounted for by all these women, this puts an Infant Mortality Rate at 86.7 infant deaths per 1000 births. Importantly, this estimated IMR remained consistent within each age category assessed with ages 12 to 27 and 28 to 49 showing an estimate of 93 and 84/1000; respectively.

Table 2. Descriptive analysis of the woman of childbearing age, according to the methylmercury exposure levels (<6.0 µg/g or ≥6.0 µg/g), *Sawré Muybu* Indigenous Land, Brazilian Amazon, 2019.

	Methylmercury Levels	
	<6.0 µg/g	≥6.0 µg/g
[MeHg]-Mean (µg/g)	4.1 (n = 20)	9.9 (n = 33)
Age Group (years)		
12–18 (n)	9	12
19–30 (n)	9	13
30–49 (n)	2	8
Sociodemographic Characteristics		
Salary Mean (US$)	281	217
Education Level (median schooling years)	6	6
Household (n)	11	8
Agriculture (n)	3	11
Student, Teacher (n)	5	6
Partner working as extractivist (n)	0	5
Dietary Characteristics		
Frequently Fruit Intake (n)	20	33
Weekly fish consumption (Median)	3	3
Nuts consumed in the wet season (n):		
Daily	10	19
Weekly	7	5
Monthly	1	8
Health Outcomes and Obstetrician History		
Hb Median (g/dL)	13.4	13.2
BMI (kg/m^2)	23.2	22.8
Depressed mood (n)	8	8
Live Births (n)	53	97
Miscarriages (n)	1	5
Infant deaths (n)	5	8

3.3. Nutritional Status Evaluation

Of the 16 infants analyzed, four (25%) were found to be moderately to severely stunted, see Figure 1. The median of height for age was −1.13 (IQR = −1.87, −1.13, and −0.24). Only one infant was found to be moderately-severely underweight. The median of weight for age was −0.58, (IQR = −1.57, −0.45, and 0.24) (Table 1).

Of infants 6–24 months (n = 12), six (50%) were found be anemic. The median of the hemoglobin levels was 10.9 g/dL (IQR = 10.3, 10.9, and 11.8). *Sawré Muybu* village was the worst affected village, where the median was 10.5 g/dL (IQR = 9.6, 10.4, and 11.4). Of the 15 mothers to infants, four (27%) were anemic (median = 12.9 g/dL, IQR = 11.9, 12.6, and 13.8). Of all women of childbearing age, data were collected for 52 (98%) women; eight (15.4%) were found to be anemic. The median of the hemoglobin levels was 13.3 g/dL (IQR = 12.3, 13.4, and 13.9). Of the five current pregnant women, one lacked data whilst the remaining women were not anemic (median = 13.1 g/dL).

In relation to weaning and with the data available, of infants described as eating foods other than breast milk daily (n = 3), no infant registered as anemic. Whilst amongst the infants registering as anemic, four out of four of the infants were recorded as weaning with alternative foods on a weekly basis.

While average BMI scores for women of childbearing age fell within the healthy range (n = 52; median = 23.0; IQR = 19.9, 22.0, and 25.8). In contrast, 20 women (38%) were found to be overweight (median = 26.8; IQR = 25.6, 26.3, and 27.1), with one woman considered obese (BMI = 32.7).

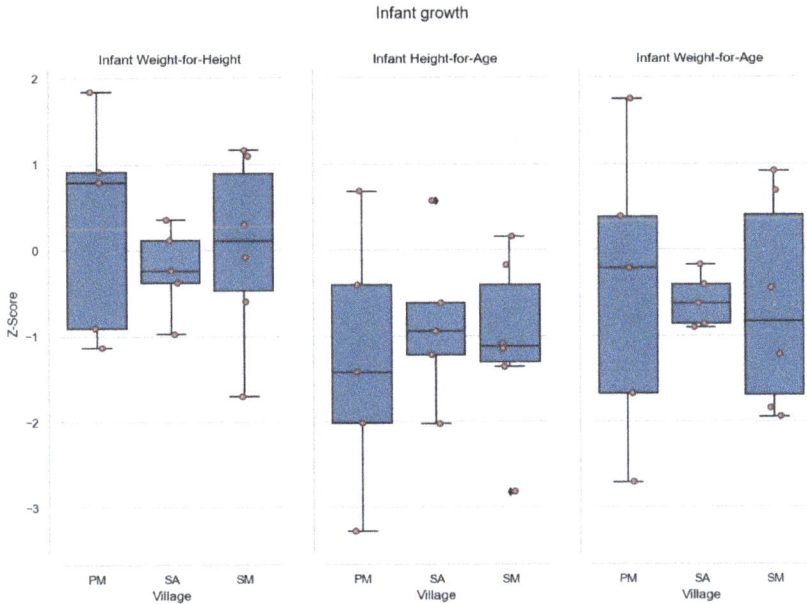

Figure 1. Infant Z Scores for measures of growth. PM corresponds to *Poxo Muybu* village; SA is *Sawré Aboy* and SM is *Sawré Muybu*. S.D. < −3 is severely deficient (severely wasted/stunted/underweight); S.D. < −3 and < −2 correspond to deficient (wasted/stunted/underweight); zero is normal; >2 is weight-for-height is overweight, *Sawré Muybu* Indigenous Land, Brazilian Amazon, 2019.

Of the 15 women, mothers of infants, no one suffered from undernutrition. In contrast two women from *Poxo Muybu* and two from *Sawré Muybu* presented as overweight (BMI ≥ 25.0). The BMI median was 23.6 kg/m^2 (IQR = 20.53, 23.92, and 25.91), with six (38%) found to be overweight (Table 1).

Moreover, the analyses showed that for three of the four stunted children, the mother was found to be overweight (BMI 26.6, 26.3 and 29.2).

A Kruskal–Wallis test did not suggest any significant differences in Infant Hb levels between villages [H (2) = 2.7, p = 0.255]. An analysis of the relationship between Mother's H-Hg level and infant's Hb level did not find any significant correlation (Spearman's r = 0.073, p = 0.831), nor was any significant correlation seen between Infant H-Hg and Hb levels (Spearman's r = −0.265, p = 0.431). In our small sample no relationship was identified between Infant growth and Infant Hb (Spearman's r = −0.146, p = 0.668).

3.4. Hair Methylmercury Levels in Women of Childbearing Age

Comparing hair methylmercury (H-Hg) in all women of childbearing age to the reference limit of 6.0 µg/g H-Hg, women's levels were significantly greater (median = 7.115, IQR = 4.678, Wilcoxon's rank = 416, p < 0.008). This group had an average of 7.71 µg/g H-Hg with a range 2.00 to 20.19 µg/g. The lowest H-Hg level (2.44 µg/g) was a 24-year-old woman from *Sawré Muybu* (SM) who described eating very little meat and fish, whilst the highest level (13.8 µg/g) recorded in a 19-year-old woman from *Sawré Aboy* (SA) was noted to consume fish frequently (≥3 times/week).

Amongst the 15 mothers who had given birth within the last two years, nine (60%) were found to have H-Hg levels above 6.0 µg/g, with an average of 7.56 µg/g, range 2.44 to 13.81.

In the worst affected region, *Sawré Aboy* (SA), the average H-Hg level in women of childbearing age was 12.67 µg/g, twice our Amazonian reference level of 6.0 µg/g. Average H-Hg amongst women of childbearing age in *Poxo Muybu* (PM) and *Sawré Muybu*

(SM) also exceeded our 6.0 µg/g reference limit, at 7.57 µg/g and 6.32 µg/g, respectively (See Figure 2).

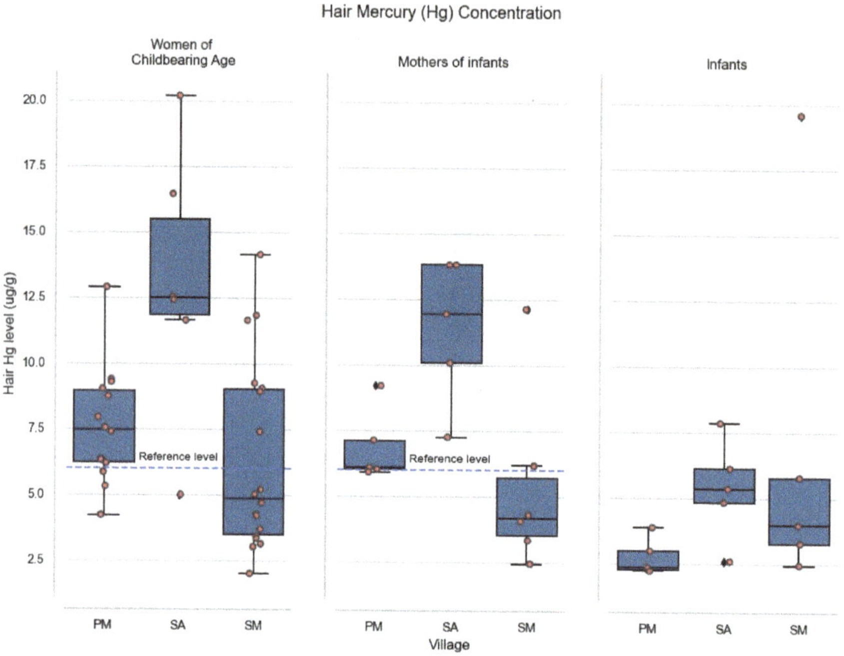

Figure 2. Methylmercury levels split by villages. PM correspond to *Poxo Muybu* village; SA is *Sawré Aboy* and SM is *Sawré Muybu*. *Sawré Muybu* Indigenous Land, Brazilian Amazon, 2019.

The five women pregnant at the time of analyses ranged in age from 15 to 39, all from the *Poxo Muybu* community. All presented with H-Hg levels above 6.0 µg/g reference level. The highest H-Hg recorded in this subsample was 12.9 µg/g in a 24-year-old woman, 12 weeks' gestation and parity two.

3.5. Hair Methylmercury Levels in Infants

Examining all infant H-Hg levels we found median levels were 3.88 (IQR = 3.05 µg/g, Wilcoxon's rank = 5, p = 0.0006). Three of the 16 infants had H-Hg levels over 6.0 µg/g. The highest level (19.6 µg/g) of mercury was found in an infant aged 11 months in the village of *Sawré Muybu* (SM) (See Table 1).

On analysis of Mother's H-Hg concentration in relation to their infant's H-Hg, we found no significant relationship between those infants solely breastfed in their first six months of life. When exploring the whole cohort those mothers with an H-Hg above 6.0 µg/g showed a positive association with their infant's H-Hg (r = 0.783, p (2-tailed) = 0.01).

3.6. Neurodevelopment Results of the Infants Studied under Two

Three of the 15 infants failed the Denver II test with two children failing on language and one on gross motor skill. These children's H-Hg levels were 2.59 µg/g, 2.44 µg/g and 19.58 µg/g with the relevant maternal H-Hg levels recording 7.25 µg/g, 4.31 µg/g and 6.18 µg/g respectively.

3.7. Comparison between Villages

Analysis with Kruskal–Wallis showed that population levels of H-Hg differed significantly between the villages, both between women of childbearing age and between infants under 2 years old [H(2) = 15.0, p = 0.0005 and H(2) = 6.2, p = 0.0455], respectively.

Post-hoc analyses of women of childbearing age suggests that *Sawré Aboy* had significantly higher H-Hg levels (median = 12.177, IQR = 3.017), than either *Poxo Muybu* (median = 7.115, IQR = 2.832; Mann-Whitney's U = 32.0, p = 0.0041), or *Sawré Muybu* (median = 4.508, IQR = 5.552; Mann-Whitney's U = 32.0, p = 0.0009). Between *Poxo Muybu* and *Sawré Muybu* villages there was no statistical differences (Mann-Whitney's U = 141.0, p = 0.0344).

Post-hoc analyses of infants under 2 years old revealed that levels of MeHg in *Sawré Aboy* (n = 5, median = 5.355, IQR = 1.284 µg/g) were significantly higher than *Poxo Muybu* (n = 5, median = 2.345, IQR = 0.720 µg/g; Mann-Whitney's U = 2.0, p = 0.0367), and *Sawré Muybu* (n = 5, median = 3.977, IQR = 2.503 µg/g; U = 10.0, p = 0.6761), whilst a trend suggests higher levels are also present in *Sawré Muybu* than *Poxo Muybu* (U = 22.0, p = 0.0601). Figure 2 shows the distribution of measurements of MeHg among the three villages that were included in the study.

4. Discussion

In response to the specific request from community leaders, this study brought together a health evaluation and an assessment of methylmercury exposure for women of childbearing age and their infants under two years old in a particular Munduruku Indigenous Land never before studied.

Our findings demonstrated that not only women of childbearing age but also their infants have been facing colossal public health challenges. These challenges are consequences of increasing illegal mining activities in their territory and due to historical abandonment by the Federal Government. Among the principal issues illustrated in this study, we highlight high levels of methylmercury exposure, stunting, anemia, poverty, and food insecurity, as well as low vaccination coverage and high infant mortality rates.

4.1. H-Hg in Women of Childbearing Age

Our study identifies a population chronically exposed to unsafe levels of MeHg, with the average hair MeHg concentration sitting above our reference limit of 6.0 µg/g. It is clear that a severe public health concern exists regarding the future generations of Munduruku, with the population of *Sawré Aboy* at greatest risk, recording an average hair MeHg level in women of 12.1 µg/g. Levels amongst these women mirror the levels found in other communities exposed to mercury released by ASGM in the Tapajos River basin [33,66–68] as well in the broader Brazilian Amazon region [69–72].

A wide range of mercury levels have been identified in different populations across the world, associated with a high fish diet. For example, Caribbean immigrants living in Brooklyn-NY [73] showed mercury levels in the blood of 2.14 µg/L, which is equivalent to 0.43 µg/g hair Hg (according to the WHO's conversion measure [61]). Bjornberg et al. [74], studying pregnant women from Sweden, found average mercury levels in hair equal to 0.35 µg/g. These groups have hair methylmercury concentrations below the limit proposed by U.S.EPA (i.e., 1.0 µg/g in hair samples which derives of the Reference Dose of 0.1 µg MeHg/kg bw/day) [45]. On the other hand, the indigenous communities from Canada investigated by Muckle et al. [75] showed hair mercury levels of 4.4 µg/g. Furthermore, a study conducted in New York by Fletcher and Gelberg [76] involving a wealthy urban population revealed mercury levels in blood of 30.8 µg/L, corresponding to 6.16 µg/g in hair. This result contrasts with our findings, where mercury levels above the reference level (i.e., 6.0 µg/g) in the Munduruku indigenous peoples of the Middle Tapajós can be explained by limited access to other animal protein sources. This dietary limitation is not a likely explanation for the mercury levels observed in investigated New Yorkers whose income is relatively high. It is possible that the high levels of mercury observed in the urban population of New York (i.e., above 6.0 µg/g) are the result of polymorphisms in genes that contribute to the toxicokinetics and toxicodynamics of mercury [77–79]. Perini et al. [80] investigated genetic polymorphisms in Munduruku indigenous people and identified two individuals with alterations in genes (*ALAD*) that hinder the elimination of mercury by the organism, who also present high levels of mercury in their hair.

The Munduruku communities represented in the present study have an elevated fish consumption as can be accessed in the recently published paper by Vasconcellos et al. [12]. This investigation concluded that women of childbearing age consume around 170 g of fish daily and consequently have a MeHg intake dose of 0.73 µg/kg bw/day (in the current exposure scenario built). This MeHg intake dose corresponds to seven times higher than the reference dose proposed by U.S.EPA [45] and three times higher than the safe dose established by FAO/WHO [46].

In line with our findings, a Metareview across 72 countries found that hair methylmercury levels largely fall below 2 µg/g and identified communities living alongside ASGM as at-risk populations for high mercury exposure [81]. Chronic MeHg exposure in adults, even at lower levels than those reported in the current study, has been associated with attention deficits and interruptions in fine-motor function as well as sleep disturbances, fatigue and depression with the impact on the aging brain the subject of recent concern [82–84].

4.2. H-Hg in Infants

Median H-Hg levels (3.80 µg/g) found amongst Munduruku infants reflect those found in other regions of the Amazon [41,43,85–87]. Santos Lima et al. [41] reported an association between MeHg exposure and lower performance in neuropsychological tests for children and adolescents, with each 10 µg/g increase of hair Hg corresponding to poorer performance by half a standard deviation. In this study, three infants failed the Denver II Developmental Screening Test, two on Language and one on Gross-Motor Skills, all these infants have high levels of H-Hg. Low-level pre-natal exposure to MeHg through maternal fish consumption has been associated with poor performance in Denver II tests [88,89] whilst other studies have found no association [90]. Due to a small sample, it is difficult to draw conclusions from our findings, collected by one pediatrician in Portuguese and not Munduruku native tongue. However, Gross Motor deficits are less subject to bias. Thus, while infant H-Hg levels are ostensibly lower than those found amongst adult women, it is important to remember the vulnerability of infants to environmental threats, given their immature immune systems and continuous growth [91,92].

4.3. Interactions between Maternal and Infant H-Hg

Studies have shown a significant relationship between maternal methylmercury levels and infant methylmercury levels from birth and during the first years of life due the intrauterine transfer and the breastfeeding [38–40,61]. Although the concentrations of mercury in breast milk are low, breastfeeding promotes continued exposure to mercury during the first months of life [38–40,61]. The intrauterine exposure is deemed a far greater risk to the developing fetus, particularly during the first trimester, since the MeHg levels in the infant blood are almost twice that of the levels found in their mothers' blood [93]. After birth, the infant MeHg levels begin to fall, suggesting that the exposure from breastmilk is lower [85,93–96]. Our study did not show a significant correlation between the methylmercury detected in mothers and their infants aged under six months who were solely breastfed. This may be in part to the limited power of our cohort to establish robust associations, but could also be explained by the reduced methylmercury exposure from the breastfeeding. This may have allowed infant methylmercury levels to fall following birth [94]. In the context of this indigenous Munduruku community, this finding could be interpreted as a positive message for the Munduruku women, that they can be less concerned about infant mercury exposure during the initial months of breastfeeding, where the health benefits of the maternal milk (including neurodevelopmental benefits) are higher compared to the risks posed by mercury during breastfeeding [85].

The statistical analyses did show a significant association between maternal and infant H-Hg levels amongst mothers with H-Hg levels above 6.0 µg/g. This association may suggest an increase in progressive methylmercury exposure for the infants the higher the mother's MeHg burden. However, additionally, the H-Hg infant levels could relate to the gradual integration of the developing infant into household eating habits [85]. So, the higher H-Hg levels in mothers represent a household more reliant on subsistence fish consumption [85].

4.4. H-Hg by Village

The average methylmercury levels detected in the studied participants varied significantly among the villages investigated. The *Sawré Aboy* village showed significantly higher levels of MeHg than the other two communities, exceeding even the highest Benchmark Dose for pregnant women found in current literature (i.e., 12 µg/g) [97]. With these higher levels, the health implications for this community could be particularly serious.

Sawré Aboy village is found near to the meeting of the Jamanxim and Tapajos Rivers. This village is the most isolated of the three villages and is furthest from any access to the largest town, Itaituba (Pará State). The habitants of this village catch the majority of fish for consumption in the Jamanxin river, which is severely impacted by the ASGM. The distance to major towns and the intense gold mining activity in this locality reduce the access to a varied diet and, at the same time, increase the exposure to mercury released by the mining [98]. These factors combined may well explain the elevated mercury detected in the indigenous living in *Sawré Aboy* village. Other studies that looked at nearby communities are consistent with our findings, showing high levels of methylmercury in the community and, in addition, a significant correlation with neurotoxicity [99].

4.5. Nutrition and Growth

The prevalence of infant anemia amongst these three Munduruku communities investigated is 50%. This value is considered a severe public health crisis by the WHO [100] and should be the target of intervention. The infants under two are known to be a high-risk group given the high demands for iron, folate and Vitamin B12 during this period of growth as well as an increased frequency of infections and parasitic disease [17]. In indigenous Brazilian children, the proportion of anemia is commonly found to be around 50% [17]. This prevalence is twice that found in comparable non-Indigenous populations [17]. This disparity is observed in indigenous communities worldwide and is often associated with preventable risk factors such as food insecurity, poor living conditions and sanitation, as well as the higher prevalence of malaria and intestinal parasites [101]. Anemia is known to negatively impact cognitive development, physical growth and immunity and is likely to further aggravate the vulnerability of this population to poverty and illness [102].

Infants identified with a slower weaning regime from six months (i.e., weekly as opposed to daily alternative foods) were found to have a higher prevalence of anemia. However, it is important to bear in mind that breastfeeding is a protective factor against neurodevelopmental delays and increases the odds of infant survival [85,103]. An exclusively breastfed child is 14 times less likely to die in the first six months of life than a non-breastfed child [104]. However, it is understood that prolonged breastfeeding without sufficient iron supplementation leaves the developing infant at risk of Iron Deficient Anemia, and it would be important to know whether the families of slow weaned infants have access to sufficient alternative foods to allow a secure and consolidated weaning regime or importantly whether we are identifying gaps in maternal awareness and understanding of this topic [86,105–107].

The prevalence of anemia in mothers and women of childbearing age sits at 24% and 15% respectively, making them of moderate and mild public health significance. Anemia during pregnancy is associated with poor pregnancy outcomes such as preterm birth and low birth weight as well as maternal and fetal mortality, and the high iron demands of pregnancy are likely to aggravate preexisting anemia [108–111]. WHO estimates of anemia amongst women of childbearing age in Brazil 2009 were 16.1%, suggesting that the findings in these Munduruku communities mirror the situation at a national level [112].

Establishing anemia through Hb levels alone makes it impossible to isolate its exact cause. These communities have limited access to a varied diet, making food insecurity and micronutrient (e.g., iron, folate) deficiencies more likely [16]. Poor sanitation and access to healthcare, alongside a high incidence of intermittent malaria, intestinal parasites and diarrhea caused by gastrointestinal infections, pose further risk factors to the development or aggravation of anemia [113,114].

The women of childbearing age from the communities investigated showed high prevalence of overweight (38%). Studies of indigenous communities in Brazil have found a wide range in the prevalence of overweight [115,116]. The First National Survey of Indigenous People's Health and Nutrition in Brazil finding the overweight prevalence of 30% [16]. The comparisons are hampered by the varied state of isolation, with some communities remaining isolated and others integrated into the local area. The Munduruku communities studied here remain semi-isolated with daily life spent within the communities and as such levels of physical inactivity and genetic predisposition should be explored [16].

On the other hand, infant Z scores showed several infants with restricted growth. Height for age (HAZ) scores showed 22% infants were moderately-severely stunted, closely mirroring the findings of the First National Survey of Indigenous People's Health and Nutrition in Brazil [16]. This is in comparison to 2.2% expected in a well-fed population. Stunting in indigenous communities has been found to reflect a combination of serious nutrient deficiencies and chronic infection such as parasitic infections, which pull on nutritional reserves and are rampant in environments where good sanitation is a challenge [117]. The prevalence of stunting within this small cohort therefore identifies serious nutritional deficits, leading to gaps in brain development and future successes in school, as well as earning capacity in adult life. In addition, there are implications for those non-stunted developing infants within a community that presents with stunting, where these infants are likely affected by under-nutrition [118]. Furthermore, for women growing up stunted there are serious consequences during childbirth, with a higher likelihood of obstetric complications, largely due to restricted pelvic growth [118].

It is worth noting that of the four infants with stunted growth, three have over-weight mothers, with the infant of the most overweight mother also considered under-weight. The so called 'double-burden of disease' where overweight and undernutrition are found within the same household, is a common finding amongst Indigenous communities experiencing food insecurity and undergoing a nutritional transition: moving away from a traditional Indigenous diet and increasingly eating a high-fat westernized diet [117–122]. This finding is surprising in a hard-to-reach region, where communities are ostensibly still reliant on Indigenous grown foods. However, this change in dietary pattern has been noted in Amazonian riverine communities (also called *ribeirinhos* in Portuguese) and as a result of the ever-increasing presence of gold miners coming from across Brazil, the rapidly increasing rates of deforestation and the Trans-Amazonian Highway making access easier from the outside, the nutritional transition seen across Brazil may be expanding [10,123,124]. It is worth noting that the pattern of overweight and undernutrition was not found for the stunted infants in *Sawré Aboy*, the most isolated of the communities, but was identified in *Poxo Muybu* and *Sawré Muybu* which have access to Itaituba and the Trans-Amazonian Highway, respectively.

It is clear that the nutritional situation in these communities is quite poor, with profound, lifelong, and irreversible consequences for the developing Munduruku infant. The implications for the developing brain of a 50% prevalence of anemia in these infants are catastrophic and likely irreversible [125,126]. Good nutrition in the first 1000 days of life is recognized globally as a key intervention to help a child's ability to grow, learn, and rise out of poverty [118,127]. An intervention is needed to support this population's long-term health, stability, and prosperity.

4.6. Infant Mortality

The Infant Mortality Rate (IMR) of 86.7/1000 live births estimated in this study for the three Munduruku villages is higher than the regional average for indigenous communities of 50.62/1000 lives births recorded in 2012, but is similar to the Kaiapó indigenous community (neighbor to the studied villages), which recorded an IMR of 85.3/1000 in 2018 [128,129]. Indeed, the research on infant mortality among indigenous children conducted by Lima et al. [128] and Teixeira et al. [129] found the majority of reported infant deaths amongst indigenous groups to be from Kaiapó and Munduruku ethnicities. This scenario suggests an ongoing burden on resources for maternal health within these communities [128,129]. With Brazil's national IMR at 12/1000 live births it has become well established that indigenous communities in South America present with a higher infant mortality rate than the national average [130].

It is important to note that the higher rates recorded within our study community may in part reflect the data collection, since our study reflects personal information gathered in fieldwork interviews. We do note that we do not have annual data to define a specific yearly incidence.

We cannot specifically comment on the causes of the infant deaths within this community, but the main causes of infant deaths in the Pará state have been identified as difficulties during birth, respiratory tract diseases and infectious and parasitic diseases [131]. All the causes are largely preventable with access to simple, affordable interventions including immunization, adequate nutrition, safe water and food and quality care by a trained health provider when needed [131]. The evidence has highlighted the difficulties in making timely interventions during the perinatal period for indigenous populations with poor access to health care [132,133]. In addition, the way of life in a village with reduced access to clean water, poor sanitation and minimal health care resources allows parasites, infectious diseases and malnutrition to persist, putting infants within our studied community at risk of increased mortality post-partum [134,135]. Furthermore, studies following the Minamata tragedy in Japan suggested that rates of miscarriage and stillbirths increased following exposure to mercury [134,136]. Benefice et al. [137] found that women living along the Beni River in Bolivia with MeHg levels over 5 µg/g presented with increased rates of infant deaths but established no causality link between MeHg exposure and infant deaths.

Our study identifies gaps in resources and infrastructure for reducing these often-reversible causes of infant death. Brazil has made good progress in reducing infant mortality but there is not the same pattern within indigenous communities only confirming major ongoing deficits in health care provision within these communities of difficulty access [22].

Another critical problem detected in our study was the insufficient vaccination coverage for this specific age group. All infants enrolled were missing vaccines. It is worth remembering that vaccination opportunity and coverage are fundamental issues for public health, especially during pandemics. Although the literature is scarce on vaccination coverage among indigenous peoples in Brazil, the consequences of low vaccination coverage on the infant mortality rates due to vaccine-preventable diseases are widely known [138,139]. At least part of the health challenges observed in the studied population may result from poor vaccination.

Within a resource depleted system, even thorough community-based intervention programs can struggle to reduce the IMR burden [140,141]. The high rates of infant mortality observed in this study are a consequence of the restricted and reduced access to secondary healthcare services, poor sanitation, and malnutrition. This study highlights the importance of thorough pre-natal care to identify women at risk of birth complications, increased training of local health care professionals in management of peri-partum care and a focus on nutritional supplementation for mothers and infants to avoid poor development and weak immune systems. Further guidance on sanitation can help reduce risks to infant mortality in their first year of life, from diarrhea and parasitic infections through clean water supplies, closed toilet systems, education regarding hygiene and wider access to anthelminthic medications.

4.7. Where Can We Go from Here?

"Women and their families should receive support to improve their diets as a general health rule, which is a basic human right" [142].

We encourage the Brazilian government to provide adequate investment to the National Unified health system (SUS) and the Special Indigenous Health Secretariat (SESAI) to screen these populations for basic needs and identify those households at greater risk of poor health outcomes. The Brazilian government committed to five pillars to improve the nutritional status of the country alongside the WHO by 2019, including commitments to focus on rural families, but these indigenous communities may be getting left behind [143].

The geography of the land and the isolated nature of living will always make service provision harder; however, evidence-based strategies can work to help improve health indicators in rural communities [141].

Finally, the Covid-19 pandemic has encouraged innovation in providing access to health through 'Telemedicine', a resource that could overcome some of the barriers to improving the social determinants of health in these communities [144].

The WHO and UNEP has described measures to communicate risk to vulnerable populations and produce an effective mercury intervention program:

"The risk manager needs to characterize the role of fish in the population of concern. Fish may play a large role in the cultural and socio-economic fabric of the country or region. The risk manager needs to evaluate whether there are alternative foods that are readily available, affordable and of equal nutritional benefit. There may be other risks associated with alternative fish or foods that should be identified and evaluated" [61].

With the above guidance in mind, we propose several evidence-based recommendations to help improve this chronic and severe public health crisis both in relation to mercury and, more broadly, nutrition. It is essential that we implement these recommendations, paying close attention to the cultural characteristics and respecting the traditional values of the investigated communities.

1. Encourage training and education in nutritional best practices with a focus on the 1000 days window;
2. Improve education around breastfeeding and encourage comprehensive weaning practices post six months;
3. Identify those infants at risk of anemia, for example those with extended breastfeeding, and provide sufficient nutritional drinks and iron supplementation;
4. Work closely with the National Unified health system and the Indigenous Special Sanitary Districts to help develop continuous, accessible, and culturally sensitive pre- (greater than four visits) and post-natal health care;
5. Help develop methods to specifically catch those fish high in Omega-3's and low in MeHg (i.e., those lower in the food chain);
6. Encourage the Brazilian government to align with the Minamata convention and Planet Gold's global initiative to reduce Mercury pollution in ASGM sites;
7. Condemn the government for its active encouragement of illegal gold mining in the Munduruku area.

4.8. Limitations

An important limitation to note is our small sample size of mothers and their infants. This reduces our power to detect any associations; however, it reinforces the need for further, more comprehensive studies in the future.

We acknowledge that in environments where one cannot control for the numerous covariates that are known to adversely influence child neurodevelopment it is not possible to accurately determine causal relationships and, therefore, we further clarify that we present only associations.

The present study is based on evidence from previous literature that mercury is passed from mother to child in utero and, although to a lesser degree, also during breastfeeding. We are limited by our dataset to analysis of the transmission from mother to child during pregnancy and at birth. While we did not have data on cord blood mercury levels, research does show hair sample levels are of correlating value.

In addition, we did not have access to sufficient data on infant birth weight, which could have helped with further analyses regarding prenatal health indicators, nutritional status and infant growth. It would also have been useful to include a control group population, however, the possibility of this has been noted in previous literature to be difficult [10].

Finally, we refer to the number of infant deaths described by the women within this population, however we do not have further details in order to establish annual changes in this figure. We also lack data regarding the mechanism of death; however, our figures are not dissimilar to the figures reported for indigenous communities within the region and rates remain consistent within age cohorts, nevertheless it is clear further investigation is warranted.

5. Conclusions

- This study was borne out of a request from the leaders of these Munduruku communities, exemplifying the experience of vulnerability within the communities;
- These already vulnerable Munduruku communities suffer chronic exposure to levels of MeHg above 6.0 µg/g reference levels, known to negatively impact on adult health and infant growth and development;
- Ongoing health inequalities are contributing to higher rates of anemia, stunting and infant mortality, preventing individuals in these Munduruku communities from reaching their full potential;
- Simple, culturally sensitive intervention is needed to reduce poor health outcomes and interrupt this cycle of poverty.

Author Contributions: Proposal design, study design and methodology, P.C.B., S.d.S.H., A.R.S.P., C.B.H., A.C.S.d.V., P.V.d.S.V. and J.W.K.; fieldwork data collection, A.R.S.P., C.B.H., J.W.K., P.V.d.S.V., A.C.S.d.V. and P.C.B.; laboratory analysis, I.M.d.J. and M.d.O.L.; writing—original draft preparation, A.R.S.P., C.B.H., J.W.K., P.V.d.S.V., S.d.S.H. and P.C.B.; writing—review and editing, P.C.B., S.d.S.H., A.R.S.P., C.B.H., A.C.S.d.V., J.W.K., P.V.d.S.V., I.M.d.J. and M.d.O.L.; supervision, obtaining resources and project management, P.C.B. and S.d.S.H. All authors have read and agreed to the published version of the manuscript.

Funding: This research was funded by the Vice-Presidency of Environment, Care and Health Promotion (VPPAS) of Fundação Oswaldo Cruz through (Fiocruz) Decentralized Execution of Resources Document No. 175/2018, Process: 25000.209221/2018-18, signed between the Fiocruz and the Special Department for Indigenous Health, both under the Ministry of Health. The non-governmental organization WWF-Brazil offered financial support to disseminate the results of the research.

Institutional Review Board Statement: This research was borne out of demand from the Pariri Indigenous Association that represents the Munduruku people of the region of the middle Tapajós river. The study was conducted in accordance with the guidelines of the Declaration of Helsinki and was approved by the Research Ethics Committee of the National School of Public Health of the Oswaldo Cruz Foundation (CEP/ENSP) and the Brazilian National Research Ethics Commission of the National Health Council (CONEP/CNS), CAAE: 65671517.1.0000.5240, with Opinion No. 2.262.686 favorable to its performance. In compliance with Convention No. 169 of the International Labor Organization (ILO), the study began with a pre-study consultation, carried out in August 2019, during a visit to the villages, in which two authors (SSH and PCB) and local indigenous leaders participated. At the time, the study objectives were presented and discussed (https://www.youtube.com/watch?v=oFEYEGxNmns&t=704s; accessed on 22 August 2019). After answering questions and approval of the proposal by the communities, we received support from the coordination of the Special Indigenous Sanitary District of the Tapajós River through the multidisciplinary indigenous health team to carry out the study. In addition, the interviews and data collection started only after the participants had their questions answered and given formal consent in the Informed Consent Form (ICF) by the children's guardians.

Informed Consent Statement: Informed consent was obtained from all subjects involved in the study. Written informed consent has been obtained from the patients to publish this paper.

Acknowledgments: Through chiefs Juarez Saw, Jairo Saw and Valdemar Poxo and the leader Alessandra Korap, we thank the Munduruku people for the trust placed in our team and the support in carrying out the research. Through coordinator Cleidiane Carvalho Ribeiro dos Santos, we thank the team from the Rio Tapajós Indigenous Special Sanitary District, who spared no efforts to support us in all stages of the fieldwork. In particular, we thank nurses Alan Marcelo Simon and Lygia Catarina de Oliveira. We thank João Paulo Goes Pereira for the mercury analysis in the hair samples. Further thanks goes to Alexander Kaula for his assistance during the stages of statistical analyses.

Conflicts of Interest: The authors declare no conflict of interest. The funders had no role in the design of the study; in the collection, analyses, or interpretation of data; in the writing of the manuscript, or in the decision to publish the results.

References

1. Darling, J.C.; Bamidis, P.D.; Burberry, J.; Rudolf, M.C.J. The First Thousand Days: Early, Integrated and Evidence-Based Approaches to Improving Child Health: Coming to a Population near You? *Arch. Dis. Child.* **2020**, *105*, 837–841. [CrossRef] [PubMed]
2. English, K.; Lau, C.; Jagals, P. The Unique Vulnerabilities of Children to Environmental Hazards. In *Early-life Environmental Exposure and Disease: Facts and Perspectives*; Xia, Y., Ed.; Springer: Singapore, 2020; pp. 103–112, ISBN 9789811537974.
3. Dórea, J.G. Environmental Exposure to Low-Level Lead (Pb) Co-Occurring with Other Neurotoxicants in Early Life and Neurodevelopment of Children. *Environ. Res.* **2019**, *177*, 108641. [CrossRef] [PubMed]
4. Woodruff, T.; Axelrad, D.; Kyle, A.; Nweke, O.; Miller, G. *America's Children and the Environment: Measures of Contaminants, Body Burdens, and Illnesses*; U.S. EPA: Cincinnati, OH, USA, 2003.
5. House of Commons Health and Social Care Committee. Parliamentary Copyright House of Commons: First 1000 Days of Life. 2019, p. 58. Available online: https://publications.parliament.uk/pa/cm201719/cmselect/cmhealth/1496/1496.pdf (accessed on 12 August 2021).
6. First 1000 Days Australia First 1000 Days Australia. Available online: https://www.first1000daysaustralia.com (accessed on 12 August 2021).
7. Thousand Days Why 1000 Days. Available online: https://thousanddays.org/why-1000-days/ (accessed on 12 August 2021).
8. United Nations Goal 2: Zero Hunger. Available online: https://www.un.org/sustainabledevelopment/hunger/ (accessed on 12 August 2021).
9. United Nations Goal 2: Health. Available online: https://www.un.org/sustainabledevelopment/health/ (accessed on 12 August 2021).
10. Crespo-Lopez, M.E.; Augusto-Oliveira, M.; Lopes-Araújo, A.; Santos-Sacramento, L.; Yuki Takeda, P.; Macchi, B.d.M.; do Nascimento, J.L.M.; Maia, C.S.F.; Lima, R.R.; Arrifano, G.P. Mercury: What Can We Learn from the Amazon? *Environ. Int.* **2021**, *146*, 106223. [CrossRef] [PubMed]
11. da Silva Brabo, E.; de Oliveira Santos, E.; de Jesus, I.M.; Mascarenhas, A.F.; de Freitas Faial, K. Mercury Contamination of Fish and Exposures of an Indigenous Community in Pará State, Brazil. *Environ. Res.* **2000**, *84*, 197–203. [CrossRef]
12. de Vasconcellos, A.C.S.; Hallwass, G.; Bezerra, J.G.; Aciole, A.N.S.; Meneses, H.N.d.M.; Lima, M.d.O.; de Jesus, I.M.; Hacon, S.d.S.; Basta, P.C. Health Risk Assessment of Mercury Exposure from Fish Consumption in Munduruku Indigenous Communities in the Brazilian Amazon. *Int. J. Environ. Res. Public Health* **2021**, *18*, 7940. [CrossRef]
13. Vega, C.M.; Orellana, J.D.Y.; Oliveira, M.W.; Hacon, S.S.; Basta, P.C. Human Mercury Exposure in Yanomami Indigenous Villages from the Brazilian Amazon. *Int. J. Environ. Res. Public Health* **2018**, *15*, 1051. [CrossRef]
14. Dórea, J.G.; de Souza, J.R.; Rodrigues, P.; Ferrari, I.; Barbosa, A.C. Hair Mercury (Signature of Fish Consumption) and Cardiovascular Risk in Munduruku and Kayabi Indians of Amazonia. *Environ. Res.* **2005**, *97*, 209–219. [CrossRef]
15. Santos, E.; de Jesus, I.; Câmara, V.; Brabo, E.; Loureiro, E.; Mascarenhas, A.; Weirich, J.; Luiz, R.; Cleary, D. Mercury Exposure in Munduruku Indians from the Community of Sai Cinza, State of Pará, Brazil. *Environ. Res.* **2002**, *90*, 98–103. [CrossRef]
16. Coimbra, C.E.; Santos, R.V.; Welch, J.R.; Cardoso, A.M.; de Souza, M.C.; Garnelo, L.; Rassi, E.; Follér, M.-L.; Horta, B.L. The First National Survey of Indigenous People's Health and Nutrition in Brazil: Rationale, Methodology, and Overview of Results. *BMC Public Health* **2013**, *13*, 1–19. [CrossRef]
17. Leite, M.S.; Cardoso, A.M.; Coimbra, C.E.; Welch, J.R.; Gugelmin, S.A.; Lira, P.C.I.; Horta, B.L.; Santos, R.V.; Escobar, A.L. Prevalence of Anemia and Associated Factors among Indigenous Children in Brazil: Results from the First National Survey of Indigenous People's Health and Nutrition. *Nutr. J.* **2013**, *12*, 1–11. [CrossRef]
18. Orellana, J.D.Y.; Coimbra, C.E.A., Jr.; Lourenço, A.E.P.; Santos, R.V. Estado nutricional e anemia em crianças Suruí, Amazônia, Brasil. *J. Pediatr. (Rio J.)* **2006**, *82*, 383–388. [CrossRef]

19. Orellana, J.D.Y.; Gatica-Domínguez, G.; Vaz, J.d.S.; Neves, P.A.R.; de Vasconcellos, A.C.S.; de Souza Hacon, S.; Basta, P.C. Intergenerational Association of Short Maternal Stature with Stunting in Yanomami Indigenous Children from the Brazilian Amazon. *Int. J. Environ. Res. Public Health* **2021**, *18*, 9130. [CrossRef] [PubMed]
20. Orellana, J.D.Y.; Marrero, L.; Alves, C.L.M.; Ruiz, C.M.V.; Hacon, S.S.; Oliveira, M.W.; Basta, P.C. Association of severe stunting in indigenous Yanomami children with maternal short stature: Clues about the intergerational transmission. *Cien Saude Colet* **2019**, *24*, 1875–1883. [CrossRef] [PubMed]
21. Manjong, F.T.; Verla, V.S.; Egbe, T.O.; Nsagha, D.S. Risk Factors of under Nutrition among Indigenous Children under Five Years in Developing Countries: A Scoping Review. *J. Public Health Epidemiol.* **2020**, *12*, 340–348. [CrossRef]
22. Cunha, M.P.L.; Marques, R.C.; Dórea, J.G. Child Nutritional Status in the Changing Socioeconomic Region of the Northern Amazon, Brazil. *Int. J. Environ. Res. Public Health* **2017**, *15*, 15. [CrossRef]
23. Santos, R.V.; Borges, G.M.; de Campos, M.B.; Queiroz, B.L.; Coimbra, C.E.A.; Welch, J.R. Indigenous Children and Adolescent Mortality Inequity in Brazil: What Can We Learn from the 2010 National Demographic Census? *SSM Popul. Health* **2020**, *10*, 100537. [CrossRef]
24. Gava, C.; Cardoso, A.M.; Basta, P.C. Infant Mortality by Color or Race from Rondônia, Brazilian Amazon. *Rev. Saúde Pública* **2017**, *51*, 3–6. [CrossRef]
25. Lobo, F.D.L.; Costa, M.; Novo, E.M.L.d.M.; Telmer, K. Distribution of Artisanal and Small-Scale Gold Mining in the Tapajós River Basin (Brazilian Amazon) over the Past 40 Years and Relationship with Water Siltation. *Remote Sens.* **2016**, *8*, 579. [CrossRef]
26. Asner, G.P.; Llactayo, W.; Tupayachi, R.; Luna, E.R. Elevated Rates of Gold Mining in the Amazon Revealed through High-Resolution Monitoring. *Proc. Natl. Acad. Sci. USA* **2013**, *110*, 18454–18459. [CrossRef]
27. Cremers, L.; De Theije, M. Small-Scale Gold Mining in the Amazon. *Small-Scale Gold Min. Amaz.* **2013**, *1*, 1–16.
28. Guimarães, J.R.D.; Roulet, M.; Lucotte, M.; Mergler, D. Mercury Methylation along a Lake–Forest Transect in the Tapajós River Floodplain, Brazilian Amazon: Seasonal and Vertical Variations. *Sci. Total Environ.* **2000**, *261*, 91–98. [CrossRef]
29. Santos-Sacramento, L.; Arrifano, G.P.; Lopes-Araújo, A.; Augusto-Oliveira, M.; Albuquerque-Santos, R.; Takeda, P.Y.; Souza-Monteiro, J.R.; Macchi, B.M.; do Nascimento, J.L.M.; Lima, R.R.; et al. Human Neurotoxicity of Mercury in the Amazon: A Scoping Review with Insights and Critical Considerations. *Ecotoxicol. Environ. Saf.* **2021**, *208*, 111686. [CrossRef]
30. Lebel, J.; Mergler, D.; Branches, F.; Lucotte, M.; Amorim, M.; Larribe, F.; Dolbec, J. Neurotoxic Effects of Low-Level Methylmercury Contamination in the Amazonian Basin. *Environ. Res.* **1998**, *79*, 20–32. [CrossRef] [PubMed]
31. Grandjean, P.; White, R.F.; Nielsen, A.; Cleary, D.; de Oliveira Santos, E.C. Methylmercury Neurotoxicity in Amazonian Children Downstream from Gold Mining. *Environ. Health Perspect.* **1999**, *107*, 587–591. [CrossRef] [PubMed]
32. Dolbec, J.; Mergler, D.; Sousa Passos, C.-J.; Sousa de Morais, S.; Lebel, J. Methylmercury Exposure Affects Motor Performance of a Riverine Population of the Tapajós River, Brazilian Amazon. *Int. Arch. Occup. Environ. Health* **2000**, *73*, 195–203. [CrossRef]
33. Khoury, E.D.T.; Souza, G.d.S.; Costa, C.A.d.; Araújo, A.A.K.d.; Oliveira, C.S.B.d.; Silveira, L.C.d.L.; Pinheiro, M.d.C.N. Somatosensory Psychophysical Losses in Inhabitants of Riverside Communities of the Tapajós River Basin, Amazon, Brazil: Exposure to Methylmercury Is Possibly Involved. *PLoS ONE* **2015**, *10*, e0144625. [CrossRef]
34. Oliveira, C.S.; Nogara, P.A.; Ardisson-Araújo, D.M.P.; Aschner, M.; Rocha, J.B.T.; Dórea, J.G. Neurodevelopmental Effects of Mercury. *Adv. Neurotoxicol.* **2018**, *2*, 27–86. [CrossRef]
35. Nyland, J.F.; Wang, S.B.; Shirley, D.L.; Santos, E.O.; Ventura, A.M.; de Souza, J.M.; Silbergeld, E.K. Fetal and Maternal Immune Responses to Methylmercury Exposure: A Cross-Sectional Study. *Environ. Res.* **2011**, *111*, 584–589. [CrossRef]
36. Cordier, S.; Garel, M.; Mandereau, L.; Morcel, H.; Doineau, P.; Gosme-Seguret, S.; Josse, D.; White, R.; Amiel-Tison, C. Neurodevelopmental Investigations among Methylmercury-Exposed Children in French Guiana. *Environ. Res.* **2002**, *89*, 1–11. [CrossRef]
37. dos Santos Freitas, J.; da Costa Brito Lacerda, E.M.; da Silva Martins, I.C.V.; Rodrigues, D.; Bonci, D.M.O.; Cortes, M.I.T.; Corvelo, T.C.O.; Ventura, D.F.; de Lima Silveira, L.C.; da Conceição Nascimento Pinheiro, M.; et al. Cross-Sectional Study to Assess the Association of Color Vision with Mercury Hair Concentration in Children from Brazilian Amazonian Riverine Communities. *NeuroToxicology* **2018**, *65*, 60–67. [CrossRef]
38. Bose-O'Reilly, S.; McCarty, K.M.; Steckling, N.; Lettmeier, B. Mercury Exposure and Children's Health. *Curr. Probl. Pediatr. Adolesc. Health Care* **2010**, *40*, 186–215. [CrossRef]
39. Bose-O'Reilly, S.; Lettmeier, B.; Matteucci Gothe, R.; Beinhoff, C.; Siebert, U.; Drasch, G. Mercury as a Serious Health Hazard for Children in Gold Mining Areas. *Environ. Res.* **2008**, *107*, 89–97. [CrossRef] [PubMed]
40. Koos, B.J.; Longo, L.D. Mercury Toxicity in the Pregnant Woman, Fetus, and Newborn Infant: A Review. *Am. J. Obstet. Gynecol.* **1976**, *126*, 390–409. [CrossRef]
41. Santos-Lima, C.d.; Mourão, D.d.S.; Carvalho, C.F.d.; Souza-Marques, B.; Vega, C.M.; Gonçalves, R.A.; Argollo, N.; Menezes-Filho, J.A.; Abreu, N.; Hacon, S.d.S. Neuropsychological Effects of Mercury Exposure in Children and Adolescents of the Amazon Region, Brazil. *NeuroToxicology* **2020**, *79*, 48–57. [CrossRef]
42. Stern, A.H.; Smith, A.E. An Assessment of the Cord Blood:Maternal Blood Methylmercury Ratio: Implications for Risk Assessment. *Env. Health Perspect.* **2003**, *111*, 1465–1470. [CrossRef]
43. Reuben, A.; Frischtak, H.; Berky, A.; Ortiz, E.J.; Morales, A.M.; Hsu-Kim, H.; Pendergast, L.L.; Pan, W.K. Elevated Hair Mercury Levels Are Associated with Neurodevelopmental Deficits in Children Living Near Artisanal and Small-Scale Gold Mining in Peru. *GeoHealth* **2020**, *4*, e2019GH000222. [CrossRef]

44. Joint, F.A.O.; WHO Expert Committee on Food Additives; World Health Organization. *Evaluation of Certain Food Additives and the Contaminants Mercury, Lead, and Cadmium: Sixteenth Report of the Joint FAO/WHO Expert Committee on Food Additives, Geneva, 4–12 April 1972*; World Health Organization: Geneva, Switzerland, 1972.
45. US EPA. *Reference Dose for Methylmercury (External Review Draft, 2000)*; U.S. Environmental Protection Agency: Washington, DC, USA, 2000.
46. WHO; FAO. *Evaluation of Certain Food Additives and Contaminants: Sixty-First Report of the Joint FAO/WHO Expert Committee on Food Additives*; World Health Organization: Geneva, Switzerland, 2004.
47. Joint, F.A.O.; WHO Expert Committee on Food Additives. *Toxicological Evaluation of Certain Food Additives and Contaminants*; Cambridge University Press: Cambridge, UK, 1989.
48. Crump, K.S.; Kjellström, T.; Shipp, A.M.; Silvers, A.; Stewart, A. Influence of Prenatal Mercury Exposure upon Scholastic and Psychological Test Performance: Benchmark Analysis of a New Zealand Cohort. *Risk Anal.* 1998, *18*, 701–713. [CrossRef]
49. Marinho, J.S.; Lima, M.O.; de Oliveira Santos, E.C.; de Jesus, I.M.; da Conceição, N.; Pinheiro, M.; Alves, C.N.; Muller, R.C.S. Mercury Speciation in Hair of Children in Three Communities of the Amazon, Brazil. *Biomed. Res. Int* 2014, *2014*, 945963. [CrossRef] [PubMed]
50. De Castro, N.S.S.; Lima, M.D.O. Hair as a Biomarker of Long Term Mercury Exposure in Brazilian Amazon: A Systematic Review. *Int. J. Environ. Res. Public Heal.* 2018, *15*, 500. [CrossRef]
51. Bastos, W.R.; Gomes, J.P.O.; Oliveira, R.C.; Almeida, R.; Nascimento, E.L.; Bernardi, J.V.E.; de Lacerda, L.D.; da Silveira, E.G.; Pfeiffer, W.C. Mercury in the Environment and Riverside Population in the Madeira River Basin, Amazon, Brazil. *Sci. Total Environ.* 2006, *368*, 344–351. [CrossRef]
52. Basta, P.C.; Viana, P.V.S.; Vasconcellos, A.C.; Perisse, A.R.S.; Hofer, C.B.; Paifa, N.S.; Kempton, J.W.; Ciampi de Andrade, D.; Oliveira, R.A.A.; Achatz, R.W.; et al. Mercury Exposure in Munduruku Indigenous Communities from Brazilian Amazon: Methodologi-Cal Background and an Overview of the Principal Results. *Int. J. Environ. Res. Public Health* 2021, *18*, 9222. [CrossRef] [PubMed]
53. Joint, F.A.O. *WHO Food Standards Programme Codex Committee on Contaminants in Foods Tenth Session Rotterdam, The Netherlands*; WHO: Geneva, Switzerland, 2016.
54. Achatz, R.W.; Vasconcellos, A.C.; Pereira, L.; Viana, P.V.S.; Basta, P.C. Impacts of the Goldmining and Chronic Methylmercury Exposure on the Good-Living and Mental Health of Munduruku Native Communities in the Amazon Basin. *Int. J. Environ. Res. Public Health* 2021, *18*, 8994. [CrossRef]
55. PNI. *Calendário Nacional de Vacinação Dos Povos Indígenas*; Secretaria de estado de saude: Goiania, Brazil, 2020.
56. Estima, N.M.; Alves, S.V. Mortes Maternas e de Mulheres Em Idade Reprodutiva Na População Indígena, Pernambuco, 2006–2012 *. *Epidemiol. E Serviços De Saúde* 2019, *28*, 2–5. [CrossRef] [PubMed]
57. Garnelo, L.; Horta, B.L.; Escobar, A.L.; Santos, R.V.; Cardoso, A.M.; Welch, J.R.; Tavares, F.G.; Coimbra, C.E.A., Jr. Avaliação da atenção pré-natal ofertada às mulheres indígenas no Brasil: Achados do Primeiro Inquérito Nacional de Saúde e Nutrição dos Povos Indígenas. *Cad. Saúde Pública* 2019, *35*, e00181318. [CrossRef] [PubMed]
58. Marrugo-Negrete, J.; Verbel, J.O.; Ceballos, E.L.; Benitez, L.N. Total Mercury and Methylmercury Concentrations in Fish from the Mojana Region of Colombia. *Env. Geochem. Health* 2008, *30*, 21–30. [CrossRef] [PubMed]
59. Kehrig, H.A.; Costa, M.; Moreira, I.; Malm, O. Total and Methylmercury in a Brazilian Estuary, Rio de Janeiro. *Mar. Pollut. Bull.* 2002, *44*, 1018–1023. [CrossRef]
60. Souza-Araujo, J.; Giarrizzo, T.; Lima, M.O.; Souza, M.B.G. Mercury and Methyl Mercury in Fishes from Bacajá River (Brazilian Amazon): Evidence for Bioaccumulation and Biomagnification. *J. Fish. Biol.* 2016, *89*, 249–263. [CrossRef] [PubMed]
61. World Health Organization. *Guidance for Identifying Populations at Risk from Mercury Exposure*; WHO: Geneva, Switzerland, 2016.
62. Berglund, M.; Lind, B.; Björnberg, K.A.; Palm, B.; Einarsson, O.; Vahter, M. Inter-Individual Variations of Human Mercury Exposure Biomarkers: A Cross-Sectional Assessment. *Env. Health* 2005, *4*, 1–11. [CrossRef]
63. Clarkson, T.W.; Magos, L. The Toxicology of Mercury and Its Chemical Compounds. *Crit. Rev. Toxicol.* 2006, *36*, 609–662. [CrossRef]
64. World Health Organization. WHO Child Growth Standards: Length/Height-for-Age, Weight-for-Age, Weight-for-Length, Weight-for-Height and Body Mass Index-for-Age: Methods and Development. Available online: https://www.who.int/publications-detail-redirect/924154693X (accessed on 14 August 2021).
65. Frankenburg, W.K.; Dodds, J.; Archer, P.; Shapiro, H.; Bresnick, B. The Denver II: A Major Revision and Restandardization of the Denver Developmental Screening Test. *Pediatrics* 1992, *89*, 91–97. [PubMed]
66. Harada, M.; Nakanishi, J.; Yasoda, E.; Pinheiro, M.d.C.N.; Oikawa, T.; de Assis Guimarâes, G.; da silva Cardoso, B.; Kizaki, T.; Ohno, H. Mercury Pollution in the Tapajos River Basin, Amazon: Mercury Level of Head Hair and Health Effects. *Environ. Int.* 2001, *27*, 285–290. [CrossRef]
67. Malm, O.; Guimarães, J.R.D.; Castro, M.B.; Bastos, W.R.; Viana, J.P.; Branches, F.J.P.; Silveira, E.G.; Pfeiffer, W.C. Follow-up of Mercury Levels in Fish, Human Hair and Urine in the Madeira and Tapajós Basins, Amazon, Brazil. *Water Air Soil Pollut.* 1997, *97*, 45–51. [CrossRef]
68. Berzas Nevado, J.J.; Rodríguez Martín-Doimeadios, R.C.; Guzmán Bernardo, F.J.; Jiménez Moreno, M.; Herculano, A.M.; do Nascimento, J.L.M.; Crespo-López, M.E. Mercury in the Tapajós River Basin, Brazilian Amazon: A Review. *Environ. Int.* 2010, *36*, 593–608. [CrossRef]

69. Barbosa, A.C.; Silva, S.R.L.; Dórea, J.G. Concentration of Mercury in Hair of Indigenous Mothers and Infants from the Amazon Basin. *Arch. Environ. Contam. Toxicol.* **1998**, *34*, 100–105. [CrossRef] [PubMed]
70. Barbosa, A.C.; Jardim, W.; Dórea, J.G.; Fosberg, B.; Souza, J. Hair Mercury Speciation as a Function of Gender, Age, and Body Mass Index in Inhabitants of the Negro River Basin, Amazon, Brazil. *Arch. Environ. Contam. Toxicol.* **2001**, *40*, 439–444. [CrossRef]
71. Oliveira, R.C.; Dórea, J.G.; Bernardi, J.V.E.; Bastos, W.R.; Almeida, R.; Manzatto, A.G. Fish Consumption by Traditional Subsistence Villagers of the Rio Madeira (Amazon): Impact on Hair Mercury. *Ann. Hum. Biol.* **2010**, *37*, 629–642. [CrossRef]
72. Vieira, S.M.; de Almeida, R.; Holanda, I.B.B.; Mussy, M.H.; Galvão, R.C.F.; Crispim, P.T.B.; Dórea, J.G.; Bastos, W.R. Total and Methyl-Mercury in Hair and Milk of Mothers Living in the City of Porto Velho and in Villages along the Rio Madeira, Amazon, Brazil. *Int. J. Hyg. Environ. Health* **2013**, *216*, 682–689. [CrossRef] [PubMed]
73. Geer, L.A.; Persad, M.D.; Palmer, C.D.; Steuerwald, A.J.; Dalloul, M.; Abulafia, O.; Parsons, P.J. Assessment of Prenatal Mercury Exposure in a Predominately Caribbean Immigrant Community in Brooklyn, NY. *J. Environ. Monit.* **2012**, *14*, 1035. [CrossRef] [PubMed]
74. Björnberg, K.A.; Vahter, M.; Petersson-Grawé, K.; Glynn, A.; Cnattingius, S.; Darnerud, P.O.; Atuma, S.; Aune, M.; Becker, W.; Berglund, M. Methyl Mercury and Inorganic Mercury in Swedish Pregnant Women and in Cord Blood: Influence of Fish Consumption. *Environ. Health Perspect.* **2003**, *111*, 637–641. [CrossRef]
75. Muckle, G.; Ayotte, P.; Dewailly, E.; Jacobson, S.; Jacobson, J. Prenatal Exposure of the Northern Québec Inuit Infants to Environmental Contaminants. *Environ. Health Perspect.* **2001**, *109*, 1291–1299.
76. Fletcher, A.M.; Gelberg, K.H. An Analysis of Mercury Exposures Among the Adult Population in New York State. *J. Community Health* **2013**, *38*, 529–537. [CrossRef]
77. Woods, J.S.; Heyer, N.J.; Echeverria, D.; Russo, J.E.; Martin, M.D.; Bernardo, M.F.; Luis, H.S.; Vaz, L.; Farin, F.M. Modification of Neurobehavioral Effects of Mercury by a Genetic Polymorphism of Coproporphyrinogen Oxidase in Children. *Neurotoxicol. Teratol.* **2012**, *34*, 513–521. [CrossRef] [PubMed]
78. Arrifano, G.P.F.; Martín-Doimeadios, R.C.R.; Jiménez-Moreno, M.; Fernández-Trujillo, S.; Augusto-Oliveira, M.; Souza-Monteiro, J.R.; Macchi, B.M.; Alvarez-Leite, J.I.; do Nascimento, J.L.M.; Amador, M.T.; et al. Genetic Susceptibility to Neurodegeneration in Amazon: Apolipoprotein E Genotyping in Vulnerable Populations Exposed to Mercury. *Front. Genet.* **2018**, *9*, 285. [CrossRef]
79. Gundacker, C.; Gencik, M.; Hengstschläger, M. The Relevance of the Individual Genetic Background for the Toxicokinetics of Two Significant Neurodevelopmental Toxicants: Mercury and Lead. *Mutat. Res.* **2010**, *705*, 130–140. [CrossRef]
80. Perini, J.A.; Silva, M.C.; Vasconcellos, A.C.S.d.; Viana, P.V.S.; Lima, M.O.; Jesus, I.M.; Kempton, J.W.; Oliveira, R.A.A.; Hacon, S.S.; Basta, P.C. Genetic Polymorphism of Delta Aminolevulinic Acid Dehydratase (ALAD) Gene and Symptoms of Chronic Mercury Exposure in Munduruku Indigenous Children within the Brazilian Amazon. *Int. J. Environ. Res. Public Health* **2021**, *18*, 8746. [CrossRef]
81. Basu, N.; Horvat, M.; Evers, D.C.; Zastenskaya, I.; Weihe, P.; Tempowski, J. A State-of-the-Science Review of Mercury Biomarkers in Human Populations Worldwide between 2000 and 2018. *Environ. Health Perspect* **2018**, *126*, 106001. [CrossRef]
82. Yokoo, E.M.; Valente, J.G.; Grattan, L.; Schmidt, S.L.; Platt, I.; Silbergeld, E.K. Low Level Methylmercury Exposure Affects Neuropsychological Function in Adults. *Environ. Health* **2003**, *2*, 1–11. [CrossRef]
83. Raposo, R.d.S.; Pinto, D.V.; Moreira, R.; Dias, R.P.; Fontes Ribeiro, C.A.; Oriá, R.B.; Malva, J.O. Methylmercury Impact on Adult Neurogenesis: Is the Worst Yet to Come from Recent Brazilian Environmental Disasters? *Front. Aging. Neurosci.* **2020**, *12*, 394. [CrossRef] [PubMed]
84. Silbernagel, S.M.; Carpenter, D.O.; Gilbert, S.G.; Gochfeld, M.; Groth, E.; Hightower, J.M.; Schiavone, F.M. Recognizing and Preventing Overexposure to Methylmercury from Fish and Seafood Consumption: Information for Physicians. *J. Toxicol.* **2011**, *2011*, e983072. [CrossRef] [PubMed]
85. Marques, R.C.; Abreu, L.; Bernardi, J.V.E.; Dórea, J.G. Traditional Living in the Amazon: Extended Breastfeeding, Fish Consumption, Mercury Exposure and Neurodevelopment. *Ann. Hum. Biol.* **2016**, *43*, 360–370. [CrossRef] [PubMed]
86. Marques, R.C.; Bernardi, J.V.E.; Dórea, J.G.; de Fatima, R.; Moreira, M.; Malm, O. Perinatal Multiple Exposure to Neurotoxic (Lead, Methylmercury, Ethylmercury, and Aluminum) Substances and Neurodevelopment at Six and 24 Months of Age. *Environ. Pollut.* **2014**, *187*, 130–135. [CrossRef] [PubMed]
87. Dórea, J.G.; Marques, R.C.; Isejima, C. Neurodevelopment of Amazonian Infants: Antenatal and Postnatal Exposure to Methyl- and Ethylmercury. *J. Biomed. Biotechnol.* **2012**, *2012*, e132876. [CrossRef]
88. Barbone, F.; Valent, F.; Pisa, F.; Daris, F.; Fajon, V.; Gibicar, D.; Logar, M.; Horvat, M. Prenatal Low-Level Methyl Mercury Exposure and Child Development in an Italian Coastal Area. *NeuroToxicology* **2020**, *81*, 376–381. [CrossRef]
89. Marques, R.C.; Dórea, J.G.; McManus, C.; Leão, R.S.; Brandão, K.G.; Marques, R.C.; Vieira, I.H.I.; Guimarães, J.-R.D.; Malm, O. Hydroelectric Reservoir Inundation (Rio Madeira Basin, Amazon) and Changes in Traditional Lifestyle: Impact on Growth and Neurodevelopment of Pre-School Children. *Public Health Nutr.* **2011**, *14*, 661–669. [CrossRef] [PubMed]
90. Golding, J.; Gregory, S.; Iles-Caven, Y.; Hibbeln, J.; Emond, A.; Taylor, C.M. Associations between Prenatal Mercury Exposure and Early Child Development in the ALSPAC Study. *Neurotoxicology* **2016**, *53*, 215–222. [CrossRef]
91. Children's Health and the Environment. *A Global Perspective: A Resource Manual for the Health Sector*; Pronczuk-Garbino, J., Ed.; World Health Organization: Geneva, Switzerland, 2005; ISBN 978-92-4-156292-8.
92. Ruggieri, F.; Majorani, C.; Domanico, F.; Alimonti, A. Mercury in Children: Current State on Exposure through Human Biomonitoring Studies. *Int. J. Environ. Res. Public Health* **2017**, *14*, 519. [CrossRef] [PubMed]

93. Santos, E.O.; Jesus, I.M.d.; Câmara, V.d.M.; Brabo, E.d.S.; Jesus, M.I.d.; Fayal, K.F.; Asmus, C.I.R.F. Correlation between Blood Mercury Levels in Mothers and Newborns in Itaituba, Pará State, Brazil. *Cad. Saude Publica* **2007**, *23*, S622–S629. [CrossRef]
94. Sakamoto, M.; Murata, K.; Nakai, K.; Satoh, H. Difference in Methylmercury Exposure to Fetus and Breast-Feeding Offspring: A Mini-Review. *J. Environ. Health Sci.* **2015**, *31*, 179–186.
95. Grandjean, P.; Jørgensen, P.J.; Weihe, P. Human Milk as a Source of Methylmercury Exposure in Infants. *Env. Health Perspect* **1994**, *102*, 74–77. [CrossRef]
96. Marques, R.C.; Dórea, J.G.; Bastos, W.R.; Malm, O. Changes in Children Hair-Hg Concentrations during the First 5 Years: Maternal, Environmental and Iatrogenic Modifying Factors. *Regul. Toxicol. Pharm.* **2007**, *49*, 17–24. [CrossRef]
97. National Research Council. Risk Characterization and Public Health Implications. In *Toxicological Effects of Methylmercury*; National Academies Press: Washington, DC, USA, 2000.
98. Passos, C.J.S.; Mergler, D.; Lemire, M.; Fillion, M.; Guimarães, J.R.D. Fish Consumption and Bioindicators of Inorganic Mercury Exposure. *Sci. Total Environ.* **2007**, *373*, 68–76. [CrossRef]
99. Dolbec, J.; Mergler, D.; Larribe, F.; Roulet, M.; Lebel, J.; Lucotte, M. Sequential Analysis of Hair Mercury Levels in Relation to Fish Diet of an Amazonian Population, Brazil. *Sci. Total Environ.* **2001**, *271*, 87–97. [CrossRef]
100. World Health Organization. *Haemoglobin Concentrations for the Diagnosis of Anaemia and Assessment of Severity*; World Health Organization: Geneva, Switzerland, 2011.
101. Khambalia, A.Z.; Aimone, A.M.; Zlotkin, S.H. Burden of Anemia among Indigenous Populations. *Nutr. Rev.* **2011**, *69*, 693–719. [CrossRef] [PubMed]
102. McCann, J.C.; Ames, B.N. An Overview of Evidence for a Causal Relation between Iron Deficiency during Development and Deficits in Cognitive or Behavioral Function. *Am. J. Clin. Nutr.* **2007**, *85*, 931–945. [CrossRef] [PubMed]
103. Allen, J.; Hector, D. Benefits of Breastfeeding. *N S W Public Health Bull.* **2005**, *16*, 42–46. [CrossRef] [PubMed]
104. UNICEF. *Breastfeeding: A Mother's Gift, for Every Child*; United Nations Children's Fund: New York, NY, USA, 2018.
105. Dube, K.; Schwartz, J.; Mueller, M.J.; Kalhoff, H.; Kersting, M. Iron Intake and Iron Status in Breastfed Infants during the First Year of Life. *Clin. Nutr.* **2010**, *29*, 773–778. [CrossRef]
106. Friel, J.K.; Aziz, K.; Andrews, W.L.; Harding, S.V.; Courage, M.L.; Adams, R.J. A Double-Masked, Randomized Control Trial of Iron Supplementation in Early Infancy in Healthy Term Breast-Fed Infants. *J. Pediatr.* **2003**, *143*, 582–586. [CrossRef]
107. Baker, R.D.; Greer, F.R.; Nutrition, T.C. on Diagnosis and Prevention of Iron Deficiency and Iron-Deficiency Anemia in Infants and Young Children (0–3 Years of Age). *Pediatrics* **2010**, *126*, 1040–1050. [CrossRef] [PubMed]
108. Sing, K.A.; Hryhorczuk, D.; Saffirio, G.; Sinks, T.; Paschal, D.C.; Sorensen, J.; Chen, E.H. Organic Mercury Levels among the Yanomama of the Brazilian Amazon Basin. *Ambio A J. Hum. Environ.* **2003**, *32*, 434–439. [CrossRef] [PubMed]
109. Bánhidy, F.; Ács, N.; Puhó, E.H.; Czeizel, A.E. Iron Deficiency Anemia: Pregnancy Outcomes with or without Iron Supplementation. *Nutrition* **2011**, *27*, 65–72. [CrossRef]
110. Haas, J.D.; Brownlie, T. Iron Deficiency and Reduced Work Capacity: A Critical Review of the Research to Determine a Causal Relationship. *J. Nutr.* **2001**, *131*, 676S–688S. [CrossRef] [PubMed]
111. Bothwell, T.H. Iron Requirements in Pregnancy and Strategies to Meet Them. *Am. J. Clin. Nutr.* **2000**, *72*, 257S–264S. [CrossRef]
112. World Health Organization. *Prevalence of Anaemia in Women of Reproductive Age (Aged 15–49) (%)*; WHO: Geneva, Switzerland, 2021.
113. Dorea, J.; Barbosa, A.C.; Ferrari, I.; de Souza, J.R. Mercury in Hair and in Fish Consumed by Riparian Women of the Rio Negro, Amazon, Brazil. *Int. J. Environ. Health Res.* **2003**, *13*, 239–248. [CrossRef] [PubMed]
114. Marques, R.C.; Bernardi, J.V.E.; Dorea, C.C.; Dórea, J.G. Intestinal Parasites, Anemia and Nutritional Status in Young Children from Transitioning Western Amazon. *Int. J. Environ. Res. Public Health* **2020**, *17*, 577. [CrossRef]
115. Oliveira, G.F.; Oliveira, T.R.R.; Ikejiri, A.T.; Galvao, T.F.; Silva, M.T.; Pereira, M.G. Prevalence of Obesity and Overweight in an Indigenous Population in Central Brazil: A Population-Based Cross-Sectional Study. *Obes. Facts* **2015**, *8*, 302–310. [CrossRef] [PubMed]
116. Capelli, J.D.C.S.; Koifman, S. Avaliação do estado nutricional da comunidade indígena Parkatêjê, Bom Jesus do Tocantins, Pará, Brasil. *Cad. Saúde Pública* **2001**, *17*, 433–437. [CrossRef] [PubMed]
117. Valeggia, C.R.; Snodgrass, J.J. Health of Indigenous Peoples. *Annu. Rev. Anthropol.* **2015**, *44*, 117–135. [CrossRef]
118. Eggersdorfer, M.; Kraemer, K.; Ruel, M.; Van Ameringen, M.; Biesalski, H.K.; Bloem, M.; Chen, J.; Lateef, A.; Mannar, V. *The Road to Good Nutrition*: Basel, Switzerland; 2013; ISBN 978-3-318-02550-7. Available online: https://www.nutri-facts.org/content/dam/nutrifacts/media/media-books/The_Road_to_Good_Nutrition.pdf (accessed on 14 August 2021).
119. Gubert, M.B.; Spaniol, A.M.; Segall-Corrêa, A.M.; Pérez-Escamilla, R. Understanding the Double Burden of Malnutrition in Food Insecure Households in Brazil. *Matern. Child Nutr.* **2017**, *13*, e12347. [CrossRef]
120. Gracey, M.; King, M. Indigenous Health Part 1: Determinants and Disease Patterns. *Lancet* **2009**, *374*, 65–75. [CrossRef]
121. Tallman, P.S.; Valdes-Velasquez, A.; Sanchez-Samaniego, G. The "Double Burden of Malnutrition" in the Amazon: Dietary Change and Drastic Increases in Obesity and Anemia over 40 Years among the Awajún. *Ecol. Food Nutr.* **2021**, *26*, 1–23. [CrossRef]
122. Ramirez-Zea, M.; Kroker-Lobos, M.F.; Close-Fernandez, R.; Kanter, R. The Double Burden of Malnutrition in Indigenous and Nonindigenous Guatemalan Populations. *Am. J. Clin. Nutr.* **2014**, *100*, 1644S–1651S. [CrossRef]
123. Piperata, B.A. Nutritional Status of Ribeirinhos in Brazil and the Nutrition Transition. *Am. J. Phys. Anthropol.* **2007**, *133*, 868–878. [CrossRef]

124. DETER-INPE. *Deforesation Warning*; Instituto Nacional de Pesquisas Espaciais: São Paulo, Brazil, 2020.
125. Christian, P.; Murray-Kolb, L.E.; Khatry, S.K.; Katz, J.; Schaefer, B.A.; Cole, P.M.; Leclerq, S.C.; Tielsch, J.M. Prenatal Micronutrient Supplementation and Intellectual and Motor Function in Early School-Aged Children in Nepal. *JAMA* **2010**, *304*, 2716–2723. [CrossRef]
126. Murray-Kolb, L.E.; Khatry, S.K.; Katz, J.; Schaefer, B.A.; Cole, P.M.; LeClerq, S.C.; Morgan, M.E.; Tielsch, J.M.; Christian, P. Preschool Micronutrient Supplementation Effects on Intellectual and Motor Function in School-Aged Nepalese Children. *Arch. Pediatr. Adolesc. Med.* **2012**, *166*, 404–410. [CrossRef] [PubMed]
127. UNICEF Office of Research the First 1000 Days of Life: The Brain's Window of Opportunity. 2013. Available online: https://www.unicef-irc.org/article/958-the-first-1000-days-of-life-the-brains-window-of-opportunity.html (accessed on 15 August 2021).
128. Lima, M.; Rego, L.; Valente Correa, P.; Trindade, L.; Rodrigues, I.; Nogueira, L. Infant Mortality among Indigenous People in the State of Pará. *Rev. Eletr. Enferm.* **2020**, *22*, 1–8.
129. Teixeira, J.J.d.M.B.; Santos, D.R.d.; Rocha, M.S.F.M.; Silva, S.C.R.d. Aspectos étnicos da mortalidade infantil: Uma contribuição para a vigilância de óbitos na população indígena e não indígena no Pará. *Para. Res. Med. J.* **2019**, *3*, e14. [CrossRef]
130. World Bank Mortality Rate, Infant (per 1000 Live Births)—Brazil | Data. Available online: https://data.worldbank.org/indicator/SP.DYN.IMRT.IN?locations=BR (accessed on 15 August 2021).
131. World Health Organization. Children: Improving Survival and Well-Being. Available online: https://www.who.int/news-room/fact-sheets/detail/children-reducing-mortality (accessed on 15 August 2021).
132. Alkema, L.; Chao, F.; You, D.; Pedersen, J.; Sawyer, C.C. National, Regional, and Global Sex Ratios of Infant, Child, and under-5 Mortality and Identification of Countries with Outlying Ratios: A Systematic Assessment. *Lancet Glob. Health* **2014**, *2*, e521–e530. [CrossRef]
133. Lansky, S.; Friche, A.A.d.L.; Silva, A.A.M.d.; Campos, D.; Bittencourt, S.D.d.A.; Carvalho, M.L.d.; Frias, P.G.d.; Cavalcante, R.S.; Cunha, A.J.L.A.d. Birth in Brazil Survey: Neonatal Mortality, Pregnancy and Childbirth Quality of Care. *Cad. Saúde Pública* **2014**, *30*, S192–S207. [CrossRef]
134. Souza, P.G.d.; Cardoso, A.M.; Sant'Anna, C.C.; March, M.d.F.B.P. Acute Lower Respiratory Infection in Guarani Indigenous Children, Brazil. *Rev. Paul Pediatr.* **2018**, *36*, 123–131. [CrossRef]
135. Da Silva, J.B.; Bossolani, G.D.P.; Piva, C.; Dias, G.B.M.; Gomes Ferreira, J.; Rossoni, D.F.; Mota, L.T.; Toledo, M.J.O. Spatial Distribution of Intestinal Parasitic Infections in a Kaingáng Indigenous Village from Southern Brazil. *Int. J. Environ. Health Res.* **2016**, *26*, 578–588. [CrossRef]
136. Itai, Y.; Fujino, T.; Ueno, K.; Motomatsu, Y. An Epidemiological Study of the Incidence of Abnormal Pregnancy in Areas Heavily Contaminated with Methylmercury. *Environ. Sci. Int. J. Environ. Physiol. Toxicol.* **2004**, *11*, 83–97.
137. Benefice, E.; Luna-Monrroy, S.; Lopez-Rodriguez, R. Fishing Activity, Health Characteristics and Mercury Exposure of Amerindian Women Living alongside the Beni River (Amazonian Bolivia). *Int. J. Hyg. Environ. Health* **2010**, *213*, 458–464. [CrossRef]
138. Shi, T.; McAllister, D.A.; O'Brien, K.L.; Simoes, E.A.F.; Madhi, S.A.; Gessner, B.D.; Polack, F.P.; Balsells, E.; Acacio, S.; Aguayo, C.; et al. Global, Regional, and National Disease Burden Estimates of Acute Lower Respiratory Infections Due to Respiratory Syncytial Virus in Young Children in 2015: A Systematic Review and Modelling Study. *Lancet* **2017**, *390*, 946–958. [CrossRef]
139. Barreto, M.L.; Teixeira, M.G.; Bastos, F.I.; Ximenes, R.A.; Barata, R.B.; Rodrigues, L.C. Successes and Failures in the Control of Infectious Diseases in Brazil: Social and Environmental Context, Policies, Interventions, and Research Needs. *Lancet* **2011**, *377*, 1877–1889. [CrossRef]
140. Boone, P.; Elbourne, D.; Fazzio, I.; Fernandes, S.; Frost, C.; Jayanty, C.; King, R.; Mann, V.; Piaggio, G.; Santos, A.d.; et al. Effects of Community Health Interventions on Under-5 Mortality in Rural Guinea-Bissau (EPICS): A Cluster-Randomised Controlled Trial. *Lancet Glob. Health* **2016**, *4*, e328–e335. [CrossRef]
141. English, R.; Peer, N.; Honikman, S.; Tugendhaft, A.; Hofman, K.J. "First 1000 Days" Health Interventions in Low- and Middle-Income Countries: Alignment of South African Policies with High-Quality Evidence. *Glob. Health Action* **2017**, *10*, 1340396. [CrossRef]
142. Villar, J.; Merialdi, M.; Gülmezoglu, A.M.; Abalos, E.; Carroli, G.; Kulier, R.; de Onis, M. Nutritional Interventions during Pregnancy for the Prevention or Treatment of Maternal Morbidity and Preterm Delivery: An Overview of Randomized Controlled Trials. *J. Nutr.* **2003**, *133*, 1606S–1625S. [CrossRef]
143. World Health Organization Commitments in Brazil | Global Database on the Implementation of Nutrition Action (GINA). Available online: https://extranet.who.int/nutrition/gina/en/commitments/1394 (accessed on 16 August 2021).
144. Saúde Indígena Specialist Doctors Assist Indigenous People of the Alto Rio Negro DSEI by Telemedicine. Available online: http://www.saudeindigena.net.br/coronavirus/en/viewNoticia.php?CodNot=4bafa5aea1 (accessed on 16 August 2021).

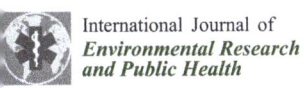

Article

Mercury Exposure in Munduruku Indigenous Communities from Brazilian Amazon: Methodological Background and an Overview of the Principal Results

Paulo Cesar Basta [1,*], Paulo Victor de Sousa Viana [2], Ana Claudia Santiago de Vasconcellos [3], André Reynaldo Santos Périssé [1], Cristina Barroso Hofer [4], Natalia Santana Paiva [5], Joseph William Kempton [6], Daniel Ciampi de Andrade [7], Rogério Adas Ayres de Oliveira [7], Rafaela Waddington Achatz [8], Jamila Alessandra Perini [9], Heloísa do Nascimento de Moura Meneses [10], Gustavo Hallwass [11], Marcelo de Oliveira Lima [12], Iracina Maura de Jesus [12], Cleidiane Carvalho Ribeiro dos Santos [13] and Sandra de Souza Hacon [1]

1. Departamento de Endemias Samuel Pessoa, Escola Nacional de Saúde Pública, Fundação Oswaldo Cruz (ENSP/Fiocruz), Rua Leopoldo Bulhões, 1480-Manguinhos, Rio de Janeiro 21041-210, Brazil; aperisse41@gmail.com (A.R.S.P.); sandrahacon@gmail.com (S.d.S.H.)
2. Centro de Referência Professor Hélio Fraga, Escola Nacional de Saúde Pública, Fundação Oswaldo Cruz (CRPHF/ENSP/Fiocruz), Estrada de Curicica, 2000-Curicica, Rio de Janeiro 22780-195, Brazil; paulovictorsviana@gmail.com
3. Laboratório de Educação Profissional em Vigilância em Saúde, Escola Politécnica de Saúde Joaquim Venâncio, Fundação Oswaldo Cruz (EPSJV/Fiocruz), Av. Brasil, 4365-Manguinhos, Rio de Janeiro 21040-900, Brazil; anacsvasconcellos@gmail.com
4. Instituto de Pediatria e Puericultura Martagão Gesteira, Faculdade de Medicina, Universidade Federal do Rio de Janeiro (UFRJ), Rua Bruno Lobo, 50-Cidade Universitária, Rio de Janeiro 21941-912, Brazil; cbhofer@hucff.ufrj.br
5. Instituto de Estudos em Saúde Coletiva (IESC), Universidade Federal do Rio de Janeiro (UFRJ), Avenida Horácio Macedo, s/n, Ilha do Fundão-Cidade Universitária, Rio de Janeiro 21941-598, Brazil; natalia_uff@hotmail.com
6. Faculty of Medicine, Imperial College London, Medical School Building, St Mary's Hospital, Norfolk Place, London W2 1PG, UK; kemptonj@hotmail.com
7. Centro de Dor, Departamento de Neurologia, Hospital das Clínicas, Faculdade de Medicina, Universidade de São Paulo (USP), Av. Dr. Enéas Carvalho de Aguiar, 255-Cerqueira César, São Paulo 05403-000, Brazil; ciampi@usp.br (D.C.d.A.); roger.adas.doc@gmail.com (R.A.A.d.O.)
8. Programa de Pós-Graduação em Psicologia Clínica do Instituto de Psicologia da Universidade de São Paulo (USP), Av. Professor Mello Moraes, 1721-Butantã, São Paulo 05508-030, Brazil; rafa.achatz@gmail.com
9. Laboratório de Pesquisa de Ciências Farmacêuticas (LAPESF), Centro Universitário Estadual da Zona Oeste (UEZO), Av. Manuel Caldeira de Alvarenga, 1.203, Rio de Janeiro 23070-200, Brazil; jamilaperini@yahoo.com.br
10. Programa de Pós-Graduação em Ciências da Saúde (PPGCSA), Universidade Federal do Oeste do Pará, Rua Vera Paz Av. Vera Paz, s/n, Bairro Salé, 1° Pavimento, Bloco Modular Tapajós, Unidade Tapajós, Santarém 68035-110, Brazil; heloisa.meneses@ufopa.edu.br
11. Programa de Pós-Graduação em Biociências (PPGBio), Universidade Federal do Oeste do Pará, Rua Vera Paz, s/n, Bairro Salé, Santarém 68035-110, Brazil; gustavo.hallwass@gmail.com
12. Seção de Meio Ambiente, Instituto Evandro Chagas, Secretaria de Vigilância em Saúde, Ministério da Saúde (SEAMB/IEC/SVS/MS), Rodovia BR-316 km 7, s/n, Levilândia 67030-000, Brazil; marcelolima@iec.gov.br (M.d.O.L.); iracinajesus@iec.gov.br (I.M.d.J.)
13. Distrito Sanitário Especial Indígena Rio Tapajós (DSEI), Secretaria Especial de Saúde Indígena Tapajós (Sesai), Av. Santa Catarina, 10° Rua, n° 96, Bairro Bela Vista, Itaituba 68180-210, Brazil; cleidiane.santos@saude.gov.br
* Correspondence: paulobasta@gmail.com

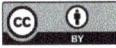

Abstract: The Amazonian indigenous peoples depend on natural resources to live, but human activities' growing impacts threaten their health and livelihoods. Our objectives were to present the principal results of an integrated and multidisciplinary analysis of the health parameters and assess the mercury (Hg) exposure levels in indigenous populations in the Brazilian Amazon. We carried out a cross-sectional study based on a census of three Munduruku indigenous villages (*Sawré Muybu*, *Poxo Muybu*, and *Sawré Aboy*), located in the *Sawré Muybu* Indigenous Land, between 29 October and 9 November 2019. The investigation included: (i) sociodemographic characterization of the participants; (ii) health assessment; (iii) genetic polymorphism analysis; (iv) hair mercury determination; and (v) fish mercury determination. We used the logistic regression model with conditional Prevalence Ratio (PR), with the respective 95% confidence intervals (CI95%) to explore factors associated with mercury exposure levels ≥ 6.0 µg/g. A total of 200 participants were interviewed. Mercury levels (197 hair samples) ranged from 1.4 to 23.9 µg/g, with significant differences between the villages (Kruskal–Wallis test: 19.9; p-value < 0.001). On average, the general prevalence of Hg exposure ≥ 6.0 µg/g was 57.9%. For participants ≥ 12 years old, the Hg exposure ≥ 6.0 µg/g showed associated with no regular income (PR: 1.3; CI95%: 1.0–1.8), high blood pressure (PR: 1.6; CI95%: 1.3–2.1) and was more prominent in *Sawré Aboy* village (PR: 1.8; CI95%: 1.3–2.3). For women of childbearing age, the Hg exposure ≥ 6.0 µg/g was associated with high blood pressure (PR: 1.9; CI95%: 1.2–2.3), with pregnancy (PR: 1.5; CI95%: 1.0–2.1) and was more prominent among residents in *Poxo Muybu* (PR: 1.9; CI95%: 1.0–3.4) and *Sawré Aboy* (PR: 2.5; CI95%: 1.4–4.4) villages. Our findings suggest that chronic mercury exposure causes harmful effects to the studied indigenous communities, especially considering vulnerable groups of the population, such as women of childbearing age. Lastly, we propose to stop the illegal mining in these areas and develop a risk management plan that aims to ensure the health, livelihoods, and human rights of the indigenous people from Amazon Basin.

Keywords: environmental pollution; mercury exposure; indigenous people; Brazilian Amazon; gold mining; fish; children health; neurological effects; genetic polymorphism; *ALAD*; illegal mining activities

1. Introduction

Mercury (Hg) is a heavy metal ubiquitously distributed in the environment [1]. Although humans have used this metal since ancient times [2], the increasing use of mercury in the last decades has caused important changes in their biogeochemical cycle and, consequently, the risk of becoming ill due to exposure to this contaminant has become a public health concern [3–6].

In Brazil, studies developed since the 1980s point out that the artisanal small-scale gold mining activities (ASGM) in the Amazon are the main cause of environmental contamination by mercury in the region [7–12]. Over the last 50 years, the ASGM have released thousands of tons of mercury into the Amazonian environment and, simultaneously, contributed to the process of soil and sediment erosion that facilitates the mobilization of natural mercury [2,13,14]. In a recent study conducted by Teixeira et al. [15], mineralogical analysis carried out on soil samples from the region of *Cachoeira do Piriá* (state of Pará) revealed high concentrations of mercury, above the limit established by Brazilian environmental legislation, despite the absence of mineral formations constituted by mercury (i.e., despite the absence of natural mercury). These results make even more evidently the contribution of the ASGM (also called *garimpo*) to environmental mercury contamination and indicate that the presence of natural mercury in the Amazon's soil is not homogenous.

Moreover, the impact of gold mining on human mercury exposure has been evaluated in several cross-sectional studies involving control groups (i.e., populations living in areas with no history of mining activity) [16–20]. These studies reveal that the mercury levels detected in hair samples collected from groups living in areas impacted by mining are considerably higher than the levels observed in control groups. Such scientific findings strengthen the hypothesis that the primary source of human mercury contamination in the Brazilian Amazon is from mining activities, despite the natural mercury in the soil.

According to a map published by RAISG (Georeferenced Social and Environmental Information Network on Amazon), there are 453 illegal mining sites in the Brazilian Amazon. In the entire Amazonian ecosystem—present in nine Latin American countries—there are more than 2500 illegal mining sites spread over a territory of 7 million km^2 [21]. This scenario of environmental destruction has had severe ramifications for the health and lives of the traditional populations living in the Amazon, especially on indigenous peoples, which are considered one of the keenest consumers of fish in the world [22–24]. As a result of the high fish consumption, these populations are at a greater risk of mercury intake above the safe limits established by the Food and Agriculture Organization/World Health Organization (FAO/WHO) [25] (i.e., 1.6 µg/kg bw/week for children, woman of childbearing age and pregnant woman, and 3.2 µg/kg bw/week for adults in general) and by the United States Environmental Protection Agency (U.S.EPA) [26] (i.e., 0.1 µg/kg bw/day). The Hg released by the ASGM undergoes methylation in the aquatic environment, mediated by microorganisms, transforming it into methylmercury (MeHg) [27]. MeHg is the most dangerous form of mercury to human health due to its deleterious effects on the central nervous system and its biomagnification up aquatic trophic chains [28–30].

The principal human exposure route to MeHg is the consumption of contaminated aquatic organisms, such as fish, shrimp, and crabs. To support this statement, numerous studies [31–44] carried out in the Amazon basin have revealed mercury concentrations in different fish species above the limits to commercialization established by FAO/WHO [45] (i.e., 0.5 µg MeHg/g for non-piscivorous fish and 1.0 µg MeHg/g for piscivorous fish). As a direct consequence of this fact, many scientific studies have been shown hair mercury concentrations from traditional Amazonian people that correspond to methylmercury intake in amounts several times greater than the safe limits recommended by FAO/WHO [25] and U.S.EPA [26], as we can see in some review papers [5,46,47].

In addition, the construction of dams for the operation of hydroelectric plants significantly affects the mercury cycle in the Amazon environment, as it facilitates the mercurial methylation process and other chemical transformations (e.g., demethylation, reduction, and oxidation) [48–50]. In general, dams have favorable physicochemical conditions (e.g., temperature, oxygenation, redox potential, dissolved organic matter) for the proliferation of bacteria that participate in mercury cycling, promoting an increase in the concentration of dissolved organic matter which serves as a carbon source for the organomercurial species, and additionally, inhibits fish migration, facilitating the bioaccumulation and biomagnification of the methylmercury produced [50–53].

Another significant challenge is mercury exposure during the prenatal period. Women's MeHg exposure during pregnancy can cause severe damage to the fetus's central nervous system, and some of these damages can be irreversible. Studies have associated prenatal MeHg exposure with cognitive delays and mild mental retardation [6,54,55]. Reuben et al. [56] observed loss of cognitive ability in ASGM mercury-exposed children in the Peruvian Amazon. In Brazil, Marques et al. [57,58] identified psychomotor alterations and mental development problems in children from Rondônia state, in the Amazon region.

Recent studies regarding the effect of mercury on adult's health revealed emotional changes, such as depression and aggressiveness, motor problems [59], and changes in the visual field [60]. Furthermore, some studies have demonstrated an association between MeHg exposure with the development of neurodegenerative diseases such as Alzheimer's and Parkinson's disease [61,62].

Considering the Tapajós River basin, an area inhabited by the Munduruku people and other indigenous groups in the Brazilian Amazon, some studies have analyzed mercury levels in environmental samples [5,13,35,41,63–65]. Almost all of the revised studies detected mercury in relevant concentrations in different environmental samples such as water, sediment, plankton, and macrophytes fish [5,13,35,41,63–65]. Nevertheless, only three studies are available on the scientific indexed bases regarding mercury exposure in the Munduruku indigenous territory [66–68].

The Munduruku indigenous that live in the *Sai Cinza* Indigenous Land, for example, have shown high mercury levels in hair samples (14.45 µg/g for children from 7 to 12 years old, 15.70 µg/g for women between 14 and 44 years old, and 14.1 µg/g for the remaining population) [67]. The average levels detected were higher than the safe limit (6 µg/g) established by WHO [69]. During an analysis of 365 samples of fish from the Tapajós basin, Dórea et al. [68] revealed that, in general, 26% of fish Hg concentrations were above

0.5 µg/g, and 11% were above 1.0 µg/g, surpassing the maximum reference limits to commercialization of the fishes by FAO/WHO [45]. Notwithstanding, the biomarker of fish consumption (Hair-Hg) was significantly higher in the Kayabi indigenous group (12.8 µg/g) that shares part of the territory with the Munduruku, who showed a mean mercury hair concentration of 3.4 µg/g. In turn, Brabo et al. [66] also pointed out that the average concentration of mercury in the carnivorous species of fish consumed in the upper Tapajós region was 0.293 µg/g.

The abovementioned studies demonstrate that mercury exposure is a long-term and persistent problem in the region, representing a severe risk for the population. Despite the undeniable relevance of this topic in the public health agenda, there is a noticeable scarcity of information about mercury exposure in the Munduruku group as well as in other indigenous people living in the Amazon. In the last two years, the Munduruku have suffered as a consequence of the anti-environmental policies proposed by the Brazilian government, especially Bill 191/2020, that aims to regulate the mining activities in protected areas of Amazon, including Indigenous Lands and Conservation Units [70]. Beyond the Munduruku, the Yanomami are also under violent attack with the invasion of the traditional territories and rights violation, but also with threats, physical attacks, setting fire to Indigenous leaders' homes, shootings, and deaths [71].

With this critical scenario in mind, the primary objective of this article is to present the methodological background, as well as to share an overview of the principal results, including the sociodemographic characterization, the general health situation in the villages, and to assess the chronic mercury exposure in the Munduruku Indigenous people, living in the Middle-Tapajos Region, Brazilian Amazon.

2. Materials and Methods

2.1. Research's Background

Given mercury's ability to contaminate the environment, as described in the previous section, and the increasing presence of *garimpeiros* (gold miners) in the area (as can be seen in Figure 1), the *Pariri* Indigenous Association (representing the Munduruku indigenous people living in the Middle-Tapajós Region) sent a letter to the Oswaldo Cruz Foundation to request an assessment of mercury contamination in their Indigenous territory. In response, a multidisciplinary, specialized team was formed to put together a comprehensive plan of action and then to deliver the fieldwork.

2.2. Population and Study Area

The Munduruku people are linked to the Tupi linguistic branch, in the Munduruku linguistic family. As people of a warrior tradition, the Munduruku have culturally dominated the Tapajós valley region, which in the early days of contact and during the 19th century was known as *Mundurukânia*. Today, the group inhabits lands located in the states of Pará, Amazonas, and Mato Grosso. These people are concentrated mainly in savanna regions of the Amazon rainforest, on the banks of navigable rivers [72,73].

The *Sawré Muybu* Indigenous Land (IL) (also known as *Pimental*), which the Munduruku people traditionally occupy, spans only 178,173 hectares and is located in the municipalities of *Itaituba* and *Trairão*, in the state of Pará (Figure 1). The area's demarcation process began in 2007, but the demarcation process remains unfinished. In the area covered by the *Sawré Muybu* IL, there are eight indigenous villages summing up almost 800 people.

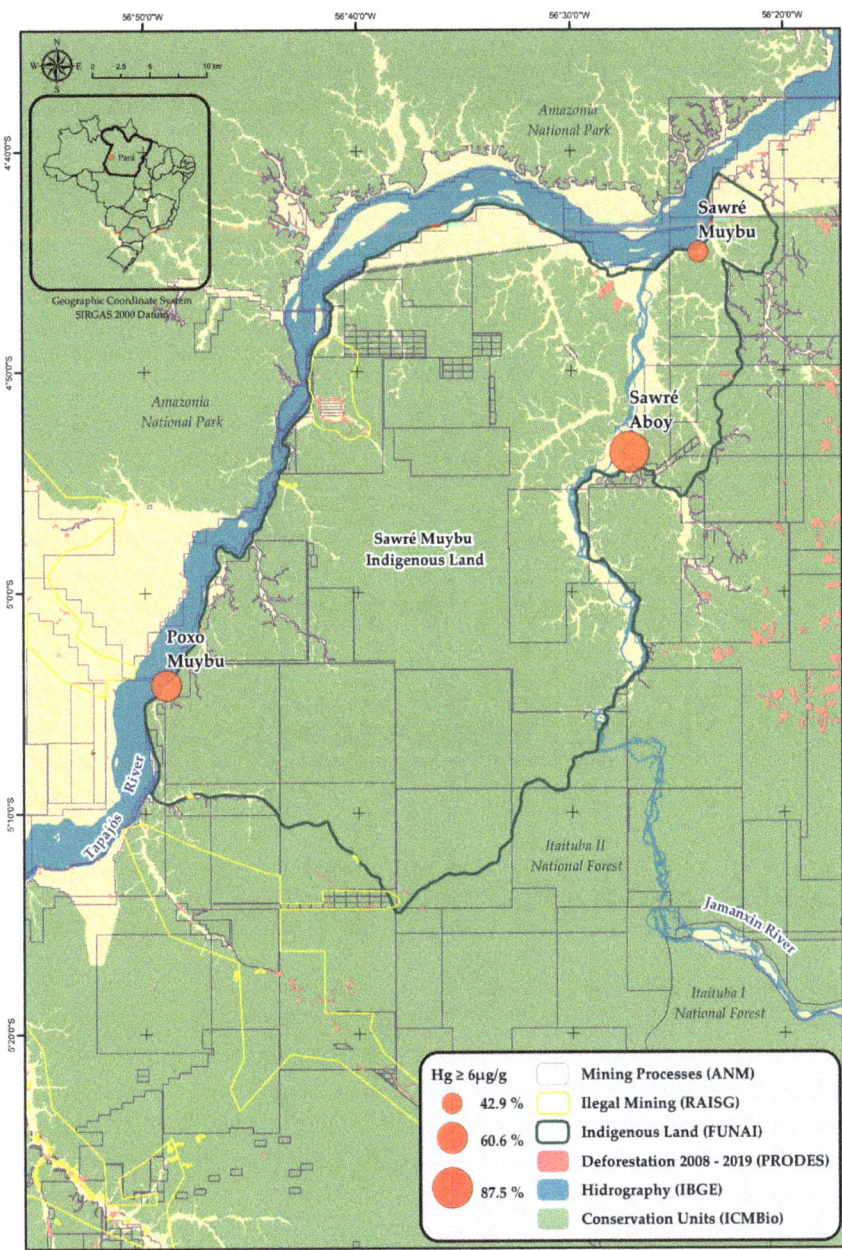

Figure 1. Study area highlighting the investigated villages: *Sawré Muybu* (downstream), and *Poxo Muybu* (upstream) on the margins of Tapajós River, and *Sawré Aboy* (downstream) on the margins of Jamanxin River. Polygons with gray lines correspond to areas with legal requirements for mining. Polygons with yellow lines correspond to illegal mining activities. *Sawré Muybu* Indigenous Land, Pará, Amazon, Brazil, 2019.

2.3. Study Design

A cross-sectional study was carried out in three villages selected from *Sawré Muybu* IL (*Sawré Muybu*, *Poxo Muybu*, and *Sawré Aboy*), according to the request of the *Pariri* Indigenous Association (Figure 1). In the designated villages, we conducted a population census, and all residents were invited to participate in the study. There was no refusal and, therefore, no probabilistic sampling methods were used to include participants.

2.4. Fieldwork Steps

The fieldwork investigation was carried out by a multidisciplinary and specialized team between 29 October and 9 November 2019, during the dry season. The investigation included: (i) sociodemographic characterization of the participants (i.e., family income, schooling, family composition, physical structure of the houses); (ii) health assessment (i.e., anthropometric indicators, estimates of the prevalence of chronic non-communicable diseases, and sexually transmitted diseases, as well as neurological and child development evaluations); (iii) genetic polymorphism analysis; (iv) hair mercury determination; and (v) fish mercury determination.

2.5. Sociodemographic Characterization

We organized the individual survey questionnaire in four sections:

(a) The first section (head of household's data) characterizes the physical and demographic structure of the homes visited, including the length of residence, materials used for building the house, sources of drinking water and presence of bathroom, occupational activities, income, social benefits, number of years in education for the head of household, and the dietary pattern of inhabitants, with an emphasis on fish consumption.
(b) The second section (family members' data) characterizes the health of the family and the community, including a history of previous hospitalizations; previous Malaria treatment, and history of contact with mercury from *garimpos*.
(c) The third section (women's health data) questionnaire addressed reproductive history, the number of children, pregnant, and breastfeeding status.
(d) The fourth section (children's data) explores the birth conditions, access to pediatric health care, previous hospitalizations, recent history of diarrhea and acute respiratory infection, and vaccination history.

The interviews were conducted based on a data collection instrument specially prepared for this study, based on previous experiences of our research group [74–76]. The questionnaire was applied with the support of Indigenous Health Agents who work in the communities and/or with the support of the local Indigenous leaders, such as chiefs and teachers.

Responses were recorded on electronic forms with the aid of portable electronic devices (tablets), and there was no use of paper forms. After conducting home visits and interviews, families were invited to participate in a standardized clinical and laboratory evaluation, described in the next section.

2.6. Health Assessment

(1) Anthropometric Measurements

All participants had their weight and height recorded. For weight measurement, an electronic scale was used (SECA®, model 770, Vogel & Halke, Hamburg, Germany), with a maximum capacity of 150 kg and accuracy of 0.1 kg. Infants had their weight measured on the mother's lap, using the electronic scale's mother-baby function. To measure height, a vertical anthropometer or stadiometer of the Alturexata® brand was used (with a dorsal adapter for infantometer and 0.1 cm precision for younger children). Children with special physical needs or suffering from problems in neuro-psychomotor development were excluded from anthropometric analyses. Finally, the body mass index

(BMI), expressed in kg/m², for those over 12 years old, and the Z-scores (adjusted for sex and age), for children from 0 to 5 years old, were calculated according to the WHO reference population [77].

(b) Hemoglobin Dosage

The measurement of capillary hemoglobin was assessed using the HemoCue® device (HemoCue®, model HB 301-System, Angelholm, Sweden) without the need to collect and store venous blood samples. Hemoglobin levels were classified as normal according to the age group and sex of the participants: (a) children aged 2 to 6 years: between 11.5 to 13.5 g/dL; (b) children from 6 to 12 years old: between 11.5 to 15.5 g/dL; (c) men > 12 years: between 14 to 18 g/dL; (d) women > 12 years: between 12 to 16 g/dL; (e) pregnant women > 11.0 g/dL. Values below the levels indicated above were considered indicators of anemia [78].

(c) Glucose Dosage

Plasma levels of casual blood glucose (measured during the interview, without considering the interval since the last meal and without fasting requirement) were taken from participants over 12 years of age. Was used the Accu-Chek Active® blood glucose monitor (Roche, Indianapolis, IN, USA), auto coded, with photometric biosensor technology (reflectance), and measurement range between 10 to 600 mg/dL, according to the manufacturer's specifications.

(d) Blood Pressure Measurement

Blood pressure was measured using an automatic pulse blood pressure monitor, Omron Model Hem-631INT (Omron Healthcare INC, Lake Forest, IL, USA). Blood pressure was measured twice, with the device placed on the left wrist of participants over 12 years of age, during the clinical evaluation. Participants remained seated with both feet flat on the floor, with the left forearm resting on the chest's anterior part, during measurements. The means of the two measures of systolic blood pressure (SBP) and diastolic blood pressure (DBP) were used to classify the participants. According to the Brazilian Guideline for Hypertension of the Brazilian Society of Cardiology [79], hypertension is considered when SBP values are $\geq$140 mmHg and/or DBP $\geq$ 90 mmHg. Individuals with an SBP between 130 and 139 and a DBP between 85 and 89 mmHg are considered as prehypertension, as this population has a consistently higher risk of CV disease, coronary artery disease, and stroke than the population with levels between 120 and 129 or 80 and 84 mmHg. For this reason, we included in this study all individuals who had an SBP $\geq$ 130 and a DBP $\geq$ 85 mmHg in the high blood pressure group [79].

(e) Prevalence of Sexually Transmitted Diseases

Rapid tests for HIV, hepatitis B and C, and syphilis were performed on indigenous people over 12 years old of both sexes. Following the Ministry of Health's testing protocol, the HIV tests used were ABON HIV® (Abon Biopharm, Hangzhou, China). In cases with differences in the results, the MEDTESTE HIV® kit (Hangzhou Biotest Biotech Co., Hangzhou, China) was used to resolve disagreements. The hepatitis B test used was BIOCLIN® (Bioclin, Belo Horizonte, MG, Brazil), and for hepatitis C the rapid test from the company ALERE® (BioMérieux, Durham, NC, USA) was used. Finally, for syphilis, the Bio Syphilis kit brand BIOCLIN® (Bioclin, Belo Horizonte, MG, Brazil) was used.

As the Ministry of Health recommended, participants were advised on testing and sexually transmitted diseases before testing. When necessary, counseling was given with results alongside referral to specialized services.

(f) Neurological Evaluation

This component of the study sought to elucidate neurological abnormalities in indigenous older than 12 years, evaluating changes in the Central Nervous System (CNS) and the Peripheral Nervous System (PNS). All participants were submitted to a systemized neurological examination protocol, specially developed for this research, to make the evaluation feasible in adverse conditions in the fieldwork in the villages. The evaluations were conducted by a neurologist (RAAO) familiar with clinical neurological semiology and duly trained to apply the protocol and use the examining instruments.

Abnormalities in the somatosensory, motor, and cognitive function were assessed by the following neurological parameters: static balance and gait assessment; examination of cranial nerves, motricity, somatic sensitivity, and cognitive assessment. The detailed methodology can be accessed elsewhere [80].

(g) Pediatric Evaluation

Indigenous children from 0 to 11 years old were submitted to a pediatric evaluation to analyze immunization coverage and growth curves. The analysis was performed from data on child vaccination registration booklets and booklets for prenatal care. Additionally, we performed an analysis of the nutritional status by weight and height/length measurements (described in the section anthropometric measurements). According to the World Health Organization, the measures of weight and height/length of children under five years old were transformed into Z-scores (adjusted for sex and age), and the weight for age (W/A), height for age (H/A), and body mass index for age (BMI/A) indices were calculated, according to the reference population proposed by the WHO [77].

Moreover, the Denver II Neurodevelopment Screening Test was carried out to evaluate children aged from 0 to 6 years without morphological abnormalities. The test is divided into four areas: (i) personal-social (aspects of the child's socialization inside and outside the family environment); (ii) fine motor skills (hand-eye coordination, manipulation of small objects, etc.); (iii) language (production of sounds, ability to recognize, understand and use language); and (iv) gross motor skills (body motor control, sitting, walking, jumping and the other movements performed by large muscles). The detailed methodology can be accessed in Hofer et al. [81].

2.7. Genetic Polymorphism Analysis

Epithelial cell samples were collected from the oral mucosa to analyze genetic polymorphisms in genes related to mercury metabolism in the human body. The cells were collected using a sterile swab (i.e., disposable cotton swab) and stored in a buffered solution (i.e., a phosphate-buffered saline solution used to prevent changes in the pH and the oral mucosa cells disruption) under refrigeration until arrival at the laboratory. The genomic DNA present in the samples was extracted with an extraction kit (Qiagen Sciences, Germantown, MD, USA), following the procedures recommended by the manufacturer.

The analyses were processed at the Laboratory of Pharmaceutical Science-LAPESF (https://lapesfuezo.wixsite.com/website, accessed on 19 June 2021) of the State University of the West Zone-UEZO, in Rio de Janeiro-RJ, using the polymerase chain reaction technique (PCR) in real-time, as previously described [82,83]. The *TNF-α* $-1031T>C$ *(rs1799964)*, -857 *C>T (rs1799724)* and -308 *G>A (rs1800629)*, *IL6* -174 *G>C (rs1800795)*, *ALAD 177 C>G (rs1800435)*, *GSTP1 A>G (rs1695)*, *VDR FokI C>T (rs2228570)* and *MMP2* -735 *C>T (rs2285053)* polymorphisms were genotyped using a validated TaqMan allelic discrimination assay obtained from Applied Biosystems (C_7514871_10, C_11918223_10, C_7514879_10, C_1839697_20, C_11495146_10, C_3237198_20, C_12060045_20 and C_26734093_20, respectively). In each reaction, two negative (blank) and two positive standardized controls of each genotype were used to guarantee the genotyping quality. The allele frequency and genotype distribution were derived by gene counting and deviations from the Hardy–Weinberg equilibrium (HWE) were assessed by the goodness-of-fit χ^2 test. The frequencies between the groups were compared using the χ^2 test or, when appropriate, the Fisher's exact test.

2.8. Determination of Mercury Levels

(a) Hair Samples

Hair samples were collected from all participants, removed close to the scalp in the occipital region with the aid of stainless-steel dissection scissors. The samples were stored in paper envelopes, individually identified, and sent for analysis of total mercury levels (THg) in the Toxicology Laboratory, in the Environment Section of the Evandro Chagas Institute (IEC), in Belém-Pará, Brazil.

In the laboratory, the samples were washed with Extran diluted 100 fold (Merck KGaA, Darmstadt, Germany) to remove any exogenous contamination. After drying, the samples were finely homogenized in glass flasks, prior to weighing. The methodology developed by Akagi [84] involves the steps of chemical opening, wet digestion, and subsequent reduction with $SnCl_2$ for quantification of THg in Cold Vapor Atomic Absorption Spectrometer (CVAAS).

Thus, approximately 10 mg of hair was weighed in 50 mL volumetric flasks and subsequently digested with a solution containing 1 mL of deionized water (Milli-Q Milipore®), 2 mL of concentrated HNO_3 and $HClO_4$ (1:1), and 5 mL of H_2SO_4 on a plate heated at 230 °C for 30 min. About 5 mL of each sample solution was used to quantify THg in the CVAAS Mercury Analyzer Hg-201 (Sanso Seisakusho Co., Nagahama, Japan). To guarantee the Quality Assurance (QA)/Quality Control (QC), for the hair mercury analysis we used the following parameters: (i) the Human Hair Certified Reference Material (IAEA-86), whose average recovery rate was 101% ($n = 8$, recovery ranging from 83.4 to 106.6%) from the International Atomic Energy Agency; (ii) a method blank; (iii) a 6-point calibration curve (concentration ranging from 0.4 to 4 ng/g); and (iv) the relative standard deviation (RSD) of 8.32%. Sample replicates ($n = 10$), whose RSD was 2.49%, were also randomly selected. The detection and quantification limits (LOD/LOQ) obtained were 0.0083 ng/mg and 0.027 ng/mg, respectively. We considered the mercury level of ≥ 6.0 µg/g in hair samples as a health risk indicator, following the safety dose recognized by WHO [69] and the parameters of previous studies carried out in the Amazon region [20,47,76,85]. This methodology for determining mercury in hair samples was previous described by Akagi [84] and Marinho et al. [20].

(b) Fish Samples

Fish samples were caught at different points at the Tapajós River (4°40′48.33″ S 56°32′35.77″ W; 4°45′21.91″ S 56°27′2.80″ W; 4°42′27.99″ S 56°37′25.62″ W; 4°44′29.18″ S; 56°27′2.79″ W), along the Jamanxin River (4°54′10.83″ S 56°28′2.02″ W; 4°53′24.34″ S; 56°27′20.33″ W) and at its mouth (4°44′56.17″ S 56°26′5.67″ W), with the help of indigenous Munduruku fishermen. A hook or gillnet was used for fishing by the studied communities. The captured fish were identified in the field, photographed, weighed, and measured for total and standard length. Then, about 10 g of muscle tissue was collected from each fish, packed and labeled in plastic bags, and stored in liquid nitrogen to be further analyzed.

Total Hg determination in the fish muscle tissue was obtained using the methodology proposed by Akagi et al. [84], using semi-automatic mercury analyzer equipment, Analyzer Model Hg-201 (Sanso Seisakusho Co., Ltd., Nagahama, Japan) [86]. The detailed methodology can be accessed in Vasconcellos et al. [87].

2.9. Health Risk Assessment

The health risk assessment was carried out according to the methodology proposed by WHO [88]. Four different scenarios of methylmercury exposure were built from the data collected for a counterfactual analysis: (i) for fish consumed in the rainy season; (ii) for fish consumed in the dry season; (iii) current, considering an empirical method to estimate fish consumption; and (iv) critical, regarding the consumption from the 95th percentile of mercury concentrations in piscivorous and non-piscivorous species. The risk ratio was calculated from the ratio between "the estimated MeHg intake" in the four different scenarios and the reference doses proposed by FAO/WHO [25] and U.S. EPA [26]. The detailed methodology can be accessed in Vasconcellos et al. [87].

2.10. Statistical Analysis

We carried out a descriptive analysis with the characterization of the study population, including household characteristics (family monthly income, infrastructure of the house, and sanitation) as well as sociodemographic characteristics (gender, age group, marital status, schooling), and clinical data of the study population (hemoglobin, glucose and blood pressure levels, as well as body mass index). Moreover, we presented the hair mercury levels of the participants according to the sociodemographic and clinical studied variables.

In order to contrast clinical and sociodemographic variables with hair mercury exposure ≥ 6.0 µg/g versus hair mercury exposure <6.0 µg/g, we used Pearson's Chi-squared test or Fisher's exact test. We also used the Kruskal–Wallis test to evaluate the differences in Hg levels between villages. To compare the hemoglobin, glucose, and blood pressure mean levels, as well as height, weight, and body mass index between the participants in the mercury exposure groups ≥ 6.0 µg/g x ≤ 6.0 µg/g, we used the F-Test.

To estimate the prevalence of human mercury exposure in the study area, we considered the number of people who presented mercury levels ≥ 6.0 µg/g as the numerator, and the denominator as the population sampled in the study region, according to the villages: *Sawré Muybu*, *Poxo Muybu*, and *Sawré Aboy*.

To explore factors associated with mercury exposure, we used the logistic regression model with conditional Prevalence Ratio (PR). In this study, PR was used as an association measure with the respective 95% confidence intervals. After the initial crude analysis, the variables with a significant association with the hair-Hg level were further adjusted in this model. According to Bastos et al. [89], the logistic regression model provides a better estimate of the prevalence ratios, representing a more significant measure of effects for cross-sectional studies. The 95% confidence intervals were obtained using the delta method and clustered bootstrap. A significance level of 5% ($p < 0.05$) was considered for all statistical tests used. The data were analyzed using the free statistical software R version 3.6.3 (http://www.r-project.org, accessed on 31 March 2021) and the package "prLogistic" [90].

3. Results

3.1. Principal Research Results

3.1.1. Sociodemographic Characterization

During fieldwork, the research team visited 35 households in the Sawré Muybu Indigenous Land: 8 in Poxo Muybu village, 7 in Sawré Aboy village, and 20 in Sawré Muybu village (Table 1).

In most families, regular incomes from salaries and or social benefits from the government were reported. The average monthly income of families was USD 294.10 ranging from USD 201.0 to USD 414.5, with averages in *Poxo Muybu* slightly higher and *Sawré Aboy* somewhat lower. Concerning physical structure, approximately 60.0% of households had dry straw-covered roofs, 65.7% had wooden or brick walls, and 80.0% had dirt floors (Table 1).

There was no bathroom for exclusive family use in any of the houses visited. Most of the heads of households reported that their family members use a collective cesspool available in the community. The vast majority of interviewers (91.4%) reported that the water consumed by the families came from rivers/streams, and 68.6% reported there is no type of water treatment in the villages. Only three homes from *Sawré Muybu* village reported an artesian well as water supply (Table 1).

Regarding the length of residence, in the *Sawré Muybu* village, most families (70.0%) had been settled for more than five years, while families had been set in the *Sawré Aboy* and *Poxo Muybu* villages up their homes within the last three years. In *Sawré Muybu*, there were between one and two adults in most households (75.0%), while in *Poxo Muybu*, half of the households were composed of more than four adults. In most of the households visited, there were between two and three children under five years old.

Table 1. Household characteristics, according to family monthly income, physical structure (flooring, walls, roofing) and sanitation, *Sawré Muybu* Indigenous Land, Pará, Amazon, Brazil, 2019.

Characteristics	Overall n = 35	Village		
		Poxo Muybu n = 8	Sawre Aboy n = 7	Sawre Muybu n = 20
Family Monthly income (USD) Median (Q1, Q3)	294.1 (201.0–414.5)	355.7 (274.5–728.4)	235.3 (203.9–485.3)	284.3 (166.7–382.0)
Regular salary				
Yes	24 (68.6%)	6 (75.0%)	6 (85.7%)	14 (75.0%)
No	11 (31.4%)	2 (25.0%)	1 (14.3%)	6 (25.0%)
Regular cash transfer				
Yes	24 (68.6%)	6 (75.0%)	6 (85.7%)	12 (60.0%)
No	11 (31.4%)	2 (25.0%)	1 (14.3%)	8 (40.0%)
Roof cover				
Dry straw	21 (60.0%)	8 (100.0%)	7 (100.0%)	6 (30.0%)
Zinc or asbestos	13 (37.1%)	0 (0.0%)	0 (0.0%)	13 (65.0%)
Clay	1 (2.9%)	0 (0.0%)	0 (0.0%)	1 (5.0%)
Wallcovering				
Wood or brick	23 (65.7%)	3 (37.5%)	1 (14.3%)	19 (95.0%)
Dry straw or canvas	12 (34.3%)	5 (62.5%)	6 (85.7%)	1 (5.0%)
Floor				
Dirt floor	28 (80.0%)	8 (100.0%)	7 (100.0%)	13 (65.0%)
Cement or ceramic	6 (17.1%)	0 (0.0%)	0 (0.0%)	6 (30.0%)
Wood	1 (2.9%)	0 (0.0%)	0 (0.0%)	1 (5.0%)
Disposal of human waste				
Collective cesspool	25 (71.4%)	6 (75.0%)	7 (100.0%)	12 (60.0%)
Forest	4 (11.4%)	1 (12.5%)	0 (0.0%)	3 (15.0%)
Individual cesspool	2 (5.7%)	0 (0.0%)	0 (0.0%)	2 (10.0%)
Bathroom outside	2 (5.7%)	0 (0.0%)	0 (0.0%)	2 (10.0%)
River/stream	2 (5.7%)	1 (12.5%)	0 (0.0%)	1 (5.0%)
Water source				
River/stream	32 (91.4%)	8 (100.0%)	7 (100.0%)	17 (85.0%)
Artesian well	3 (8.6%)	0 (0.0%)	0 (0.0%)	3 (15.0%)
Water treatment				
Yes	11 (31.4%)	1 (12.5%)	4 (57.1%)	6 (30.0%)
No	24 (68.6%)	7 (87.5%)	3 (42.9%)	14 (70.0%)

Two hundred participants were interviewed and clinically evaluated, 66 from *Poxo Muybu*, 40 from *Sawré Aboy*, and 94 from the *Sawré Muybu* village. The study population was predominantly young, with an average age of 18 (median: 14; IQR: 6, 14, and 25 years old). Adults over 45 years old represented only 7.0% of all study population. In general, the presence of female participants was more evident, except for *Sawré Aboy* village, where 48.0% were women (Table 2).

Almost three-quarters (71%) of the participants had only 1 to 9 years of schooling, with more years spent in education (10 years or more) observed in the *Poxo Muybu* village (21%). The most frequent marital status was married (39% of the participants), being more frequent in the *Sawré Muybu* village (41%) (Table 2).

Considering the principal occupational activities, participants above 12 years old (n = 112) reported working as a farmer (38.7%), carrying out activities at home (37.8%), student (32.4%), fisherman (18.9%), teacher (10.8%), extractors of natural forest products/hunter (9.9%), bricklayer (5.4%), retired (3.6%). Only one participant designated themself as unemployed. It is worth remembering that participants can do more than one activity simultaneously.

Table 2. Sociodemographic and clinical characteristics of the study population, according to villages of residence, *Sawré Muybu* Indigenous Land, Pará, Amazon, Brazil, 2019.

Characteristics	Overall n = 200	Village			p-Value [1]
		Poxo Muybu n = 66	Sawre Aboy n = 40	Sawre Muybu n = 94	
Age mean (in years)	18	16	17	18	0.820
Minimum–Maximum	(0–73)	(0–59)	(0–72)	(0–73)	
Sex					0.570
Female	109 (55.0%)	36 (55.0%)	19 (48.0%)	54 (57.0%)	
Male	91 (45.0%)	30 (45.0%)	21 (52.0%)	40 (43.0%)	
Age group					0.100
Under 12 years	88 (44.0%)	31 (47.0%)	16 (40.0%)	41 (44.0%)	
13–19 years	38 (19.0%)	15 (23.0%)	12 (30.0%)	11 (12.0%)	
20–29 years	39 (20.0%)	8 (12.0%)	5 (12.0%)	26 (28.0%)	
30–44 years	21 (10.0%)	8 (12.0%)	5 (12.0%)	8 (8.5%)	
45 years and over	14 (7.0%)	4 (6.1%)	2 (5.0%)	8 (8.5%)	
Schooling					0.390
Illiterate	4 (2.0%)	1 (1.5%)	1 (2.5%)	2 (2.1%)	
1–9 years	142 (71.0%)	42 (64.0%)	31 (78.0%)	69 (73.0%)	
≥10 years	26 (13.0%)	14 (21.0%)	3 (7.5%)	9 (9.6%)	
Not applicable	28 (14.0%)	9 (14.0%)	5 (12.0%)	14 (15.0%)	
Marital status					0.049
Single	30 (15.0%)	15 (23.0%)	9 (22.0%)	6 (6.4%)	
Married	78 (39.0%)	23 (35.0%)	16 (40.0%)	39 (41.0%)	
Widow(er)	6 (3.0%)	1 (1.5%)	1 (2.5%)	4 (4.3%)	
Not applicable	86 (43.0%)	27 (41.0%)	14 (35.0%)	45 (48.0%)	
Anemia					0.054
Yes	66 (33.0%)	22 (33.0%)	19 (48.0%)	25 (27.0%)	
No	129 (64.0%)	42 (64.0%)	19 (48.0%)	68 (72.0%)	
Missing	5 (2.5%)	2 (3.0%)	2 (5.0%)	1 (1.0%)	
Body Mass Index [2]					0.827
<18.5	4 (3.5%)	2 (5.4%)	1 (4.2%)	1 (1.9%)	
18.5–24.9	73 (63.5%)	22 (59.5%)	17 (70.8%)	34 (63.0%)	
25.0–29.9	34 (29.6%)	11 (29.7%)	5 (20.8%)	18 (33.3%)	
≥30.0	4 (3.5%)	2 (5.4%)	1 (4.2%)	1 (1.9%)	

[1] Pearson's Chi-squared test; Fisher's exact test; [2] Only to indigenous ≥12 years old.

Ten men (seven from *Sawré Muybu*, two from *Poxo Muybu*, and one from *Sawré Aboy*) aged 26 to 67 years (mean 38 years) reported working previously in mining activities. Half of them reported having worked at mining for less than five years. Seven participants had between 1 and 9 years of schooling, and three had more than ten years. The median mercury level in the hair samples of these participants was 6.8 µg/g (mean: 8.8; standard deviation: 4.9; range: 3.5 to 18.7), and 6 of them had levels above 6.0 µg/g.

Interviews regarding diet revealed that almost all families (96%) eat fish frequently (average three times per week). Moreover, the study participants related that fish consumption varies according to the season (dry or rainy) and fish availability in the region's rivers. During the rainy season, the most consumed fish species are *aracu* (family *Anostomidae*), *surubim* (*Pseudoplatystoma* spp.), *barbado* (*Pinirampus pirinampu*), *matrincha* (*Brycon* spp.), *tucunaré* (*Cichla* spp.), and *caratinga* (*Geophagus* spp.). During the dry season, the most consumed species are *caratinga*, *curimata* (*Prochilodus nigricans*), *surubim*, *pacu* (family *Serrasalmidae*), *barbado*, *mandiá* (*Pimelodina flavipinnis*), *aracu*, *aruana* (*Osteoglossum bicirrhosum*), *piranha* (family *Serrasalmidae*), and *matrincha*.

3.1.2. Health Assessment

Regarding the self-reported morbidities, in the month before our team's visit, we highlight the high frequency of flu/colds, fever, and diarrhea that were mentioned by 44.8%, 17.2%, and 12.0% of the participants, respectively.

Considering previous hospitalizations, 69 individuals (35.0% of the study population) reported at least one hospitalization throughout their lives. The highest frequencies were reported in *Sawré Muybu* (53.2%) and *Sawré Aboy* (35.0%) villages. While in *Poxo Muybu*, only 10.6% of the participants reported previous hospitalization. Sixty-six participants (31.0% of all interviews) reported at least one previous treatment for Malaria. The highest proportions of previous treatment for Malaria were identified in *Sawré Muybu* (41.5%) and *Sawré Aboy* (32.5%) villages. In *Poxo Muybu*, 21.2% of participants had previous treatment for Malaria.

There were 53 women of childbearing age in the study area. Two-thirds of women reported having given birth at least once. For them, the number of completed pregnancies ranged from 1 to 14, and almost 70% reported they have less than seven children. Five women were pregnant, and 17 reported were breastfeeding. For all women within the study population, including those aged above 49 years old, three-quarters having given birth at least once, one-fifth reported previous spontaneous abortion, while almost half mentioned at least one fetal death. For more details, see Kempton et al. [91].

3.1.3. Anthropometric Measurements

The body mass index (BMI) analysis shows that 63.5% of the adults are within normal ranges of weight and height (BMI range 18.5 to 24.9 Kg/m^2). However, the analysis by village reveals that the population of *Sawré Muybu* represents most cases of being overweight (BMI range 25.0 to 29.9 kg/m^2), while *Poxo Muybu* reported the highest rate of obesity (BMI $\geq$ 30.0 km/m^2) (Table 2).

3.1.4. Hemoglobin Levels

The analysis of hemoglobin levels reveals that one-third (33.0%) of the participants had anemia. The prevalence varies between the villages, with the most challenging scenario was observed in the *Sawré Aboy* village, where 48% of the participants had anemia (Table 2).

Anemia was present in 21.1% of the children under five years old, more evident among children aged 6 to 12 months, whose 66.7% had hemoglobin levels under 11.5 g/dL. This index suggests a prominent micronutrient deficit when exclusive breastfeeding is interrupted. Despite the variations of the hemoglobin levels between the studied villages, there were no associations with Hg levels.

3.1.5. Glucose Levels

Due to logistical and operational problems, the dosage of glucose levels was carried out only among 36 adults living in the *Poxo Muybu* village. Plasma levels of casual blood glucose ranged from 94.0 to 197.0 mg/dL (median: 110.0 mg/dL; standard deviation: 18.4 mg/dL), not exceeding the 200 mg/dL limit established as a reference to indicate a diagnostic suspicion of diabetes mellitus. Moreover, the glucose levels were not associated with Hg levels.

3.1.6. Blood Pressure Levels

Looking at the blood pressure levels of those over 12 years old, we observed that only 13 participants presented hypertension or pre-hypertension, understood as systolic blood pressure (SBP) above 130 mmHg, and diastolic blood pressure (DBP) above 85 mmHg. Thus, on average, the prevalence of hypertension was 11.3%. Again, there was variation between the villages, and the problem was more prominent in the *Sawré Muybu* village, where 14.5% of the participants have high blood pressure levels. In addition, the highest levels of systolic blood pressure and diastolic blood pressure have been associated with hair mercury levels above 6.0 µg/g (F-Test: 4.157, *p*-value: 0.044; and F-Test: 4.363, *p*-value: 0.039, for SBP and DBP, respectively).

3.1.7. Sexually Transmitted Diseases

One hundred and twenty-three rapid tests were carried out to investigate hepatitis B infection. A 10-year-old girl living in the *Poxo Muybu* village presented a positive result (0.8%). Following the Brazilian Ministry of Health guidelines, our team repeated the test, and in the end, the test proved to be non-reactive. One hundred and twenty rapid tests were carried out to investigate infection by the hepatitis C virus. All of them proved to be non-reactive.

One hundred and twenty-three rapid HIV tests were carried out. Of these, five showed positive results in the first test (4.1%): a 19-year-old woman, a 23-year-old man, and a 39-year-old man, living in the *Sawré Aboy* village, and two men (one is 27 and the other is 30 years old), living in *Sawré Muybu* village. Following the Brazilian Ministry of Health guidelines, our team repeated the tests twice, using kits from different manufacturers. In the end, only the 19-year-old woman from the *Sawré Aboy* village remained undetermined. We referred all participants who presented problems in the tests to the Unified Health System (SUS) for follow-up. Moreover, 123 tests were carried out to investigate infection of Treponema pallidum, the causative agent of syphilis, all of which proved to be non-reactive.

3.1.8. Neurological Evaluation

Somatosensory, motor, and cognitive abnormalities were investigated in indigenous over 12 years old in the three studied villages. The principal abnormalities—which correspond to somatosensory dysfunctions and alterations in verbal fluency—were more prevalent in participants with mercury exposure levels above 10 µg/g who live in the *Sawré Aboy* and *Sawré Muybu* villages. Moreover, participants with higher levels of mercury exposure presented the highest prevalence of cognitive development deficits, in addition to motor signs such as cerebellar ataxia. These findings suggest a worsened motor and cognitive function resulting from neurotoxicity due to chronic Hg exposure. Further details can be seen in Oliveira et al. [80].

3.1.9. Pediatric Evaluation

The pediatric evaluation revealed that less than half of the children had a complete vaccination schedule. Nine of the 55 eligible children under six years old showed problems in the neurodevelopment tests. The main observed problems include limitations in the language, fine motor and gross motor skills, and personal-social components of the test. Among the nine children who presented problems in the neurodevelopment tests, the average mercury levels in hair samples were 7.34 µg/g (median: 6.2; range from 2.4 to 19.6; standard deviation: 5.4 µg/g). In contrast, the average mercury levels for all children under 11 years were 6.9 (median: 5.5; range from 1.4 to 23.9; standard deviation: 4.8 µg/g).

We measured the weight and height/length of 42 children under 5 years old. The analysis of the Z-scores (adjusted for sex and age) revealed that on average, 26.2% presented with stunting (Z-scores < -2.0 to height for age), and 7.1% were underweight (Z-scores < -2.0 to weight for age), while 16.0% were at risk of being overweight (Z-scores > 1.0 to weight for height. Additional information can be seen in Hofer et al. [81].

3.1.10. Genetic Polymorphism Analysis

Polymorphisms in genes involved in mercury toxicity were analyzed and the efficiency of the genotyping ranged between 96.5% to 100% (192 participants). The distribution of studied polymorphisms was in Hardy–Weinberg equilibrium in the overall study population. The minor allele frequencies (MAF) of the *TNF-α* (rs1799964, rs1799724 and rs1800629), *IL-6* (rs1800795), *ALAD* (rs1800435), *GSTP1* (rs1695), *VDR* (rs2228570) and *MMP2* (rs2285053) in the population was 13.1%, 28.9%, 2.3%, 0.3%, 0.5%, 35.9%, 34.2%, and 12.4%, respectively. Table 3 shows the genotype distribution of the eight polymorphisms among the three villages. There were significant differences (*p*-value < 0.05) in the genotypic distribution among the three villages for the *TNF-α* rs1799964 and rs1800629, *GSTP1* rs1695, *VDR* rs2228570 and *MMP2* rs2285053 polymorphisms.

Table 3. Genotypic distribution of polymorphisms in villages, *Sawré Muybu* Indigenous Land, Pará, Amazon, Brazil, 2019.

Gene/SNP	Village	n *	Genotypic Distribution n (%)			p-Value **
TNF-α (Chromossome 6) rs1799964			TT	TC	CC	
	Poxo Muybu	61	56 (91.8)	4 (6.6)	1 (1.6)	
	Sawre Aboy	40	25 (62.5)	13 (32.5)	2 (5.0)	0.008
	Sawre Muybu	97	70 (72.1)	25 (25.8)	2 (2.1)	
rs1799724			CC	CT	TT	
	Poxo Muybu	62	31 (50.0)	27 (43.5)	4 (6.5)	
	Sawre Aboy	40	15 (37.5)	24 (60.0)	1 (2.5)	0.34
	Sawre Muybu	97	50 (51.5)	40 (41.3)	7 (7.2)	
rs1800629			GG	GA	AA	
	Poxo Muybu	56	56 (100)	0	0	
	Sawre Aboy	40	39 (97.5)	1 (2.5)	0	0.050
	Sawre Muybu	97	89 (91.8)	8 (8.2)	0	
IL6 (Chromosome 7) rs1800795			GG	GC	CC	
	Poxo Muybu	62	62 (100)	0	0	
	Sawre Aboy	40	40 (100)	0	0	0.59
	Sawre Muybu	97	96 (99.0)	1 (1.0)	0	
ALAD (Chromosome 9) rs1800435			CC	CG	GG	
	Poxo Muybu	56	56 (100)	0	0	
	Sawre Aboy	40	40 (100)	0	0	0.36
	Sawre Muybu	96	94 (97.9)	2 (2.1)	0	
GSTP1 (Chromosome 11) rs1695			AA	AG	GG	
	Poxo Muybu	62	37 (59.7)	24 (38.7)	1 (1.6)	
	Sawre Aboy	40	30 (75.0)	10 (25.0)	0	<0.0001
	Sawre Muybu	97	13 (13.4)	61 (62.9)	23 (23.7)	
VDR (Chromosome 12) rs2228570			CC	CT	TT	
	Poxo Muybu	62	27 (43.5)	29 (46.8)	6 (9.7)	
	Sawre Aboy	40	9 (22.5)	22 (55)	9 (22.5)	0.01
	Sawre Muybu	97	49 (50.5)	41 (42.3)	7 (7.2)	
MMP2 (Chromosome 16) rs2285053			CC	CT	TT	
	Poxo Muybu	62	58 (93.5)	4 (6.5)	0	
	Sawre Aboy	40	34 (85.0)	6 (15.0)	0	<0.0001
	Sawre Muybu	96	58 (60.4)	37 (38.5)	1 (1.1)	

* *n* is the number of examined samples of the participants for each polymorphism. Differences in sample sizes are due to available data from PCR amplification for each polymorphism. ** *p*-value from Chi-square test (Pearson *p*-value) or Fisher's exact test.

Each gene/polymorphism will be evaluated in the context of chronic mercury exposure and on the health situation of the Munduruku population in further publications. Firstly, regarding *ALAD* (rs1800435) polymorphism, two individuals from the *Sawré Muybu* village were heterozygous and presented high mercury concentrations, as well as severe symptoms of chronic mercury exposure. For more details, see Perini et al. [92].

3.2. Determination of Mercury Levels

3.2.1. Hair Samples

Hair samples analysis showed mercury levels ranging from 1.42 to 23.9 µg/g. The median mercury level for the entire population was 6.6 µg/g (mean: 7.7; standard deviation: 4.5, Q1: 4.5; Q3: 9.5). There were statistically significant variations between the villages: *Sawré Muybu* (5.2 µg/g), *Poxo Muybu* (6.6 µg/g), and *Sawré Aboy* (11.5 µg/g) (Kruskal–Wallis = 42.2; p-value < 0.001); and between adults and children (Kruskal–Wallis = 10.4; p-value = 0.001) (Table 4, Figure 2).

Table 4. Hair Mercury levels (mean, standard deviation, median, minimum, maximum, and prevalence % of ≥ 6 µg/g), according to the villages of residence (*Sawré Muybu, Poxo Muybu, Sawré Aboy*), by age group and sex, *Sawré Muybu* Indigenous Land, Pará, Amazon, Brazil, 2019.

Villages	n	Mean	Standard Deviation	Median	Minimum	Maximum	≥ 6.0 µg/g
Sawré Muybu							
Children < 12 years	38	5.9	4.7	4.3	1.6	22.1	28.9
Adults $\geq$ 12 years							
Male	24	7.3	3.2	6.9	2.6	16.0	66.7
Female	29	6.3	3.5	4.7	2.0	14.1	41.4
Total	91	6.4	4.0	5.2	1.6	22.1	42.9
Poxo Muybu							
Children < 12 years	28	5.9	2.6	5.8	1.4	11.8	46.4
Adults $\geq$ 12 years							
Male	18	7.1	2.3	7.3	2.8	11.9	61.1
Female	20	7.6	2.2	7.3	4.2	12.9	80.0
Total	66	6.8	2.5	6.6	1.4	12.9	60.6
Sawré Aboy							
Children < 12 years	15	11.0	5.7	10.1	2.6	23.9	80.0
Adults $\geq$ 12 years							
Male	14	13.6	5.4	14.2	4.8	22.8	92.9
Female	11	12.1	4.1	11.9	5.0	20.2	90.9
Total	40	12.2	5.3	11.5	2.6	23.9	87.5
All Villages							
Children < 12 years	81	6.9	4.8	5.5	1.4	23.9	44.4
Adults $\geq$ 12 years							
Male	56	8.8	4.6	7.5	2.6	22.8	71.4
Female	60	7.8	3.8	7.3	2.0	20.2	63.3
Total	197	7.7	4.5	6.6	1.4	23.9	57.9

On average, the prevalence of exposure above 6.0 µg/g for all villages was 57.9%. In the *Sawré Muybu* village, we observed the lowest prevalence (42.9%), while in the *Sawré Aboy* village, was reported the highest (87.5%).

In addition, the mercury average levels among children (5.9 µg/g) were slightly lower than adults (7.3 and 6.3 µg/g for men and women, respectively), in the *Sawré Muybu* village. It is worth remembering that the highest mercury level (22.1 µg/g), in the *Sawré Muybu*, was reported in a 5-year-old girl (Table 4).

Within the *Poxo Muybu* village, the prevalence of mercury exposure above 6.0 µg/g was 60.6%. The average mercury levels among children (5.9 µg/g) and adults (7.1 and 7.6 µg/g for men and women, respectively) were similar when compared to *Sawré Muybu* (Table 4).

In contrast, in the *Sawré Aboy* village, the prevalence of mercury exposure reached 87.5% (Table 4). Moreover, the average mercury levels among children (11.0 µg/g) and adults (13.6 and 12.1 µg/g for men and women, respectively) were almost two-fold, compared to those observed in *Sawré Muybu*. It is worth noting that the highest level of mercury in our study population (23.9 µg/g) was registered in a 10-year-old boy living in *Sawré Aboy* (Table 4).

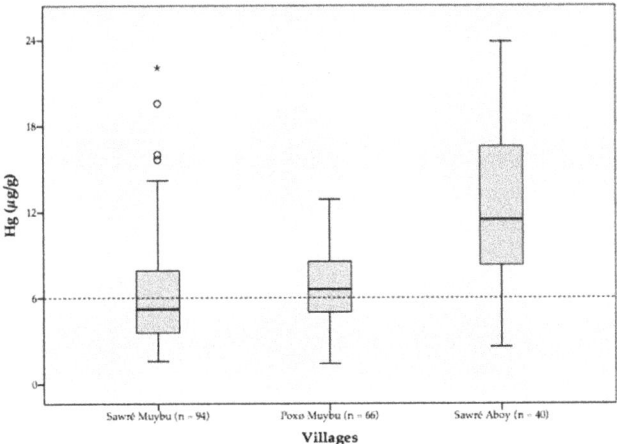

Figure 2. Boxplot with total hair mercury concentrations (µg/g), according to the investigated villages. *Sawré Muybu* Indigenous Land, Pará, Amazon, Brazil, 2019. Obs: The dashed line corresponds to the safe Hg exposure level adopted in this study (6.0 µg/g). The circles correspond to the cases that showed hair mercury levels that surpassed the superior limit of the interquartile (IQR). The asterisk corresponds to an outlier case in the *Sawré Muybu* village from one indigenous who presented a hair mercury level equal to 22.1 µg/g.

Considering the sociodemographic characteristics among indigenous older than 12 years, only "income" and "village of residence" were associated with the prevalence of mercury exposure $\geq$ 6.0 µg/g (p-values equal to 0.042 and 0.002, respectively) (Table 5). This means that the prevalence of hair mercury levels above 6.0 ug/g was higher among individuals who declared had no income (73.1%), in contrast to those who had income (26.7%). Similarly, the prevalence of hair mercury levels above 6.0 ug/g was higher among individuals living in the *Sawré Aboy* village (73.7%), compared to they were living in *Poxo Muybu* (71.1%) and *Sawré Muybu* (52.8%) (p-value: 0.002). The other variables did not show statistically significant differences.

Table 5. Sociodemographic and clinical characteristics of the participants $\geq$ 12 years old, according to hair mercury exposure ($\geq$6.0 µg/g x < 6.0 µg/g), *Sawré Muybu* Indigenous Land, Pará, Amazon, Brazil, 2019.

	Hair Mercury Levels						p-Value *
	<6.0 µg/g		$\geq$6.0 µg/g		Total		
	Sociodemographic Characteristics						
Sex	n	% #	n	% #	n	% †	
Female	22	36.7	38	63.3	60	51.7	0.353
Male	16	28.6	40	71.4	56	48.3	
Total	38	32.8	78	67.2	116		
Age range (years)							
12 to 19	13	29.5	31	70.5	44	37.9	0.843
20 to 29	13	34.2	25	65.8	38	32.8	
30 and +	12	35.3	22	64.7	34	29.3	
Total	38		78		116		

Table 5. Cont.

	Hair Mercury Levels						
	<6.0 µg/g		≥6.0 µg/g		Total		p-Value *
Marital Status							
Married	25	33.3	50	66.7	75	64.7	0.980
Single	11	31.4	24	68.6	35	30.2	
Widow(er)	2	33.3	4	66.7	6	5.2	
Total	38		78		116		
Income							
Yes	18	45.0	22	55.0	40	34.5	0.042
No	20	26.3	56	73.7	76	65.5	
Total	38		78		116		
Schooling (years)							
≥10	11	45.8	13	54.2	24	20.7	0.170
5 to 9	23	31.5	50	68.5	73	62.9	
1 to 4	2	13.3	13	86.7	15	12.9	
Iliterate	2	50.0	2	50.0	4	3.4	
Total	38		78		116		
Villages							
Sawré Muybu	25	47.2	28	52.8	53	45.7	0.002
Poxo Muybu	11	28.9	27	71.1	38	32.8	
Sawré Aboy	2	8.0	23	92.0	25	21.6	
Total	38		78		116		
Clinical characteristics							
BMI (kg/m²)	n	%	n	%	n	%	
18.5–24.9	24	33.3	48	66.7	72	63.7	0.972
<18.5	1	25.0	3	75.0	4	3.5	
25.0–29.9	11	33.3	22	66.7	33	29.2	
≥30.0	1	25.0	3	75.0	4	3.5	
Total	37		76		113		
Blood Pressure							
Normal	37	36.3	65	63.7	102	88.7	0.039
Hypertension	1	7.7	12	92.3	13	11.3	
Total	38		77		115		
Anemia							
No	32	34.8	60	65.2	92	80.0	0.428
Yes	6	26.1	17	73.9	23	20.0	
Total	38		77		115		
Glucose							
<100.0 mg/dL	2	50.0	2	50.0	4	11.1	0.293
≥100.0 mg/dL	8	25.0	24	75.0	32	88.9	
Total	10		26		36		
Previous Hospitalization							
No	22	32.4	46	67.6	68	58.6	0.912
Yes	16	33.3	32	66.7	48	41.4	
Total	38		78		116		

* Pearson's Chi-Square; # % in row; † % in column.

Regarding the clinical characteristics, only indigenous with high blood pressure levels, classified as "hypertension", showed a statistically significant association (p-value < 0.20) with mercury levels ≥ 6.0 ug/g. In this case, 92.3% of the indigenous older than 12 years diagnosed with hypertension have mercury levels in hair samples greater than or equal to 6.0 µg/g (Table 5).

Concerning the women of childbearing age, only the variable "pregnancy" showed a statistically significant association with the prevalence of contamination ≥ 6.0 µg/g at the level of 10% (p-value, 0.067). All pregnant investigated women showed hair mercury levels above 6.0 µg/g. The variables "number of children" and "breastfeeding" showed no significant association (Table 6).

Table 6. Hg levels in women of childbearing age, according to the number of children, pregnancy, and breastfeeding status, *Sawré Muybu* Indigenous Land, Pará state, Brazilian.

Women Features	Hair Mercury Levels						p-Value *
	<6.0 µg/g		≥6.0 µg/g		Total		
Number of children	n	% #	n	% #	n	% †	
1 to 2	4	28.6	10	71.4	14	26.4	0.531
3 to 6	8	50.0	8	50.0	16	30.2	
7 or +	1	20.0	4	80.0	5	9.4	
No children	7	38.9	11	61.1	18	34.0	
Total	20	37.7	33	62.3	53		
Pregnant							
No	20	41.7	28	58.3	48	90.6	0.067
Yes	0	0.0	5	100.0	5	9.4	
Total	20		33		53		
Breastfeeding							
No	13	36.1	23	63.9	36	67.9	0.723
Yes	7	41.2	10	58.8	17	32.1	
Total	20		33		53		

* Pearson's Chi-Square; # % in row; † % in column. Obs: Hg mean level in pregnant = 8.86 µg/g; Hg mean level in non-pregnant = 7.59 µg/g (F-test: 1.94; p-value: 0.169).

Table 7 shows the comparison between the mean values of the variables that make up the clinical characterization of individuals older than 12 years. The means of the "SBP" and "DBP" variables were higher in the group with mercury exposure ≥ 6.0 µg/g, with p-values equal to 0.044 and 0.039, respectively. The other tested variables did not reveal any differences between the groups, considering the mercury exposure groups.

Table 7. Clinical characteristics of Munduruku adults ≥ 12 years old, including height (cm), weight (kg), SBP and DBP (mmHg), glucose level (mg/dL), and hemoglobin level (g/dL), according to mercury exposure (<6.0 µg/g x ≥ 6,0µg/g), *Sawré Muybu* Indigenous Land, Pará, Amazon, Brazil, 2019.

Clinical Characteristics	Hg Detected	Participants	Mean	SD #	SE †	F-Test	p-Value
Height (cm)	<6.0 µg/g	37	150.6	6.7916	1.1165	0.065	0.799
	≥6.0 µg/g	76	151.2	7.2156	0.8277		
Weight (kg)	<6.0 µg/g	37	53.7	9.5022	1.5621	1.189	0.278
	≥6.0 µg/g	77	52.8	9.7792	1.1144		
BMI (kg/m²)	<6.0 µg/g	37	23.6	3.38	0.5557	1.936	0.167
	≥6.0 µg/g	76	23.1	3.6339	0.4168		
SBP * (mmHg)	<6.0 µg/g	38	110.5	9.42	1.528	4.157	0.044
	≥6.0 µg/g	77	113.2	15.557	1.773		
DBP ** (mmHg)	<6.0 µg/g	38	67.8	7.577	1.229	4.363	0.039
	≥6.0 µg/g	77	69.3	11.225	1.279		
Glucose level (mg/dL)	<6.0 µg/g	10	115.2	16.858	5.331	0.075	0.786
	≥6.0 µg/g	26	115.4	19.438	3.812		
Hemoglobin level (g/dL)	<6.0 µg/g	38	13.8	1.2437	0.2018	0.175	0.677
	≥6.0 µg/g	77	13.8	1.3299	0.1516		

* Systolic Blood Pressure; ** Diastolic Blood Pressure; # Standard Deviation; † Standard Error.

The logistic regression model applied to all adult participants (men and women ≥ 12 years old) pointed out that the prevalence of mercury exposure ≥ 6.0 µg/g was significantly higher among participants living in the *Sawré Aboy* village (adjusted PR: 1.8; 95% CI: 1.3–2.3; *p*-value: 0.001), among participants who had no regular income (adjusted PR: 1.3; 95% CI: 1.0–1.8; *p*-value: 0.031) and among participants who have had hypertension on clinical evaluation (adjusted PR: 1.6; 95% CI: 1.3–2.1; *p*-value: 0.01).

For the women of childbearing age, the logistic regression model revealed that the prevalence of mercury exposure ≥6.0 µg/g was 2.5 times higher in women living in the *Sawré Aboy* village (adjusted PR: 2.5; 95% CI: 1.4–4.4; *p*-value: 0.001), 1.9 times higher in women living in the *Poxo Muybu* village (adjusted PR: 1.9; 95% CI: 1.0–3.4; *p*-value: 0.044), 1.9 times higher among women with hypertension (adjusted PR: 1.9; 95% CI: 1.2–3.3; *p*-value: 0.012) and 1.5 times higher among pregnant women (adjusted PR: 1.5; 95% CI: 1.0–2.1; *p*-value: 0.029) (Table 8).

Table 8. Logistic regression model based on prevalence ratios (PR) crude and adjusted (confidence interval 95%), according to the mercury exposure (≥6.0 µg/g), to indigenous ≥12 years old, and to women of childbearing age, *Sawré Muybu* Indigenous Land, Pará, Amazon, Brazil, 2019.

Characteristics	Crude PR	95%CI	*p*-Value	Adjusted PR	95%CI	*p*-Value
Indigenous ≥ 12 Years-Old Both Sex						
Villages						
Sawré Muybu	1			1		
Poxo Muybu	1.3	(0.9–1.9)	0.074	1.3	(0.9–1.8)	0.098
Sawré Aboy	1.7	(1.3–2.3)	0.001	1.8	(1.3–2.3)	0.001
Income						
Yes	1			1		
No	1.3	(0.9–1.8)	0.065	1.3	(1.0–1.8)	0.031
Schooling (years)						
≥10	1					
5 to 9	1.3	(0.9–1.9)	0.250	–		
1 to 4	1.6	(1.0–2.4)	0.028	–		
Illiterate	0.9	(0.3–2.6)	0.881	–		
Blood Pressure						
Normal	1					
Hypertension	1.4	(1.2–1.8)	0.001	1.6	(1.3–2.1)	0.001
Women of Childbearing Age						
Characteristics	Crude PR	95%CI	*p*-Value	Adjusted PR	95%CI	p-Value
Villages						
Sawré Muybu	1			1		
Poxo Muybu	2.1	(1.2–3.7)	0.010	1.9	(1.0–3.4)	0.044
Sawré Aboy	2.4	(1.4–4.2)	0.002	2.5	(1.4–4.4)	0.001
Income						
Yes	1			–		
No	1.3	(0.8–2.3)	0.273	–		
Blood Pressure						
Normal	1			1		
Hypertension	1.7	(1.3–2.1)	0.001	1.9	(1.2–3.3)	0.012
Pregnant status						
No	1			1		
Yes	1.7	(1.4–2.2)	0.001	1.5	(1.0–2.1)	0.029

3.2.2. Fish Samples

In total, 88 fish specimens were captured, distributed in 17 species and 4 trophic levels. Three piscivorous species showed average mercury levels above 0.5 µg/g. The Hg-biomagnification in the fish trophic chain was confirmed, as there was a significant difference in the THg concentration in muscle tissues between trophic levels.

The highest level of mercury in muscle samples (1.95 µg/g) was observed in the *Serrasalmus rhombeus* (also known as *piranha preta*), a fish located on the top of the food chain. All results on the capture and determination of mercury in fish samples can be accessed in Vasconcellos et al. [87].

3.3. Health Risk Assessment

With dietary patterns in mind, estimates of fish mercury levels place daily methylmercury consumption above the safe limits recommended by the FAO/WHO [25], and the U.S.EPA [26] in all scenarios and in all studied population strata (i.e., children, childbearing women, and men).

Estimates of Hg ingestion, performed here, indicated that the daily methylmercury intake surpasses up to 11 times the FAO/WHO [25] and exceeds the U.S. EPA [26] reference dose from 3- to 25-fold. In all scenarios analyzed (dry season, rainy season, current, and critical), the risk ratio estimates were above 1.0, meaning that the studied Munduruku villages are at severe risk of harm due to ingestion of mercury-contaminated fish. Detailed findings can be accessed in Vasconcellos et al. [87].

4. Discussion

This is the first time a research group has prepared a multidisciplinary and inter-institutional study to meet the demand of an indigenous association in order to clarify the consequences and assess the impacts of illegal mining in their territory.

Through this investigation, it was possible to better understand the impact and magnitude of decades of illegal economic activities within the *Sawré Muybu* Indigenous Land and adjacent areas, with emphasis on direct and indirect health impacts caused by the ASGM. Without exception, we detected relevant mercury levels in all hair samples analyzed, including adults, elderly, men, childbearing women, and children. In fact, all of the indigenous Munduruku who participated in the study showed hair mercury levels above the safe limits established by the most varied international health agencies [25,26,88]. Considering the safety parameter adopted by the present study (i.e., 6 µg Hg/g in hair), on average, 6 out of 10 participants had mercury levels above this limit. However, human mercury exposure was not homogeneous in the three villages investigated and was directly associated with the intensity and extent of mining activity in each location. The *Sawré Aboy* village, located downstream from the Jamanxin River, was the closest to the mining activities (see Figure 1). In its surroundings, the environmental effects of the mining activity were easily observed. Since there were many floats for gold extracting from the river sediment, the river's water quality was compromised, and deforestation areas in the riverbanks for the excavation could be noted. In that village, 9 out of 10 participants had Hg exposure levels greater than 6.0 µg/g, with median levels of 11.5 µg/g. The second village most impacted by gold mining was *Poxo Muybu*. According to data published by the RAISG [21], there are many illegal mining points in the vicinity of that village (Figure 1). The median levels of mercury in hair samples collected from residents of that village reflected the intensity of mining activity in that area (6.6 µg/g). Finally, the least impacted village by mining was *Sawré Muybu*, and as a consequence, its residents showed median levels of mercury in hair equal to 5.2 µg/g. In order to support these findings, the abovementioned variations seemed not to be random, once they were statistically significant.

Mercury has been a valuable metal in various industrial processes, particularly in gold mining activities and especially in developing countries surrounding the Amazon basin. This apparent economic benefit is insignificant compared to its severe environmental and neurotoxicological health impact [4–6,15–20,93]. The present study provides evidence that communities living in the Tapajos River basin in the Munduruku indigenous territories have a mean level of Hg exposure surpassing the safety limit (6.0 µg/g) recognized by the World Health Organization [69].

It is essential to clarify that health agencies do not define safe levels of mercury exposure from concentrations detected in hair samples or other exposure biomarkers. In fact, the limits recommended by the health agencies consist of a definition of a maximum methylmercury intake dose (daily or weekly) that does not cause observable health effects. However, as there is a well-defined correlation between MeHg intake and levels detected in hair and blood, it is possible to establish correspondences. Remarkably, the intake recommendations vary significantly from one agency to another, and that occurs because the data used for the estimations are collected from different studies, including different populations and regions of the planet.

The present study used 6.0 µg/g of mercury in hair samples as a threshold for toxic effects, according to other research studies developed in the Amazon [20,47,76,85]. Kjellstrom et al. [94,95] and Crump et al. [96] adopted this concentration during the New Zealand cohort study to identify women with high mercury exposure.

This hair mercury level is derived from calculations for safe intake defined in 1972 by the Joint FAO/WHO Expert Committee on Food Additives (JECFA) [97], which were ratified in 1989 [98] and 2000 [99]. The basis for these estimates was the poisoning episodes of Minamata and Niigata, in Japan, that occurred in the 1950s. From the health endpoints related to poisoning, the JEFCA established a Provisional Tolerable Weekly Intake (PTWI) of 3.3 µg/kg bw/week as a safe intake dose (that corresponds to 6.0 µg MeHg/g in hair).

With the same purpose, the U.S. EPA [26] defined the reference dose (RfD) of 0.1 µg/kg bw/day based on studies carried out in Iraq. This dose was revised from the Faroes Island cohort study's findings and confirmed in the year 2000. In this case, the hair mercury levels correspond to 1.0 µg MeHg/g. Nowadays, the FAO/WHO [25] recommends doses of 1.6 µg/kg bw/week for vulnerable groups (such as women of childbearing age and pregnant), which correspond to mercury hair levels of 2.3 µg/g. In contrast, for the general population, the PTWI recommended is 3.2 µg/kg bw/week, which corresponds to a hair level of 4.5 µg/g [25].

The variety of safe limits reveals the challenges in developing global monitoring and surveillance instruments to identify populations at risk of mercury exposure. It occurs because the proposed doses result from observing the health mercury effects in different population groups and from very different exposure scenarios (e.g., chronic exposure observed in cohort studies and poisoning episodes in Iraq and Japan). Besides that, this limitation reinforces the need to develop longitudinal studies in native populations from the Amazon, such as indigenous and riverine populations, that consume large amounts of fish. These groups share a unique exposure scenario worldwide, where there is a combination of natural mercury present in the soil and different anthropic actions that increase the supply of mercury to the Amazon ecosystem, which then affect the biogeochemical cycle of this element, such as gold mining, the construction of dams, hydroelectric plants and forest fires [27,48,50].

In our study, the logistic regression model revealed that sociodemographic variables such as "income" and "village"; clinical variables, such as "hypertension," as well as pregnancy in women of childbearing age showed a significant association with hair mercury levels above 6.0 µg/g. Focusing on the findings related to "income," the prevalence of mercury exposure above 6.0 µg/g was 30% higher among indigenous who had no source of regular income, for example, salary, cash transfer, pension, retirement, among others. The absence of regular income to some families can impair the access to other protein sources in the diet besides fish, such as meat, chicken, pork, and other products that came from markets in the nearest municipalities. Consequently, these families potentially increase their ingestion of mercury-contaminated fish and become more prone to illness due to contamination, worsening the scenario of social and environmental vulnerability in the villages. Theoretically, the consumption of other protein sources would ensure a more diversified diet as well as less dependence on the protein obtained from fish consumption. Therefore, the lowest hair mercury levels would be observed in individuals who have a regular income.

Another important finding revealed that the indigenous living in the *Sawré Aboy* village had had 80% more prone to have mercury levels above 6.0 µg/g. When we analyzed the women of childbearing age who live in that village, the prevalence of mercury levels above 6.0 µg/g is 2.5-fold higher. As previously mentioned, in that community, the proximity to the ASGM is more significant than in other villages, contributing to the detection of higher levels of contamination in humans.

Among the studied clinical variables, it was observed that the prevalence of mercury exposure above 6.0 µg/g was 1.6 times higher in adults (including men and women) who presented with hypertension. In women of childbearing age, the prevalence of mercury exposure above 6.0 µg/g was 1.9-fold higher in women with hypertension. Different authors have studied the association between mercury exposure and the incidence of cardiovascular diseases in different contexts [100–105]. Fillion et al. [106] investigated the association between mercury exposure with hypertension in riverside dwellers living on the banks of the Tapajós River. The mentioned study enrolled 250 people from six different communities and used a linear regression model, which pointed out a significant association between mercury levels above 10 µg/g and an increase of systolic blood pressure levels in adults (Odds Ratio: 2.91; CI95%: 1.26–7.28), in harmony with our findings.

On the other hand, Dórea et al. [68] did not reported a significant relationship between mercuric exposure and hypertension in an investigation carried out among Kayabi and Munduruku indigenous peoples, 15 years ago. We might suppose that environmental contamination and mercury exposure have worsened in that region over the last two decades, putting the local population at a new risk rate.

In addition, these indigenous communities maintain their cultural and linguistic distinctiveness with substantial genetic distance from other non-indigenous populations. So, it is essential to verify the genetic profile ascribed to inter-populational diversity because data on genetic polymorphisms associated with mercury toxicokinetics and toxicodynamics cannot be extrapolated from other populations. In this study, we identified two individuals with the *ALAD* gene polymorphism which has previously been associated with low enzyme activity and, consequently, with high mercury levels in blood samples [107]. Detailed findings can be found in Perini et al. [92]. Moreover, indigenous people keep consistently underrepresented in genetics databases [82].

There is a long and ongoing history of gold mining activities in the Tapajos River basin and its impacts are well documented [5,13,14,41,43,63,64,66,67,108–110]. It is widely known that artisanal gold mining activities are responsible for emitting 200 metric tons of mercury annually; approximately 27% of global emissions are discarded annually without any control [111,112], constituting a potential risk to human health and the environment. It is important to note that, in general, the Munduruku people living in their traditional territories are not involved in gold mining activities, and yet they are victims of this controversial and doubtful development process, suffering the consequences of mercury contamination.

As well as being described by Khoury et al. [16], Santos Freitas et al. [17], Domingues et al. [18], Pinheiro et al. [19], Marinho et al. [20], Vega et al. [76], Barbieri and Gardon [113], our findings suggest that the proximity of the investigated communities with the gold mining activities is related to higher levels of methylmercury in hair samples. The comparative analyses performed on the communities revealed that in the *Sawré Aboy* village, which is located closer to gold mining operations, the greater hair Hg concentrations were reported. According to the WHO [88], human hair is an excellent biomarker for MeHg exposure, because MeHg deposited in the hair remains stable for a long time.

In the Amazon, hair-Hg levels in indigenous communities vary considerably. For instance, the mean Hg concentration in the hair of Munduruku people from Teles Pires (Pará, Brazil) was 3.4 µg/g [64], whereas, in ethnic groups from 19 villages at the Yanomami reserve, these varied between 0.4 and 22.1 µg/g ($n = 239$) [76]. The mean of the T-Hg value reported here (7.7 µg/g) was below that registered for indigenous communities living at the upper Tapajos River basin (14.7 µg/g) [67]. Nevertheless, it was above those found in other Amazonian municipalities where artisanal gold extraction has been established as the primary source of Hg-contamination, such as Belmont (Rondônia) (2.71 µg/g), Cunia (Rondônia) (0.9 µg/g) [114], Novo Airão (Amazonas) (5.67 µg/g) [115], Porto Velho (Rondônia) (0.60 µg/g) [116], and Manaus (Amazonas) (1.93 µg/g) [117].

There is a well-established relationship between human mercury exposure and fish consumption, not only in our study area but also in other parts of the Amazon region [37]. Amazon fish are the most important protein source for the local riverine populations, and fishing is a significant and traditional economic activity throughout the region [118,119]. Traditional communities in this study are likely exposed through the consumption of contaminated fish from the Tapajos River, based on extensive prior evidence of fish as the primary source of human MeHg exposure [41,63,64,66,87].

In addition to high levels of mercury exposure, our study revealed that families live in vulnerable conditions, since the average monthly income does not exceed USD 300.00, and most of it comes from social benefits. Households have a precarious structure, with no bathrooms for the families' exclusive use, nor potable water for people's consumption. The level of education is also low, there are not enough jobs available, nor sustainable development projects, and most adults work in informal or subsistence activities. Even some adults end up being enticed to work in mining activities due to an absolute lack of work opportunities.

The precarious scenario experienced in the villages results in other health challenges, which can be observed in the high rates of illness such as diarrhea, influenza, and Malaria, high rates of hospital admissions, and the high number of abortions and fetal deaths, revealing gaps in health services. Additionally, the lack of sanitation plays a significant role in nutritional deviations and in the high rates of anemia recorded in children under five years old [120–123].

Despite the illustrative findings of this investigation, it is necessary to reflect on some limitations. Our first challenge was bearing in mind the diversity of approaches on chronic mercury exposure in the Amazon territories. We start from a biomedical perspective with a focus on neurological and pediatric evaluations, including the estimation of the burden of infectious disease as well as non-communicable diseases and the analysis of genetic polymorphisms, while considering the fish ecology in the region, and the social context in which the illegal mining activities are performed in that territory. In all approaches, we thought of the appropriate statistical treatment to the cross-sectional source data.

After that, we were faced with the challenge of choosing validated and simplified data collection instruments for use in fieldwork conditions and how these instruments would be used in a differentiated sociocultural context. In this sense, we cannot fail to mention the difficulties faced in conducting extensive interviews with families, who in some situations did not speak Portuguese fluently, requiring the presence of interpreters.

In addition, we handled the challenge of applying child neurodevelopment tests, such as Denver II [124], which has been validated for use in urban contexts in Brazil, therefore, requiring some adaptations from researchers, especially in the language component.

It was also complex to carry out neurological evaluations in adults. In general, other authors value complaints and symptoms reported by participants to assess the harm caused by mercury contamination in adults [88,125]. Our study chose to prioritize the clinical evaluation directed in elements already considered in the literature and focus on identifying signs of somatosensory, motor, and cognitive impairment in young people and adults. Detailed results of this approach can be reached in Oliveira et al. [80].

Furthermore, due to the limited time of contact with the communities and the linguistic difficulties already mentioned, we could not accurately assess the exact amount of fish consumed nor characterize other elements of the families' diet. To address part of this limitation, we developed an empirical method to estimate household fish consumption, found in the manuscript lead by Vasconcellos et al. [87].

Our study covered only three villages in the region of the Middle-Tapajós River, including a total of 200 participants. The entire Munduruku population is estimated at approximately 12,000 people, distributed in more than 120 villages, primarily concentrated in the region of the upper Tapajós River, where more intensive illegal mining activity is concentrated. Therefore, it is possible that despite robust estimates, our findings are underestimated and do not reveal the true impact on the majority of the Munduruku people from mercury exposure.

Finally, our team could not collect longitudinal data to assess possible changes in the health situation over time (for example, related to seasonality, typical in the Amazon region). Given the limitations mentioned above, it is impossible to make more robust causal inferences about mercury exposure in the region. Therefore, more in-depth studies are needed, with a longitudinal approach, focusing mainly on pregnant women and children under five years old. In our opinion, this is the only way to measure the actual extension of health impacts related to chronic mercury exposure in traditional communities in the Amazon.

On the other hand, this study's strengths lie in the census of indigenous populations living in the three studied villages, and the use of prevalence ratios in the multivariate analyses, making a sound basis for planning public health interventions.

5. Conclusions

In conclusion, the time spent in the communities, the observation of the environmental impacts resulting from illegal mining, and the analysis of the collected data in the fieldwork allows us to make some reflections and therefore propose the following recommendations:

(a) The immediate interruption of illegal mining activities and cessation of invasion of traditional and protected lands of the Amazon.
(b) In parallel, to develop a national plan to discontinue mercury use in artisanal mining to achieve the goals of the Minamata Convention on Mercury.
(c) To develop a risk management plan (RMP) for populations chronically exposed to mercury. The plan should contain a set of integrated guidelines and actions, such as:
   (i) to expand the monitoring of mercury levels in fish consumed not only in traditional territories but also in urban areas of the Amazon.
   (ii) to develop educational material for the population of the affected areas, containing clear information on safe fish consumption, respecting cultural aspects related to different ethnic groups.
   (iii) to include testing of mercury levels in hair samples in the routine of the prenatal care program and in the program for monitoring child growth and development, in the Brazilian Unified Health System (SUS).
   (iv) to develop a Basic Care Protocol for Contaminated People to be equally incorporated into the SUS.
   (v) to promote a research and scientific development program to carry out more in-depth studies to enhance the knowledge about the health impacts of Amazon populations chronically exposed to mercury.
   (vi) to formulate public policies to create sustainable economic alternatives for indigenous communities affected by illegal mining in order to guarantee food security, sovereignty, and respect for ancestral traditions.

Lastly, as a signatory of the 2013 Minamata Convention, the Brazilian Government should commit to combatting environmental contamination and exposure to mercury. It is of particular importance given that, currently, the ASGM is the main responsible for increased levels of mercury in the Amazonian environment. Additionally, the ASGM has been promoted conflicts and attacks within these traditional territories. Summing up, the indigenous populations are looking to the Brazilian authorities to ban and control gold mining in their sacred territories.

Author Contributions: Proposal design, study design, and methodology, P.C.B., A.C.S.d.V., P.V.d.S.V., A.R.S.P., C.B.H., D.C.d.A., R.A.A.d.O., M.d.O.L., I.M.d.J., J.A.P., G.H., H.d.N.d.M.M., C.C.R.d.S. and S.d.S.H.; fieldwork data collection, A.R.S.P., C.B.H., J.W.K., P.V.d.S.V., A.C.S.d.V., R.A.A.d.O., R.W.A. and P.C.B.; laboratory analysis, I.M.d.J. and M.d.O.L.; writing—original draft preparation, A.C.S.d.V., P.V.d.S.V., S.d.S.H. and P.C.B.; writing—review and editing, P.C.B., A.C.S.d.V., P.V.d.S.V., S.d.S.H., A.R.S.P., C.B.H., J.W.K., I.M.d.J., M.d.O.L., N.S.P., D.C.d.A., R.A.A.d.O., R.W.A., J.A.P., G.H., H.d.N.d.M.M., M.d.O.L. and I.M.d.J.; supervision, obtaining resources, and project management, P.C.B. and S.d.S.H. All authors have read and agreed to the published version of the manuscript.

Funding: This research was funded by the Vice-Presidency of Environment, Care and Health Promotion (VPPAS) of Fundação Oswaldo Cruz (Fiocruz) through Decentralized Execution of Resources Document No. 175/2018, Process: 25000.209221/2018-18, signed between the Fiocruz and the Special Department for Indigenous Health, both under the Ministry of Health. The non-governmental organization WWF-Brazil offered financial support to disseminate the results of the research.

Institutional Review Board Statement: The study was conducted in accordance with the guidelines of the Declaration of Helsinki and was approved by the Research Ethics Committee of the National School of Public Health at Fiocruz (REC/ENSP) and the Brazilian National Research Ethics Commission of the National Health Council (CONEP/CNS), CAAE: 65671517.1.0000.5240, with Opinion No. 2.262.686 favorable to its performance. In compliance with Convention No. 169 of the International Labor Organization (ILO), the study began with a pre-study consultation, carried out in August 2019, during a visit to the villages, in which two authors (SSH and PCB) and local indigenous leaders participated. At the time, the study objectives were presented and discussed (https://www.youtube.com/watch?v=oFEYEGxNmns&t=704s, accessed on 20 September 2019). After answering questions and approval of the proposal by the communities, we received support from the coordination of the Special Indigenous Sanitary District of the Tapajós River through the multidisciplinary indigenous health team to carry out the study. In addition, the interviews and data collection started only after the participants had their questions answered and were given formal consent in the Informed Consent Form (ICF) by the children's guardians.

Informed Consent Statement: Informed consent was obtained from all subjects involved in the study. Written informed consent has been obtained from the patients to publish this paper.

Data Availability Statement: Data sharing not applicable.

Acknowledgments: Through chiefs Juarez Saw, Jairo Saw, and Valdemar Poxo, and the leader Alessandra Korap, we thank the Munduruku people for the trust placed in our team and the support in carrying out the research. We thank the team from the Rio Tapajós Indigenous Special Sanitary District, who spared no efforts to support us in all stages of the fieldwork. In particular, we thank nurses Alan Marcelo Simon and Lygia Catarina de Oliveira. We thank João Paulo Goes Pereira for the mercury analysis in the hair and fish samples. We also thank Marcelo Oliveira-da-Costa from World-Wide Fund for Nature (WWF-Brazil) for technical and financial support to this scientific communication. Finally, we thank Daniel de Oliveira d'El Rei Pinto, who made the study area map.

Conflicts of Interest: The authors declare no conflict of interest. The funders had no role in the design of the study; in the collection, analyses, or interpretation of data; in the writing of the manuscript, or in the decision to publish the results.

References

1. Morel, F.M.; Kraepiel, A.M.; Amyot, M. The chemical cycle and bioaccumulation of mercury. *Annu. Rev. Ecol. Syst.* **1998**, *29*, 543–566. [CrossRef]
2. Malm, O. Gold mining as a source of mercury exposure in the Brazilian Amazon. *Environ. Res.* **1998**, *77*, 73–78. [CrossRef]
3. Mason, R.P.; Fitzgerald, W.F.; Morel, F.M. The biogeochemical cycling of elemental mercury: Anthropogenic influences. *Geochim. Cosmochim. Acta* **1994**, *58*, 3191–3198. [CrossRef]
4. Clifton II, J.C. Mercury exposure and public health. *Pediatr. Clin. N. Am.* **2007**, *54*, 237.e1–237.e45. [CrossRef] [PubMed]
5. Passos, C.J.; Mergler, D. Human mercury exposure and adverse health effects in the Amazon: A review. *Cad. Saúde Pública* **2008**, *24*, s503–s520. [CrossRef] [PubMed]

6. Bose-O'Reilly, S.; McCarty, K.M.; Steckling, N.; Lettmeier, B. Mercury exposure and children's health. *Curr. Probl. Pediatr. Adolesc. Health Care* **2010**, *40*, 186–215. [CrossRef]
7. Pfeiffer, W.C.; de Lacerda, L.D. Mercury inputs into the Amazon region, Brazil. *Environ. Technol.* **1988**, *9*, 325–330. [CrossRef]
8. Martinelli, L.A.; Ferreira, J.R.; Forsberg, B.R.; Victoria, R.L. Mercury contamination in the Amazon: A gold rush consequence. *Ambio* **1988**, *17*, 252–254.
9. Cleary, D. An Anatomy of a Gold Rush: Garimpagem in the Brazilian Amazon. Ph.D. Thesis, University of Oxford, Oxford, UK, 1989.
10. Lacerda, L.D.; Pfeiffer, W.C. Mercury from gold mining in the Amazon environment: An overview. *Química Nova* **1992**, *15*, 155–160.
11. Pfeiffer, W.C.; Lacerda, L.D.; Salomons, W.; Malm, O. Environmental fate of mercury from gold mining in the Brazilian Amazon. *Environ. Rev.* **1993**, *1*, 26–37. [CrossRef]
12. Akagi, H.; Naganuma, A. Human exposure to mercury and the accumulation of methylmercury that is associated with gold mining in the Amazon Basin, Brazil. *J. Health Sci.* **2000**, *46*, 323–328. [CrossRef]
13. Roulet, M.; Lucotte, M.; Canuel, R.; Farella, N.; Courcelles, M.; Guimaraes, J.R.; Mergler, D.; Amorim, M. Increase in mercury contamination recorded in lacustrine sediments following deforestation in the central Amazon. *Chem. Geol.* **2000**, *165*, 243–266. [CrossRef]
14. Lino, A.S.; Kasper, D.; Guida, Y.S.; Thomaz, J.R.; Malm, O. Total and methyl mercury distribution in water, sediment, plankton and fish along the Tapajós River basin in the Brazilian Amazon. *Chemosphere* **2019**, *235*, 690–700. [CrossRef]
15. Teixeira, R.A.; da Silveira Pereira, W.V.; de Souza, E.S.; Ramos, S.J.; Dias, Y.N.; de Lima, M.W.; de Souza Neto, H.F.; de Oliveira, E.S.; Fernandes, A.R. Artisanal gold mining in the eastern Amazon: Environmental and human health risks of mercury from different mining methods. *Chemosphere* **2021**, *284*, 131220. [CrossRef]
16. Khoury, E.D.; Souza, G.D.; da Costa, C.A.; de Araújo, A.A.; de Oliveira, C.S.; Silveira, L.C.; Pinheiro, M.D. Somatosensory psychophysical losses in inhabitants of riverside communities of the Tapajós River Basin, Amazon, Brazil: Exposure to methylmercury is possibly involved. *PLoS ONE* **2015**, *10*, e0144625. [CrossRef]
17. dos Santos Freitas, J.; Lacerda, E.M.; da Silva Martins, I.C.; Rodrigues, D., Jr.; Bonci, D.M.; Cortes, M.I.; Corvelo, T.C.; Ventura, D.F.; de Lima Silveira, L.C.; Pinheiro, M.D.; et al. Cross-sectional study to assess the association of color vision with mercury hair concentration in children from Brazilian Amazonian riverine communities. *Neurotoxicology* **2018**, *65*, 60–67. [CrossRef]
18. Domingues, M.M.; Cury, E.D.; de Araújo, A.A.; Junior, J.M.; Pinheiro, M.D. Somatosensory psychophysic losses in inhabitants of riverside communities of the Tapajós river basin, Amazonas, Brazil: The possible involvement of exposure to methylmercury. *J. Neurol. Sci.* **2019**, *405*, 255–256. [CrossRef]
19. Pinheiro, M.D.; Oikawa, T.; Vieira, J.L.; Gomes, M.S.; Guimarães, G.D.; Crespo-López, M.E.; Müller, R.C.; Amoras, W.W.; Ribeiro, D.R.; Rodrigues, A.R.; et al. Comparative study of human exposure to mercury in riverside communities in the Amazon region. *Braz. J. Med. Biol. Res.* **2006**, *39*, 411–414. [CrossRef]
20. Marinho, J.S.; Lima, M.O.; Santos, E.C.; de Jesus, I.M.; Pinheiro, M.D.; Alves, C.N.; Muller, R.C. Mercury speciation in hair of children in three communities of the Amazon, Brazil. *BioMed. Res. Int.* **2014**, *2014*, 945963. [CrossRef]
21. Mapa inédito Indica Epidemia de Garimpo Ilegal na Panamazônia—RAISG. Available online: https://www.amazoniasocioambiental.org/pt-br/radar/mapa-inedito-indica-epidemia-de-garimpo-ilegal-na-panamazonia/ (accessed on 14 June 2021).
22. Cerdeira, R.G.P.; Ruffino, M.L.; Isaac, V.J. Consumo de Pescado e Outros Alimentos Pela População Ribeirinha do Lago Grande de Monte Alegre, PA-Brasil. *Acta Amaz.* **1997**, *27*, 213–227. [CrossRef]
23. Santos, G.M.D.; Santos, A.C.M.D. Sustentabilidade da pesca na Amazônia. *Estud. Avançados* **2005**, *19*, 165–182. [CrossRef]
24. Arruda, M.C.F.D. Avaliação dos Indicadores da Política de pesca do Programa Zona Franca Verde: Perspectivas Econômicas e Ambientais. Dissertação de Mestrado, Programa de Pós-Graduação em Engenharia de Produção, Universidade Federal do Amazonas (UFAM), Manaus, Brasil, 2017. Available online: https://tede.ufam.edu.br/handle/tede/6068 (accessed on 19 June 2021).
25. Joint FAO/WHO Expert Committee on Food Additives, Meeting, & World Health Organization. Evaluation of Certain Food Additives and Contaminants: Sixty First Report of the Joint FAO/WHO Expert Committee on Food Additives), Rome 10, 19 June 2003. 2003. Available online: ftp://ftp.org/es/esn/jecfa/jecfa61sc.pdf (accessed on 17 June 2021).
26. U.S. EPA. *Reference Dose for Methylmercury (External Review Draft, 2000)*; NCEA-S-0930; U.S. Environmental Protection Agency: Washington, DC, USA. Available online: https://www.regulations.gov/document/EPA-HQ-OAR-2018-0794-0006 (accessed on 18 June 2021).
27. Crespo-Lopez, M.E.; Augusto-Oliveira, M.; Lopes-Araújo, A.; Santos-Sacramento, L.; Takeda, P.Y.; Macchi, B.D.M.; Nascimento, J.L.M.D.; Maia, C.S.; Lima, R.R.; Arrifano, G.P. Mercury: What Can We Learn Amazon? *Environ. Int.* **2021**, *146*, 106223. [CrossRef]
28. Bakir, F.; Damluji, S.F.; Amin-Zaki, L.; Murtadha, M.; Khalidi, A.; Al-Rawi, N.Y.; Tikriti, S.; Dhahir, H.I.; Clarkson, T.W.; Smith, J.C.; et al. Methylmercury poisoning in Iraq. *Science* **1973**, *181*, 230–241. [CrossRef]
29. Akagi, H.; Grandjean, P.; Takizawa, Y.; Weihe, P. Methylmercury dose estimation from umbilical cord concentrations in patients with Minamata disease. *Environ. Res.* **1998**, *77*, 98–103. [CrossRef]
30. Ceccatelli, S.; Daré, E.; Moors, M. Methylmercury-induced neurotoxicity and apoptosis. *Chem.-Biol. Interact.* **2010**, *188*, 301–308. [CrossRef]

31. Lechler, P.J.; Miller, J.R.; Lacerda, L.D.; Vinson, D.; Bonzongo, J.C.; Lyons, W.B.; Warwick, J.J. Elevated mercury concentrations in soils, sediments, water, and fish of the Madeira River basin, Brazilian Amazon: A function of natural enrichments? *Sci. Total Environ.* **2000**, *260*, 87–96. [CrossRef]
32. Rodríguez Martín-Doimeadios, R.C.; Berzas Nevado, J.J.; Guzmán Bernardo, F.J.; Jiménez Moreno, M.; Arrifano, G.P.F.; Herculano, A.M.; Nascimento, J.L.M.D.; Crespo-López, M.E. Comparative study of mercury speciation in commercial fishes of the Brazilian Amazon. *Environ. Sci. Pollut. Res.* **2014**, *21*, 7466–7479. [CrossRef] [PubMed]
33. Souza-Araujo, J.; Giarrizzo, T.; Lima, M.O.; Souza, M.B.G. Mercury and methyl mercury in fishes from Bacajá River (Brazilian Amazon): Evidence for bioaccumulation and biomagnification. *J. Fish Biol.* **2016**, *89*, 249–263. [CrossRef]
34. Lino, A.S.; Kasper, D.; Guida, Y.S.; Thomaz, J.R.; Malm, O. Mercury and selenium in fishes from the Tapajós River in the Brazilian Amazon: An evaluation of human exposure. *J. Trace Elements Med. Biol.* **2018**, *48*, 196–201. [CrossRef]
35. Guimaraes, J.R.D.; Roulet, M.; Lucotte, M.; Mergler, D. Mercury methylation along a lake–forest transect in the Tapajós river floodplain, Brazilian Amazon: Seasonal and vertical variations. *Sci. Total Environ.* **2000**, *261*, 91–98. [CrossRef]
36. Albuquerque, F.E.A.; Minervino, A.H.H.; Miranda, M.; Herrero-Latorre, C.; Barrêto Júnior, R.A.; Oliveira, F.L.C.; Sucupira, M.C.A.; Ortolani, E.L.; López-Alonso, M. Toxic and essential trace element concentrations in fish species in the Lower Amazon, Brazil. *Sci. Total Environ.* **2020**, *732*, 138983. [CrossRef] [PubMed]
37. Hacon, S.D.S.; Oliveira-Da-Costa, M.; Gama, C.D.S.; Ferreira, R.; Basta, P.C.; Schramm, A.; Yokota, D. Mercury exposure through fish consumption in traditional communities in the Brazilian Northern Amazon. *Int. J. Environ. Res. Public Health* **2020**, *17*, 5269. [CrossRef] [PubMed]
38. Azevedo, L.S.; Pestana, I.A.; Almeida, M.G.; Ferreira da Costa Nery, A.; Bastos, W.R.; Magalhães Souza, C.M. Mercury biomagnification in an ichthyic food chain of an amazon floodplain lake (Puruzinho Lake): Influence of seasonality and food chain modeling. *Ecotoxicol. Environ. Saf.* **2021**, *207*, 111249. [CrossRef] [PubMed]
39. Akagi, H.; Malm, O.; Branches, F.J.P.; Kinjo, Y.; Kashima, Y.; Guimaraes, J.R.D.; Oliveira, R.B.; Haraguchi, K.; Pfeiffer, W.C.; Takizawa, Y.; et al. Human exposure to mercury due to goldmining in the Tapajos River Basin, Amazon, Brazil: Speciation of mercury in human hair, blood and urine. *Water Air Soil Pollut.* **1995**, *80*, 85–94. [CrossRef]
40. Lebel, J.; Roulet, M.; Mergler, D.; Lucotte, M.; Larribe, F. Fish diet and mercury exposure in a riparian Amazonian population. *Water Air Soil Pollut.* **1997**, *97*, 31–44. [CrossRef]
41. Malm, O.; Branches, F.J.; Akagi, H.; Castro, M.B.; Pfeiffer, W.C.; Harada, M.; Bastos, W.R.; Kato, H. Mercury and methylmercury in fish and human hair from the Tapajos river basin, Brazil. *Sci. Total Environ.* **1995**, *175*, 141–150. [CrossRef]
42. de Souza Lima, A.P.; Müller, R.C.S.; de Souza Sarkis, J.E.; Alves, C.N.; da Silva Bentes, M.H.; Brabo, E.; de Oliveira Santos, E. Mercury contamination in fish from Santarém, Pará, Brazil. *Environ. Res.* **2000**, *83*, 117–122. [CrossRef]
43. Passos, C.J.S.; Da Silva, D.S.; Lemire, M.; Fillion, M.; Guimaraes, J.R.D.; Lucotte, M.; Mergler, D. Daily mercury intake in fish-eating populations in the Brazilian Amazon. *J. Expo. Sci. Environ. Epidemiol.* **2008**, *18*, 76–87. [CrossRef]
44. Gimenes, T.C.; Penteado, J.O.; dos Santos, M.; da Silva Júnior, F.M.R. Methylmercury in Fish from the Amazon Region—A Review Focused on Eating Habits. *Water Air Soil Pollut.* **2021**, *232*, 1–9. [CrossRef]
45. FAO/WHO. Joint FAO/WHO Expert Committee on Food Additives (JECFA), Report of the Tenth Section, Rotterdam, The Netherlands 4 to 8 April 2016. Available online: http://www.fao.org/fao-who-codexalimentarius/sh-proxy/en/?lnk=1&url=https%253A%252F%252Fworkspace.fao.org%252Fsites%252Fcodex%252FMeetings%252FCX-735-10%252FReport%252FREP16_CFe.pdf (accessed on 22 June 2020).
46. Berzas Nevado, J.J.; Rodríguez Martín-Doimeadios, R.C.; Guzmán Bernardo, F.J.; Jiménez Moreno, M.; Herculano, A.M.; do Nascimento, J.L.M.; Crespo-López, M.E. Mercury in the Tapajós River basin, Brazilian Amazon: A review. *Environ. Int.* **2010**, *36*, 593–608. [CrossRef]
47. Santos Serrão de Castro, N.; de Oliveira Lima, M. Hair as a biomarker of long term mercury exposure in Brazilian Amazon: A systematic review. *Int. J. Environ. Res. Public Health* **2018**, *15*, 500. [CrossRef]
48. Arrifano, G.P.; Martín-Doimeadios, R.C.; Jiménez-Moreno, M.; Ramírez-Mateos, V.; da Silva, N.F.; Souza-Monteiro, J.R.; Augusto-Oliveira, M.; Paraense, R.S.; Macchi, B.M.; do Nascimento, J.L.; et al. Large-scale projects in the amazon and human exposure to mercury: The case-study of the Tucuruí Dam. *Ecotoxicol. Environ. Saf.* **2018**, *147*, 299–305. [CrossRef]
49. Kelly, C.A.; Rudd, J.W.M.; Bodaly, R.A.; Roulet, N.P.; StLouis, V.L.; Heyes, A.; Moore, T.R.; Schiff, S.; Aravena, R.; Scott, K.J.; et al. Increases in fluxes of greenhouse gases and methyl mercury following flooding of an experimental reservoir. *Environ. Sci. Technol.* **1997**, *31*, 1334–1344. [CrossRef]
50. Gomes, V.M.; dos Santos, A.; Zara, L.F.; Ramos, D.D.; Forti, J.C.; Ramos, D.D.; Santos, F.A. Study on mercury methylation in the Amazonian rivers in flooded areas for hydroelectric use. *Water Air Soil Pollut.* **2019**, *230*, 211. [CrossRef]
51. Palermo, E.F.A.; Kasper, D.; Reis, T.S.; Nogueira, S.; Branco, C.W.C.; Malm, O. Mercury level increase in fish tissues downstream the Tucuruí reservoir, Brazil. *RMZ-M&G* **2004**, *51*, 1292–1294.
52. Forsberg, B.R.; Melack, J.M.; Dunne, T.; Barthem, R.B.; Goulding, M.; Paiva, R.C.D.; Sorribas, M.V.; Silva, U.L., Jr.; Weisser, S. The potential impact of new Andean dams on Amazon fluvial ecosystems. *PLoS ONE* **2017**, *12*, e0182254. [CrossRef] [PubMed]
53. Pestana, I.A.; Azevedo, L.S.; Bastos, W.R.; de Souza, C.M.M. The impact of hydroelectric dams on mercury dynamics in South America: A review. *Chemosphere* **2019**, *219*, 546–556. [CrossRef]

54. Vasconcellos, A.C.; Barrocas, P.R.; Ruiz, C.M.; Mourão, D.D.; Hacon, S.D. Burden of mild mental retardation attributed to prenatal methylmercury exposure in amazon: Local and regional estimates. *Cienc E Saude Coletiva* **2018**, *23*, 3535–3545. [CrossRef] [PubMed]
55. Poulin, J.; Gibb, H.; Prüss-Üstün, A.; World Health Organization. *Mercury: Assessing the Environmental Burden of Disease at National and Local Levels*; World Health Organization: Geneva, Switzerland, 2008; 60p.
56. Reuben, A.; Frischtak, H.; Berky, A.; Ortiz, E.J.; Morales, A.M.; Hsu-Kim, H.; Pendergast, L.L.; Pan, W.K. Elevated Hair Mercury Levels Are Associated With Neurodevelopmental Deficits in Children Living Near Artisanal and Small-Scale Gold Mining in Peru. *GeoHealth* **2020**, *4*, e2019GH000222. [CrossRef]
57. Marques, R.C.; Bernardi, J.V.E.; Abreu, L.; Dórea, J.G. Neurodevelopment Outcomes in Children Exposed to Organic Mercury from Multiple Sources in a Tin-Ore Mine Environment in Brazil. *Arch Environ. Contam. Toxicol.* **2015**, *68*, 432–441. [CrossRef]
58. Marques, R.C.; Bernardi, J.V.E.; Cunha, M.P.L.; Dórea, J.G. Impact of organic mercury exposure and home delivery on neurodevelopment of Amazonian children. *Int. J. Hyg. Environ. Health* **2016**, *219*, 498–502. [CrossRef] [PubMed]
59. Junior, J.M.F.C.; Da Silva Lima, A.A.; Junior, D.R.; Khoury, E.D.T.; Da Silva Souza, G.; De Lima Silveira, L.C.; Pinheiro, M.D.C.N. Manifestações emocionais e motoras de ribeirinhos expostos ao mercúrio na Amazônia. *Rev. Bras. Epidemiol.* **2017**, *20*, 212–224. [CrossRef]
60. Lacerda, E.M.D.C.B.; Souza, G.D.S.; Cortes, M.I.T.; Rodrigues, A.R.; Pinheiro, M.C.N.; Silveira, L.C.D.L.; Ventura, D.F. Comparison of Visual Functions of Two Amazonian Populations: Possible Consequences of Different Mercury Exposure. *Front. Neurosci.* **2020**, *13*, 1428. [CrossRef]
61. Aaseth, J.; Wallace, D.R.; Vejrup, K.; Alexander, J. Methylmercury and developmental neurotoxicity: A global concern. *Curr. Opin. Toxicol.* **2020**, *19*, 80–87. [CrossRef]
62. Kishi, R. Impacts of Developmental Exposure to Environmental Chemicals on Human Health with Global Perspectives. In *Health Impacts of Developmental Exposure to Environmental Chemicals*; Springer: Singapore, 2020; pp. 3–22. [CrossRef]
63. Da Silva Brabo, E.; De Oliveira Santos, E.; Maura De Jesus, I.; Fernando Silva Mascarenhas, A.; De Freitas Faial, K. Mercury contamination of fish and exposures of an indigenous community in Para state, Brazil. In *Environmental Research*; Academic Press Inc.: Cambridge, MA, USA, 2000; pp. 197–203.
64. Dórea, J.G.; Barbosa, A.C.; Ferrari, Í.; de Souza, J.R. Fish consumption (hair mercury) and nutritional status of Amazonian Amer-Indian children. *Am. J. Hum. Biol.* **2005**, *17*, 507–514. [CrossRef]
65. Telmer, K.; Costa, M.; Angélica, R.S.; Araujo, E.S.; Maurice, Y. The source and fate of sediment and mercury in the Tapajós River, Pará, Brazilian Amazon: Ground- and space-based evidence. *J. Environ. Manag.* **2006**, *81*, 101–113. [CrossRef]
66. Brabo, E.D.; Santos, E.D.; Jesus, I.M.; Mascarenhas, A.F.; Faial, K.F. Mercury levels in fish consumed by the Sai Cinza indigenous community, Munduruku Reservation, Jacareacanga County, State of Pará, Brazil. *Cad Saúde Pública/Ministério Da Saúde Fundação Oswaldo Cruz Esc Nac Saúde Pública* **1999**, *15*, 325–331. [CrossRef]
67. de Oliveira Santos, E.C.; de Jesus, I.M.; Camara, V.D.; Brabo, E.; Loureiro, E.C.; Mascarenhas, A.; Weirich, J.; Luiz, R.R.; Cleary, D. Mercury exposure in Munduruku Indians from the community of Sai Cinza, State of Pará, Brazil. *Environ. Res.* **2002**, *90*, 98–103. [CrossRef]
68. Dórea, J.G.; De Souza, J.R.; Rodrigues, P.; Ferrari, Í.; Barbosa, A.C. Hair mercury (signature of fish consumption) and cardiovascular risk in Munduruku and Kayabi Indians of Amazonia. *Environ. Res.* **2005**, *97*, 209–219. [CrossRef]
69. WHO. *Toxicological Evaluation of Certain Food Additives and Contaminants*; WHO Food Additives Series, No. 24; Cambridge University Press: Cambridge, UK, 1989.
70. Siqueira-Gay, J.; Soares-Filho, B.; Sanchez, L.E.; Oviedo, A.; Sonter, L.J. Proposed Legislation to Mine Brazil's Indigenous Lands Will Threaten Amazon Forests and Their Valuable Ecosystem Services. *One Earth* **2020**, *3*, 356–362. [CrossRef]
71. The Guardian. Brazilian Wildcat Miners Attack Police and Burn Indigenous Homes in Amazon [Internet]. 2021. Available online: https://www.theguardian.com/world/2021/may/28/brazil-wildcat-miners-police-indigenous-amazon (accessed on 31 May 2021).
72. Henrique, M.C.; Oliveira RM, D. Os 'cortadores de cabeças': A memória como patrimônio dos Munduruku. Boletim do Museu Paraense Emílio Goeldi. *Ciências Hum.* **2021**, *16*, e20200049. [CrossRef]
73. Munduruku—Povos Indígenas no Brasil. Available online: https://pib.socioambiental.org/pt/Povo:Munduruku (accessed on 14 June 2021).
74. Hacon, S.; Rochedo, E.R.; Campos, R.R.; Lacerda, L.D. Mercury exposure through fish consumption in the urban area of Alta Floresta in the Amazon Basin. *J. Geochem. Explor.* **1997**, *58*, 209–216. [CrossRef]
75. Hacon, S.; Yokoo, E.; Valente, J.; Campos, R.; Da Silva, V.; De Menezes, A.; De Moraes, L.; Ignotti, E. Exposure to mercury in pregnant women from Alta Floresta—Amazon Basin, Brazil. *Environ. Res.* **2000**, *84*, 204–210. [CrossRef] [PubMed]
76. Vega, C.M.; Orellana, J.D.Y.; Oliveira, M.W.; Hacon, S.S.; Basta, P.C. Human Mercury Exposure in Yanomami Indigenous Villages from the Brazilian Amazon. *Int. J. Environ. Res. Public Health* **2018**, *15*, 1051. [CrossRef]
77. WHO. WHO Child Growth Standards: Length/Height-for-Age, Weight-for-Age, Weight-for-Length, Weight-for-Height and Body Mass Index-for-Age: Methods and Development. 2006. Available online: https://www.who.int/publications/i/item/924154693X (accessed on 14 June 2021).

78. Rosenfeld, L.G.; Malta, D.C.; Szwarcwald, C.L.; Bacal, N.S.; Cuder, M.A.; Pereira, C.A.; Figueiredo, A.W.; Silva, A.G.; Machado, Í.E.; Silva, W.A.; et al. Reference values for blood count laboratory tests in the Brazilian adult population, national health survey. *Rev. Bras. Epidemiol.* **2019**, *22*, E190003-SUPL.
79. Barroso, W.K.; Rodrigues, C.I.; Bortolotto, L.A.; Mota-Gomes, M.A.; Brandão, A.A.; Feitosa, A.D.; Machado, C.A.; Poli-de-Figueiredo, C.E.; Amodeo, C.; Mion, D.; et al. Diretrizes Brasileiras de Hipertensão Arterial–2020. *Arq. Bras. Cardiol.* **2021**, *116*, 516–658. [CrossRef]
80. Oliveira, R.; Pinto, B.; Resende, B.; Ciampi de Andrade, D.; Basta, P. Neurological impacts of chronic methylmercury exposure in Munduruku indigenous adults: Somatosensory, motor and cognitive abnormalities. *Int. J. Environ. Res. Public Health* **2021**, *18*, in press.
81. Hofer, C.B.; Périssé, A.R.S.; Vasconcellos, A.C.S.; Viana, P.V.; Kempton, J.W.; Lima, M.O.; Jesus, I.M.; Hacon, S.S.; Basta, P.C. Munduruku Indigenous children health's in the Tapajos River basin: Situational diagnosis and impacts of chronic mercury exposure. *Int. J. Environ. Res. Public Health* **2021**, *18*, in press.
82. Perini, J.A.; Petzl-Erler, M.L.; Tsuneto, L.T.; Suarez-Kurtz, G. VKORC1 polymorphisms in Amerindian populations of Brazil. *Pharmacogenomics* **2008**, *9*, 1623–1629. [CrossRef] [PubMed]
83. Lopes, L.R.; de Miranda, V.A.R.; Guimarães, J.A.M.; Souza, G.G.D.A.; Wainchtock, V.S.; Neto, J.A.G.; Goes, R.D.A.; Perini, J.A. Association of TNF-α-308G > A polymorphism with susceptibility to tendinopathy in athletes: A case–control study. *BMC Sports Sci. Med. Rehabil.* **2021**, *13*, 51. [CrossRef]
84. Akagi, H.; Suzuki, T.; Arimura, K.; Ando, T.; Sakamoto, M.; Satoh, H.; Matsuyama, A. *Mercury Analysis Manual*, 105th ed.; Ministry of the Environmental: Tokyo, Japan, 2004. Available online: http://nimd.env.go.jp/kenkyu/docs/march_mercury_analysis_manual(e).pdf (accessed on 21 November 2019).
85. Bastos, W.R.; Gomes, J.P.O.; Oliveira, R.C.; Almeida, R.; Nascimento, E.L.; Bernardi, J.V.E.; de Lacerda, L.D.; da Silveira, E.G.; Pfeiffer, W.C. Mercury in the environment and riverside population in the Madeira River Basin, Amazon, Brazil. *Sci Total Environ.* **2006**, *368*, 344–351. [CrossRef]
86. Ferreira da Silva, S.; de Oliveira Lima, M. Mercury in fish marketed in the Amazon Triple Frontier and Health Risk Assessment. *Chemosphere* **2020**, *248*, 125989. [CrossRef] [PubMed]
87. Vasconcellos, A.C.S.; Hallwass, G.; Bezerra, J.G.; Aciole, A.N.S.; Meneses, H.N.M.; Lima, M.O.; Jesus, I.M.; Hacon, S.S.; Basta, P.C. Health Risk Assessment of Mercury Exposure from Fish Consumption in Munduruku Indigenous Communities in the Brazilian Amazon. *Int. J. Environ. Res. Public Health* **2021**, *18*, 7940. [CrossRef]
88. WHO. *Guidance for Identifying Populations at Risk from Mercury Exposure*; WHO: Geneva, Switzerland, 2008. Available online: https://wedocs.unep.org/.../IdentifyingPopnatRiskExposuretoMercury2008Web.pdf (accessed on 20 March 2021).
89. Bastos, L.S.; Oliveira, R.D.V.C.D.; Velasque, L.D.S. Obtendo razões de chance prevalentes de modelos de regressão logística em estudos transversais. *Cad Saude Publica* **2015**, *31*, 487–495. [CrossRef]
90. Ospina, R.; Amorim, L. prLogisticDelta: Estimation of Prevalence Ratios using Logistic Models. 2013. Available online: https://rdrr.io/cran/prLogistic/man/prLogisticDelta.html (accessed on 14 June 2021).
91. Kempton, J.W.; Hofer, C.B.; Périssé, A.R.S.; Vasconcellos, A.C.S.; Viana, P.V.S.; Lima, M.O.; Jesus, I.M.; Hacon, S.S.; Basta, P.C. An assessment of health outcomes and methylmercury exposure in Munduruku indigenous women of childbearing age and their children under 2 years old. *Int. J. Environ. Res. Public Health* **2021**, *18*. in press.
92. Perini, J.A.; Silva, M.C.; Vasconcellos, A.C.S.; Viana, P.V.S.; Lima, M.O.; Jesus, I.M.; Kempton, J.W.; Oliveira, R.A.A.; Hacon, S.S.; Basta, P.C. Genetic polymorphism of Delta Aminolevulinic Acid Dehydratase (ALAD) Gene and Symptoms of Chronic Mercury Exposure in Munduruku Indigenous Children from within the Brazilian Amazon. *Int. J. Environ. Res. Public Health* **2021**, *18*, 8746. [CrossRef]
93. Afrifa, J.; Opoku, Y.K.; Gyamerah, E.O.; Ashiagbor, G.; Sorkpor, R.D. The clinical importance of the mercury problem in artisanal small-scale gold mining. *Front. Public Health* **2019**, *7*, 1–9. [CrossRef]
94. Kjellstrom, T.; Kennedy, P.; Wallis, S.; Mantell, C. *Physical and Mental Development of Children with Prenatal Exposure to Mercury from Fish. Stage 1: Preliminary Tests at Age 4*; Report 3080; National Swedish Environmental Board: Solna, Sweden, 1986.
95. Kjellstrom, T.; Kennedy, P.; Wallis, S.; Mantell, C. *Physical and Mental Development of Children with Prenatal Exposure to Mercury from Fish. Stage 2. Interviews and Psychological Tests at Age 6*; Report 3642; National Swedish Environmental Board: Solna, Sweden, 1989.
96. Crump, K.S.; Kjellström, T.; Shipp, A.M.; Silvers, A.; Stewart, A. Influence of prenatal mercury exposure upon scholastic and psychological test performance: Benchmark analysis of a New Zealand cohort. *Risk Anal.* **1998**, *18*, 701–713. [CrossRef]
97. Joint FAO/WHO Expert Committee on Food Additives. Evaluation of Mercury, Lead, Cadmium and the Food Additives Amaranth, Diethylpyrocarbonate and Octyl Gallate. FAO Nutrition Meetings Report Series, No. 51A; WHO Food Additives Series No. 4. 1972. Available online: https://apps.who.int/iris/handle/10665/40985 (accessed on 15 May 2021).
98. Joint FAO/WHO Expert Committee on Food Additives. *Evaluation of Certain Food Additives and Contaminants*; Technical Report Series No. 776; World Health Organization: Geneva, Switzerland, 1989.
99. Joint FAO/WHO Expert Committee on Food Additives. *Safety Evaluation of Certain Food Additives and Contaminants*; WHO Food Additives Series 44; World Health Organization: Geneva, Switzerland, 2000.
100. Houston, M.C. The role of mercury in cardiovascular disease. *J. Cardiovasc. Dis. Diagn* **2014**, *2*, 1–8. [CrossRef]
101. Virtanen, J.K.; Rissanen, T.H.; Voutilainen, S.; Tuomainen, T.P. Mercury as a risk factor for cardiovascular diseases. *J. Nutr. Biochem.* **2007**, *18*, 75–85. [CrossRef]

102. Hu, X.F.; Lowe, M.; Chan, H.M. Mercury exposure, cardiovascular disease, and mortality: A systematic review and dose-response meta-analysis. *Environ. Res.* **2021**, *193*, 110538. [CrossRef]
103. Kim, D.S.; Yu, S.D.; Cha, J.H.; Ahn, S.C.; Lee, E.H. Heavy metal as risk factor of cardiovascular disease-an analysis of blood lead and urinary mercury. *J. Prev. Med. Public Health* **2005**, *38*, 401–407. [PubMed]
104. Virtanen, J.K.; Voutilainen, S.; Rissanen, T.H.; Mursu, J.; Tuomainen, T.-P.; Korhonen, M.; Valkonen, V.-P.; Seppänen, K.; Laukkanen, J.; Salonen, J.T. Mercury, fish oils, and risk of acute coronary events and cardiovascular disease, coronary heart disease, and all-cause mortality in men in eastern Finland. *Arterioscler. Thromb. Vasc. Biol.* **2005**, *25*, 228–233. [CrossRef]
105. Salonen, J.T.; Seppänen, K.; Nyyssönen, K.; Korpela, H.; Kauhanen, J.; Kantola, M.; Tuomilehto, J.; Esterbauer, H.; Tatzber, F.; Salonen, R. Intake of mercury from fish, lipid peroxidation, and the risk of myocardial infarction and coronary, cardiovascular, and any death in eastern Finnish men. *Circulation* **1995**, *91*, 645–655. [CrossRef] [PubMed]
106. Fillion, M.; Mergler, D.; Passos CJ, S.; Larribe, F.; Lemire, M.; Guimarães JR, D. A preliminary study of mercury exposure and blood pressure in the Brazilian Amazon. *Environ. Health* **2006**, *5*, 1–9. [CrossRef]
107. Barcelos, G.R.M.; de Souza, M.F.; de Oliveira, A.; Ávila, S.; Lengert, A.V.H.; de Oliveira, M.T.; Camargo, R.B.D.O.G.; Grotto, D.; Valentini, J.; Garcia, S.; et al. Effects of genetic polymorphisms on antioxidant status and concentrations of the metals in the blood of riverside Amazonian communities co-exposed to Hg and Pb. *Environ. Res.* **2015**, *138*, 224–232. [CrossRef]
108. Faial, K.; Deus, R.; Deus, S.; Neves, R.; Jesus, I.; Santos, E.; Alves, C.N.; Brasil, D. Mercury levels assessment in hair of riverside inhabitants of the Tapajós River, Pará State, Amazon, Brazil: Fish consumption as a possible route of exposure. *J. Trace Elem. Med. Biol.* **2015**, *30*, 66–76. [CrossRef]
109. Freitas, J.S.; Lacerda, E.M.D.C.B.; Júnior, D.R.; Corvelo, T.C.O.; Silveira, L.C.L.; Pinheiro, M.D.C.N.; Souza, G.S. Mercury exposure of children living in amazonian villages: Influence of geographicalocation where they lived during prenatal and postnatal development. *Acad. Bras. Cienc.* **2019**, *91*, e20180097. [CrossRef]
110. Hacon, S.; Barrocas, P.R.; Vasconcellos, A.C.S.D.; Barcellos, C.; Wasserman, J.C.; Campos, R.C.; Ribeiro, C.; Azevedo-Carloni, F.B. An overview of mercury contamination research in the Amazon basin with an emphasis on Brazil Uma revisão das pesquisas sobre contaminação por mercúrio na Amazônia com ênfase no território brasileiro. *Cad Saude Publica.* **2008**, *24*, 1479–1492. [CrossRef]
111. Galvis, S.R. The Amazon Biome in the face of Mercury Contamination. *WWF Gaia Amaz* **2020**, *168*. Available online: https://d2ouvy59p0dg6k.cloudfront.net/downloads/reporte_eng.pdf (accessed on 19 March 2021).
112. WWF. Factsheet: Garimpos—Gold Mines in the Amazon. 2006. Available online: https://wwf.panda.org/?72800/Factsheet-Garimpos-Gold-mines-in-the-Amazon (accessed on 22 June 2021).
113. Barbieri, F.L.; Gardon, J. Hair mercury levels in Amazonian populations: Spatial distribution and trends. *Int. J. Health Geogr.* **2009**, *8*, 71. [CrossRef]
114. Carvalho, L.V.B. *Avaliação dos Níveis de Estresse Oxidativo Induzido por Exposição ao Mercúrio em População Ribeirinha Infantojuvenil do rio Madeira (RO)*; Fundação Oswaldo Cruz: Rio de Janeiro, Brazil, 2016.
115. de Bortoli, M.C. Avaliação dos Níveis Sanguíneos do Hormônio Tireoidiano Ativo (T3) e do Estado Nutricional Relativo ao Selênio de Mulheres Residentes em área de Exposição ao Mercúrio. Ph.D. Thesis, Universidade de São Paulo, São Paulo, Brazil, 2010. [CrossRef]
116. Rocha, A.V.; Cardoso, B.R.; Zavarize, B.; Almondes, K.; Bordon, I.; Hare, D.; Favaro, D.I.T.; Cozzolino, S.M.F. GPX1 Pro198Leu polymorphism and GSTM1 deletion do not affect selenium and mercury status in mildly exposed Amazonian women in an urban population. *Sci. Total Environ.* **2016**, *571*, 801–808. [CrossRef]
117. Farias, L.A.; Fávaro, D.I.T.; Pessoa, A.; Aguiar, J.P.L.; Yuyama, L.K.O. Mercury and methylmercury concentration assessment in children's hair from Manaus, Amazonas state, Brazil. *Acta Amaz.* **2012**, *42*, 279–286. [CrossRef]
118. Begossi, A.; Salivonchyk, S.V.; Hallwass, G.; Hanazaki, N.; Lopes, P.; Silvano, R.A.M.; Dumaresq, D.; Pittock, J. Fish consumption on the amazon: A review of biodiversity, hydropower and food security issues. *Braz. J Biol.* **2019**, *79*, 345–357. [CrossRef] [PubMed]
119. Dórea, J.G. Mercury and lead during breast-feeding. *Br. J. Nutr.* **2004**, *92*, 21–40. [CrossRef] [PubMed]
120. Freeman, M.C.; Garn, J.V.; Sclar, G.D.; Boisson, S.; Medlicott, K.; Alexander, K.T.; Penakalapati, G.; Anderson, D.; Mahtani, A.G.; Grimes, J.E.T.; et al. The impact of sanitation on infectious disease and nutritional status: A systematic review and meta-analysis. *Int. J. Hyg. Environ. Health* **2017**, *220*, 928–949. [CrossRef] [PubMed]
121. Dangour, A.D.; Watson, L.; Cumming, O.; Boisson, S.; Che, Y.; Velleman, Y.; Cavill, S.; Allen, E.; Uauy, R. Interventions to improve water quality and supply, sanitation and hygiene practices, and their effects on the nutritional status of children. *Cochrane Database Syst. Rev.* **2013**, *8*, CD009382. [CrossRef]
122. Horta, B.L.; Santos, R.V.; Welch, J.R.; Cardoso, A.M.; dos Santos, J.V.; Assis, A.M.; Lira, P.C.; Coimbra, C.E., Jr. Nutritional status of indigenous children: Findings from the First National Survey of Indigenous People's Health and Nutrition in Brazil. *Int. J. Equity Health* **2013**, *12*, 23. [CrossRef]
123. Santos, A.P.; Mazzeti, C.M.D.S.; Franco, M.D.C.P.; Santos, N.L.G.O.; Conde, W.L.; Leite, M.S.; Pimenta, A.M.; Villela, L.C.M.; Castro, T.G. Estado nutricional e condições ambientais e de saúde de crianças Pataxó, Minas Gerais, Brasil [Nutritional status and environmental and health conditions of Pataxó indigenous children, Minas Gerais State, Brazil]. *Cad Saude Publica* **2018**, *34*, e00165817. [CrossRef]

124. Frankenburg, W.K.; Dodds, J.; Archer, P.; Shapiro, H.; Bresnick, B. The Denver II: A Major Revision and Restandardization of the Denver Developmental Screening Test. *Pediatrics* **1992**, *89*, 91–97. Available online: https://pediatrics.aappublications.org/content/89/1/91 (accessed on 21 April 2021).
125. Santos-Sacramento, L.; Arrifano, G.P.; Lopes-Araújo, A.; Augusto-Oliveira, M.; Albuquerque-Santos, R.; Takeda, P.Y.; Souza-Monteiro, J.R.; Macchi, B.M.; Nascimento, J.L.M.D.; Lima, R.R.; et al. Human neurotoxicity of mercury in the Amazon: A scoping review with insights and critical considerations. *Ecotoxicol. Environ. Saf.* **2021**, *208*, 111686. [CrossRef] [PubMed]

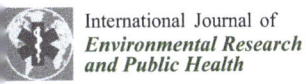

Article

Intergenerational Association of Short Maternal Stature with Stunting in Yanomami Indigenous Children from the Brazilian Amazon

Jesem Douglas Yamall Orellana [1], Giovanna Gatica-Domínguez [2], Juliana dos Santos Vaz [2,3], Paulo Augusto Ribeiro Neves [2], Ana Claudia Santiago de Vasconcellos [4], Sandra de Souza Hacon [5] and Paulo Cesar Basta [5,*]

1. Leônidas e Maria Deane Institute, Oswaldo Cruz Foundation, Rua Teresina, 476, Adrianópolis, Manaus 69057-070, Brazil; jesem.orellana@gmail.com
2. Postgraduate Program in Epidemiology, Faculty of Medicine, Federal University of Pelotas, Rua Marechal Deodoro, 1160-3° Piso, Centro, Pelotas 96020-220, Brazil; giovagatica@gmail.com (G.G.-D.); juliana.vaz@gmail.com (J.d.S.V.); paugustorn@gmail.com (P.A.R.N.)
3. Faculty of Nutrition, Federal University of Pelotas, Rua Gomes Carneiro, 1, Centro, Pelotas 96010-610, Brazil
4. Laboratory of Professional Education in Health Surveillance, Joaquim Venâncio Polytechnic School of Health, Oswaldo Cruz Foundation, Av. Brasil, 4365-Manguinhos, Rio de Janeiro 21040-900, Brazil; anacsvasconcellos@gmail.com
5. Samuel Pessoa Department of Endemics, National School of Public Health, Oswaldo Cruz Foundation, Rio de Janeiro 21041-210, Brazil; sandrahacon@gmail.com
* Correspondence: paulobasta@gmail.com; Tel.: +55-21-2598-2503

Abstract: To describe the factors associated to stunting in <5-year-old Yanomami Brazilian children, and to evaluate the association of short maternal stature to their offspring's stunting. A cross-sectional study carried out in three villages in the Yanomami territory. We performed a census, in which all households with children < 5-years-old were included. The length/height-for-age z-score <−2 standard deviations was used to classify the children as stunted. Short maternal height was defined as <145 cm for adult women, and <−2 standard deviations of the height-for-age z-score for adolescent women. We used adjusted Poisson regression models to estimate prevalence ratios (PR) along the 90% confidence interval. We evaluated 298 children. 81.2% of children suffered from stunting and 71.9% of the mothers from short stature. In the bivariate analysis, a significant association of stunting with short maternal stature, gestational malaria and child's place of birth were observed. Considering the variables of the children under five years of age, there were significant associations with age group, the child's caregiver, history of malaria, pneumonia, and malnutrition treatment. In the adjusted hierarchical model, stunting was 1.22 times greater in the offspring of women with a short stature (90% CI: 1.07–1.38) compared to their counterparts. Brazilian Amazonian indigenous children living in a remote area displayed an alarming prevalence of stunting, and this was associated with short maternal height, reinforcing the hypothesis of intergenerational chronic malnutrition transmission in this population. In addition, children above 24 months of age, who were born in the village healthcare units and who had had previous treatment in the past for stunting presented higher rates of stunting in this study.

Keywords: poverty areas; undernutrition; indigenous populations; intergenerational relations; epidemiologic determinants

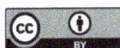

1. Introduction

Stunting, defined as the height-for-age deficit, not only raises the risk of mortality and incapacity in childhood [1], but is also associated with short stature in adulthood, neurocognitive development impairment, and long-term reduction in human capital [2–4]. The 2030 Agenda for sustainable development aims to eliminate all forms of malnutrition in children under 5 years of age (Goal 2.2) and reduce inequalities, ensuring no one is left behind (Goal 10) [5]. Unfortunately, it is expected that the Covid-19 pandemic will not only affect the discreet advancements towards eliminating all forms of malnutrition in children under 5 years of age, but it will also widen already existing socioeconomic inequalities [6,7].

In general, the indigenous peoples of Latin America have been an ethnical group disproportionately less favored [8]. Indigenous children present high prevalence of stunting when compared to non-indigenous children [9,10]. In Brazil, it is estimated that stunting affects approximately 6% of children under 5 years of age [11], with important regional inequalities, since stunting prevalence reaches 8.5% and 3.9% in non-indigenous children living in the North and South regions, respectively [11]. In indigenous people the situation is even worst, as stunting occurs in approximately 26% of indigenous Brazilian children, especially in the North region (nearly 41% of children experiencing stunted growth) [12]. The comparative analysis reveals deep inequalities between Brazilian macro-regions and different ethnical groups in the country.

There is evidence that short maternal height negatively influences the growth of linear offspring [13], which persists through adulthood [13–15]. Recent studies showed that growth-faltering begins during pregnancy [14]. Therefore, the need for measures to intervene and prevent the intergenerational effects (e.g., epigenetics, metabolic programming due to alterations, amongst others) associated with short maternal stature is crucial, especially during the "first 1000 days window". The interventions must seek to break the poverty cycle and the consequential intergenerational deficits in adult human capital [14].

Recognizing the worrisome nutritional situation in indigenous children, the investigation of its determinants remains an important challenge not only for sanitary authorities, but also for healthcare workers and professionals [16]. Therefore, the objective of this study was to describe the factors associated with stunting in <5-year-old Yanomami Brazilian children, and to evaluate the association of short maternal stature to their offspring's stunting.

2. Materials and Methods

2.1. Study Area and Population

In Brazil, the Yanomami population is comprised of nearly 28,000 individuals, distributed over 360 villages. The Yanomami Indigenous Territory (YIT) covers 9,664,975 hectares, bordering with Venezuela. This study was conducted with children under 5 years of age and their mothers, in the administrative regions *Auaris* and *Maturacá* in the Brazilian Amazon. Two villages in the *Maturacá* region were included in the study, namely *Ariabú* and *Maturacá* (Figure 1).

The *Auaris* region is located in the extreme north of the state of Roraima, one of the areas with the highest population density of the YIT (Figure 1). It is exclusively accessed by air from the state capital, *Boa Vista*. In turn, *Maturacá* is based in the Amazonas state and can be accessed by air from *Boa Vista* or *São Gabriel da Cachoeira*, Amazonas, or by land and boat from *São Gabriel da Cachoeira*.

2.2. Study Design

A cross-sectional census study was conducted between 9 and 22 December 2018 in the *Auaris* region and between 6 and 27 February 2019 in *Ariabú* and *Maturacá* villages. For this study, semi-structured interviews were conducted by key-informants (women/mothers or people responsible for the household) using data collection questionnaires. When key-informants did not speak Portuguese, a local translator mediated the interviews. The consent to participate was obtained through signature (or fingerprint) of the informed consent.

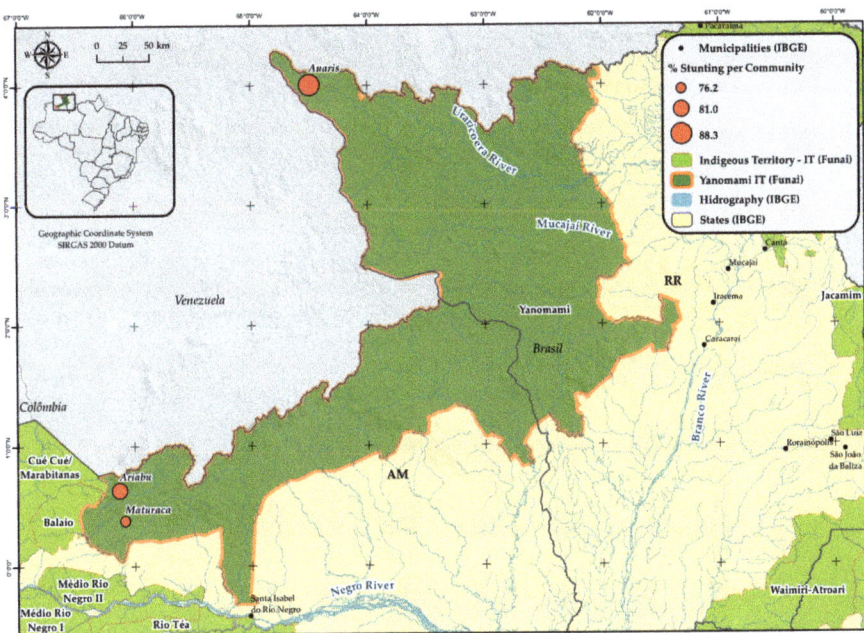

Figure 1. Studied villages in the Yanomami Indigenous Territory (YIT), according to the prevalence of stunting. Roraima and Amazonas states, Brazilian Amazon, 2018–2019.

2.3. Maternal and Child Anthropometry

To measure the height and weight of participants we used the following equipment: vertical anthropometer or Alturexata® stadiometer with an infantometer adaptor with a precision of 0.1 cm (length measure) and a Seca® portable digital scale (model 877) with maximum capacity of 150 kg and a precision of 0.1 kg.

We used the WHO-Anthro® [17] and WHO-Anthro Plus® [18] programs to build the anthropometric length/height-for-age index in z-scores of children under 5 years of age and adolescent women, respectively.

We classified children as stunted and adolescent women with a short stature if they presented a length/height-for-age z-score less than −2 standard deviations of the median population of reference, according to the WHO Growth Charts.

Anthropometric information of six children was excluded from the analysis due to congenital malformations and implausible values of the length/height-for-age z-scores. No adolescent mother showed implausible z-score values [17,18]. For women older than 18 years of age, we considered a height of less than 145 cm as constituting a short stature [19].

2.4. Sociodemographic, Maternal and Child Characteristics

The following sociodemographic characteristics were considered: (i) region/village of residence (*Auaris; Maturacá; Ariabú*); (ii) parent knowledge (read or write) in Portuguese (yes; no); (iii) home source of income (Federal, Statal/Municipal Governments, Others or No Income); (iv) household water source for human consumption (well; river/stream); (v) waste management (thrown in the forest/river; burnt/buried); (vi) household wall-type (wood/brick; clay; straw/no wall); (vii) household density (1 to 6; 7 to 9; ≥10 people).

The maternal characteristics considered were: (i) age group (13 to 24; 25 years or older); (ii) short stature (yes; no); (iii) number of antenatal consultations (0 to 3; 4 to 6; 7

to 9); (iv) gestational malaria history (yes; no); (v) children's place of birth (house/forest; village's healthcare units; Casa de Saúde do Índio—CASAI/Hospital).

With respect to the children, we considered the following characteristics: (i) sex (male; female); (ii) age group ($\leq$23; 24 to 59 months); (iii) child's main caregiver (mother or father, other family member); (iv) weight at birth (<2500 g; $\geq$2500 g); (v) previous pneumonia treatment (yes; no); (vi) previous malnutrition treatment (yes; no); (vii) previous malaria treatment (yes; no).

2.5. Statistical Analysis

Differences between proportion were assessed using the Pearson chi-square test. The Crude-Poisson regression, adjusted to covariables with consistent covariance matrix estimator type HC2, was used to estimate the Prevalence Ratio (PR) for stunting [20].

In the crude analysis, we selected variables with a p value < 0.20 to further adjust the analysis, using an hierarchical framework based on previous studies [21]. The conceptual hierarchical framework, established a priori, was structured into four levels and the introduction of variables in the models obeyed a hierarchical sequence. The hierarchical levels included were: 1st level (sociodemographic characteristics): region/village of residence and type of wall; 2nd level (maternal characteristics): gestational malaria and child's place of birth; 3rd level (child characteristics): age group and child main caregiver; 4th level (health history of the child): child's previous malaria treatment.

After the first selection, we used the backward method to select variables associated at p-values < 0.10 in each level to the final adjust model. Pre-selected variables in each level were retained in the subsequent models, independent of their p-value. Additionally, the interaction between household wall-type and place of birth was tested in the final adjusted model, considering a p-value < 0.10.

The villages included in the present study were based in hard-to-reach areas of the Brazilian Amazon. Due to the small sample size (n = 298), we adopted p-values of 0.10 and 0.20 as statistically significant in order to guarantee that any effects from the studied variables could be tested. However, it is worth remembering that we carried out a census in the investigated villages, and all children under 5 years of age were included in the study.

Data analysis was performed using the statistical software R, version 3.3.2 [22].

3. Results

The prevalence of stunting among indigenous children under 5 years of age was 81.2% (Table 1), varying greatly across villages, with the highest burden in *Auaris* (88.3%) and the lowest in *Ariabú* (76.2%). Considering only children older than 12 months of age, stunting prevalence was superior to 85%, and in the age-group ranging from 24 to 59 months of age stunting was superior to 90%, regardless of region/village. The prevalence of short maternal stature was 71.9% (mean maternal height of 143.0 cm; standard deviation = 4.3) (Table 2). Similarly to stunting in children, the highest burden of short maternal height was seen in *Auaris* (87.7%) and the lowest in mothers in *Ariabú* (65.0%) regions/villages.

When comparing the sociodemographic characteristics between the villages, we observed that most fathers in *Auaris* did not know how to read and write in Portuguese (44.9%). Similarly, the stunting frequencies were higher among families that dispose household waste in the river or the forest (92.4%), households with no regular income (65.4%), and households with clay walls (74.4%) (Table 2). Furthermore, regarding maternal and perinatal variables, only 1.7% of mothers in *Auaris* attended between 7 and 9 antenatal visits, and only 6.4% of mothers in *Auaris* gave birth in a healthcare facility (hospital/CASAI).

Regarding sociodemographic variables, only household wall-type was shown to be significantly associated with stunting (Table 3). We found a significant association between stunting with short maternal stature, gestational malaria, and the child's place of birth. Lastly, for variables related to child health, stunting was associated with age, the child's caregiver, previous malaria, pneumonia, and previous undernutrition treatment.

Table 1. Stunting characterization in children under 5 years of age, according to the villages of residence. Yanomami Indigenous Territory, Brazilian Amazon, 2018–2019.

Age Group (Months)	Stunting											
	Auaris			*Maturacá*			*Ariabú*			Total		
	N	n	%	N	n	%	N	n	%	N	n	%
≤11	12	7	58.3	24	9	37.5	25	7	28.0	61	23	37.7
12 to 23	16	16	100.0	18	16	88.9	20	17	85.0	54	49	90.7
24 to 35	12	12	100.0	22	22	100.0	17	17	100.0	51	51	100.0
36 to 59	37	33	89.2	52	47	90.4	43	39	90.7	132	119	90.2
Total	77	68	88.3	116	94	81.0	105	80	76.2	298	242	81.2

N—total number of children in the evaluated age group; n—number of children with stunting.

Table 2. Sociodemographic, maternal and children under five years of age characteristics, according to the village of residence. Yanomami Indigenous Territory, Brazilian Amazon, 2018–2019.

	Villages of Residence			
	Ariabú n (%)	*Auaris* n (%)	*Maturacá* n (%)	*p*-Value *
Sociodemographic variables				
Read or write in Portuguese				<0.001
No	11 (10.7%)	35 (44.9%)	16 (14.0%)	
Yes	92 (89.3%)	43 (55.1%)	98 (86.0%)	
Source of Income				<0.001
Federal	12 (11.4%)	18 (23.1%)	11 (9.3%)	
Municipal/Statal	24 (22.9%)	4 (5.1%)	25 (21.2%)	
Other	8 (7.6%)	5 (6.4%)	26 (22.0%)	
No income	61 (58.1%)	51 (65.4%)	56 (47.5%)	
Drinking water source				<0.001
River or stream	82 (78.1%)	55 (70.5%)	17 (14.4%)	
Well	23 (21.9%)	23 (29.5%)	101 (86.6%)	
Household waste destination				<0.001
Burnt or buried	38 (36.2%)	6 (7.6%)	90 (76.9%)	
Forest or river	67 (63.8%)	73 (92.4%)	27 (23.1%)	
Household wall type				<0.001
Wood/brick	40 (38.1%)	7 (9.0%)	46 (49.5%)	
Clay	52 (49.5%)	58 (74.4%)	61 (35.7%)	
Straw/no wall	13 (12.4%)	13 (16.6%)	09 (25.7%)	
Household density (number of people)				0.035
1 to 6	32 (30.5%)	18 (23.7%)	40 (33.9%)	
7 to 9	27 (25.7%)	27 (35.5%)	47 (39.8%)	
10 or more	46 (43.8%)	31 (40.8%)	31 (26.3%)	
Maternal and perinatal variables				
Age group (years)				0.118
13.0 to 24.9	42 (40.0%)	20 (27.7%)	49 (41.5%)	
25.0 or more	63 (60.0%)	53 (72.6%)	69 (58.5%)	
Short maternal stature				0.002
No	35 (35.0%)	9 (12.3%)	37 (32.2%)	
Yes	65 (65.0%)	64 (87.7%)	78 (67.8%)	
Number of antenatal consultations				<0.001
0 to 3	19 (21.1%)	31 (52.5%)	22 (20.2%)	
4 to 6	50 (55.6%)	27 (45.8%)	71 (65.1%)	
7 to 9	21 (23.3%)	1 (1.7%)	16 (14.7%)	
Gestational malaria				0.205
No	89 (84.8%)	68 (93.2%)	100 (85.5%)	
Yes	16 (15.2%)	5 (6.8%)	17 (14.5%)	

Table 2. Cont.

	Villages of Residence			
	Ariabú	Auaris	Maturacá	p-Value *
	n (%)	n (%)	n (%)	
Place of birth				<0.001
Household/Forest	57 (53.8%)	71 (91.0%)	68 (59.6%)	
Primary Healthcare Center (villages)	27 (25.5%)	2 (2.6%)	23 (20.2%)	
Hospital/CASAI [1]	22 (20.8%)	5 (6.4%)	23 (20.2%)	
Child's variables				
Sex				<0.001
Female	69 (65.7%)	26 (32.9%)	81 (68.6%)	
Male	36 (34.3%)	53 (67.1%)	37 (31.4%)	
Age group (months)				0.534
≤23	46 (43.4%)	29 (36.2%)	44 (37.3%)	
24 to 59	60 (56.6%)	51 (63.8%)	74 (62.7%)	
Child's caregiver				<0.001
Mother or father	80 (75.5%)	40 (50.6%)	101 (87.8%)	
Another family member	26 (24.5%)	39 (49.4%)	14 (12.2%)	
Low weight at birth				0.977
No	93 (89.4%)	61 (88.4%)	103 (88.8%)	
Yes	11 (10.6%)	8 (11.6%)	13 (11.2%)	
Pneumonia treatment				0.069
No	70 (66.7%)	39 (50.0%)	66 (56.9%)	
Yes	35 (33.3%)	39 (50.0%)	50 (43.1%)	
Undernutrition treatment				0.127
No	93 (87.7%)	60 (76.9%)	94 (79.7%)	
Yes	13 (12.3%)	18 (23.1%)	24 (20.3%)	
Malaria treatment				0.239
No	97 (91.5%)	67 (84.8%)	108 (91.5%)	
Yes	9 (8.5%)	12 (15.2%)	10 (8.5%)	
Stunting prevalence				0.118
No	25 (23.8%)	9 (11.7%)	22 (19.0%)	
Yes	80 (76.2%)	68 (88.3%)	94 (81.0%)	

n = number of cases observed in each variable, according to the village of residence; * p-value refers to Pearson's chi-square test; [1] CASAI (*Casa de Saúde do Índio*): Unit of support to the indigenous people who live in villages during healthcare attendance in urban centers.

Table 3. Proportion of children under five years of age with and without stunting according to sociodemographic, maternal and child variables. Yanomami Indigenous Territory, Brazilian Amazon, 2018–2019.

	Stunting		
	No	Yes	p-Value *
	n (%)	n (%)	
Sociodemographic variables			
Parent knows how to read or write in Portuguese			0.877
No	11 (20.0%)	49 (20.9%)	
Yes	44 (80.0%)	185 (79.1%)	
Source of Income			0.305
Federal	11 (19.6%)	30 (12.6%)	
Municipal/Statal	12 (21.4%)	41 (17.2%)	
Other	8 (14.3%)	30 (12.6%)	
No income	25 (44.6%)	138 (57.7%)	
Drinking water source			0.799

Table 3. Cont.

	Stunting		p-Value *
	No	Yes	
	n (%)	n (%)	
River or stream	28 (50.0%)	124 (51.9%)	
Well	28 (50.0%)	115 (48.1%)	
Household waste destination			0.409
Burnt or buried	28 (50.0%)	105 (43.9%)	
Forest or river	28 (50.0%)	134 (56.1%)	
Household wall type			0.063
Wood/brick	25 (44.6%)	68 (28.7%)	
Clay	27 (48.2%)	141 (59.5%)	
Straw/no wall	4 (7.1%)	28 (11.8%)	
Household density (number of people)			0.770
1 to 6	17 (30.4%)	71 (30.0%)	
7 to 9	17 (30.4%)	83 (35.0%)	
10 or more	22 (39.3%)	83 (35.0%)	
Maternal and perinatal variables			
Age group (years)			0.390
13.0 to 24.9	17 (32.1%)	91 (38.4%)	
25.0 or more	36 (67.9%)	146 (61.6%)	
Short maternal stature			<0.001
No	28 (52.8%)	53 (23.1%)	
Yes	25 (47.2%)	176 (76.9%)	
Number of antenatal consultations			0.797
0 to 3	16 (31.4%)	54 (26.7%)	
4 to 6	28 (54.9%)	117 (57.9%)	
7 to 9	7 (13.7%)	31 (15.3%)	
Gestational malaria			0.071
No	52 (94.5%)	201 (85.5%)	
Yes	3 (5.5%)	34 (14.5%)	
Place of birth			0.027
House/Forest	33 (62.3%)	158 (66.1%)	
Primary Healthcare Center (villages)	5 (9.4%)	46 (19.2%)	
Hospital/CASAI [1]	15 (28.3%)	35 (14.6%)	
Child variables			
Sex			0.479
Female	30 (54.5%)	144 (59.8%)	
Male	25 (45.5%)	97 (40.2%)	
Age group (months)			<0.001
≤23	43 (76.8%)	72 (29.8%)	
24 to 59	13 (23.2%)	170 (70.2%)	
Child's caregiver			0.089
Mother or father	45 (83.3%)	170 (70.8%)	
Another family member	9 (16.7%)	70 (29.2%)	
Low weight at birth			0.779
No	46 (90.2%)	207 (88.8%)	
Yes	5 (9.8%)	26 (11.2%)	
Pneumonia treatment			<0.001
No	43 (78.2%)	126 (52.9%)	
Yes	12 (21.8%)	112 (47.1%)	
Undernutrition treatment			0.002
No	54 (96.4%)	189 (78.8%)	
Yes	2 (3.6%)	51 (21.2%)	
Malaria treatment			0.072
No	54 (96.4%)	213 (88.4%)	
Yes	2 (3.6%)	28 (11.6%)	

n = number of cases observed; * p-value refers to Poisson regression; [1] *Casa de Saúde do Índio*: Unit of support to the indigenous people who live in villages during healthcare attendance in urban centers.

In the hierarchical multiple regression analysis, which included the interactive term between household wall-type and child's place of birth, the final model indicated a stunting risk of 22% (7–38%) higher in children whose mothers with a short stature, compared to those with normal stature (Table 4).

Table 4. Crude and adjusted hierarchical models of the association between stunting in Yanomami children under five years old and short maternal height. Yanomami Indigenous Territory, Brazilian Amazon, 2018–2019.

Level	Variable	Crude PR (CI 80%)	p-Value	Adjusted PR (CI 90%)	p-Value
1	Region/village of residence				
	Ariabú	1		1	
	Auaris	1.07 (1.06–1.27)	0.032	1.09 (0.97–1.22)	0.222
	Maturacá	1.07 (0.97–1.16)	0.385	1.04 (0.93–1.17)	0.563
	Household wall type				
	Wood/brick	1		1	
	Clay	1.15 (1.05–1.26)	0.055	1.13 (1.01–1.26)	0.088
	Straw/no wall	1.20 (1.06–1.35)	0.053	1.19 (1.01–1.40)	0.082
2	Gestational malaria				
	No	1		1	
	Yes	1.06 (1.07–1.25)	0.014	1.12 (1.01–1.25)	0.070 [a]
	Place of birth				
	Hospital/Casai	1		1	
	Forest	1.10 (1.04–1.34)	0.092	1.17 (0.99–1.38)	0.118 [b]
	Primary Healthcare Center (in the villages)	1.11 (1.13–1.47)	0.015	1.26 (1.05–1.51)	0.041 [b]
3	Age group (months)				
	≤23	1		1	
	24 to 59	1.08 (1.35–1.63)	0.001	1.48 (1.30–1.67)	0.001 [c]
	Child's caregiver				
	Mother or father	1		1	
	Other family member	1.06 (1.05–1.20)	0.034	1.10 (1.01–1.20)	0.080 [d]
4	Malaria treatment				
	No	1		1	
	Yes	1.06 (1.09–1.26)	0.007	1.05 (0.95–1.17)	0.412 [e]
	Child stunting (outcome)				
	No	1		1	
	Yes	1.34 (1.20–1.49)	0.001	1.22 (1.07–1.38)	0.012 [f]

PR = Prevalence Ratio; [a] Adjusted by wall-type. [b] Adjusted by wall-type and gestational malaria. [c] Adjusted by wall-type, gestational malaria and place of birth. [d] Adjusted by wall-type, gestational malaria, place of birth and age group. [e] Adjusted by wall-type, gestational malaria, place of birth, age group and child's caregiver. [f] Adjusted by wall-type, gestational malaria, place of birth, age group and child's caregiver to the interaction between wall-type and place of birth.

4. Discussion

We described an alarming prevalence of stunting among Brazilian indigenous children living in the Amazon. Additionally, we found a significant association between short maternal stature and stunting in the offspring. Such findings reinforce the hypothesis of intergenerational transmission of stunting in Yanomami indigenous people, highlighting the precarity of health and nutrition conditions in these settings.

Stunting prevalence varies markedly across regions of the world. Recent evidence suggests that stunting occurs in 39.0% and 55.0% of African and Asian children under five, respectively [6,23]. In Brazil, a nationwide survey showed that 40.8% of indigenous children under five years of age, living in the North region, suffered from stunting [12]. In contrast, stunting prevalence of 6.3% and 5.7% were reported in the same period for non-indigenous boys and girls under 5 years of age in the same area, respectively [11], revealing huge inequalities in the nutritional status of indigenous children in Brazil. Despite the chronic patterns of stunting among indigenous people globally, a prevalence of stunting above 80% have only been reported among Yanomami children, highlighting the critical nutritional status of this group [24,25].

Scientific research on the determinants of the nutritional status in indigenous children under five years of age can improve public policies and reduce social inequalities in health, fostering social protection mechanisms. At the same time, the association between short maternal stature and stunting in our study showed not only an intergenerational effect but reinforces previous findings of the high burden of stunting in Yanomami children, as well as the need for interventions aimed at breaking down the cycle of sickness and death that remain for decades [24–30].

The critical scenario revealed in this study confirms that the high rates of stunting persist for a long time in the Yanomami Indigenous territory as a result of not only a permanent state of food insecurity but also due to structural racism historically imposed by the Government. In contrast with the goals of the 2030 Agenda for sustainable development [5], which aim to eliminate all forms of malnutrition in children under five years of age and reduce inequalities, leaving no one behind, and the United Nations Declaration on the Rights of Indigenous Peoples (UNDRIP) [31,32], the Brazilian Government has not fulfilled its duty.

Throughout history, the indigenous people have been marginalized, discriminated against, and exploited by Western society. In turn, the Government has not implemented inclusive and sustainable public policies to reduce poverty and starvation and promote reparation for the violations suffered by these peoples. In addition, the Government continues to deny them access to essential public services, such as health, sanitation, education, employment, and income, as well as the rights to self-determination and the control over natural resources existing on their traditional territories. Moreover, in the last couple of years, several bills have been presented to the parliament in order to reduce rights assured in the Brazilian Federal Constitution.

Therefore, we consider that the path to sovereignty should be built in another way, putting on the indigenous people at the center of the debate, valorizing their culture and their traditional knowledge, in order to attain a fairer and equitable society, where no child, no citizen and no nations will be left behind.

A recent analysis regarding ethnic inequalities in the prevalence of stunting in children under 5 years of age in 13 Latin American countries showed a highly unfavorable situation for indigenous populations. The polled prevalence ratio of stunting for all countries was 1.34 (CI 95% 1.28 to 1.39) for indigenous children compared to non-indigenous children, even after adjustments were made to household wealth and place of residence [9]. Furthermore, another study conducted in Latin American countries showed a low coverage of healthcare services for indigenous women and children when compared to non-indigenous people, independent of wealth or place of residence [33]. Although these studies did not capture the specific space-temporal contextual particularities, they reinforce social inequality and precarious access to healthcare and sanitary services by indigenous people, even though such items are considered part of universal rights [32,33]. In Brazil, indigenous people are a minority, and they represent less than 0.5% of the country's population, which makes the adoption and implementation of a broad intercultural healthcare model crucial [34].

The well-known intergenerational transmission of poverty and some critical prenatal determinants play a significant role in the high burden of stunting in many parts of the world. The more precarious the living conditions, the worse the malnutrition indicators in children, notably the stunting cases [35]. This phenomenon is consistent with the social determinants of the child malnutrition model developed by UNICEF [36], that states that the precarious conditions of health and maternal diet, before conception and during pregnancy, as well as a persistent exposure to a poor diet, considering quantity and quality of the food (i.e., food with low energy, protein, and micronutrients content), in addition, recurrent infections of infancy are each among the leading causes of stunting. On the other hand, other causes of stunting include food insecurity, inadequate feeding practices, an unhealthy domestic environment, inadequate healthcare service access, and poverty [36].

Food insecurity leads to the reduction in quantity and quality of consumed foods, as well as changing eating habits, due to lack of money or the absence of other material resources. This combination of factors acting together negatively affects the nutritional status, health and welfare of families [36]. There is evidence that indigenous children between 6 and 23 months of age in Latin American countries receive maternal milk for a longer period of time, however, the complementary foods available for these children are low in quality. Therefore, the availability of maternal milk for a longer period of time does not seem sufficient to meet the nutritional needs of the children in this age group. Consequently, these children are more susceptible to catch-up delays in growth [9].

It is important to point out that, historically, indigenous people have been exposed to high loads of infectious and parasitic diseases, both in terms of frequency and seriousness of the reported clinical conditions [37,38]. In this sense, parasitic infestation, gastrointestinal infections, and enteric environmental disfunctions are especially important due to negative effects in nutrient digestion and absorption, threatening not only the growth potential, but also raising the risk of death in indigenous children [39–41]. The precarious sanitary conditions in the indigenous villages in Latin America [42], as well as those observed in the studied Yanomami children—including the limited access to potable drinking water and inadequate household waste destination—help to understand not only the elevated and permanent exposure of these children to infectious and parasitic diseases [30], but the severity of the nutritional situation. The precarious nutritional status of the Yanomami children living in Brazil and Venezuela [24–29] has been systematically denounced for at least three decades.

One of the long-term consequences of stunting in childhood is the short stature in adulthood [43]. Mothers with a short stature in adulthood can give birth to tiny babies due to an insufficient supply of nutrients or due to an unfavorable intrauterine environment—due to lack of food—for adequate fetal growth [44]. Our findings reinforce another record from Orellana et al. [24] that shows an association between short maternal stature and severe stunting in Yanomami children under five years of age who reside in other regions of the YIT in Brazil. In the same study, the authors also revealed a stunting prevalence of 83.8%, and that children of mothers with height < 145 cm presented higher prevalence of stunting (PR: 2.1; CI 95%: 1.2–3.6) compared to children of mothers with stature $\geq$145 cm.

In turn, a study using data from birth cohorts carried out in five low- or middle-income countries (Brazil, Guatemala, India, Philippines, and South Africa) showed that mothers with a stature shorter than 150.1 cm presented a 3.2 times higher probability of having children with stunting at 2 years of age (CI 95%: 2.8–3.6) and 4.7 times higher in the adulthood (CI 95%: 4.1–5.4), when compared to mothers with a higher stature [13].

Other potential threats help explain the precarious nutritional conditions of the Yanomami Brazilian children, such as the invasions of the traditional territories by illegal miners, loggers, grabbing, and other criminals searching of wealth in the Amazon Forest [45,46]. All factors previously mentioned can simultaneously increase the risks of food insecurity and the maintenance of stunting in children under five years of age and all family members living in the region.

Despite the illustrative findings of this investigation, consistent with the specialized literature, it is important to consider the limitations. It was not possible to evaluate children who were receiving healthcare treatments outside of the villages at the time of our visits. On the one hand, this could have contributed to underestimation of stunting prevalence in our study. On the other hand, the reduced number of villages included in this study does not represent the nutritional status of all the children who live in the YIT, thus requiring caution in the generalizations of the results. Although all of the house visits were conducted with a local translator, the information bias cannot be disregarded, as well as memory bias, especially in questions related to healthcare services access and former sickness in older children.

Aside the aforementioned limitations, it is worth highlighting that although the number of Yanomami children evaluated ($n = 298$) could be considered small, it was expressive since these children live in regions with difficult access and that, in certain circumstances, these children can pass months without regular visits by healthcare teams. Under the methodological point of view, the exposure and the outcome evaluated in this study were measured following quality recommendations standards by WHO. Despite the cross-sectional nature of our data, we can say that the reverse causality phenomenon did not affect our association estimates, since the short maternal stature exposure was already defined before pregnancy and childbirth, which eliminates the exposure-outcome temporality dilemma in our data. Finally, even without excluding the possibility of residual confusion, we adopted robust data analysis methods by a hierarchical approach, using a measure of appropriate association to sectional studies.

5. Conclusions

The high prevalence of stunting recorded in children under 5 years of age in the Yanomami Indigenous territory, especially those living in the *Auaris* region, reveals an alarming and unprecedented situation of health neglect. Therefore, it is essential to remember that Article 21 of the United Nations Declaration on the Rights of Indigenous Peoples assures that: "Indigenous peoples have the right, without discrimination, to the improvement of their economic and social conditions, including, among other things, in the areas of education, employment, vocational training and retraining, housing, sanitation, health and social security" [33].

In conclusion, even if the birth of many generations is necessary to eliminate the effects of intergenerational short stature, it is vital to understand that specific, broad, and inclusive nutritional interventions and programs are essential to prevent stunting in an ethnic and culturally differentiated context, especially if they are addressed in the first 1000 days of a child's life. This period is considered a unique window of opportunity, especially in indigenous children, seriously affected by stunting. Therefore, effective multisectoral measures must be implemented to eradicate stunting in the Yanomami Territory.

Finally, we consider it equally essential to create sustainable projects by the Federal Government in close collaboration with non-governmental organizations and indigenous associations. These projects must propose strategies to assure regular income generation with the participation of local society in managing the resources, assuring self-identification patterns, cultural valorizing, respect to ancient knowledge, and traditional foods. The ultimate goal should be to reach food sovereignty and social inclusion, guaranteeing basic water supply services, sanitation in villages, and regular access to health services.

Author Contributions: Conceptualization, J.D.Y.O. and P.C.B.; methodology, J.D.Y.O.; A.C.S.d.V.; S.d.S.H. and P.C.B.; formal analysis, J.D.Y.O.; G.G.-D.; J.d.S.V.; P.A.R.N. and P.C.B.; investigation, J.D.Y.O.; A.C.S.d.V. and P.C.B.; resources, J.D.Y.O. and P.C.B.; writing—original draft preparation, J.D.Y.O.; G.G.-D.; J.d.S.V. and P.A.R.N.; writing—review and editing, J.D.Y.O. and P.C.B.; project administration, J.D.Y.O. and P.C.B.; funding acquisition, P.C.B. All authors have read and agreed to the published version of the manuscript.

Funding: This research was funded by the United Nations International Children's Emergency Fund (UNICEF), contract number 43246507/2018.

Institutional Review Board Statement: The study was conducted in accordance with the guidelines of the Declaration of Helsinki and the study protocol was submitted and approved by the Research Ethics Committee of the National School of Public Health at Fiocruz (REC/ENSP) and the Brazilian National Research Ethics Commission of the National Health Council (CONEP/CNS) (CAAE: 91612218.8.0000.5240, Opinion number 2.896.403). In addition, the research team requested authorization to the *Fundação Nacional do Índio* (FUNAI) for entrance in the Yanomami Indigenous Territory and a previous consultation of the studied communities was conducted before the fieldwork. The data collection instruments were applied only after expressed consent in the informed consent forms.

Informed Consent Statement: Informed consent was obtained from all subjects involved in the study. Written informed consent has been obtained from the mothers and/or caregivers of the children to publish this paper.

Data Availability Statement: Data sharing not applicable.

Acknowledgments: Through chiefs Davi Kopenawa Yanomami, Francisco Xavier da Silva, and Floriza da Cruz Pinto which represented of Hutukara Yanomami Association (HAY), Association of Yanomami Women (Kumirãyõma), and Yanomami of Cauaburis River and Tributaries Association (AYRCA) at the fielwork, we thank the Yanomami indigenous people for the trust placed in our team and the support in carrying out the research. We would thank Cristina Albuquerque and the technical team from UNICEF Brazil for funding this research. We thank the Yanomami Indigenous Special Sanitary District (DSEI-Y) coordination, which spared no effort to support us in all stages of the fieldwork. On behalf of all teams that work for DSEI-Y, we thank the nurses Eliane Sanches Henriques and Geovanny Ribeiro Carvalho. We also thank Anderson Vasconcelos, Clarisse do Carmo Jabur and Túlio Caio Binotti from National Indian Foundation (FUNAI) to the logistic and legal support. Finally, we thank Daniel de Oliveira d'El Rei Pinto, who made the study area map. We appreciate the Joênia Wapichana Federal Deputy for her support for publication fee costs through the parliamentary amendment number 41510004.

Conflicts of Interest: The authors declare no conflict of interest. The funders had no role in the design of the study; in the collection, analyses, or interpretation of data; in the writing of the manuscript, or in the decision to publish the results.

References

1. World Health Organization (WHO). *WHO Child Growth Standards: Length/Height-for-Age, Weight-for-Age, Weight-for-Length, Weight-for-Height and Body Mass Index-for-Age*; Methods and Development; WHO (Nonserial Publication); WHO: Geneva, Switzerland, 2006.
2. Black, R.E.; Allen, L.H.; Bhutta, Z.A.; Caulfield, L.E.; De Onis, M.; Ezzati, M.; Mathers, C.; Rivera, J.; Maternal and Child Undernutrition Study Group. Maternal and child undernutrition: Global and regional exposures and health consequences. *Lancet* **2008**, *371*, 243–260. [CrossRef]
3. Ozaltin, E.; Hill, K.; Subramanian, S.V. Association of maternal stature with offspring mortality, underweight, and stunting in low- to middle-income countries. *JAMA* **2010**, *303*, 1507–1516. [CrossRef] [PubMed]
4. Stein, A.D.; Wang, M.; Martorell, R.; Norris, S.A.; Adair, L.S.; Bas, I.; Sachdev, H.S.; Bhargava, S.K.; Fall, C.H.D.; Gigante, D.; et al. Growth patterns in early childhood and final attained stature: Data from five birth cohorts from low- and middle-income countries. *Am. J. Hum. Biol.* **2010**, *22*, 353–359. [CrossRef] [PubMed]
5. United Nations (UN). *Transforming Our World: The 2030 Agenda for Sustainable Development*; Division for Sustainable Development Goals: New York, NY, USA, 2021.
6. UNICEF; WHO; World Bank Group. *Levels and Trends in Child. Malnutrition*; UNICEF-WHO-World Bank Group Joint Child Malnutrition Estimates: Key Findings of the 2019 Edition; UNICEF: New York, NY, USA; WHO: Geneva, Switzerland; World Bank Group: Washington, DC, USA, 2019.
7. Victora, C.G.; Christian, P.; Vidaletti, L.P.; Gatica-Domínguez, G.; Menon, P.; Black, R.E. Revisiting maternal and child undernutrition in low-income and middle-income countries: Variable progress towards an unfinished agenda. *Lancet* **2021**, *397*, 1388–1399. [CrossRef]
8. World Bank Group. Indigenous Latin America in the Twenty-First Century: The First Decade. World Bank. © World Bank. 2015. Available online: https://openknowledge.worldbank.org/handle/10986/23751 (accessed on 23 June 2021).
9. Gatica-Domínguez, G.; Victora, C.; Barros, A.J. Ethnic inequalities and trends in stunting prevalence among Guatemalan children: An analysis using national health surveys 1995–2014. *Int. J. Equity Health* **2019**, *18*, 1–11. [CrossRef] [PubMed]
10. Amarante, V.; Figueroa, N.; Ullman, H. Inequalities in the reduction of child stunting over time in Latin America: Evidence from the DHS 2000–2010. *Oxf. Dev. Stud.* **2018**, *46*, 519–535. [CrossRef]
11. Instituto Brasileiro de Geografia e Estatística (IBGE). *Pesquisa de Orçamentos Familiares (POF): Antropometria e Estado Nutricional de Crianças, Adolescentes e Adultos no Brasil*; IBGE: Rio de Janeiro, Brazil, 2010.
12. Horta, B.L.; Santos, R.V.; Welch, J.R.; Cardoso, A.M.; dos Santos, J.V.; Assis, A.M.; Lira, P.C.; Coimbra, C.E., Jr. Nutritional status of indigenous children: Findings from the First National Survey of Indigenous People's Health and Nutrition in Brazil. *Int. J. Equity Health* **2013**, *12*, 23. [CrossRef]
13. Addo, O.Y.; Stein, A.D.; Fall, C.H.; Gigante, D.P.; Guntupalli, A.M.; Horta, B.L.; Kuzawa, C.W.; Lee, N.; Norris, S.A.; Consortium on Health Orientated Research in Transitional Societies (COHORTS) Group; et al. Maternal height and child growth patterns. *J. Pediatrics* **2013**, *163*, 549–554. [CrossRef]
14. De Onis, M.; Branca, F. Childhood stunting: A global perspective. *Matern. Child. Nutr.* **2016**, *12*, 12–26. [CrossRef]

15. Prendergast, A.J.; Humphrey, J.H. The stunting syndrome in developing countries. *Paediatr. Int. Child. Health* **2014**, *34*, 250–265. [CrossRef]
16. Ferreira, A.A.; Welch, J.R.; Cunha, G.M.; Júnior, C.C.E.A. Physical growth curves of indigenous Xavante children in Central Brazil: Results from a longitudinal study (2009–2012). *Ann. Hum. Biol.* **2016**, *43*, 293–303. [CrossRef]
17. WHO. *WHO-Anthro for Personal Computers, Version 3.2.2, 2011: Software for Assessing Growth and Development of the World's Children*; WHO: Geneva, Switzerland, 2010.
18. WHO. *WHO-AnthroPlus for Personal Computers, Manual: Software for Assessing Growth of the World's Children and Adolescents*; WHO: Geneva, Switzerland, 2009.
19. Nestel, P.; Rutstein, S. Defining nutritional status of women in developing countries. *Public Health Nutr.* **2002**, *5*, 17–27. [CrossRef] [PubMed]
20. Cribari Neto, F.; Ferrari, S.L.; Cordeiro, G.M. Improved heteroscedasticity consistent covariance matrix estimators. *Biometrika* **2000**, *87*, 907–918. [CrossRef]
21. Victora, C.G.; Huttly, S.R.; Fuchs, S.C.; Olinto, M. The role of conceptual frameworks in epidemiological analysis: A hierarchical approach. *Int. J. Epidemiol.* **1997**, *26*, 224–227. [CrossRef]
22. The R Foundation. *The R Project for Statistical Computing [Internet]*; The R Foundation: Vienna, Austria, 2021; Available online: http://www.r-project.org (accessed on 31 May 2021).
23. Manjong, F.T.; Verla, V.S.; Egbe, T.O.; Nsagha, D.S. Undernutrition among under-five indigenous Mbororo children in the Foumban and Galim health districts of Cameroon: A cross-sectional study. *Pan. Afr. Med. J.* **2021**, *38*. [CrossRef]
24. Orellana, J.D.Y.; Marrero, L.; Alves, C.L.M.; Ruiz, C.M.V.; Hacon, S.S.; Oliveira, M.W.; Basta, P.C. Associação de baixa estatura severa em crianças indígenas Yanomami com baixa estatura materna: Indícios de transmissão intergeracional. *Ciência Saúde Coletiva* **2019**, *24*, 1875–1883. [CrossRef]
25. Pantoja, L.N.; Orellana, J.D.Y.; Leite, M.S.; Basta, P.C. Cobertura do Sistema de Vigilância Alimentar e Nutricional Indígena (SISVAN-I) e prevalência de desvios nutricionais em crianças Yanomami menores de 60 meses, Amazônia, Brasil. *Rev. Bras. Saúde Matern. Infant.* **2014**, *14*, 53–63. [CrossRef]
26. Verhagen, L.M.; Incani, R.N.; Franco, C.R.; Ugarte, A.; Cadenas, Y.; Sierra Ruiz, C.I.; Hermans, P.W.; Hoek, D.; Campos Ponce, M.; de Waard, J.H.; et al. High malnutrition rate in Venezuelan Yanomami compared to Warao Amerindians and Creoles: Significant associations with intestinal parasites and anemia. *PLoS ONE* **2013**, *8*, e77581. [CrossRef]
27. Hidalgo, G.; Marini, E.; Sanchez, W.; Contreras, M.; Estrada, I.; Comandini, O.; Buffa, R.; Magris, M.; Dominguez-Bello, M.G. The nutrition transition in the Venezuelan Amazonia: Increased overweight and obesity with transculturation. *Am. J. Hum. Biol.* **2014**, *26*, 710–712. [CrossRef]
28. Pithan, O.A.; Confalonieri, U.E.; Morgado, A.F. A situação de saúde dos índios Yanomámi: Diagnóstico a partir da Casa do Índio de Boa Vista, Roraima, 1987–1989. *Cad. Saúde Pública* **1991**, *7*, 563–580. [CrossRef]
29. Grenfell, P.; Fanello, C.I.; Magris, M.; Goncalves, J.; Metzger, W.G.; Vivas-Martínez, S.; Vivas, L.; Curtis, C. Anaemia and malaria in Yanomami communities with differing access to healthcare. *Trans. R. Soc. Trop. Med. Hyg.* **2008**, *102*, 645–652. [CrossRef] [PubMed]
30. Caldart, R.V.; Marrero, L.; Basta, P.C.; Orellana, J.D.Y. Fatores associados à pneumonia em crianças Yanomami internadas por condições sensíveis à atenção primária na região norte do Brasil. *Ciência Saúde Coletiva* **2016**, *21*, 1597–1606. [CrossRef] [PubMed]
31. International Labour Organization (ILO), Indigenous and Tribal Peoples Convention, C169, 27 June 1989, C169. Available online: https://www.refworld.org/docid/3ddb6d514.html (accessed on 7 June 2021).
32. UN. *UN Document A/61/L.67 12 September 2007: The United Nations Declaration on the Rights of Indigenous Peoples, Adopted by the UN General Assembly on 13 September 2007*; UN: New York, NY, USA, 2007.
33. Mesenburg, M.A.; Restrepo-Mendez, M.C.; Amigo, H.; Balandrán, A.D.; Barbosa-Verdun, M.A.; Caicedo-Velásquez, B.; Carvajal-Aguirre, L.; Coimbra, C.E., Jr.; Ferreira, L.Z.; del Pilar Flores-Quispe, M.; et al. Ethnic group inequalities in coverage with reproductive, maternal and child health interventions: Cross-sectional analyses of national surveys in 16 Latin American and Caribbean countries. *Lancet Glob. Health* **2018**, *6*, e902–e913. [CrossRef]
34. Mignone, J.; Bartlett, J.; O'Neil, J.; Orchard, T. Best practices in intercultural health: Five case studies in Latin America. *J. Ethnobiol. Ethnomedicine* **2007**, *3*, 31. [CrossRef]
35. Svefors, P.; Sysoev, O.; Ekstrom, E.C.; Persson, L.A.; Arifeen, S.E.; Naved, R.T.; Rahman, A.; Khan, A.I.; Selling, K. Relative importance of prenatal and postnatal determinants of stunting: Data mining approaches to the MINIMat cohort, Bangladesh. *BMJ* **2019**, *9*, e025154. [CrossRef]
36. United Nations Children's Fund (UNICEF). *Improving Child. Nutrition: The Achievable Imperative for Global Progress*; UNICEF: New York, NY, USA, 2013.
37. Anderson, I.; Robson, B.; Connolly, M.; Al-Yaman, F.; Bjertness, E.; King, A.; Tynan, M.; Madden, R.; Bang, A.; Coimbra, C.E., Jr.; et al. Indigenous and tribal peoples' health (The Lancet–Lowitja Institute Global Collaboration): A population study. *Lancet* **2016**, *388*, 131–157. [CrossRef]
38. Basnayake, T.L.; Morgan, L.C.; Chang, A.B. The global burden of respiratory infections in indigenous children and adults: A review. *Respirology* **2017**, *22*, 1518–1528. [CrossRef]
39. Valeggia, C.R.; Snodgrass, J.J. Health of indigenous peoples. *Annu. Rev. Anthropol.* **2015**, *44*, 117–135. [CrossRef]
40. Gracey, M.; King, M. Indigenous health part 1: Determinants and disease patterns. *Lancet* **2009**, *374*, 65–75. [CrossRef]

41. Tickell, K.D.; Atlas, H.E.; Walson, J.L. Environmental enteric dysfunction: A review of potential mechanisms, consequences and management strategies. *BMC Med.* **2019**, *17*, 1–9. [CrossRef]
42. Jiménez, A.; Cortobius, M.; Kjellén, M. Water, sanitation and hygiene and indigenous peoples: A review of the literature. *Water Int.* **2014**, *39*, 277–293. [CrossRef]
43. FAO; FIDA; OPS; WFP; UNICEF. *Panorama de la Seguridad Alimentaria y Nutrición en América Latina y el Caribe 2020*; FAO: Rome, Italy; OPS: Washington, DC, USA; WFP: Rome, Italy; UNICEF: New York, NY, USA, 2020; Available online: http://www.fao.org/documents/card/en/c/cb2242es/ (accessed on 30 June 2021). [CrossRef]
44. Martorell, R.; Zongrone, A. Intergenerational influences on child growth and undernutrition. *Paediatr. Perinat. Epidemiol.* **2012**, *26*, 302–314. [CrossRef] [PubMed]
45. The Guardian. Brazilian wildcat miners attack police and burn indigenous homes in Amazon [Internet]. 2021. Available online: https://www.theguardian.com/world/2021/may/28/brazil-wildcat-miners-police-indigenous-amazon (accessed on 31 May 2021).
46. Fellows, M.; Paye, V.; Alencar, A.; Nicácio, M.; Castro, I.; Coelho, M.E.; Silva, C.V.J.; Bandeira, M.; Lourival, R.; Basta, P.C. Under-Reporting of COVID-19 Cases Among Indigenous Peoples in Brazil: A New Expression of Old Inequalities. *Front. Psychiatry* **2021**, *12*, 638359. [CrossRef] [PubMed]

Article

Impacts of the Goldmining and Chronic Methylmercury Exposure on the Good-Living and Mental Health of Munduruku Native Communities in the Amazon Basin

Rafaela Waddington Achatz [1], Ana Claudia Santiago de Vasconcellos [2], Lucia Pereira [3], Paulo Victor de Sousa Viana [4] and Paulo Cesar Basta [5,*]

[1] Programa de Pós-Graduação em Psicologia Clínica do Instituto de Psicologia, Universidade de São Paulo (USP), Av. Professor Mello Moraes, 1721-Butantã, São Paulo 05508-030, Brazil; rafa.achatz@gmail.com
[2] Laboratório de Educação Profissional em Vigilância em Saúde, Escola Politécnica de Saúde Joaquim Venâncio, Fundação Oswaldo Cruz (EPSJV/Fiocruz), Av. Brasil, 4365-Manguinhos, Rio de Janeiro 21040-900, Brazil; anacsvasconcellos@gmail.com
[3] Programa de Pós-Graduação em Antropologia, Universidade Federal da Grande Dourados (UFGD), Rodovia Dourados, Km 12, Unidade II, 364, Itahum, Dourados 79804-970, Brazil; luciakaiova@gmail.com
[4] Centro de Referência Professor Hélio Fraga, Escola Nacional de Saúde Pública, Fundação Oswaldo Cruz (CRPHF/ENSP/Fiocruz), Estrada de Curicica, 2000, Curicica, Rio de Janeiro 22780-195, Brazil; paulovictorsviana@gmail.com
[5] Departamento de Endemias Samuel Pessoa, Escola Nacional de Saúde Pública, Fundação Oswaldo Cruz (ENSP/Fiocruz), Rua Leopoldo Bulhões, 1480, Manguinhos, Rio de Janeiro 21041-210, Brazil
* Correspondence: paulobasta@gmail.com

Abstract: This paper is an exploratory study that examines the illegal goldmining impacts on Munduruku communities' "Good-Living" (*Xipan Jewewekukap*) and explores the possible relationship between chronic methylmercury (MeHg) exposure and the worsening mental health conditions in three villages in the Middle-Tapajós River, Brazilian Amazon. The region has been experiencing a long-lasting threat of goldminers' invasions. A total of 109 people were interviewed and evaluated. Total mercury (THg) exposure levels were evaluated through hair samples analysis, from which MeHg exposure levels were calculated. The Geriatric Depression Scale—Short Form (GDS-SF) was used as a screening tool in order to assess mental health indicators. Brief non-structured interviews were carried out to investigate how goldmining is impacting the communities Good-Living. A Poisson regression model was used to estimate the possible association between mental health indicators (assessed through the GDS-SF) and the following independent variables: (i) mercury exposure level (<10.0 µg/g vs. ≥10.0 µg/g), (ii) self-reported nervousness, (iii) self-reported irritability, (iv) age group, and (v) monthly income. The analysis revealed high levels of mercury in hair samples (median: 7.4 µg/g, range 2.0–22.8; 70% and 28% of the participants had THg levels ≥6.0 and ≥10.0 µg/g, respectively) and pointed to a tendency in which higher levels of methylmercury exposure (Hg ≥ 10.0 µg/g) could be linked to worse mental health indicators. Although the GDS-SF has presented limitations due to the Munduruku sociocultural context, our findings suggest a tendency of worse mental health indicators in participants presenting high levels of MeHg exposure. Despite this limitation, the qualitative approach indicates an evident association between the impacts of goldmining and the Munduruku people's decreasing autonomy to maintain a Good-Living on their own terms, pointing to the importance of carrying out new investigations, especially considering longitudinal studies with qualitative methodologies and ethnographic approaches.

Keywords: illegal mining activities; methylmercury exposure; Good-Living; mental health; Munduruku; Amerindian people; Brazilian amazon; environmental pollution; cosmopolitics

1. Introduction

The Munduruku are Amerindian people who are part of the Munduruku linguistic family and integrate the Tupi linguistic trunk. They are traditionally located at the

Tapajós Valley, in Brazil. Currently, the majority live on the banks of navigable rivers, in savanna regions of the Amazon rainforest located in the states of Pará, Amazonas, and Mato Grosso [1,2]. Presently, the Munduruku population is estimated at approximately 12,000 people distributed in more than 120 villages. The contemporary battles fought by the Munduruku are still focused on guaranteeing the integrity of their territory, permanently threatened by pressures not only from illegal goldmining activities, land grabbing, and logging but also from large government projects that include the expansion of agribusiness over traditional territories as well as the construction of hydroelectric dams and a large waterway in the Tapajós River. Furthermore, like other native people in Brazil, the Munduruku people have also been striving against colonial and environmental racism [3,4].

Since the 19th century, Munduruku people have been struggling to protect their territory from the invasion of the economic and missionary expansion fronts. Between 1880 and 1920, the rubber exploitation and the religious missions' proselytism played an important role in the Munduruku territory's invasion. In the late 1950s, after the fall of rubber prices on the international market, a gold rush took place in the Tapajós valley. The gold rush was intensified during the civil–military dictatorship, mostly after 1972 (when the *Transamazônica* highway began its construction) and had its peak in the period between 1975 and 1990. Highly profitable for non-Amerindian people, the exploitation of gold left a noxious legacy for the local population, not only related to the harm it caused to the environment and its inhabitants (such as uncontrolled deforestation, major excavations, and contamination of waters by mercury) [5–9] but also due to the psychosocial impacts that, since then, have been contributing to making Munduruku communities vulnerable.

At the beginning of the 21st century, with the developmentalist policies of the Brazilian Workers Party's governments and the impacts of the global economic crisis in Brazil, there was a further expansion in the search for gold in the Tapajós region, which was intensified by the current extreme right-wing Brazilian government agenda. Illegal small-scale goldmining (ASGM) has significantly expanded in the Amazon in recent decades [10], being an important cause of deforestation and environmental degradation [11–13]. The mercurial form used in artisanal and small-scale mining is metallic mercury, also known as elemental mercury (Hg0). During the extraction process, a large part of the mercury used is released into rivers and undergoes a methylation process (mediated by aquatic microorganisms), producing methylmercury, which is extremely harmful to human health and the ecosystem.

Much of the danger attributed to methylmercury (MeHg) refers to its capacity for bioaccumulation and biomagnification in aquatic food chains and due to its highly neurotoxic potential. Since it is highly fat-soluble, it can cross the blood–brain barrier and reach the central nervous system. Most traditional peoples of the Amazon are large consumers of fish, and in many cases, it represents the main or the only source of animal protein in their diet [14,15]. As such, the presence of goldmines in traditional territories converts the consumption of fish, which was once considered to be healthy, into a risky behavior, since the mercury used in the process contaminates the rivers and is incorporated into the food chain, contaminating humans [16–18].

In the literature, mercury exposure is linked to the manifestation of psychological symptoms, which differ in extent and severity according to multiple etiological factors, such as the mercurial chemical form (organic or inorganic), the duration and levels of exposure (acute or chronic), and the pathway of contamination. Most of the studies on the relationship between mercury exposure and the manifestation of psychological symptomatology report on cases of acute contamination by methylmercury or occupational exposure to inorganic mercury. Among other health problems, acute MeHg exposure has been related to the manifestation of psychological symptoms such as depression, anxiety, insomnia, irritability, and decreased attention and memory [19,20]. Some studies suggest that chronic MeHg exposure can produce neuropsychological impacts, affecting cognition, memory, IQ, verbal fluency, and psychomotor performance [21–23]. However, there is still little research focusing specifically on the psychological effects of chronic exposure to methylmercury through diet [24].

Be that as it may, the impacts of goldmining on the Munduruku people's mental health indicators go far beyond chronic exposure to methylmercury, since it undermines their possibilities to maintain a *Xipan Jewewekukap*, a Munduruku concept that could be translated as "Good-Living". Good-Living ("*Bem Viver*" in Portuguese) is a translation of Amerindian concepts such as *Teko Porã* (in Guarani-Mbya), *Suma Qamaña* (in Aymara), and *Sumak Kawsay* (in Quechua), only to mention some examples. The definition of what is a Good-Living is different for each Amerindian people and may vary from generation to generation. However, there are some common points between those concepts translated as Good-Living: they belong to philosophical systems that propose an ecological conception of reality and consider that nature is a living being (and not an object or a source of resources). Thus, these philosophical systems recognize that the lives of all beings that inhabit the Earth (including human beings) are deeply intertwined. In the last decades, the possibilities of non-capitalistic definitions of what may be Good-Living have been an important topic of debate for Latin American social movements, public health agents, psychologists, and social scientists [25–28].

Many Munduruku leaders have been tireless in warning about how the goldmining is radically damaging their *Xipan Jewewekukap*. In an interview given in 2016, Maria Leusa Munduruku, an important leader in the fight to protect Munduruku territory, said [29]:

> For us, the river is the place where we take our food from. We drink the river, we bathe in the river. For us the breast milk, as we say, is the riverbed. The same river also runs in people's veins. Without the river, there will be no "us". Without water, nobody can live. Our river is our mother. So it is with the forest. They are sacred because they came from a story in which our ancestors made the Tapajós River with water squeezed from tucumã *woodworms*.

In 2016, the Pariri Amerindian Association (representing the Munduruku people living in the Middle-Tapajós Region) sent a letter to the Oswaldo Cruz Foundation to request an assessment of mercury contamination in Amerindian people, given the increasing presence of goldminers in the area. This work is an exploratory study that integrates a broader effort to follow this request and investigate the impacts of goldmining in the Amazon on human health and the environment, focusing on the exposure to methylmercury (for more details, see Basta et al. [30]).

With this requesting in mind, the purpose of the present paper is (i) to examine the impacts of illegal goldmining on the Munduruku Amerindian communities' Good-Living and (ii) to explore the possible relationship between MeHg exposure and the worsening mental health conditions reported by the residents living in the studied communities. The following analysis is based on data collected through home visits and interviews with the participating families during fieldwork at Munduruku communities.

2. Materials and Methods

This study integrates quantitative and qualitative approaches, the latter being predominantly ethnographic. We consider that the qualitative approach enables (i) a more symmetrical dialogue with Munduruku knowledge regimes and (ii) the research team to ask questions and pay attention to variables that escape what was foreseen in the initial methodological design. In other words, it enables accessing variables that cannot be evaluated using psychometric or psychiatric scales, which nonetheless are fundamental variables to be considered in the study.

2.1. Sampling

A cross-sectional study was carried out seeking to investigate mental health indicators in Munduruku people over 12 years of age living in the *Sawré Muybu*, *Poxo Muybu*, and *Sawré Aboy* Munduruku villages, which are located in the Middle-Tapajós region. Those villages were included in the sample following the request of the *Pariri* Indigenous Association, which represents the Munduruku People living in the Middle-Tapajós River. Those communities are located in the *Sawré Muybu* Indigenous Land (IL) and are chronically exposed to methylmercury as a result of the increasing illegal goldmining activity in the region. The *Sawré Muybu* IL is located in the Southwest of Pará State, in an area of 173,178 hectares situated between the municipalities of Itaituba and Trairão. The demarcation process of *Sawré Muybu* IL, which is traditionally occupied by the Munduruku people, started in 2007 and remains uncompleted. For the Munduruku people, the territory where the *Sawré Muybu* IL is located is extremely important since it is known as *Daje Kapap Eipi*—the place where the Tapajós River emerged according to Munduruku cosmogony.

A population census was carried out in those communities, and all residents aged 12 years or over were invited to participate in the study. Therefore, probabilistic sampling methods were not used to select participants. In total, 109 people were included in the study. Two residents of the *Sawré Muybu* community were excluded: a 73-year-old woman who had speech and mobility difficulties due to a stroke and a 15-year-old boy who had congenital chronic non-progressive encephalopathy due to perinatal complications and neurological symptoms resulting from cerebral palsy.

2.2. Fieldwork

The fieldwork was held over 11 days between October and November 2019. The data that support the following analysis were obtained through home visits, interviews with the participating families, and the collection of hair samples, used as a biomarker of total mercury (THg) exposure. Four researchers participated in home visits and interviews with families: an Amerindian anthropologist (L.P.), a biologist (A.C.S.V.), a nurse (P.V.S.V.), and a psychologist (R.W.A.). The interviews were conducted based on a questionnaire specially prepared for this research, based on previous experiences of our research group [30].

2.3. Data Collection Instruments

The data collection instrument was a questionnaire structured in thematic modules, through which we sought to (a) characterize the physical and demographic structure of the visited households; (b) characterize the health situation in the family and in the community, searching for psychological self-reported symptoms; and (c) characterize the dietary pattern of families, with emphasis on the fish consumption. Concerning mental health indicators, the Geriatric Depression Scale—Short Form (GDS-SF) was used to screen depressive symptoms. Brief non-structured interviews were carried out to investigate how the participants perceived the goldmining impacts on their right to self-determinatively maintain a Good-Living.

The meaning of each question was carefully explained to participants and, if necessary, translated into Munduruku. The questionnaire was applied with the help of Munduruku health agents who work in the communities and/or with the help of village leaders, including chiefs (*caciques*) and teachers. Answers were recorded on electronic forms with the help of portable electronic devices (tablets), and there was no use of paper forms.

2.3.1. Geriatric Depression Scale—Short Form

The GDS-SF (Figure 1) is a reduced version of the original scale (which is composed of 30 questions) and aims to screen depressive symptoms [31,32]. The scale ranges from zero (absence of depressive symptoms) to fifteen points (maximum score for depressive symptoms).

Even though the GDS-SF is designed to evaluate depressive symptoms in the elderly, it can be applied to a younger population for the following reasons: it is composed of easily understood questions, it has small variation in answer possibilities (yes/no), it can be applied by any trained interviewer, and it requires little time for application. Additionally, research indicates that the GDS-SF shows good diagnostic sensitivity and specificity for young and middle-aged adults [33]. It is worth remembering that the GDS-SF has widespread use in clinical practice and is commonly used to assess young adults in Brazil, especially those with little access to formal education.

According to Abas M. et al. [34] experience and considering culture-specific criteria, a cutoff score ≥4 was employed to screen the presence of depressive symptoms. It is important to emphasize that for the present analysis, this cutoff score was employed only to access mental health indicators and not to diagnose any kind of mental disorder.

> The interviewer asks the participant to choose the answers that best describe how she/he/they felt over the past week:
>
> 1. Are you basically satisfied with your life?
> 2. Have you dropped many of your activities and interests?
> 3. Do you feel that your life is empty?
> 4. Do you often get bored?
> 5. Are you in good spirits most of the time?
> 6. Are you afraid that something bad is going to happen to you?
> 7. Do you feel happy most of the time?
> 8. Do you often feel helpless?
> 9. Do you prefer to stay at home, rather than going out and doing things?
> 10. Do you feel that you have more problems with memory than most?
> 11. Do you think it is wonderful to be alive now?
> 12. Do you feel worthless the way you are now?
> 13. Do you feel full of energy?

Figure 1. Geriatric Depression Scale—Short Form (Sheikh J.I., Yesavage J.A., 1986).

2.3.2. Brief Non-Structured Interviews

Brief non-structured interviews were performed to access the goldmining impacts on the Good-Living of the communities. The interviewers asked the participants how they had been feeling in the last months. If the person answered that she/he had not been feeling well, the interviewer asked if she/he would like to specify how they had been feeling and which were their complaints about it. If necessary, the interviewer gave examples of uncomfortable emotional states (such as nervousness, irritability, sadness, anxiety, fear, grief, and outbreaks of rage), which were usually translated into the Munduruku language. Some of these interviews triggered testimonies from the participants, who detailed how they understood the impacts of goldmining in their territory. These extended interviews were fundamental to access how the impacts of goldmining on Munduruku people's Good-Living go far beyond the impacts of methylmercury contamination.

Hearing Munduruku leaders' testimonials is a fundamental step in order to better understand the scale of the noxious impacts promoted by goldmining in their territory. These impacts go beyond the impacts on mental health, affecting the socio-cosmological organization of the Munduruku people. We assume that Amerindian knowledge systems are different and no less legitimate than Western knowledge systems [35], and we consider that it is necessary to acknowledge ontoepistemological legitimacy to non-Western people [36,37]. As such, in order to take Munduruku people seriously and to reduce the misunderstandings that are inherent to cultural translation [38], it is necessary to listen carefully to their analyses and experiences about how goldmining and methylmercury exposure affect them.

2.3.3. Mercury Exposure Biomarker

Hair samples were collected from the occipital region of all participants using stainless steel dissection scissors. The samples were packed in paper envelopes and individually identified. Analyses of THg levels in the participants' hair samples were performed at the

Environment Section of the Evandro Chagas Institute of the Ministry of Health, located in Belém-PA. The health risk assessment was carried out according to the methodology proposed by WHO [39]. For more details on the analysis of hair samples and the discussion about safe levels of methylmercury exposure standards, see Basta et al. [30].

There is no consensus on the thresholds of lower levels of mercury in hair samples that may impact the onset of psychological effects. The World Health Organization and some studies carried out in the Amazon region [40–42] propose a level of mercury in hair samples ≥ 6.0 µg/g as an indicator of general health risk. Concerning specifically neurological abnormalities associated with the consumption of methylmercury contaminated fish, some studies propose a level of mercury in hair samples ≥ 10.0 µg/g as an indicator of neurological alteration risk. Research performed in the Amazon since the 1990s has identified adult individuals with neurological alterations associated with THg levels in hair samples varying between 10 and 20 µg/g [43–46]. According to Oliveira et al. [47], Munduruku indigenous adults with Hg exposure level ≥ 10µg/g presented twice as high chances of cognitive development deficits (Prevalence Ratio-PR: 2.2; CI 95%:1.13–4.26) in Brief Cognitive Screening Battery as well as in the verbal fluency test (PR: 2.0; CI 95%:1.18–3.35). Similar findings were reported in riparian populations in Bolivia and Suriname [48,49].

2.4. Statistical Analysis

A descriptive analysis of the participants was conducted according to clinical and sociodemographic variables of interest, including gender (female/male), age group (12–19; 20–29, or ≥ 30 years old), schooling (0 to 4 years, 5 to 9 years, or >9 years of formal education), marital status (married or single/widow), village of residence (*Sawré Muybu*, *Poxo Muybu*, or *Sawré Aboy*), regular monthly income (yes/no), psychological self-reported symptoms, such as nervousness (yes/no), irritability (yes/no), besides school failure (yes/no), physical activity restriction (yes/no), previous treatment for Malaria (yes/no), previous hospitalization (yes/no), and MeHg exposure (<10.0 µg/g vs. ≥ 10.0 µg/g). Moreover, the mental health indicators (assessed through the GDS-SF <4 vs. ≥ 4) were compared according to the abovementioned variables.

To estimate the prevalence of exposure, the proportion of people over 12 years of age who had mercury levels ≥ 10.0 µg/g in the sampled population in the study region was considered. The prevalence was presented for the three studied villages: *Sawré Muybu*, *Poxo Muybu*, and *Sawré Aboy*.

In order to contrast clinical and sociodemographic variables with mental health indicators (assessed through the GDS-SF <4 vs. ≥ 4), we used Pearson's Chi-squared test or Fisher's exact test. We also used the Kruskal–Wallis test to evaluate the differences in Hg levels between villages.

A Poisson regression model was used to estimate the possible association between mental health indicators (assessed through the GDS-SF <4 vs. ≥ 4) and the following independent variables: (i) mercury exposure level (<10.0 µg/g vs. ≥ 10.0 µg/g), (ii) self-reported nervousness, (iii) self-reported irritability, (iv) age group, and (v) monthly income. Prevalence ratio (PR), with the respective confidence interval of 95%, was used as an association measure.

Variables with p-value < 0.10 in the simple analysis were selected and included in the model. Variables that presented significance levels of 5% (p-value < 0.05) remained in the final model. Age group and income also remained in the final model in order to control the effects of the sociodemographic variables on the mental health indicators.

The data were analyzed using SPSS (Statistical Package for the Social Sciences), version 9.0 (Chicago, IL, USA).

3. Results

During fieldwork, 109 people over 12 years old provided hair samples and answered the mental health questionnaires: 46 from the *Sawré Muybu* village, 39 from *Poxo Muybu* and 24 from *Sawré Aboy* (Table 1). A total of 35 households were visited in the *Sawré Muybu*

IL, 20 in *Sawré Muybu* village, 8 in *Poxo Muybu* village, and 7 in *Sawré Aboy* village. Most families reported having regular incomes from social benefits and or salaries. A total of 53 women (48.6%) and 56 men (51.4%) participated in the study. The age of participants ranged from 12 to 72 years old (mean: 27.4 years old; standard deviation: 13.8 years old).

The distribution of participants according to age group was heterogeneous among the studied villages. There was a predominance of people aged from 12 to 19 years old in *Sawré Aboy* and *Poxo Muybu* villages, with the presence of 12 (50%) and 18 (46%) participants, respectively, in contrast to only 7 (15%) in the *Sawré Muybu* village. On the other hand, the *Sawré Muybu* village had the highest concentration of people aged between 20 and 29 years old, with the presence of 25 participants (54%), in relation to only 5 (21%) and 8 (21%) in the *Sawré Aboy* and *Poxo Muybu* villages, respectively. There was a similar concentration of people aged 30 years or more in the three villages: 7 (29%) in *Sawré Aboy*, 13 (33%) in *Poxo Muybu*, and 14 (30%) in *Sawré Muybu*.

Table 1. Sociodemographic and clinical variables of the study participants, according to GDS-SF. *Sawré Muybu* Indigenous Land, Pará, Brazilian Amazon, 2019.

	GDS-SF						
	<4		≥4		Total		
	Sociodemographic Features						
Sex	n	%	n	%	n	%	p-value
Male	39	69.6	17	30.4	56	51.4	0.416
Female	33	62.3	20	37.7	53	48.6	
Total	72		37		109		
Age range							
≥30 years	23	67.6	11	32.4	34	31.2	0.376
20 to 29 years	22	57.9	16	42.1	38	34.9	
12 to 19 years	27	73.0	10	27.0	37	33.9	
Total	72		37		109		
Schooling							
>9 years	17	68.0	8	32.0	25	22.9	0.339
5 to 9 years	47	69.1	21	30.9	68	62.4	
0 to 4 years	8	50.0	8	50.0	16	14.7	
Total	72		37		109		
Marital Status							
Married	49	64.5	27	35.5	76	69.7	0.597
Single/Widow	23	69.7	10	30.3	33	30.3	
Total	72		37		109		
Villages							
Sawré Muybu	24	52.2	22	47.8	46	42.2	0.002
Poxo Muybu	34	87.2	5	12.8	39	35.8	
Sawré Aboy	14	58.3	10	41.7	24	22.0	
Total	72		37		109		
Regular Income							
Yes	27	67.5	13	32.5	40	36.7	0.808
No	45	65.2	24	34.8	69	63.3	
Total	72		37		109		

Table 1. Cont.

		GDS-SF					
		<4		≥4		Total	
		Clinical Features					
	n	%	n	%	n	%	p-value
Nervousness							
No	61	74.4	21	25.6	82	75.2	0.001
Yes	11	40.7	16	59.3	27	24.8	
Total	72		37		109		
School failure							
No	41	74.5	14	25.5	55	51.9	0.055
Yes	29	56.9	22	43.1	51	48.1	
Total	70		36		106		
Irritability							
No	69	71.9	27	28.1	96	88.1	0.001
Yes	3	23.1	10	76.9	13	11.9	
Total	72		37		109		
Physical Activity restriction							
No	68	68.0	32	32.0	100	91.7	0.153
Yes	4	44.4	5	55.6	9	8.3	
Total	72		37		109		
Previous Malaria							
No	38	73.1	14	26.9	52	47.7	0.139
Yes	34	59.6	23	40.4	57	52.3	
Total	72		37		109		
Previous hospitalization							
No	44	68.8	20	31.3	64	58.7	0.479
Yes	28	62.2	17	37.8	45	41.3	
Total	72		37		109		

3.1. Mercury Exposure

The analysis of mercury levels for the 109 participants who provided hair samples revealed that the average concentration level was 8.4 (±4.2) µg/g and the median was 7.4 µg/g, ranging between 2.0 and 22.8 µg/g. In general, the prevalence of exposure reported, considering THg hair levels ≥10.0 µg/g, was 28%.

The prevalence of methylmercury exposure, considering THg hair levels ≥10.0 µg/g, was uneven among the investigated communities (p-value = 0.001). In the *Poxo Muybu* village, 13.3% (n = 4) of the sampled residents had THg hair levels ≥10.0 µg/g, while in *Sawré Muybu* and *Sawré Aboy* villages, respectively, 30% (n = 9) and 57% (n = 17) of the residents had THg hair levels ≥10.0 µg/g. In other words, the prevalence of methylmercury exposure considering the limit of 10.0 µg/g was 2.3 times higher in *Sawré Muybu* and 4.3 times higher in *Sawré Aboy* when compared to the exposure rates observed in *Poxo Muybu*.

3.2. GDS-SF

Out of the 109 participants who answered the GDS-SF, 32% scored zero or one points, 34% scored two or three points, 17% scored four or five points, 12% scored six or seven points, and 6% scored between eight and ten points. Even though the scale reached up to 15 points, no participant obtained a score higher than 10 points. Therefore, 35% of the participants (n = 37) scored ≥4 points.

When considering the scores obtained in each item by the 109 participants as a whole, the lowest scores refer to Items 11 (since only 2% of the participants answered "no" to the question "Do you think it is wonderful to be alive now?") and 1 (since only 6% of the participants answered "no" to the question "Are you basically satisfied with your life?"), and the highest scores refer to Items 6 (since 34% of the participants answered "yes" to the question "Are you afraid that something bad is going to happen to you?") and 14 (since 32% of the participants answered "yes" to the question "Do you feel that your situation is hopeless?").

The prevalence of scores ≥4 did not vary significantly according to gender (*p*-value = 0.416), schooling (*p*-value = 0.339), income (*p*-value = 0.540), marital status (*p*-value = 0.597), or age group (*p*-value = 0.376) (Table 1). Nevertheless, it is noteworthy that only participants aged between 20 and 25 years old scored 9 or 10 points and only participants aged between 20 and 35 years old scored ≥8 points (Table 2).

Table 2. Clinical and sociodemographic variables, according to GDS-SF scores ≥ 4 (Crude Poisson Regression Model). *Sawré Muybu* Indigenous Land, Pará, Amazon, Brazil, 2019.

Variables	GDS-SF ≥ 4	
	PR Crude (CI 90%)	*p*-Value
Hg Level		
Hg < 10 µg/g	1.0	
Hg ≥ 10 µg/g	1.6 (1.0–2.5)	0.072
Nervousness		
No	1.0	
Yes	2.3 (1.5–3.5)	0.001
Irritability		
No	1.0	
Yes	2.7 (1.9–3.9)	0.001
Regular Income		
Yes	1.0	
No	1.1 (0.7–1.7)	0.809
Villages		
Sawré Muybu	1.0	
Poxo Muybu	0.3 (0.1–0.6)	0.003
Sawré Aboy	0.9 (0.5–1.4)	0.630
Age range		
≥30 years	1.0	
20 to 29 years	1.3 (0.8–2.2)	0.399
12 to 19 years	0.8 (0.5–1.5)	0.624
Gender		
Male	1.0	
Female	1.2 (0.8–1.9)	0.418
Schooling		
>9 years	1.0	
5 to 9 years	1.0 (0.6–1.7)	0.918
0 to 4 years	1.6 (0.8–2.9)	0.245
School Failure		
No	1.0	
Yes	1.7 (1.1–2.7)	0.061
Marital Status		
Married	1.0	
Single/Widow	0.9 (0.5–1.4)	0.603

In the multivariate analysis (PR adjusted), the presence of depressive symptoms (indicated by the score ≥4 on the GDS-SF) appears to be associated with THg hair levels ≥ 10 µg/g (PR = 1.8; CI 95%: 1.1–3.0), complaints of irritability (PR = 3.0; CI 95%:1.9–4.9), and nervousness (PR = 2.1; CI 95%: 1.3–3.3), even when controlling the income effect

(PR = 1.1; CI 95%: 0.6–1.9) and age group effect (PR = 0.7; CI 95%: 0.4–1.5; (PR = 1.4; CI 95%: 0.8–2.5) (Table 3).

In other words, people with THg levels $\geq$10 µg/g are 1.8 times more likely to manifest depressive symptoms according to the GDS $\geq$ 4, when compared to people with THg levels < 10 µg/g. Participants who reported feeling excessive irritability are 3.0 times more likely to manifest depressive symptoms according to the GDS $\geq$ 4, in contrast to participants who did not complain of irritability. In addition, people who complained of excessive nervousness are 2.1 times more likely to manifest depressive symptoms according to the GDS $\geq$ 4, when compared to people who did not report feeling nervous, even when controlling the effect of the income and the age group.

Table 3. Clinical and sociodemographic variables, according to GDS-SF scores $\geq$ 4 (adjusted Poisson regression model). Sawré Muybu Indigenous Land, Pará, Amazon, Brazil, 2019.

Variables	GDS-SF $\geq$ 4	
	PR-Adjusted (CI 95%)	*p*-Value
Hg Level		
Hg < 10 µg/g	1.0	
Hg $\geq$ 10 µg/g	1.8 (1.1–3.0)	0.024
Nervousness		
No	1.0	
Yes	2.1 (1.3–3.3)	0.003
Irritability		
No	1.0	
Yes	3.0 (1.9–4.9)	0.001
Regular Income		
Yes	1.0	
No	1.1 (0.6–1.9)	0.766
Age range		
$\geq$30 years	1.0	
20 to 29 years	1.4 (0.8–2.5)	0.219
12 to 19 years	0.7 (0.4–1.5)	0.400

3.3. Brief Non-Structured Interviews

Besides the individual mental health indicators assessed through the GDS-SF, the non-structured interviews triggered testimonials about how goldmining is affecting these Munduruku villages collectively.

The conversations held with Munduruku people during fieldwork suggest that there is a close relationship between the impacts of illegal goldmining and Munduruku people's decreasing Good-Living. This is mainly related to the fact that goldmining activities in Munduruku territory undermine the Munduruku people's possibility to maintain Good-Living on their own terms. The Munduruku elders and leaders explained that, in order to cultivate the Good-Living of each community and each person, it is necessary to take care of the relationships between the different inhabitants of the forest. As one of the villages' leaders said:

The forest (auadip) is beautiful to me; it makes me joyful and makes me recognize who I am. If I am not in the forest, I feel strange, unfocused, and shattered. And if the forest is being assaulted and hurt, I get hurt. I get sick if the forest gets sick, because my body and my speech are also made of the forest.

4. Discussion

4.1. Methylmercury Exposure and Mental Health Impacts

The relationship between mercury exposure and psychological disorders is determined by multiple etiological factors, such as the mercurial form (organic or inorganic), the duration and levels of exposure, and the pathway of contamination [50,51].

Cases of acute inorganic mercury contamination have been associated with symptoms such as hallucinations, delusions, insomnia, suicidal tendencies, loss of memory, and manic-depressive behavior [52]. Chronic inorganic mercury contamination is usually due to occupational exposure to the metal and has been related to anxiety, irritability, depression, memory problems, and erethism (popularly known as "mad hatter disease") [53–55]. Cases of chronic inorganic mercury exposure were also discussed by studies on the mental health of individuals with mercury dental amalgam, which suggested that long-term exposure to small amounts of inorganic mercury can produce devastating effects after several years without the onset of symptoms [56].

Cases of acute organic mercury exposure were also related to the manifestation of depressive symptoms. Several outbreaks of methylmercury contamination have been reported around the world since 1956, when an outbreak of acute methylmercury contamination took place in Minamata Bay, Japan [57]. Another well-known episode took place in Iraq in the 1970s when thousands of people were hospitalized due to the consumption of grains treated with methylmercury or ethylmercury fungicides [58]. Mayhazati [59] reported on the psychological effects of acute methylmercury contamination in patients in Iraq whose total blood levels of mercury ranged between 320 and 4260 ng/mL, with an average of 2118 ng/mL. Of the 43 patients studied, 32 (74.4%) showed depressive symptoms and 19 (44.2%) manifested irritability. The average blood levels of mercury (both organic and inorganic) were considerably higher in depressed patients than in non-depressed patients. Nevertheless, the author highlights that mercury poisoning may be one of the various contributory factors in causing depression in the patients, who were also suffering physically and financially and handling the stress and grief produced by the disruption of their lives.

However, there is still little research on the impacts of methylmercury exposure in cases of chronic toxicity, especially considering its psychological impacts. Most of the studies focus on the neuropsychological impacts of chronic MeHg exposure, such as cognition, memory, sleep, and psychomotor performance [21–23]. It is not consensual that chronic exposition to methylmercury by diet has direct impacts on mental health indicators. Junior et al. [20] analyzed emotional and motor symptoms of riverside dwellers exposed to methylmercury by diet in the municipalities of Itaituba and Acará, in Pará, Brazil. The mean levels of THg in Itaituba (9.15 µg/g) were significantly higher than in Acará (0.67 µg/g), but emotional symptoms were identified in 26 (26.5%) participants from Itaituba and in 24 (52.2%) from Acará, suggesting that the exposure to Hg may not be the causal factor of these emotional symptoms.

Tracing the relationship between MeHg chronic exposure and psychological symptomatology is difficult for some reasons, for example: (1) Chronic methylmercury exposure may be a silent pandemic. It is considered by some authors as a silent damage [60]—unlike cases of acute contamination, chronic exposure to lower doses of methylmercury usually produces subclinical manifestations, which are insidiously and cumulatively manifested over a long period of time; (2) Multiple factors contribute to the manifestation of psychological symptoms. Mental health indicators are never determined by a single factor but are produced by a multifactorial combination. For instance, besides methylmercury exposure, goldmining in the Tapajós river produces several other negative impacts on the communities' mental health and Good-Living, as it undermines environmental relations that are imperative to provide the conditions for Good-Living on the terms of the Munduruku people and other native people from the Amazon.

4.2. Methylmercury Exposure and Mental Health Indicators

Data suggest that the variation on the scores obtained in the GDS-SF according to the levels of THg concentration in hair samples is statistically significant. Even though the sampled population is predominantly young, these results may point to a tendency in which higher levels of methylmercury exposure could be linked to worse mental health indicators. The highest scores are concentrated in *Sawré Aboy* village, where there is the highest prevalence of MeHg exposure, and in *Sawré Muybu*, where the population is older. Additionally, the prevalence of participants who scored ≥4 points in the GDS-SF is higher in participants who had mercury levels above 10.0 µg/g, in comparison to participants who had mercury levels under 10.0 µg/g—according to GDS-SF scores, people with THg ≥ 10 µg/g are 1.8 times more likely to manifest depressive symptomatology, when compared to people with THg levels < 10 µg/g.

The variations considering the overall points scored in each item of the GDS-SF are also relevant. Most of the participants answered that they felt happy and that they were satisfied with their lives. Nevertheless, many participants also answered in the GDS-SF that they felt hopeless and that they were afraid that something bad could happen to them or their relatives. Such data may suggest that the greatest sources of anguish and anxiety are related to future prospects. Given the situation of the progressive invasion and destruction of the Munduruku territories, the future presents itself as full of uncertainties and daunting prospects.

It is noteworthy that such data can only point to tendencies since the instruments of data collection should be better adapted to Munduruku sociocultural specificities. Moreover, it is possible that psychological symptoms are not manifesting since these are cases of chronic contamination by methylmercury that could be described as a "silent pandemic". Considering that the entire population is exposed to considerable levels of mercury, it is difficult to establish relationships between the prevalence of methylmercury exposure and the results of the scales and reported symptoms. The goldmining itself has devastating impacts on Munduruku people's mental health conditions, whether mercury exposure is ≥10.0 µg/g or not. Therefore, MeHg exposure may be increasing the negative impacts of goldmining activities on the Good-Living of the Munduruku people and other inhabitants of the forest.

4.3. Limitations

The limitations of this study are mostly related to the data collection instruments employed, the limited size of the sample considering the Munduruku population, and the context of the application of the questionnaires. Such limitations point to the importance of carrying out new investigations, especially considering longitudinal studies with qualitative methodologies articulated to ethnographic research.

Since the interviews were conducted at the participants' homes, in most cases, the entire family was present during the interview. The lack of privacy, combined with the lack of intimacy between interviewer and interviewee, may have contributed to people being embarrassed to answer about issues that could be sensitive. Additionally, some questions can be perceived as invasive to participants if asked without well-established trust bonds.

Linguistic and cultural translation was also a challenge in conducting the interviews. Like other Amerindian people, Munduruku knowledge and medical practices are based on onto-epistemological assumptions that differ from those postulated by biomedical or psychological knowledge. As such, it is inaccurate to translate Munduruku nosological categories into categories like "depressive symptomatology", "psychological disorder", or "mental health" [61]. Therefore, the instruments utilized in this research may produce equivocal comprehension [38] regarding Munduruku ontological and sociocultural specificities, since the GDS-SF is not validated for Munduruku people.

There is no consensus on the reliability of the GDS-SF in different cultural contexts. Some studies support that the GDS-SF is reliable for the cultural contexts investigated, despite cultural differences [62,63]. Some authors argue that the GDS-SF cutoff score may vary according to ethnocultural specificities. Almeida and Almeida [64] propose a cutoff score ≥ 5 to determine the presence of depressive symptoms in elderly Brazilian people. In turn, Abas M. et al. [34] recommend a cutoff score of ≥ 4 to detect significant forms of depression in older African–Caribbean people living in south London.

On the other hand, other studies support that GDS-SF results are not equivalent in different cultures, since the concept of depression and the forms of expression of positive and negative emotions may vary in each culture [65]. The same may occur with concepts such as "worthlessness" and "hopelessness" [66]. Moreover, the clinical presentation of depression and anxiety is also culturally variable [67]. Jang Y. et al. [68] argue that cultural differences may affect the participants understanding of the GDS-SF questions, highlighting, for example, that a positive response to the question "Do you prefer to stay at home, rather than going out and doing new things?" does not necessarily indicate a depressive symptom as it does for an older adult in the United States. This may be the case for Munduruku people as well.

We did not establish a cutoff score to diagnose depression in this study because the Munduruku have sociocultural specificities and the GDS-SF was applied in a predominantly young population. The GDS-SF was used as a research screening tool and not as a diagnostic tool. Therefore, the scores obtained in the scale can only provide partial indicators of the participants' mental health status. In other words, the scores obtained on the scale can only provide "clues" about the mental health conditions and Good-Living in the communities; it is not possible to establish any diagnosis or conclusive statement about it.

To our knowledge, there are no quantitative instruments to assess mental health indicators that were validated for Amerindian populations. This may be due to the scarcity of research on this subject but also to the fact that Amerindian people have medical systems and concepts of personhood, health, and territory that differ from those postulated in biomedical or psychological sciences. Additionally, in biomedical or psychological sciences, there is no consensus on concepts and research instruments to assess "well-being", "happiness", or "sadness", for example [69].

From a clinical point of view, the conversations held with the participants during fieldwork provided exceptional data. However, there was no time available to conduct such conversations or non-structured interviews in a systematic way in order to produce robust qualitative data. Hereupon, qualitative research based on ethnographic and participative methodology may be interesting to investigate the relationship between methylmercury exposure and "mental health" indicators in Amerindian communities. Articulating quantitative and qualitative research may produce more substantial data. For example, based on this experience, it could be interesting to build a semi-structured questionnaire together with people from the Munduruku communities. It could also be interesting if, in addition to participating in the elaboration of the questionnaires, Munduruku people were the ones to apply it.

4.4. Impacts of Goldmining on Munduruku People Good-Living (Xipan Jewewekukap)

As was discussed above, the concepts of "well-being", "happiness", and "sadness" vary greatly between different cultures, as well as the symbolic forms used to represent it. For the Munduruku people, what biomedical and psychological sciences define as "mental health" is deeply intertwined with the maintenance of a Good-Living. As such, to understand how goldmining is affecting Munduruku people beyond the impacts of methylmercury contamination, it is important to understand what makes a Good-Living—a *Xipan Jewewekukap*—according to the Munduruku people that live in the villages where the research took place.

Elders and leaders that were interviewed talked about the complexity of the problems caused by mining. A village leader explained to the team that the ecological problems caused by goldmining are not limited to factors that non-Amerindian people tend to consider but are also related to cosmopolitical dynamics [70]:

Pajés [traditional healers] learned what they know from snakes. They learned that human diseases come from antiquity, from the first times of the world—times when abysses were open. Many other diseases remained at the bottom of the earth when these abysses closed. Nowadays, since pariwat (non-Amerindian people) are rummaging deep in the earth, these diseases are rising. If pariwat continue to rummage where they shouldn't, all of us, Munduruku and pariwat, will have serious problems.

The goldmining activities, as well as logging, grabbing, and the construction of hydroelectric dams, have been destroying places that are sacred for the Munduruku [71]. Leaders and elders report that some of the affected places are the homes of powerful entities, which are becoming angry at the destruction of their dwelling-place. Enraged with such disrespect, those entities can cause many diseases and deaths among the Munduruku. Such cosmopolitical imbalance caused by goldmining activities at the Munduruku territory is intertwined with the phenomena of methylmercury contamination. A *pajé* that works and lives in one of the communities visited explained:

I am a pajé, *but I don't know how to cure problems caused by mercury contamination. This is new to me. Nevertheless, I know how to take care of illnesses that are caused by the fact that* pariwat *are messing with places they shouldn't. They are messing with other beings' houses and those beings are getting very angry. That is why we need to combine Munduruku medicines with* pariwat *medicines. And that is why we have to combine efforts to stop* pariwat *from messing with the other being's houses.*

In addition to damaging the relationships that Munduruku people carefully maintain with other forest-dwelling beings, the goldmining activities affect structural aspects of the Munduruku cosmos. A Munduruku Health Agent of the *Poxo Muybu* and *Sawré Muybu* communities told the team stories about the beginning of the world. He explained:

Everything in this world has a mother: the fish, the water, the stone... When we mess with the mothers' offspring, they get angry and attack us, making us ill. Making these mothers mad is very dangerous for the Munduruku. Unfortunately, the destruction of the forest brings even more serious problems than those illnesses. I have learned from the elders that, since the beginning of the world, there is an enormous tree that supports the sky, preventing it from falling to the earth. The miners and loggers are cutting the nails that are at the roots of this tree. If that tree falls, the sky will fall and this world we live in will end.

In this regard, this Munduruku Health Agent emphasizes that fighting against the destruction of the forest is a matter of life or death not only for the Munduruku people but for non-Amerindian people as well. Consequently, it is urgent to combine efforts to prevent an ecological collapse or the fall of the sky [72–74]. The invasion of Munduruku territory by non-Amerindian people brought several problems that did not exist before. Since those problems are increasing at great speed, the Munduruku people are calling on *pariwat* to take responsibility and to collaborate in facing those problems.

5. Conclusions

This research team has made the effort to examine the impacts of illegal goldmining on Amerindian villages' Good-Living and explore the possible relationship between methylmercury exposure and the worsening mental health conditions in areas under the long-lasting threat of invaders.

Our data point to a tendency in which higher levels of methylmercury exposure could be linked to worse mental health indicators. Nevertheless, the GDS-SF does not seem to be a reliable data collection instrument regarding the Munduruku sociocultural context. However, qualitative research indicates an evident relationship between the impacts of illegal goldmining, Munduruku people's worsening mental health conditions, and an increasing difficulty in maintaining a self-determined Good-Living. Such results, thus, point to the importance of carrying out new investigations, especially considering longitudinal studies with qualitative methodologies articulated to ethnographic research.

Author Contributions: Proposal design, study design, and methodology, P.C.B., A.C.S.d.V., P.V.d.S.V. and R.W.A.; fieldwork data collection, L.P., P.V.d.S.V., A.C.S.d.V., P.C.B. and R.W.A.; data curation, R.W.A. and P.C.B.; writing—review and editing, R.W.A., P.C.B. and A.C.S.d.V.; supervision, obtaining resources, and project management, P.C.B. All authors have read and agreed to the published version of the manuscript.

Funding: This research was funded by the Vice-Presidency of Environment, Care, and Health Promotion (VPPAS) of Fundação Oswaldo Cruz (Fiocruz) through Decentralized Execution of Resources Document No. 175/2018, Process: 25000.209221/2018-18, signed between the Fiocruz and the Special Department for Indigenous Health, both under the Ministry of Health. The non-governmental organization WWF-Brasil offered financial support to disseminate the results of the research.

Institutional Review Board Statement: The study was conducted in accordance with the guidelines of the Declaration of Helsinki and was approved by the Research Ethics Committee of the National School of Public Health at Fiocruz (REC/ENSP) and the Brazilian National Research Ethics Commission of the National Health Council (CONEP/CNS), CAAE: 65671517.1.0000.5240, with Opinion No. 2.262.686 favorable to its performance. In compliance with Convention No. 169 of the International Labor Organization (ILO), the study began with a pre-study consultation, carried out in August 2019, during a visit to the villages, in which one author (PCB) and local indigenous leaders participated. At the time, the study objectives were presented and discussed (https://www.youtube.com/watch?v=oFEYEGxNmns&t=704s, accessed on 30 June 2021). After answering questions and the approval of the proposal by the communities, we received support from the coordination of the Special Indigenous Sanitary District of the Tapajós River through the multidisciplinary indigenous health team to carry out the study. In addition, the interviews and data collection started only after the participants had their questions answered and had given formal consent in the Informed Consent Form (ICF) by the children's guardians.

Informed Consent Statement: Informed consent was obtained from all subjects involved in the study. Written informed consent has been obtained from the patients to publish this paper.

Data Availability Statement: Data sharing not applicable.

Acknowledgments: Through chiefs Juarez Saw, Jairo Saw, and Valdemar Poxo and the leader Alessandra Korap, we thank the Munduruku people for the trust placed in our team and the support in carrying out the research. We thank the team from the Rio Tapajós Indigenous Special Sanitary District, who spared no efforts to support us in all stages of the fieldwork. In particular, we thank the coordination Cleidiane Santos and the nurses Alan Marcelo Simon and Lygia Catarina de Oliveira. We also thank to Marcelo O. Lima, Iracina M. Jesus, and João Paulo Goes Pereira who performed the mercury laboratory analysis.

Conflicts of Interest: The authors declare no conflict of interest. The funders had no role in the design of the study; in the collection, analyses, or interpretation of data; in the writing of the manuscript; or in the decision to publish the results.

References

1. Ramos, A.R.F. Entre a Cruz e a Riscadeira: Catequese e Empresa Extrativista Entre os Munduruku (1910 a 1957). Master's Thesis, Universidade Federal de Goiás (UFG), Goiânia, Brasil, 2000.
2. Ramos, A.R.F. Munduruku. In *Enciclopédia dos Povos Indígenas No Brasil*; Instituto Socioambiental: São Paulo, Brazil, 2003. Available online: http://www.socioambiental.org/pib/epi/munduruku/munduruku.shtm (accessed on 10 October 2020).
3. Quijano, A. Colonialidad del poder, eurocentrismo y America Latina. In *A Colonialidade do Saber: Eurocentrismo e Ciências Sociais. Perspectivas Latino-Americanas*, 1st ed.; Lander, E., Ed.; CLACSO: Buenos Aires, Argentina, 2000; pp. 117–142.
4. dos Santos, O.A.; Massola, G.M.; da Silva, G.L.G.; Svartman, B.P. Racismo ambiental e lutas por reconhecimento dos povos de floresta da Amazônia. *Glob. J. Community Psychol. Pract.* **2016**, *7*, 1–20.
5. Brabo, E.D.S.; Santos, E.D.O.; Jesus, I.M.D.; Mascarenhas, A.F.; Faial, K.F. Mercury levels in fish consumed by the sai cinza indigenous community, Munduruku reservation, Jacareacanga county, state of Para, Brazil. *Cad. Saude Publica* **1999**, *15*, 325–332. [CrossRef]
6. Barbosa, A.C.; Dórea, J.G. Indices of mercury contamination during breast feeding in the Amazon Basin. *Environ. Toxicol. Pharmacol.* **1998**, *6*, 71–79. [CrossRef]
7. Roulet, M.; Lucotte, M.; Canuel, R.; Rheault, I.; Tran, S.; De Freitos Gog, Y.G.; Farella, N.; do Vale, R.S.; Passos, C.J.S.; da Silva, E.D.J.; et al. Distribution and partition of total mercury in waters of the Tapajos River Basin, Brazilian Amazon. *Sci. Total Environ.* **1998**, *213*, 203–211. [CrossRef]

8. Lacerda, L.; Pfeiffer, W. Mercury from gold mining in the Amazon environment-an overview. *Química Nova* **1992**, *15*, 155–160.
9. Akagi, H.; Malm, O.; Kinjo, Y.; Harada, M.; Branches, F.J.P.; Pfeiffer, W.C.; Kato, H. Methylmercury pollution in the Amazon, Brazil. *Sci. Total Environ.* **1995**, *175*, 85–95. [CrossRef]
10. RAISG. *Mapa Inédito Indica Epidemia de Garimpo Ilegal na Panamazônia*; Rede Amazônica de Informação Socioambiental Georreferenciada: Manaus, Brasil, 2018. Available online: https://www.amazoniasocioambiental.org/pt-br/radar/mapa-inedito-indica-epidemia-de-garimpo-ilegal-na-panamazonia/ (accessed on 11 October 2020).
11. Alvarez-Berríos, N.L.; Aide, T.M. Global demand for gold is another threat for tropical forests. *Environ. Res. Lett.* **2015**, *10*, 014006. [CrossRef]
12. Rahm, M.; Jullian, B.; Lauger, A.; de Carvalho, R.; Vale, L.; Totaram, J.; Cort, K.A.; Djojodikromo, M.; Hardjoprajitno, M.; Neri, S.; et al. *Monitoring the Impact of Gold Mining on the Forest Cover and Freshwater in the Guiana Shield. Reference Year 2014*; WWF-France: French Guiana, France, 2015; 60p.
13. Legg, E.D.; Ouboter, P.E.; Wright, M.A.P. *Small-Scale Gold Mining Related to Mercury Contamination in the Guianas: A Review*; WWF Guianas: Paramaribo, Suriname, 2015.
14. Brabo, E.; Santos, O.E.C.; Jesus, I.M.; Mascarenhas, A.F.S.; Faial, K.F. Mercury contamination of fish and exposures of an indigenous community in Para state, Brazil. *Environ. Res.* **2000**, *84*, 197–203. [CrossRef]
15. Santos, E.C.; de Jesus, I.M.; Câmara, V.M.; Brabo, E.; Loureiro, E.C.; Mascarenhas, A.; Weirich, J.; Luiz, R.R.; Cleary, D. Mercury exposure in Munduruku Indians from the community of Sai Cinza, State of Pará, Brazil. *Environ. Res.* **2002**, *90*, 98–103. [CrossRef]
16. FAO; WHO. *Expert Committee on Food Additives. Sixty-First Meeting. Summary and Conclusions*; World Health Organization: Geneva, Switzerland, 2008.
17. FAO; WHO. Evaluation of Certain Food Additives and Contaminants: Sixty-first Report of the Joint FAO/WHO Expert Committee on Food Additives. In Proceedings of the Joint FAO/WHO Expert Committee on Food Additives (JECFA), Rome, Italy, 10–19 June 2003.
18. Zahir, F.; Rizwi, S.J.; Haq, S.K.; Khan, R.H. Low dose mercury toxicity and human health. *Environ. Toxicol. Pharmacol.* **2005**, *20*, 351–360. [CrossRef] [PubMed]
19. Ekino, S.; Susa, M.; Ninomiya, T.; Imamura, K.; Kitamura, T. Minamata disease revisited: An update on the acute and chronic manifestations of methyl mercury poisoning. *J. Neurol. Sci.* **2007**, *262*, 131–144. [CrossRef] [PubMed]
20. Chuu, Y.Y.; Liu, S.H.; Lin-Shiau, S. Differential neurotoxic effects of methylmercury and mercuric sulfide in rats. *Toxicol. Lett.* **2007**, *169*, 109–120. [CrossRef] [PubMed]
21. Chang, J.W.; Pai, M.C.; Chen, H.L.; Guo, H.R.; Su, H.J.; Lee, C.C. Cognitive function and blood methylmercury in adults living near a deserted chloralkali factory. *Environ. Res.* **2008**, *108*, 334–339. [CrossRef] [PubMed]
22. Dolbec, J.; Mergler, D.; Passos, S.C.J.; De Morais, S.S.; Lebel, J. Methylmercury exposure affects motor performance of a riverine population of the Tapajós river, Brazilian Amazon. *Int. Arch. Occup. Environ. Health* **2000**, *73*, 195–203. [CrossRef]
23. Santos-Lima, C.D.; Mourão, D.S.; Carvalho, C.F.; Souza-Marques, B.; Vega, C.M.; Gonçalves, R.A.; Argollo, N.; Mene-zes-Filho, J.A.; Abreu, N.; Hacon, S.S. Neuropsychological effects of mercury exposure in children and adolescents of the Amazon region, Brazil. *Neurotoxicology* **2020**, *79*, 48–57. [CrossRef]
24. Junior, J.M.F.C.; Lima, A.A.S.; Junior, D.R.; Khoury, E.D.T.; Souza, G.S.; Silveira, L.C.L.; Pinheiro, M.C.N. Manifestações emocionais e motoras de ribeirinhos expostos ao mercúrio na Amazônia. *Rev. Bras. Epidemiol.* **2017**, *20*, 212–224. [CrossRef] [PubMed]
25. Belaunde, L.E. *Viviendo Bien: Género y Fertilidad Entre los Airo-Pai de la Amazonía Peruana*; CAAAP: Lima, Peru, 2001.
26. McCallum, C. Intimidade com estranhos: Uma perspectiva Kaxinawá sobre confiança e a construção de pessoas na Amazônia. *Mana* **2013**, *19*, 123–155. [CrossRef]
27. Costa, A. *O Bem Viver—Uma Oportunidade Para Imaginar Outros Mundos*; Autonomia Literária e Editora Elefante: São Paulo, Brazil, 2015.
28. Baniwa, A.F. *Bem Viver e Viver Bem: Segundo o Povo Baniwa no Noroeste Amazônico Brasileiro*; UFPR: Curitiba, Brazil, 2019.
29. Munduruku, M.L. Vamos continuar guerreando. Interview given to Patricia Bonilha. *Rev. Porantim* **2016**, *390*, 6–7.
30. Basta, P.C.; Viana, P.V.S.; Vasconcellos, A.C.S.; Périssé, A.R.S.; Hofer, C.B.; Paiva, N.S.; Kempton, J.W.; Ciampi de Andrade, D.; Oliveira, R.A.A.; Achatz, R.W.; et al. Mercury exposure in Munduruku indigenous communities from Brazilian Amazon: Methodological background and an overview of the principal results. *Int. J. Environ. Res. Public Health* **2021**, *18*. in press.
31. Sheikh, J.I.; Yesavage, J.A.; Brooks, J.O.; Friedman, L.; Gratzinger, P.; Hill, R.D.; Zadeik, A.; Crook, T. Proposed factor structure of the Geriatric Depression Scale. *Int. Psychogeriatr.* **1991**, *3*, 23–28. [CrossRef]
32. Sheikh, J.I.; Yesavage, J.A.; Scale, G.D. Recent evidence and development of a shorter version. *Clin. Gerontol.* **1986**, *5*, 165–172.
33. Guerin, J.M.; Copersino, M.L.; Schretlen, D.J. Clinical utility of the 15-item geriatric depression scale (GDS-15) for use with young and middle-aged adults. *J. Affect Disord.* **2018**, *241*, 59–62. [CrossRef]
34. Abas, M.; Phillips, C.; Carter, J.; Walter, J.; Banerjee, S.; Levy, R. Culturally sensitive validation of screening questionnaires for depression in older African–Caribbean people living in south London. *Br. J. Psychiatry* **1998**, *173*, 249–254. [CrossRef]
35. Latour, B. *Nous N'avons Jamais été Modernes: Essai D'anthropologie Symétrique*; La Découverte: Paris, France, 1991.
36. de Castro, V.E. O nativo relativo. *Rev. Mana* **2002**, *8*. [CrossRef]
37. Silva, D.F. *Toward a Global Idea of Race*; University of Minnesota Press: Minneapolis, MN, USA, 2007.
38. de Castro, V.E. Perspectival Anthropology and the Method of Controlled Equivocation. *Tipití J. Soc. Anthropol. Lowl. South Am.* **2004**, *2*. Available online: https://digitalcommons.trinity.edu/tipiti/vol2/iss1/1 (accessed on 30 June 2021).

39. World Health Organization (WHO). *Guidance for Identifying Populations at Risk from Mercury Exposure*; WHO: Geneva, Switerzeland, 2008. Available online: https://wedocs.unep.org/bitstream/handle/20.500.11822/11786/IdentifyingPopnatRiskExposuretoMercury_2008Web.pdf?sequence=1&isAllowed=y (accessed on 30 June 2021).
40. Marinho, J.S.; Lima, M.O.; de Oliveira Santos, E.C.; de Jesus, I.M.; da Conceição, N.; Pinheiro, M.; Alves, C.N.; Muller, R.C. Mercury speciation in hair of children in three communities of the Amazon, Brazil. *Biomed. Res. Int.* **2014**, 945963. [CrossRef] [PubMed]
41. de Castro, S.S.N.; de Oliveira Lima, M. Hair as a biomarker of long term mercury exposure in Brazilian Amazon: A systematic review. *Int. J. Environ. Res. Public Health* **2018**, *15*, 500. [CrossRef] [PubMed]
42. Vega, C.M.; Orellana, J.D.; Oliveira, M.W.; Hacon, S.S.; Basta, P.C. Human mercury exposure in Yanomami indigenous villages from the Brazilian Amazon. *Int. J. Environ. Res. Public Health* **2018**, *15*, 1051. [CrossRef]
43. Lebel, J.; Mergler, D.; Lucotte, M.; Amorim, M.; Dolbec, J.; Miranda, D.; Pichet, P. Evidence of early nervous system dysfunction in Amazonian populations exposed to low-levels of methylmercury. *Neurotoxicology* **1996**, *17*, 157–167.
44. Lebel, J.; Mergler, D.; Branches, F.; Lucotte, M.; Amorim, M.; Larribe, F.; Dolbec, J. Neurotoxic effects of low-level methylmercury contamination in the Amazonian Basin. *Environ. Res.* **1998**, *79*, 20–32. [CrossRef]
45. Harada, M.; Nakanishi, J.; Yasoda, E.; da Conceicâo, M.N.P.; Oikawa, T.; de Assis Guimarâes, G.; Ohno, H. Mercury pollution in the Tapajos river basin, Amazon: Mercury level of head hair and health effects. *Environ. Int.* **2001**, *27*, 285–290. [CrossRef]
46. Lacerda, E.M.D.C.B.; Souza, G.D.S.; Cortes, M.I.T.; Rodrigues, A.R.; Pinheiro, M.C.N.; Silveira, L.C.D.L.; Ventura, D.F. Comparison of visual functions of two Amazonian populations: Possible consequences of different mercury exposure. *Front. Neurosci.* **2020**, *13*, 1428. [CrossRef] [PubMed]
47. Oliveira, R.A.A.; Pinto, B.D.; Rebouças, B.H.; Ciami de Andrade, D.; Vasconcellos, A.C.S.; Basta, P.C. Neurological impacts of chronic methylmercury exposure in Munduruku indigenous adults: Somatosensory, motor and cognitive abnormalities. *Int. J. Environ. Res. Public Health* (under review).
48. Benefice, E.; Luna-Monrroy, S.; Lopez-Rodriguez, R. Fishing activity, health characteristics and mercury exposure of Amerindian women living alongside the Beni River (Amazonian Bolivia). *Int. J. Hyg. Environ. Health* **2010**, *213*, 458–464. [CrossRef] [PubMed]
49. Peplow, D.; Augustine, S. Neurological abnormalities in a mercury exposed population among indigenous Wayana in Southeast Suriname. *Environ. Sci. Process. Impacts* **2014**, *16*, 2415–2422. [CrossRef] [PubMed]
50. Gochfeld, M. Cases of mercury exposure, bioavailability and absorption. *Ecotoxicol. Environ. Saf.* **2003**, *56*, 174–179. [CrossRef] [PubMed]
51. Bernhoft, R.A. Mercury toxicity and treatment: A review of the literature. *J. Environ. Public Health* **2012**, *2012*, 460508. [CrossRef]
52. Park, J.D.; Zheng, W. Human exposure and health effects of inorganic and elemental mercury. *J. Prev. Med. Public Health* **2012**, *45*, 344–352. [CrossRef]
53. O'Carroll, R.; Masterton, G.; Dougall, N.; Ebmeier, K.; Goodwin, G. The neuropsychiatric sequelae of mercury poisoning: The mad hatter's disease revisited. *Br. J. Psychiatry* **1995**, *167*, 95–98. [CrossRef]
54. Wojcik, D.P.; Godfrey, M.E.; Christie, D.; Haley, B.E. Mercury toxicity presenting as chronic fatigue, memory impairment and depression: Diagnosis, treatment, susceptibility, and outcomes in a New Zealand general practice setting (1994–2006). *Neuroendocrinol. Endocrinol. Lett.* **2006**, *27*, 415–423.
55. Uzzell, B.P.; Oler, J. Chronic low-level mercury exposure and neuropsychological functioning. *J. Clin. Experim. Neuropsychol.* **1986**, *8*, 581–593. [CrossRef] [PubMed]
56. Siblerud, R.L. The relationship between mercury from dental amalgam and mental health. *Am. J. Psychother.* **1989**, *43*, 575–587. [CrossRef]
57. World Health Organization. *Environmental Health Criteria 1. Mercury*; WHO: Geneva, Switerzeland, 1976.
58. Bakir, F.; Damluji, S.F.; Amin-Zaki, L.; Murtadha, M.; Khalidi, A.; Al-Rawi, N.Y.; Tikriti, S.; Dahahir, H.I.; Clarkson, T.W.; Smith, J.C.; et al. Methylmercury poisoning in Iraq. *Science* **1973**, *181*, 230–241. [CrossRef]
59. Maghazaji, H.I. Psychiatric aspects of methyl mercury poisoning. *J. Neurol. Neurosurg. Psychiatry* **1974**, *37*, 954–958. [CrossRef] [PubMed]
60. Grant, C.A. Pathology of experimental methylmercury intoxication: Some problems of exposure and response. In *Mercury, Mercurials and Mercaptans*; Miller, M.W., Clarkson, T.W., Eds.; Charles C Thomas Publisher, Ltd.: Springfield, IL, USA, 1973; Volume 111, pp. 294–310.
61. Batista, Q.M.; Zanello, V. Saúde mental em contextos indígenas: Escassez de pesquisas brasileiras, invisibilidade das diferenças. *Estud. Psicol.* **2016**, *21*, 403–414. [CrossRef]
62. Pedraza, O.; Dotson, V.M.; Willis, F.B.; Graff-Radford, N.R.; Lucas, J.A. Internal consistency and test-retest stability of the geriatric depression scale-short form in African American older adults. *J. Psychopathol. Behav. Assess.* **2009**, *31*, 412–416. [CrossRef] [PubMed]
63. Mui, A.C.; Kang, S.-Y.; Chen, L.M.; Domanski, M.D. Reliability of the geriatric depression scale for use among elderly Asian immigrants in the USA. *Int. Psychogeriatr.* **2003**, *15*, 253–271. [CrossRef]
64. Almeida, O.P.; Almeida, S.A. Confiabilidade da versão brasileira da escala de depressão em geriatria (GDS) versão reduzida. *Arq. Neuro-Psiquiatr.* **1999**, *57*, 421–426. [CrossRef]
65. Jang, Y.; Kim, J.; Chiriboga, D. Acculturation and manifestation of depressive symptoms among Korean-American older adults. *Aging Ment. Health* **2005**, *9*, 500–507. [CrossRef]

66. Flacker, J.M.; Spiro, L. Does question comprehension limit the utility of the Geriatric Depression Scale in older African Americans? *J. Am. Geriatr. Soc.* **2003**, *51*, 1511–1512. [CrossRef]
67. Kirmayer, L.J. Cultural variations in the clinical presentation of depression and anxiety: Implications for diagnosis and treatment. *J. Clin. Psychiatry* **2001**, *62*, 22–30.
68. Jang, Y.; Small, B.J.; Haley, W.E. Cross-cultural comparability of the Geriatric Depression Scale: Comparison between older Koreans and older Americans. *Aging Ment. Health* **2001**, *5*, 31–37. [CrossRef] [PubMed]
69. Hallal, P.C.; Dumith, S.C.; Bertoldi, A.D.; Scalco, D.L.; Menezes, A.M.; Araújo, C.L. Well-being in adolescents: The 11-year follow-up of the 1993 Pelotas (Brazil) birth cohort study. *Cad. Saude Publica* **2010**, *26*, 1887–1894. [CrossRef] [PubMed]
70. Stengers, I. *Cosmopolitics*; University of Minnesota Press: Minneapolis, MN, USA, 2010; Volume I.
71. Tosold, L. Por uma vida sem barragens: Corpos, território e o papel da autodeterminação na desnaturalização da violência. *Rev. Antropol.* **2020**, *63*, e178182. [CrossRef]
72. Weir, J.A.Q. Del 'Giro Ontológico' al Tiempo de Vuelta del Nosotrxs. *Amaz. Latit.* **2021**, *26*. Available online: https://amazonialatitude.com/2021/04/08/del-giro-ontologico-al-tiempo-de-vuelta-del-nosotrxs/ (accessed on 30 June 2021).
73. Krenak, A. *Ideias Para Adiar o Fim do Mundo*; Companhia das Letras: São Paulo, Brazil, 2019.
74. Kopenawa, D.; Albert, B. *La Chute du Ciel. Paroles d'un Chaman Yanomami*; Terre Humain, Plon: Paris, France, 2014.

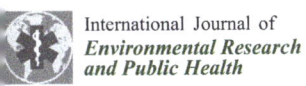

Article

Genetic Polymorphism of Delta Aminolevulinic Acid Dehydratase (*ALAD*) Gene and Symptoms of Chronic Mercury Exposure in Munduruku Indigenous Children within the Brazilian Amazon

Jamila Alessandra Perini [1], Mayara Calixto Silva [1], Ana Claudia Santiago de Vasconcellos [2], Paulo Victor Sousa Viana [3], Marcelo Oliveira Lima [4], Iracina Maura Jesus [4], Joseph William Kempton [5], Rogério Adas Ayres Oliveira [6], Sandra Souza Hacon [7] and Paulo Cesar Basta [7,*]

1. Laboratório de Pesquisa de Ciências Farmacêuticas (LAPESF), Centro Universitário Estadual da Zona Oeste (UEZO), Av. Manuel Caldeira de Alvarenga, 1.203, Rio de Janeiro 23070-200, RJ, Brazil; jamilaperini@yahoo.com.br (J.A.P.); mayaracx_2010@hotmail.com (M.C.S.)
2. Laboratório de Educação Profissional em Vigilância em Saúde, Escola Politécnica de Saúde Joaquim Venâncio, Fundação Oswaldo Cruz (EPSJV/Fiocruz), Av. Brasil, 4365-Manguinhos, Rio de Janeiro 21040-900, RJ, Brazil; anacsvasconcellos@gmail.com
3. Centro de Referência Professor Hélio Fraga, Escola Nacional de Saúde Pública, Fundação Oswaldo Cruz (CRPHF/ENSP/Fiocruz), Estrada de Curicica, 2000-Curicica, Rio de Janeiro 22780-195, RJ, Brazil; paulovictorsviana@gmail.com
4. Seção de Meio Ambiente, Instituto Evandro Chagas, Secretaria de Vigilância em Saúde, Ministério da Saúde (SEAMB/IEC/SVS/MS), Rodovia BR-316 km 7 s/n-Levilândia, Ananindeua 67030-000, PA, Brazil; marcelolima@iec.gov.br (M.O.L.); iracinajesus@iec.gov.br (I.M.J.)
5. Faculty of Medicine, Imperial College London, Medical School Building, St Mary's Hospital, Norfolk Place, London W2 1PG, UK; kemptonj@hotmail.com
6. Faculdade de Medicina, Universidade de São Paulo—USP, São Paulo 01246-903, SP, Brazil; roger.adas.doc@gmail.com
7. Departamento de Endemias Samuel Pessoa, Escola Nacional de Saúde Pública, Fundação Oswaldo Cruz (ENSP/Fiocruz), Rua Leopoldo Bulhões, 1480-Manguinhos, Rio de Janeiro 21041-210, RJ, Brazil; sandrahacon@gmail.com
* Correspondence: paulobasta@gmail.com; Tel.: +55-21-2598-2503

Abstract: Genetic polymorphisms involved in mercury toxicokinetics and toxicodynamics may be associated with severe mercury toxicity. This study aimed to investigate the impact of an *ALAD* polymorphism on chronic mercury exposure and the health situation of indigenous children from the Brazilian Amazon. One-hundred-and-three indigenous children (under 15 years old) were included and genotyped (rs1800435) using a TaqMan validated assay. The mean age was 6.6 ± 4.5 years old, 60% were female, 49% presented with anemia, and the mean hair mercury concentration was 7.0 ± 4.5 (1.4–23.9) µg/g, with 49% exceeding the reference limit (≥6.0 µg/g). Only two children were heterozygous *ALAD*, while the others were all wild type. Minor allele frequency (*ALAD* G) and heterozygous genotype (*ALAD* CG) were 1% and 2%, respectively. The two children (12 and 14 years old) with the *ALAD* polymorphism had mercury levels above the average as well as had neurological symptoms related to chronic mercury exposure, such as visual field alterations, memory deficit, distal neuropathy, and toe amyotrophy. Both children also reported frequent consumption of fish in the diet, at least three times a week. In conclusion, our data confirm that an *ALAD* polymorphism can contribute to mercury half-life time, harmful effects, and neuropsychological disorders in indigenous children with chronic mercury exposure to gold mining activity.

Keywords: mercury exposure; *ALAD*; genetic polymorphism; neurotoxicity; environmental health; indigenous people

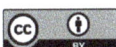

1. Introduction

Our society has long made use of Mercury (Hg) in industry and technology. However, mercury exposure is a global public health concern due to its adverse effects on human health and the environment. The three forms of mercury, elemental, inorganic, and organic, induce toxic effects with different transport and metabolic mechanisms [1,2]. The organic form of mercury, methylmercury (MeHg), is the most toxic to humans due to toxicokinetic features: fast absorbed; extensively distributed to all tissues, including the hematoencephalic and placental barriers; and slowly eliminated. In addition, mercury exposure has already been associated with developmental disorders and impaired growth, as well as behavioral, immunological, hormonal, reproductive, and neurological changes [1,3–5].

Polymorphisms in genes that encode proteins involved in mercury toxicokinetics and toxicodynamics may be valuable for a personalized response to detrimental mercury toxicity, especially among vulnerable population groups with significant mercury exposure [6,7]. The indigenous communities of the Brazilian Amazon are one of these vulnerable groups owing to the high levels of MeHg found in the food staples they rely on, including fish and hunted animals. This makes it environmentally relevant [5,8].

The delta aminolevulinic acid dehydratase (*ALAD*) enzyme is required in heme synthesis and plays an important role in metal toxicokinetics, mainly transporting metals through the body. *ALAD* polymorphism rs1800435 in exon 4 (chromosome 9q34) is characterized by a C > G allele change (*177 C > G*), which results in a Lys-Asn variation in position 59 of the protein. This Lys-Asn variation, therefore, creates a different functional isozyme with different protein binding affinity for metals [9,10]. This *ALAD* polymorphism was associated with higher Hg concentrations in blood and lower enzyme activity than non-variant subjects from riverside Amazonian communities [11]. In addition, it has already been observed that in similar mercury exposures, children have a higher susceptibility to adverse neurological effects than adults [7,12]. Neuropsychological disturbances were associated with exposure to mercury in children from the Amazon region [13].

Thus, the objectives of this study were (1) to identify the presence of this *ALAD* polymorphism in the Munduruku indigenous communities of the Brazilian Amazon and (2) to evaluate the effects of this polymorphism on the chronic exposure to mercury and on the health situation of them.

2. Materials and Methods

2.1. Study Population and Clinical Evaluation

This study is part of a major project entitled "Mercury exposure in Munduruku indigenous communities from Brazilian Amazon: Methodological background and an overview of the principal results" [14]. Here, a case study was carried out involving indigenous children (under 15 years old) from *Sawré Muybu*, *Poxo Muybu*, and *Sawré Aboy* villages (Munduruku people of the middle Tapajós River) between October and November 2019. The National Ethics Committee of Human Research approved this study (protocol number 65671517.1.0000.5240). After presenting the research protocol to the community and clarifying doubts, the guardian of each participant provided written informed consent and answered a questionnaire, as previously described [14]. All residents under 15 years old were invited to participate in the study and there was no refusal. Furthermore, no probabilistic sampling methods were used to select the participants.

The research team collected data through (i) home visits and interviews with participating families; (ii) clinical and laboratory evaluation; (iii) collection of hair samples for mercury exposure analysis; and (iv) collection of epithelial cells from the oral mucosa collected by swab for DNA extraction and genotyping analysis of an *ALAD* polymorphism.

The body mass index (BMI) was calculated as the weight (kg) divided by the square of height (m^2) for those over 6 years old ($n = 60$), and the Z-scores (BMI for age) for children from 0 to 5 years old, were calculated according to the World Health Organization [15]. The hemoglobin levels were assessed using the Hemocue device, and anemia was considered when the levels were below 11.5 g/dL. The blood pressure of participants over 12 years of age (n = 22) was measured twice using an automatic pulse blood pressure monitor (Omron Model Hem-631INT). The means of the two measures of systolic blood pressure (SBP) and diastolic blood pressure (DBP) were used to classify the participants [16], and hypertension was considered when SBP values were $\geq$140 mm Hg and DBP were $\geq$90 mm Hg.

2.2. Neurological Assessment

Participants aged 12 years or older (n = 15) underwent a systematized neurological examination protocol, specially developed for this research. The assessments were carried out by one of the authors (RAAO), and the other two neurologists (BDP, BHR) familiarized with neurological semiology and trained in the application of the protocol and the assessment scales. We assessed the balance and gait, coordination, Achilles deep tendon reflex test, and complete cranial nerve evaluation, including visual campimetry by confrontation, pupillary and extrinsic ocular motricity, facial motility and sensitivity, and elevation of the palate and vomiting reflex. Moreover, we tested the painful nociceptive as well as the tactile and thermal sensitivity to cold in the upper and lower limbs in the respective proximal and distal segments with standardized instruments. For cognitive assessments, we applied the Short Battery of Cognitive Screening Instrument [17], which includes the following domains: (i) immediate memory; (ii) learning; (iii) interference task; and (iv) long-term memory. Verbal Fluency Test in the animal category [18] and Stick Design Test [19] were also used to assess cognition. For further details on neurological assessment, see Oliveira et al. (2021) [20].

A neurodevelopment assessment was performed with the Denver II neurodevelopment screening test in children aged 0 to 6 years (n = 56), without morphological changes. The Denver II test assesses and identifies children at risk for developmental impairment. The test is divided into four areas: (i) personal-social: aspects of the child's socialization inside and outside the family environment; (ii) fine motor skills: hand-eye coordination and manipulation of small objects; (iii) language: production of sounds, ability to recognize, understand, and use language; (iv) gross motor skills: body motor control, sitting, walking, jumping, and the other movements performed by large muscles, as previously described [21].

2.3. Hair Mercury Analysis

Hair samples (n = 102) were collected from the occipital area and mercury speciation analysis was performed based on a previously optimized procedure [14,22]. The hair mercury detection method was previously described [22–24]. For quality assurance and control of the method we used: (i) a 6-point calibration curve with concentrations ranging from 0.4 to 4 ng/g; (ii) the Human Hair Certified Reference Material (IAEA-86), whose average recovery rate was 101% (n = 8, recovery ranging from 83.4 to 106.6%) from the International Atomic Energy Agency; and (iii) the relative standard deviation (RSD) of 8.32%. The detection and quantification limits (LOD/LOQ) obtained were 0.0083 ng/mg and 0.027 ng/mg, respectively. Sample replicates (n = 10), whose RSD was 2.49%, were also randomly selected. The level of $\geq$6.0 µg/g of mercury in hair samples was considered as a health risk limit indicator, as previously described in the Amazon region [23–25].

2.4. ALAD Genotyping

Genomic DNA obtained from oral mucosa and collected by swab was extracted using an extraction kit (Qiagen) following the procedures recommended by the manufacturer. The genotyping analysis of *ALAD* (chr9:113391611) *177 C > G* (rs1800435) missense variant was performed using a *TaqMan* allelic discrimination assay (C_11495146_10) by 7500 Real-Time System (Applied Biosystems, Foster City, CA, USA), and the genotypes were directly determined. PCR amplification was performed in 8 µL reactions with 1 µL of template DNA (3–23 ng/µL), 1 × TaqMan Universal Master Mix, 1 × each primer, and probe assay. Thermal cycling was initiated with a first denaturation step of 10 min at 95 °C, followed by

40 cycles of denaturation at 92 °C for 15 s and annealing at 60 °C for 1 min. *ALAD* allele frequency and genotype distribution were derived by gene counting.

2.5. Data Analysis

Continuous variables were reported as mean ± standard deviation (SD), range, median, and interquartile range (IQR). Categorical data were shown as number (n) and frequency (%). Deviations from Hardy–Weinberg equilibrium (HWE) in *ALAD* polymorphism frequency were assessed by the goodness-of-fit χ^2 test. The Kruskal–Wallis test was performed to evaluate the differences in Hg-levels between groups. All analyses were performed using the IBM SPSS 20.0 Statistics for Windows (SPSS Inc., Chicago, IL, USA).

3. Results

The present study comprised 103 children under 15 years old, from which 46 (44.7%) reside in *Sawré Muybu*, 38 (36.9%) in *Poxo Muybu*, and 19 (18.4%) in *Sawré Aboy* villages. The mean age of all indigenous children was 6.6 ± 4.5 years old and 62 (60.2%) were female. The anthropometric measurements are shown according to the age group: 29 (28.2%) were over 10 years old, 31 (30.1%) were between 6 to 10 years old, and 43 (41.7) children were between 0 to 5 years old (Table 1).

Table 1. Epidemiological features and *ALAD* genotypes of the study population (n = 103), *Sawré Muybu* Indigenous Land, Pará, Amazon, Brazil, 2019.

Variables	Case 1	Case 2	Children Population n = 101 (%)
Munduruku indigenous group	Sawré Muybu	Sawré Muybu	Sawré Muybu, n = 44 (43.6%) Poxo Muybu, n = 38 (37.6%) Sawré Aboy, n = 19 (18.8%)
Sex	Male	Female	Female, n = 61 (60.4%) Male, n = 40 (39.6%)
ALAD genotypes	CG	CG	Wild-type (CC)
			Mean ± SD (range) median
Age (years)	12	14	6.4 ± 4.4 (0–14) 6.0 IQR = 3; 6 and 10
BMI (Over 10 years old) [a]	18.9	21.7	18.8 ± 1.9 (15–22) 18.9 IQR = 17; 19 and 20
BMI (6 to 10 years old) [b]	-	-	16.0 ± 1.3 (14–22) 15.6 IQR = 15; 16 and 17
Anthropometric measurements (0 to 5 years old) [c]	-	-	0.16 ± 0.8 (−1.7–1.8) 0.17 IQR = −0.4; 0.2 and 0.8

BMI: Body mass index (Kg/m^2). SD: standard deviation. IQR: interquartile range. [a] Data were obtained from 29 children over 10 years old. [b] Data was obtained from 31 children between 6 to 10 years old. [c] Z-score was obtained from 42 children between 0 to 5 years old (missing n = 1).

The rate of successful genotyping of the *ALAD* C > G was 100%, and the distribution of polymorphism was in Hardy–Weinberg equilibrium (*p*-value = 0.92). Of the 103 indigenous children, only two from *Sawré Muybu* village were heterozygous *ALAD* CG. Minor allele frequency (MAF) of *ALAD* G, wild-type (*ALAD* CC), and heterozygous (*ALAD* CG) frequency genotypes in all subjects was 0.97%, 98.1%, and 1.9%, respectively. Table 1 displays the sociodemographic and genetic characteristics of the studied population (n = 101) compared with the two children with *ALAD* polymorphism.

All indigenous children's mean hair mercury concentration was 7.0 ± 4.5 (1.4–23.9) μg/g. The prevalence of mercury exposure above 6.0 μg/g was 49.0% in all studied population (n = 102) and 66.7% in children between 12 to 14 years old (n = 21).

Both heterozygous (*ALAD CG*) genotype children from *Sawré Muybu* had mercury levels above the average and third interquartile of the studied population (n = 100), considering only *Sawré Muybu* or *Poxo Muybu* villages. In addition, the mercury levels of *ALAD CG* children were considered as a health risk indicator (≥ 6.0 µg/g). There were statistically significant variations between the three villages (Kruskal–Wallis = 17.9; p-value < 0.0001). The *Sawre Aboy* people showed the highest risk of mercury contamination compared with other villages (Table 2). One wild-type *ALAD* child from *Sawré Aboy* (10-year-old boy, BMI 17.2) showed the highest mercury concentration (23.9 µg/g), according to the high levels of the village. For all participants under 15 years old, the median level of mercury in girls (n = 61) was 5.35 µg/g (IQR: 3.93, 5.35 and 9.17; range 1.60–22.07) and in boys (n = 41) it was 6.12 µg/g (IQR: 4.28, 6.12 and 8.94; variation 1.42–23.87) (p-value = 0.835). Considering the participants between 12 to 14 years old, the median level of mercury in girls (n = 13) was 6.19 µg/g (IQR: 4.24, 6.19 and 10.55; range 2.00–16.44) and in boys (n = 8) it was 8.13 µg/g (IQR: 5.76, 8.13 and 8.96; variation 5.76–9.13) (p-value = 0.515).

Table 2. Hair mercury levels (µg/g) in the study population (n = 102) *Sawré Muybu* Indigenous Land, Pará, Amazon, Brazil, 2019.

Variables	Case 1	Case 2	Children Population (n = 100) Mean ± SD (Range) Median
Mercury (µg/g) [a]	11.8	9.1	7.0 ± 4.5 (1.4–23.9) 5.8 IQR = 4.0; 5.8 and 8.8
	Sawré Muybu [b] (n = 45)	*Poxo Muybu* (n = 38)	*Sawré Aboy* (n = 19)
Mercury (µg/g) [c]	5.9 ± 4.5 (1.6–22.1) 4.4 IQR = 3.2; 4.4 and 7.3	6.3 ± 2.5 (1.4–11.8) 6.4 IQR = 4.5; 6.4 and 7.9	10.9 ± 5.6 (2.6–23.9) 10.1 IQR = 6.1; 10.1 and 15.2

IQR: interquartile range. [a] Data were obtained from 102 children. [b] Data were obtained from 44 children. [c] Significant different between the three villages (Kruskal–Wallis = 17.9; p-value < 0.0001).

Regarding blood pressure levels, 22 (21.4%) adolescents over 12 years old from whom we had this data, were classified as normal. Systolic blood pressure (SBP) mean level was 105 ± 6.8 (92–116), and diastolic blood pressure (DBP) mean level was 63 ± 6.8 (54–76). Peripheral blood samples were assessed for children from over 6 months old to 14-year-old adolescents (n = 99). For all participants, the hemoglobin levels vary from 9.2 to 16.1 g/dL (mean 12.4 ± 1.2). The prevalence of anemia (Hb level $\leq$ 11.5 g/dL) was 48.5% for all participants and 23.8% for adolescents between 12 to 14 years old (n = 21).

Table 3 displays the clinical characteristics and occurrence of mercury exposure symptoms of the studied population compared with two children with *ALAD* polymorphism. Both heterozygous genotype (*ALAD CG*) children had adverse neurological symptoms associated with chronic mercury exposure. The first case is a 12-year-old male that, from the 15 individuals able to be tested (aged 12–14 years old), was the only one that presented visual field alterations such as loss of differential light sensitivity and leukocoria in his right eye. In addition, the 14-year-old girl had the highest number of neurological manifestations (three of the four observed symptoms), including cognitive, somatosensory, and motor symptoms, such as memory deficit (evidenced by the verbal fluency test), distal neuropathy, and toe amyotrophy. The 12-year-old boy also reported recurrent diarrhea and acute respiratory infections, including an event of hospitalization for pneumonia. The boy's mother reported that his birth weight was 2000 g. Both children reported frequent consumption of fish in the diet, at least three times a week. Regarding the age group and neurological tests, 56 children (54.4%) aged between 0 to 6 years old had Denver II test results. Amongst them, nine children had a risk for developmental impairment (Table 3), from which one presented three symptoms (*Poxo Muybu*), one presented two symptoms (*Sawré Muybu*), and the other seven presented only one symptom (4 *Sawré Muybu* and

3 *Sawré Aboy*). However, this children's median mercury level was 6.2 μg/g (IQR: 3.2, 6.2, and 9.9), therefore, lower than in the two heterozygous *ALAD CG* children (Table 2).

Table 3. Clinical characteristics of the study population *Sawré Muybu* Indigenous Land, Pará, Amazon, Brazil, 2019.

Variables	Case 1	Case 2	Children Population Mean ± SD (Range) Median
Blood pressure [a] SBP (mmHg)	107	112	105 ± 6.9 (92–116) 106 IQR = 98; 106 and 110
DBP (mmHg)	69	73	62 ± 6.6 (54–76) 61 IQR = 56; 61 and 69
Hemoglobin level (g/dL) [b]	14.8	14.2	12.4 ± 1.2 (9–16) 12.3 IQR = 11.8; 12.3 and 13.1
Symptoms of chronical mercury exposure [c]			(n = 13)
Visual Field	Yes	No	Yes (n = zero)
Toe extensor amyotrophy	No	Yes	Yes (n = 2)
Distal neuropathy	No	Yes	Yes (n = 3)
Cognitive deficit	No	Yes	Yes (n = 4)
Denver neurodevelopment test [d]			n = 56 (%)
Deficit language	-	-	8 (14.3)
Fine motor skills	-	-	2 (3.6)
Gross motor skills	-	-	2 (3.6)

SBP: systolic blood pressure. DBP: diastolic blood pressure. IQR: interquartile range. [a] Data were obtained from 22 children over 12 years old. [b] Data were obtained from 99 children. [c] Data were obtained from 15 children aged 12 years or older. [d] Data were obtained from 56 children aged between 0 to 6 years old.

4. Discussion

In this study, we described the effects of chronic exposure to mercury in 103 indigenous children living in the Brazilian Amazon, who face the burden of long-term impacts from illegal mining activities. Genetic analysis identified two children with the *ALAD* polymorphism who had high levels of mercury in their hair samples and severe symptoms of chronic mercury exposure. Although there is a growing number of studies investigating the effects of chronic exposure to mercury on population health [5,8,25,26], little is known about the influence of the individual's genetic susceptibility on mercury toxicokinetics and toxidinamics, thus gaps remain in our knowledge about the role that genetic variability plays.

As far as we know, only one study has evaluated the effects of *ALAD* polymorphism on mercury-exposed individuals from the Brazilian Amazon. As previously described, heterozygous individuals *ALAD CG* had significant lower ALAD activity and higher Hg levels in blood compared with non-variant genotype subjects [11]. In the present study, both *ALAD CG* individuals had a mercury concentration even higher than the average, which suggests that the polymorphism is also contributing to mercury half-life time. The amino acid change caused by the *ALAD 177 C > G* polymorphism, resulted in a more negatively charged ALAD isozyme, which makes it more attracted to inorganic metals, such as lead (Pb) for example, and therefore, promotes higher levels of metal and free erythrocyte protoporphyrin in blood and tissues [27]. Since lead and mercury have similar atomic radii (1.76 and 1.81 Å, respectively) [28], and the ALAD enzyme may interact with other metals besides Pb [29,30], it is possible that Hg is capable of binding to the same sites in ALAD, also resulting in higher Hg levels in total blood [11]. *ALAD* polymorphisms and levels of essential (iron, copper, selenium, and manganese) and toxic trace elements (lead, cadmium, Hg, and arsenic) were tested in a Kyrgyz-stan population of uranium legacy sites. Lead blood variability was associated with *ALAD* polymorphisms with a slight influence on Hg, arsenic, and selenium levels also observed [31].

The average concentration of hair mercury in all studied population exceeds the reference limit (≥6.0 μg/g), which is in agreement with other studies from the Amazon region [24,25,32]. Recently our group evaluated Hg levels of 197 hair samples (ranging from 1.4 to 23.9 µg/g) and observed significant differences between the three villages (*Sawré Muybu*, *Poxo Muybu* and *Sawré Aboy*), with the residents of *Sawre Aboy* village at highest risk of mercury contamination [14], according to the present study. Once ingested through contaminated food, the digestive tract easily absorbs MeHg and it reaches the bloodstream, affecting various tissues in the human body, including the nervous system, due to its highly lipophilic nature [33]. In pregnant women, MeHg has the capacity to cross the placental barrier and to contaminate breast milk, exposing both fetuses and infants to this toxic compound [34,35].

The higher possibility of absorption through the digestive tract and the immaturity of the blood–brain barrier and metabolic excretory pathways, makes children one of the demographics most vulnerable to the effects of mercury exposure [13,36]. In line with this, children have a higher susceptibility to adverse neurological symptoms caused by chronic mercury exposure compared to adults with similar levels [7]. Chronic mercury exposure can cause serious neurological damage such as decrements in memory, attention, language, and visual-motor skills in childhood [13,33]; this is in accordance with what was observed in our present study, especially with the two children with the heterozygous *ALAD* CG genotype, who had a high risk of mercury contamination. *ALAD* polymorphism may modulate the burden of mercury exposure in the body and, consequently, induce metal toxicity [11]. Despite little evidence, Santos-Lima et al. (2020) identified in 263 children aged 6–14 years old from the Amazon region, several changes in neuropsychological functions, related to mercury exposure [13]; however, the children's genetic profile was not evaluated.

There is evidence that maternal-fetal genetic background can modulate fetal exposure to these neurotoxicants [37]; however, studies focused on the association between Hg exposure and *ALAD* polymorphism are very scarce. From the 103 children in our study population, two presented *ALAD* polymorphism. Both these children were the same children that presented the most significant burden of neurological and clinical abnormalities, including toe extensor amyotrophy, distal polyneuropathy, cognitive and memory deficits, visual field changes, and leukocoria. Although the symptoms were different between the two cases, both children shared genetic backgrounds, had very high levels of mercury, and resided in the same village. *Sawré Muybu* village presented the lowest average mercury level and, therefore, had the same environmental exposure to mercury. Since it was the village with the lowest level of mercury and cases exceed the reference limit (≥ 6.0 µg/g), we hypothesize that the presence of the variant *ALAD* allele influences the occurrence of these disturbances by increasing the association between ALAD protein and Hg molecules and, consequently, raising blood Hg levels. Nevertheless, in addition to the *ALAD* polymorphism, there may be other genetic influences, making individuals more predisposed to certain conditions influencing the occurrence of neurological symptoms [38–42]. Visual field defects, for instance, have already been associated with a mutation on the *OPA 1* (*OPA1 Mitochondrial Dynamin Like GTPase*) gene [39] and a polymorphism near the *TGFBR3* (*Transforming Growth Factor Beta Receptor (3) gene* [38]. Another example is the *COMT* gene (*Catechol-O-Methyltransferase*), whose SNPs have been associated with lower chances of developing memory impairment [41] and higher odds of developing distal neuropathic pain [40]. A review study published in 2020 showed that epigenetic alterations such as miRNA expression and DNA methylation could cause impaired memory and neuronal development, depression-like behavior, visual deficits, and hyperactivity, in experimental models [42].

In addition, several studies have investigated the influence of mercury exposure on visual function [43–45] and sensorimotor polyneuropathy [46], symptoms here that were observed in the child with the *ALAD* polymorphism. A recent study, conducted in two Amazonian populations, investigated the visual functions of riverine individuals exposed to MeHg through food intake. The authors observed that all riverine subjects had a perimetric area smaller than the reference value and loss in color vision [45]. Another study, involving children from Turkey, showed that, besides the visual field defects, peripheral neuropathy was also a consequence of acute mercury exposure [43]. As previously described, mercury can cross the blood–retina barrier, accumulating in the cells and layers of the retina, inducing changes in the photoreceptors and, consequently, causing visual field defects [47].

Another neuropsychological function that can be disrupted for mercury exposure is the memory [48,49], also observed in one of the studied children with *ALAD* polymorphism. Grandjean and cols. (2014) conducted a cohort study with 694 individuals born in 1986 and 1987 in the Faroe Islands, investigating the association between postnatal exposures to MeHg and neurobehavioral performance at the age of 7. The study demonstrated that, from the 17 supposed outcomes, only the visuospatial memory measure showed a clear negative association after the adjusted analysis [49]. Furthermore, there is evidence that mercury exposure can also be a cause of Alzheimer's disease [50]. A recent study reported a case of an old man diagnosed with Alzheimer's disease, presenting with high levels of mercury due to MeHg-containing fish consumption. After a detoxification dietary regime, his body mercury levels dropped and his memory partially improved [51].

Almost half of the studied population had anemia (Hb level ≤ 11.5 g/dL). There is little evidence in the literature regarding this matter [26], however, a few recent studies showed an inverse association between hemoglobin levels and mercury exposure in the last decade [52–54]. A study from 2017, conducted with 83 children from the Peruvian Amazon region, demonstrated that MeHg exposure was associated with toxicant-induced anemia [54]. Nevertheless, Hb levels of two *ALAD* polymorphism children were within the normal range. Regarding the blood pressure, both SBP and DBP in the present study were found to be normal considering all indigenous children or specifically the *ALAD CG* individuals. High concentrations of Hg may play a role in blood pressure measurements since subclinical vascular changes start at an early age, even though studies investigating the relationship between Hg exposure and altered blood pressure provide conflicting results [55]. In addition, it is important to highlight the complexity of identifying effects related to long-term Hg exposure due to the absence of accurate diagnosis and the ability of Hg to deposit in different parts of the body, modifying many molecular pathways [7].

Within the Brazilian population, the MAF of *ALAD 177 C > G* polymorphism is low (approximately 1–7%) [56–58], with the majority being found in riverside communities of the Brazilian Amazon (2.7%) [11], an observation also seen in the present study, with only two subjects being heterozygous for the *ALAD CG* genotype (1.9%). Although an obvious limitation was the small sample size, the strengths of this study included the accurate analyses of the indigenous children's genetic profile and individual mercury exposure levels alongside thorough assessment of neuropsychological function, general health status, and the sociodemographic characterization of the families. The results can be used to build a database from different populations chronically exposed to mercury in order to help identify the health impacts of illegal mining activities.

5. Conclusions

Despite the low frequency of *ALAD 177 C > G* polymorphism in the study population, both children with the heterozygous *ALAD* genotype presented with the health risk indicators of high mercury concentration levels, exceeding the reference limit, and severe neurological symptoms associated with chronic mercury exposure. It is worth mentioning that this is the first time an analysis of genetic polymorphism, focusing on mercury toxicokinetics and toxicodynamics, has been carried out among an indigenous children population living in remote areas of the Brazilian Amazon. Therefore, the knowledge regarding possible individual predisposing factors to the effects of heavy metals exposure is essential to understand the health situation of a hard-to-reach population and to inform public policy to help mitigate the extensive impact of gold mining activity in exposed communities within the Amazon region.

Author Contributions: Proposal design, study design and methodology, J.A.P., A.C.S.d.V., P.V.S.V., S.S.H. and P.C.B.; fieldwork data collection, A.C.S.d.V., P.V.S.V., J.W.K., R.A.A.O. and P.C.B.; laboratory analysis, J.A.P., M.C.S., I.M.J. and M.O.L.; writing original draft preparation, J.A.P., M.C.S. and P.C.B.; writing—review and editing, J.W.K., R.A.A.O., S.S.H. and P.C.B.; supervision, obtaining resources and project management, P.C.B. and S.S.H. All authors have read and agreed to the published version of the manuscript.

Funding: This research was funded by the Vice-Presidency of Environment, Care and Health Promotion (VPPAS) of Fundação Oswaldo Cruz through Decentralized Execution of Resources Document No. 175/2018, Process: 25000.209221/2018-18, signed between the Fundação Oswaldo Cruz and the Special Department for Indigenous Health, both under the Ministry of Health. The nongovernmental organization WWF-Brasil offered financial support to disseminate the results of the research. This study was supported by the Brazilian agency Fundação Carlos Chagas Filho de Amparo à Pesquisa do Estado do Rio de Janeiro—FAPERJ, Brazil. Funding body contributed to acquisition of research inputs.

Institutional Review Board Statement: The study was conducted in accordance with the guidelines of the Declaration of Helsinki and was approved by the Research Ethics Committee of the National School of Public Health at Fundação Oswaldo Cruz (REC/ENSP) and the Brazilian National Research Ethics Commission of the National Health Council (CONEP/CNS), CAAE: 65671517.1.0000.5240, with Opinion No. 2.262.686 favorable to its performance. In compliance with Convention No. 169 of the International Labor Organization (ILO), the study began with a pre-study consultation, carried out in August 2019, during a visit to the villages, in which two authors (SSH and PCB) and local indigenous leaders participated. At the time, the study objectives were presented and discussed (https://www.youtube.com/watch?v=oFEYEGxNmns&t=704s, accessed on 22 August 2020). After answering questions and approval of the proposal by the communities, we received support from the coordination of the Special Indigenous Sanitary District of the Tapajós River through the multidisciplinary indigenous health team to carry out the study. In addition, the interviews and data collection started only after the participants had their questions answered and given formal consent in the Informed Consent Form (ICF) by the children's guardians.

Informed Consent Statement: Informed consent was obtained from all subjects involved in the study. Written informed consent has been obtained from the patients to publish this paper.

Data Availability Statement: Data sharing not applicable.

Acknowledgments: Through Juarez Saw, Jairo Saw, Valdemar Poxo, and Alessandra Korap, we thank the Munduruku people for the trust placed in our team and the support in carrying out the research. We thank the team from the Rio Tapajós Indigenous Special Sanitary District, who spared no efforts to support us in all stages of the fieldwork. In particular, we thank nurses Alan Marcelo Simon and Lygia Catarina de Oliveira. We thank João Paulo Goes Pereira for mercury analysis in the fish samples. We also thank Marcelo Oliveira da Costa from World-Wide Fund for Nature (WWF-Brazil) for technical and financial support to this scientific communication. The authors thank the technical assistance of Jessica Vilarinho Cardoso from Laboratório de Pesquisa de Ciências Farmacêuticas (https://lapesfuezo.wixsite.com/website, accessed on 13 Mays 2021)) of Centro Universitário Estadual da Zona Oeste (UEZO).

Conflicts of Interest: The authors declare no conflict of interest. The funders had no role in the design of the study; in the collection, analyses, or interpretation of data; in the writing of the manuscript, or in the decision to publish the results.

References

1. WHO (World Health Organization). Mercury and Health. 2017. Available online: https://www.who.int/news-room/factsheets/detail/mercury-and-health (accessed on 13 May 2021).
2. Yang, L.; Zhang, Y.; Wang, F.; Luo, Z.; Guo, S.; Strähle, U. Toxicity of mercury: Molecular evidence. *Chemosphere* **2020**, *245*, 125586. [CrossRef]
3. Scheuhammer, A.M.; Meyer, M.W.; Sandheinrich, M.B.; Murray, M.W. Effects of environmental methylmercury on the health of wild birds, mammals, and fish. *AMBIO J. Hum. Environ.* **2007**, *36*, 12–19. [CrossRef]
4. Rice, K.M.; Walker, E.M., Jr.; Wu, M.; Gillette, C.; Blough, E.R. Environmental mercury and its toxic effects. *J. Prev. Med. Public Health* **2014**, *47*, 74. [CrossRef] [PubMed]

5. Crespo-Lopez, M.E.; Augusto-Oliveira, M.; Lopes-Araújo, A.; Santos-Sacramento, L.; Takeda, P.Y.; Macchi, B.D.M.; Nascimento, J.L.M.D.; Maia, C.S.; Lima, R.R.; Arrifano, G.P. Mercury: What can we learn from the Amazon? *Environ. Int.* **2021**, *146*, 106223. [CrossRef] [PubMed]
6. Branco, V.; Caito, S.; Farina, M.; Da Rocha, J.B.T.; Aschner, M.; Carvalho, C. Biomarkers of mercury toxicity: Past, present, and future trends. *J. Toxicol. Environ. Health Part B* **2017**, *20*, 119–154. [CrossRef]
7. Andreoli, V.; Sprovieri, F. Genetic Aspects of Susceptibility to Mercury Toxicity: An Overview. *Int. J. Environ. Res. Public Health* **2017**, *14*, 93. [CrossRef] [PubMed]
8. Hacon, S.D.S.; Oliveira-Da-Costa, M.; Gama, C.D.S.; Ferreira, R.; Basta, P.C.; Schramm, A.; Yokota, D. Mercury Exposure through Fish Consumption in Traditional Communities in the Brazilian Northern Amazon. *Int. J. Environ. Res. Public Health* **2020**, *17*, 5269. [CrossRef]
9. Battistuzzi, G.; Petrucci, R.; Silvagni, L.; Urbani, F.R.; Caiola, S. δ-aminolevulinate dehydrase: A new genetic polymorphism in man. *Ann. Hum. Genet.* **1981**, *45*, 223–229. [CrossRef]
10. Smith, C.M.; Wang, X.; Hu, H.; Kelsey, K.T. A polymorphism in the delta-aminolevulinic aciddehydratase gene may modify the pharmacokinetics and toxicity of lead. *Environ. Health Perspect.* **1995**, *103*, 248–253.
11. Barcelos, G.R.M.; de Souza, M.F.; de Oliveira, A.Á.S.; van Helvoort Lengert, A.; de Oliveira, M.T.; Camargo, R.B.D.O.G.; Barbosa, F., Jr. Effects of genetic polymorphisms on antioxidant status and concentrations of the metals in the blood of riverside Amazonian communities co-exposed to Hg and Pb. *Environ. Res.* **2015**, *138*, 224–232. [CrossRef]
12. Karagas, M.R.; Choi, A.L.; Oken, E.; Horvat, M.; Schoeny, R.; Kamai, E.M.; Cowell, W.; Grandjean, P.; Korrick, S. Evidence on the Human Health Effects of Low-Level Methylmercury Exposure. *Environ. Health Perspect.* **2012**, *120*, 799–806. [CrossRef] [PubMed]
13. dos Santos-Lima, C.; Mourão, D.D.S.; de Carvalho, C.F.; Souza-Marques, B.; Vega, C.M.; Gonçalves, R.A.; Argollo, N.; Menezes-Filho, J.A.; Abreu, N.; Hacon, S.D.S. Neuropsychological Effects of Mercury Exposure in Children and Adolescents of the Amazon Region, Brazil. *Neurotoxicology* **2020**, *79*, 48–57. [CrossRef] [PubMed]
14. Basta, P.C.; Viana, P.V.S.; Vasconcellos, A.; Périssé, A.; Hofer, C.; Paiva, N.S.; Kempton, J.W.; de Andrade, D.C.; Oliveira, R.A.A.; Achatz, R.W.; et al. Mercury exposure in Munduruku indigenous communities from Brazilian Amazon: Methodological background and an overview of the principal results. *Int. J. Environ. Res. Public Health* **2021**, *18*, in press.
15. World Health Organization (WHO). *WHO Child Growth Standards: Length/Height-for-Age, Weight-for-Age, Weight-for-Length, Weight-for-Height and Body Mass Index-for-Age. Methods and Development*; WHO (Nonserial Publication): Geneva, Switzerland, 2006.
16. Malachias, M.V.B.; Barbosa, E.C.D.; Martim, J.F.V.; Rosito, G.B.A.; Toledo, J.Y.; Júnior, O.P. 7ª Diretriz Brasileira de Hipertensão Arterial: Capítulo 14–Crise Hipertensiva. *Arq. Bras. Cardiol.* **2016**, *107*, 79–83. [CrossRef] [PubMed]
17. Nitrini, R.; Caramelli, P.; Herrera, E.; Porto, C.S.; Charchat-Fichman, H.; Carthery-Goulart, M.T.; Takada, L.; Lima, E.P. Performance of illiterate and literate nondemented elderly subjects in two tests of long-term memory. *J. Int. Neuropsychol. Soc.* **2004**, *10*, 634–638. [CrossRef]
18. Brucki, S.; Malheiros, S.M.F.; Okamoto, I.H.; Bertolucci, P. Dados normativos para o teste de fluência verbal categoria animais em nosso meio. *Arq. Neuro-Psiquiatr.* **1997**, *55*, 56–61. [CrossRef] [PubMed]
19. Baiyewu, O.; Unverzagt, F.W.; Lane, K.A.; Gureje, O.; Ogunniyi, A.; Musick, B.; Gao, S.; Hall, K.S.; Hendrie, H.C. The Stick Design test: A new measure of visuoconstructional ability. *J. Int. Neuropsychol. Soc.* **2005**, *11*, 598–605. [CrossRef]
20. Oliveira, R.A.A.; Pinto, B.D.; Resende, B.H.; Andrade, D.C.A.; Basta, P.C. Neurological impacts of chronic methylmercury exposure in Munduruku indigenous adults: Somatosensory, motor and cognitive abnormalities. *Int. J. Environ. Res. Public Health* **2021**, *18*, in press.
21. Hofer, C.B.; Périssé, A.R.S.; Vasconcellos, A.C.S.; Viana, P.V.S.; Kempton, J.W.; Lima, M.O.; Jesus, I.M.; Hacon, S.S.; Basta, P.C. Munduruku Indigenous children health's in the Tapajos river basin: Situational diagnosis and possible impacts of chronic mercury exposure. *Int. J. Environ. Res. Public Health* **2021**, *18*, in press.
22. Suzuki, T.; Akagi, H.; Arimura, K.; Ando, T.; Sakamoto, M.; Satoh, H.; Matsuyama, A. *Mercury Analysis Manual*; Ministry of the Environment: Tokyo, Japan, 2004.
23. Marinho, J.S.; Lima, M.O.; Santos, E.C.D.O.; De Jesus, I.M.; Pinheiro, M.D.C.N.; Alves, C.N.; Müller, R.C.S. Mercury Speciation in Hair of Children in Three Communities of the Amazon, Brazil. *BioMed Res. Int.* **2014**, *2014*, 1–9. [CrossRef]
24. Vega, C.M.; Orellana, J.D.; Oliveira, M.W.; Hacon, S.S.; Basta, P.C. Human Mercury Exposure in Yanomami Indigenous Villages from the Brazilian Amazon. *Int. J. Environ. Res. Public Health* **2018**, *15*, 1051. [CrossRef] [PubMed]
25. de Castro, N.S.S.; de Oliveira Lima, M. Hair as a biomarker of long term mercury exposure in Brazilian Amazon: A systematic review. *Int. J. Environ. Res. Public Health* **2018**, *15*, 500. [CrossRef] [PubMed]
26. Vianna, A.D.S.; De Matos, E.P.; De Jesus, I.M.; Asmus, C.I.R.F.; Câmara, V.D.M. Human exposure to mercury and its hematological effects: A systematic review. *Cad. Saúde Pública* **2019**, *35*, e00091618. [CrossRef] [PubMed]
27. Onalaja, A.O.; Claudio, L. Genetic susceptibility to lead poisoning. *Environ. Health Perspect.* **2000**, *108* (Suppl. S1), 23–28.
28. Flora, S.J.S.; Mittal, M.; Mehta, A. Heavy metal induced oxidative stress & its possible reversal by chelation therapy. *Indian J. Med. Res.* **2008**, *128*, 501.
29. Bernard, A.; Lauwerys, R. Metal-Induced Alterations of δ-Aminolevulinic Acid Dehydratase. *Ann. N. Y. Acad. Sci.* **1987**, *514*, 41–47. [CrossRef] [PubMed]
30. Rocha, J.B.T.; Saraiva, R.A.; Garcia, S.C.; Gravina, F.S.; Nogueira, C.W. Aminolevulinate dehydratase (δ-ALA-D) as marker protein of intoxication with metals and other pro-oxidant situations. *Toxicol. Res.* **2012**, *1*, 85–102. [CrossRef]

31. Stajnko, A.; Tuhvatshin, R.; Suranova, G.; Mazej, D.; Šlejkovec, Z.; Falnoga, I.; Krušič, Ž.; Lespukh, E.; Stegnar, P. Trace elements and ALAD gene polymorphisms in general population from three uranium legacy sites—A case study in Kyrgyzstan. *Sci. Total Environ.* **2020**, *719*, 134427. [CrossRef] [PubMed]
32. Ashe, K. Elevated Mercury Concentrations in Humans of Madre de Dios, Peru. *PLoS ONE* **2012**, *7*, e33305. [CrossRef]
33. Cariccio, V.L.; Samà, A.; Bramanti, P.; Mazzon, E. Mercury Involvement in Neuronal Damage and in Neurodegenerative Diseases. *Biol. Trace Elem. Res.* **2018**, *187*, 341–356. [CrossRef]
34. De Vasconcellos, A.C.S.; Barrocas, P.; Ruiz, C.M.V.; Mourão, D.D.S.; Hacon, S.D.S. Burden of Mild Mental Retardation attributed to prenatal methylmercury exposure in Amazon: Local and regional estimates. *Ciência Saúde Coletiva* **2018**, *23*, 3535–3545. [CrossRef] [PubMed]
35. Pajewska-Szmyt, M.; Sinkiewicz-Darol, E.; Gadzała-Kopciuch, R. The impact of environmental pollution on the quality of mother's milk. *Environ. Sci. Pollut. Res.* **2019**, *26*, 7405–7427. [CrossRef] [PubMed]
36. Bauer, J.A.; Fruh, V.; Howe, C.G.; White, R.F.; Henn, B.C. Associations of Metals and Neurodevelopment: A Review of Recent Evidence on Susceptibility Factors. *Curr. Epidemiol. Rep.* **2020**, *7*, 237–262. [CrossRef]
37. Gundacker, C.; Gencik, M.; Hengstschläger, M. The relevance of the individual genetic background for the toxicokinetics of two significant neurodevelopmental toxicants: Mercury and lead. *Mutat. Res. Mutat. Res.* **2010**, *705*, 130–140. [CrossRef]
38. Trikha, S.; Saffari, E.; Nongpiur, M.; Baskaran, M.; Ho, H.; Li, Z.; Tan, P.-Y.; Allen, J.; Khor, C.-C.; Perera, S.A.; et al. A Genetic Variant in TGFBR3-CDC7 Is Associated with Visual Field Progression in Primary Open-Angle Glaucoma Patients from Singapore. *Ophthalmology* **2015**, *122*, 2416–2422. [CrossRef]
39. Gaier, E.D.; Boudreault, K.; Nakata, I.; Janessian, M.; Skidd, P.; Delbono, E.; Allen, K.F.; Pasquale, L.R.; Place, E.; Cestari, D.M.; et al. Diagnostic genetic testing for patients with bilateral optic neuropathy and comparison of clinical features according to OPA1 mutation status. *Mol. Vis.* **2017**, *23*, 548–560. [PubMed]
40. Xu, J.; Umlauf, A.; Letendre, S.; Franklin, D.; Bush, W.; Atkinson, J.H.; Keltner, J.; Ellis, R.J. Catechol-O-methyltransferase polymorphism Val158Met is associated with distal neuropathic pain in HIV-associated sensory neuropathy. *AIDS* **2019**, *33*, 1575–1582. [CrossRef]
41. Li, W.; Zhao, J.; Ding, K.; Chao, H.H.; Li, C.-S.R.; Cheng, H.; Shen, L. Catechol-O-Methyltransferase Gene Polymorphisms and the Risk of Chemotherapy-Induced Prospective Memory Impairment in Breast Cancer Patients with Varying Tumor Hormonal Receptor Expression. *Med. Sci. Monit.* **2020**, *26*, e923567-1. [CrossRef]
42. Ijomone, O.M.; Ijomone, O.K.; Iroegbu, J.D.; Ifenatuoha, C.W.; Olung, N.F.; Aschner, M. Epigenetic influence of environmentally neurotoxic metals. *Neurotoxicology* **2020**, *81*, 51–65. [CrossRef]
43. Carman, K.B.; Tutkun, E.; Yilmaz, H.; Dilber, C.; Dalkiran, T.; Cakir, B.; Arslantaş, D.; Cesaretli, Y.; Aykanat, S.A. Acute mercury poisoning among children in two provinces of Turkey. *Eur. J. Nucl. Med. Mol. Imaging* **2013**, *172*, 821–827. [CrossRef]
44. Feitosa-Santana, C.; Souza, G.D.S.; Sirius, E.V.P.; Rodrigues, A.R.; Côrtes, M.I.T.; Silveira, L.C.D.L.; Ventura, D.F.; Pupo, E.S.V. Color vision impairment with low-level methylmercury exposure of an Amazonian population—Brazil. *Neurotoxicology* **2018**, *66*, 179–184. [CrossRef] [PubMed]
45. Lacerda, E.M.D.C.B.; Souza, G.D.S.; Cortes, M.I.T.; Rodrigues, A.R.; Pinheiro, M.C.N.; Silveira, L.C.D.L.; Ventura, D.F. Comparison of Visual Functions of Two Amazonian Populations: Possible Consequences of Different Mercury Exposure. *Front. Neurosci.* **2020**, *13*, 1428. [CrossRef] [PubMed]
46. Franzblau, A.; D'Arcy, H.; Ishak, M.B.; Werner, R.A.; Gillespie, B.W.; Albers, J.W.; Hamann, C.; Gruninger, S.E.; Chou, H.-N.; Meyer, D.M. Low-level mercury exposure and peripheral nerve function. *Neurotoxicology* **2012**, *33*, 299–306. [CrossRef] [PubMed]
47. Mela, M.; Groetzner, S.R.; Legeay, A.; Mesmer-Dudons, N.; Massabuau, J.-C.; Ventura, D.; Ribeiro, C.O. Morphological evidence of neurotoxicity in retina after methylmercury exposure. *Neurotoxicology* **2012**, *33*, 407–415. [CrossRef] [PubMed]
48. Freire, C.; Ramos, R.T.; Lopez-Espinosa, M.-J.; Díez, S.; Vioque, J.; Ballester, F.; Fernandez, M.F. Hair mercury levels, fish consumption, and cognitive development in preschool children from Granada, Spain. *Environ. Res.* **2010**, *110*, 96–104. [CrossRef]
49. Grandjean, P.; Weihe, P.; Debes, F.; Choi, A.L.; Budtz-Jørgensen, E. Neurotoxicity from prenatal and postnatal exposure to methylmercury. *Neurotoxicol. Teratol.* **2014**, *43*, 39–44. [CrossRef] [PubMed]
50. Siblerud, R.; Mutter, J.; Moore, E.; Naumann, J.; Walach, H. A Hypothesis and Evidence That Mercury May be an Etiological Factor in Alzheimer's Disease. *Int. J. Environ. Res. Public Health* **2019**, *16*, 5152. [CrossRef]
51. Foley, M.M.; Seidel, I.; Sevier, J.; Wendt, J.; Kogan, M. One man's swordfish story: The link between Alzheimer's disease and mercury exposure. *Complement. Ther. Med.* **2020**, *52*, 102499. [CrossRef]
52. Mathee, A.; Naicker, N.; Kootbodien, T.; Mahuma, T.; Nkomo, P.; Naik, I.; De Wet, T. A cross-sectional analytical study of geophagia practices and blood metal concentrations in pregnant women in Johannesburg, South Africa. *S. Afr. Med. J.* **2014**, *104*, 568–573. [CrossRef] [PubMed]
53. Ekawanti, A.; Krisnayanti, B.D. Effect of Mercury Exposure on Renal Function and Hematological Parameters among Artisanal and Small-scale Gold Miners at Sekotong, West Lombok, Indonesia. *J. Heal. Pollut.* **2015**, *5*, 25–32. [CrossRef]
54. Weinhouse, C.; Ortiz, E.J.; Berky, A.J.; Bullins, P.; Hare-Grogg, J.; Rogers, L.; Morales, A.-M.; Hsu-Kim, H.; Pan, W.K. Hair Mercury Level is Associated with Anemia and Micronutrient Status in Children Living Near Artisanal and Small-Scale Gold Mining in the Peruvian Amazon. *Am. J. Trop. Med. Hyg.* **2017**, *97*, 1886–1897. [CrossRef] [PubMed]
55. Farzan, S.F.; Howe, C.G.; Chen, Y.; Gilbert-Diamond, D.; Korrick, S.; Jackson, B.P.; Weinstein, A.R.; Karagas, M.R. Prenatal and postnatal mercury exposure and blood pressure in childhood. *Environ. Int.* **2021**, *146*, 106201. [CrossRef] [PubMed]

56. Montenegro, M.F.; Barbosa Jr, F.; Sandrim, V.C.; Gerlach, R.F.; Tanus-Santos, J.E. Ethnicity affects the distribution of δ-aminolevulinic acid dehydratase (ALAD) genetic variants. *Clin. Chim. Acta* **2006**, *367*, 192–195. [CrossRef] [PubMed]
57. da Cunha Martins, A., Jr.; Mazzaron Barcelos, G.R.; Jacob Ferreira, A.L.B.; de Souza, M.F.; de Syllos Cólus, I.M.; Greggi Antunes, L.M.; Barbosa, F., Jr. Effects of lead exposure and genetic polymorphisms on ALAD and GPx activities in Brazilian battery workers. *J. Toxicol. Environ. Health Part A* **2015**, *78*, 1073–1081. [CrossRef] [PubMed]
58. Bah, H.A.; Dos Anjos, A.L.S.; Gomes-Júnior, E.A.; Bandeira, M.J.; de Carvalho, C.F.; Dos Santos, N.R.; Menezes-Filho, J.A. Delta-Aminolevulinic Acid Dehydratase, Low Blood Lead Levels, Social Factors, and Intellectual Function in an Afro-Brazilian Children Community. *Biol. Trace Elem. Res.* **2011**, 1–11. [CrossRef]

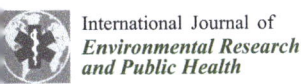

Article

Health Risk Assessment of Mercury Exposure from Fish Consumption in Munduruku Indigenous Communities in the Brazilian Amazon

Ana Claudia Santiago de Vasconcellos [1,*], Gustavo Hallwass [2], Jaqueline Gato Bezerra [2], Angélico Nonato Serrão Aciole [2], Heloisa Nascimento de Moura Meneses [3], Marcelo de Oliveira Lima [4], Iracina Maura de Jesus [4], Sandra de Souza Hacon [5] and Paulo Cesar Basta [5,*]

[1] Laboratory of Professional Education in Health Surveillance, Joaquim Venâncio Polytechnic School of Health, Oswaldo Cruz Foundation, 21040-900 Rio de Janeiro, Brazil
[2] Laboratory of Human Ecology, Fish, Fisheries and Conservation, Postgraduate Program in Biosciences, Federal University of West Para, 68270-000 Oriximiná, Brazil; gustavo.hallwass@gmail.com (G.H.); jaqlinegb@gmail.com (J.G.B.); angelico.aciole@bol.com.br (A.N.S.A.)
[3] Laboratory of Molecular Epidemiology, Postgraduate Program in Health Sciences, Federal University of West Para, 68040-470 Santarém, Brazil; heloisa.meneses@ufopa.edu.br
[4] Environment Section, Evandro Chagas Institute, Health Surveillance Secretariat, Ministry of Health, 67030-000 Ananindeua, Brazil; marcelolima@iec.gov.br (M.O.L.); iracinajesus@iec.gov.br (I.M.J.)
[5] Samuel Pessoa Department of Endemics, National School of Public Health, Oswaldo Cruz Foundation, 21041-210 Rio de Janeiro, Brazil; sandrahacon@gmail.com
* Correspondence: ana.vasconcellos@fiocruz.br (A.C.S.V.); paulobasta@gmail.com (P.C.B.); Tel.: +55-21-2598-2503 (P.C.B.)

Abstract: Fish serves as the principal source of animal protein for the indigenous people of the Amazon, ensuring their food and nutritional security. However, gold mining causes mercury (Hg) contamination in fish, and consequently increases health risks associated with fish consumption. The aim of this study was to assess the health risk attributed to the consumption of mercury-contaminated fish by Munduruku indigenous communities in the Middle-Tapajós Region. Different fish species were collected in the *Sawré Muybu* Indigenous Land to determine mercury levels. The health risk assessment was carried out according to the World Health Organization (WHO 2008) methodology and different scenarios were built for counterfactual analysis. Eighty-eight fish specimens from 17 species and four trophic levels were analyzed. Estimates of Hg ingestion indicated that the methylmercury daily intake exceeds the U.S. EPA (United States Environmental Protection Agency) (2000) reference dose from 3 to 25-fold, and up to 11 times the FAO (Food and Agriculture Organization)/WHO (2003) dose recommendation. In all situations analyzed, the risk ratio estimates were above 1.0, meaning that the investigated Munduruku communities are at serious risk of harm as a result of ingestion of mercury-contaminated fish. These results indicate that, at present, fish consumption is not safe for this Munduruku population. This hazardous situation threatens the survival of this indigenous population, their food security, and their culture.

Keywords: mercury; indigenous; health risk assessment; Munduruku; fish; Brazilian Amazon

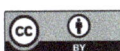

1. Introduction

Fish has an important role in food security, since 17% of all animal protein consumed in the world is provided by fish [1]. In addition, fish consumption contributes to nutritional security, given its high content of essential nutrients (i.e., vitamins and minerals) and polyunsaturated fatty acids (e.g., omega-3 and omega-6) [2,3]. The food and nutritional security attributed to fish consumption is especially important for low-income populations in developing countries where over 90% of inland water caught fish are directed for local human consumption [4,5]. Indeed, fish is often the only quality protein accessible to poor people [6,7]. These reasons make fish a vital element for Amazonian populations, especially for indigenous and riverine populations.

The Amazon is the largest freshwater ecosystem and displays the greatest diversity of freshwater fish in the world [8,9]. Therefore, it is not surprising that Amazonian people have one of the highest fish consumption rates in the world [10–12]. An archaeological study found that fish was the species of vertebrates most consumed (>75% of total) in an ancient settlement of indigenous populations in the Central Brazilian Amazon. Fish consumption is historically related to culture and to food security of the original peoples from the Amazon [13,14]. However, several anthropogenic activities threaten the survival of Amazonian peoples, such as deforestation promoted by agribusiness (e.g., soybean cultivate and cattle), construction of hydroelectric dams, and artisanal gold mining [15–22]. The indigenous populations are particularly affected by the impact of these activities because they live in socially and environmentally vulnerable conditions caused by historical government neglect.

In this sense, the artisanal gold mining (also called *garimpos*) can be considered one of the most harmful economic activities in the Amazon, because it causes not only deforestation, river siltation, and soil erosion, but also releases large amounts of mercury into the environment. Mercury is a toxic heavy metal that contaminates the atmosphere, waters, sediments, and organisms [23,24].

Nevertheless, the current policies of the Brazilian federal government aim to allow oil and natural gas extraction, agribusiness, mining, and other economic activities in protected areas and indigenous lands. These policies are responsible for the highest rate of deforestation in the past 10 years, weakening the environmental protection legislation and human rights of traditional and indigenous populations [20,25,26].

In addition, recent studies carried out in the Amazon region indicate that illegal gold mining has had a sharp increase in the past years due to incentives from the federal government, mainly due to Bill 191/2020 presented by President Jair Bolsonaro to Parliament. The situation becomes even more serious because this increase is largely concentrated in indigenous areas, mainly affecting the Yanomami and Munduruku traditional territories [20,25].

The mercury used in *garimpos* is converted into methylmercury (MeHg), the most dangerous mercurial form to human health. Methylmercury undergoes bioaccumulation and biomagnification through aquatic trophic chains and, consequently, the consumption of contaminated fish and other organisms (e.g., crabs, shrimp, turtle, etc.) provides the main route of human exposure to this persistent environmental contaminant [27]. Ingested methylmercury is rapidly absorbed by the human gastrointestinal tract, principally affecting the central nervous and cardiovascular systems [28–30]. This mercurial form is especially harmful to pregnant women because the fetal brain is more sensitive to the action of methylmercury, causing many neurodevelopment problems to occur, including mental retardation, learning delays, visual and auditory alterations, and other harmful effects [31–33].

Considering this critical situation of mercury contamination within the Amazon and the consequences of human exposure to this contaminant, the present study aimed to assess the health risks from consumption of fish by mercury-exposed Munduruku indigenous communities in the Middle-Tapajós Region, in the state of Pará, one of the areas most threatened by illegal mining in the Brazilian Amazon. Risk assessment studies are of fundamental importance to identify population groups with a higher risk of exposure to a certain contaminant and can be the basis for the development of public policies to mitigate contamination.

2. Materials and Methods

2.1. Study Area

The present study was developed in the *Sawré Muybu* Indigenous Land (also known as Pimental), where a proportion of the Munduruku indigenous people live. This indigenous land is in the municipalities of Itaituba and Trairão, in the state of Pará, Brazil. The data collection and the fish capture were carried out between 29 October and 9 November 2019, in the villages *Poxo Muybu*, *Sawré Aboy*, and *Sawré Muybu* (see Basta et al. [34] to access the map and more details).

2.2. Fish Capture

The fish samplings were conducted in the mornings (8:00 to 12:00 a.m.) for seven consecutive days. All fish catches were conducted by the indigenous Munduruku themselves using their own fishing gears (i.e., gillnets and handlines) accompanied by field researchers. Indigenous fishermen employed gillnets with different sized mesh, one of them with 25 mm between opposite knots to catch bait to handline and other gillnets with 35 and 45 mm between opposite knots aiming to catch their target fish species. All fish caught were measured to standard length (cm), weighed (g), and the popular names recorded by researchers. Each fish specimen caught was identified to a species level in the field with further analyses in the laboratory, and the trophic level was recorded based on Santos et al. [35,36]. After the measurement and identification of the fish species, samples of 2 to 5 g of dorsal muscle tissue without skin or scales were collected from each specimen and stored in liquid nitrogen.

2.3. Mercury Analysis

The total mercury (THg) determined in the fish muscle tissue was obtained using the methodology proposed by Akagi et al. [37]. For each sample, 0.3 to 0.5 g of muscle tissue was weighed (wet weight) in a 50 mL Pyrex® volumetric flask (Corelle Brands, Charleroi, Belgium). Then, 1 mL of deionized water, 2 mL of HNO_3 and $HClO_4$ (1:1), and 5 mL of H_2SO_4 were added for digestion. The vials were exposed to a hot plate (200 to 230 °C) for 30 min. After cooling to room temperature, the flasks were measured with deionized water and the digested samples were homogenized. The THg determination was made by cold vapor atomic absorption system (CVAAS), using semi-automatic mercury analyzer equipment Analyzer Model Hg-201 (Sanso Seisakusho Co. Ltd., Tokyo, Japan) [38]. To guarantee the Quality Assurance (QA)/ Quality Control (QC), we used for the mercury analysis in fish samples the following parameters: (i) reference materials dogfish liver certified reference material for trace metals (DOLT-4) (% of recovery: 92.24 ± 7.73; 70.92 to 100) and fish protein certified reference material for trace metals (DORM-3) (% of recovery: 96.22 ± 4.69; 87.16 to 100) from the National Research Council of Canada; (ii) a method blank; (iii) a 6-point calibration curve; and (iv) the relative standard deviation (RSD) of 8.32%. The detection and quantification limits (LOD/LOQ) obtained were 0.0083 ng/mg and 0.027 ng/mg, respectively.

Based on chemical analysis results, the mercury potential for biomagnification (between different trophic levels) and bioaccumulation (between different fish sizes of the same trophic level) was evaluated. The mercury biomagnification between four trophic levels sampled (i.e., piscivorous, omnivorous, herbivorous, and detritivorous) was checked by Kruskal–Wallis tests (residuals were not normal and variance non-homogeneous), with a post-hoc Dunn test. Bioaccumulation was analyzed using linear regression between THg levels and different fish sizes (standard length in cm) inside each trophic level. The linear regression was run due to expected relation of cause–effect between fish size and THg level. The residuals of regressions were checked, and one outlier, an individual of Piranha-preta (*Serrasalmus rhombeus*), was excluded from the analysis to ensure normality of the data and homogeneity of variances.

2.4. Data Collection: Participants' Weight, Family Composition and Fish Consumption

To perform the health risk assessment related to consumption of mercury-contaminated fish, it was necessary to collect data about participants' average weight (i.e., women, men, and children), fish consumption by Munduruku indigenous families (i.e., most consumed species and frequency), and family composition (i.e., number of individuals, age, and gender). The access to the amount of fish consumed (in grams) by the family members is described in the next section.

Data about diet were obtained through interviews with the head of households (husband/father), followed by weight measurements of all individuals living in the three investigated villages. The interview answers were recorded on electronic forms with the aid of portable devices (i.e., tablets). To measure weight, a portable digital scale from Seca® (model 877) (Seca GmbH, Hamburg, Germany) was used, with a maximum capacity of 150 kg and precision of 0.1 kg.

2.5. Potential Fish Consumption Estimative from Catch Effort

The average amount of fish captured in one fishing day by the Munduruku indigenous was used to estimate the fish consumption by a family.

For the calculation of the family members' fish consumption, we assumed as a premise that the effort of the Munduruku fishermen to catch fish during this fieldwork was similar to the fishing effort usually devoted by the heads of households. Due to this assumption, the average quantity of fish obtained could be a proxy for the quantity of fish available at home to feed a family for a week.

Taking into consideration that the amount of fish consumed varies according to the gender and age of the family member, we assumed that adult men consume 45% of the fish captured, adult women consume 35%, children aged 5 to 12 years consume 15%, while children from 2 to 5 years old consume only 5%.

2.6. Health Risk Assessment

The health risk assessment was carried out according to the methodology proposed by World Health Organization (WHO) [39]. We made two assumptions to calculate the daily mercury intake: (i) 100% of the mercury detected in the fish sample is in the form of methylmercury; (ii) 100% of the methylmercury available in the fish muscle tissue is absorbed in the human's gastrointestinal tract. The amount of mercury ingested was estimated from the equation:

$$MI = \frac{FI \times MC}{KBW} \qquad (1)$$

where MI is methylmercury intake per kilogram body weight per day (µg methylmercury per kg body weight per day); FI is amount of fish ingested per day (g/day); MC is mercury concentration in the fish ingested (µg/g); KBW is kilogram body weight (kg bw).

We created different scenarios of methylmercury exposure from the data collected: (1) Rainy Season, (2) Dry Season, (3) Current, and (4) Critical. Scenarios 1 and 2 were constructed from the average mercury levels detected in fish species most consumed by the indigenous in the different seasons of the year, based on interview data. Scenario 3 was constructed from the weighted average of medium mercury concentrations detected in piscivorous and non-piscivorous species. The percentages of piscivorous and non-piscivorous species caught by the fishermen (34% and 66%, respectively) were multiplied by the average mercury levels detected. Scenario 4 was constructed from the 95th percentile of mercury concentrations in piscivorous and non-piscivorous species (1.42 and 0.29 µg/g, respectively). The 95th percentile was multiplied by the occurrence of the fish species, similarly to the previous scenario.

The risk ratio was calculated from the ratio between "the methylmercury estimated intake" and the reference doses proposed by U.S. EPA (United States Environmental Protection Agency) [40] and by FAO (Food and Agriculture Organization)/WHO [41]. According to U.S. EPA, the safe daily intake, also known as Reference Dose (RfD), is equal to 0.1 µg Hg/Kg bw/day. With the same purpose, FAO/WHO limits of 0.23 µg Hg/Kg bw/day for childbearing age women and for children and 0.45 µg Hg/Kg bw/day for adults in general.

When the risk ratio is less than 1, the risk of exposure is below the reference levels and, consequently, the risk of becoming ill is low. On the other hand, when the risk ratio is equal to or greater than 1, the risk of becoming ill due to mercury exposure must be considered. Therefore, the higher the risk ratio, the greater the risk of becoming ill due to mercury exposure.

3. Results

3.1. Fish Catch and Mercury Contamination

In total, 88 fish specimens were captured, distributed across 17 species and four trophic levels, as described in Table 1 showing the general characterization of the fish caught by the Munduruku fishermen during the fieldwork. Three piscivorous species showed average mercury levels above 0.5 µg/g. The biomagnification in the trophic chain of fish was confirmed, as there was a significant difference in the concentration of total mercury in muscle tissues among trophic levels ($H = 60.2$; $df = 3$; $p < 0.0001$) (Figure 1a). The average mercury levels in samples of non-piscivorous fish ($n = 57$) was 0.10 µg/g (SD = 0.09) and the average for piscivorous fish ($n = 31$) was 0.44 µg/g (SD = 0.34). In addition, bioaccumulation was found only in piscivorous species, where there was a positive and significant relationship between the size of the fish and the THg concentration in the muscle tissues ($y = -0.041 + 0.0151X$; $R^2 = 0.36$; $F = 15.4$; $df = 27$; $p = 0.0005$) (Figure 1b). On the other hand, among other analyzed trophic levels (i.e., omnivorous, detritivorous, and herbivorous), there was no significant relationship between size and concentration of mercury ($p > 0.05$).

3.2. Weight Measurement, Family Composition and Fish Consumption

During the fieldwork, our team visited 35 domiciles: 20 in the *Sawré Muybu* village, 8 in the *Poxo Muybu* village, and 7 in the *Sawré Aboy* village. Among the participants, 53 were women of childbearing age (12 to 49 years old), 58 were adult men ($\geq$12 years old), 24 were children aged 5 to 12 years old, and 42 were children aged 2 to 5 years. The interviews revealed that families are composed on average of 4 members (i.e., two adults and two children). According to the data collected in the fieldwork, the women of childbearing age had an average weight of 49.89 kg, adult men were 56.45 kg, children over 5 years old were 24.45 kg, and children under 5 years old were 14.07 kg (Table 2).

Table 1. Characterization of the species of fish caught, Sawré Muybu Indigenous Land, Pará, Amazon, Brazil, 2019.

Fish Species	Popular Name	N	Size (cm)	Weight (g)	Trophic Level	Hg (µg/g) (SD)	Min-Max (Hg)
Serrasalmus rhombeus	Piranha Preta	6	17–34.5	140–1305	Piscivorous	0.71 (±0.61)	0.33–1.95
Pseudoplatystoma fasciatum	Surubim	6	23.8–45	141–907	Piscivorous	0.24 (±0.15)	0.13–0.45
Pinirampus pirinampu	Barbado	8	17.3–42	109–961	Piscivorous	0.49 (±0.14)	0.31–0.75
Cichla ocellaris	Tucunaré	6	25–29	347–571	Piscivorous	0.33 (±0.06)	0.22–0.41
Rhaphiodon vulpinus	Peixe Cachorro	2	39–41	328–469	Piscivorous	0.66 (±0.48)	0.32–1.00
Ageneiosus inermis	Mandubé	1	33	550	Piscivorous	0.6	-
Pachyurus junki	Corvina	1	20.5	148	Piscivorous	0.14	-
Geophagus proximus	Caratinga	10	10.5–18.5	36–171	Omnivorous	0.07 (±0.03)	0.03–0.10
Pimelodus blochii	Mandii	7	14.5–17.3	60–84	Omnivorous	0.20 (±0.05)	0.13–0.28
Leporinus fasciatus	Aracu Flamengo	5	17.7–23.3	102–244	Omnivorous	0.09 (±0.02)	0.05–0.11
Caenotropus labyrinthicus	João Duro	6	13.7–14.8	63–73	Omnivorous	0.28 (±0.07)	0.17–0.39
Hemiodus unimaculatus	Charuto	1	17.5	95	Omnivorous	0.02	-
Schizodon vittatus	Aracu	4	21.3–27.3	163–351	Herbivorous	0.03 (±0.01)	0.02–0.04
Myloplus rubripinnis	Pacu Branco	7	12.5–20.5	89–390	Herbivorous	0.02 (±0.03)	0.01–0.07
Semaprochilodus insignis	Jaraqui Escama Grossa	6	21–23.5	223–329	Detritivorous	0.11 (±0.05)	0.05–0.16
Prochilodus nigricans	Curimatá	6	20.5–24	253–369	Detritivorous	0.07 (±0.02)	0.04–0.10
Curimata sp.	Branquinha	6	12.7–14	64–85	Detritivorous	0.09 (±0.03)	0.06–0.13

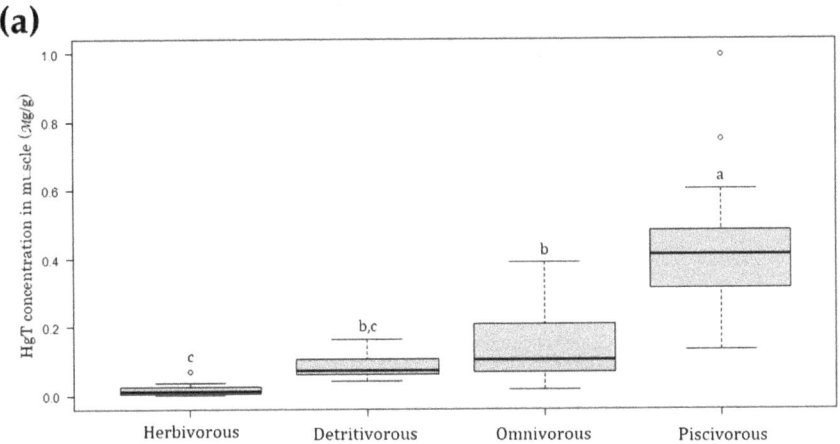

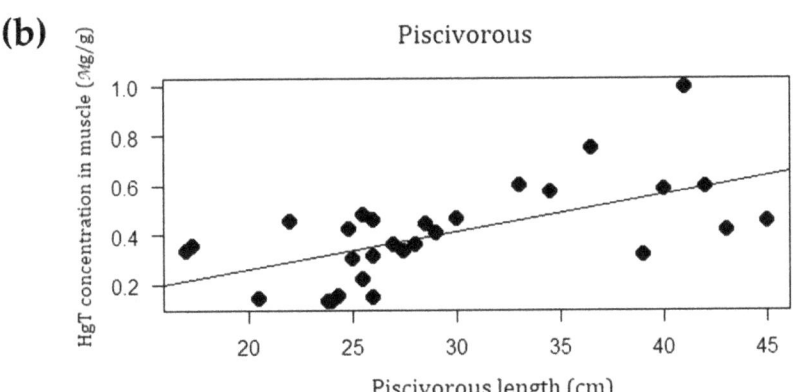

Figure 1. (a) Concentrations of mercury total (µg/g) in the muscle tissue of fish sampled (n = 88) compared among different trophic levels. Median (darker line in the box plot), minimum and maximum values (vertical lines), and outer lines of boxplot (25% and 75%). Dunn test: a > b > c, $p < 0.05$. Circles are outliers. (b) Linear regression between standard length (cm) of piscivorous fish (n = 29) and the concentration of mercury total (µg/g) in the muscle tissue of fish ($y = -0.041 + 0.0151X$; $R^2 = 0.36$; $F = 15.4$; df = 27; $p = 0.0005$). One individual of Piranha-preta (*Serrasalmus rhombeus*) was excluded from the analysis to maintain normality and homogeneity of variances.

Table 2. Data collected and estimates, *Sawré Muybu* Indigenous Land, Pará, Amazon, Brazil, 2019.

Fish Catch		
Total fish caught ($n°$)		88
Catch period (days)		7
Fish caught per day ($n°$)		12.6
Average weight of fish (grams)		268.2
Amount of fish per family (grams)		3371.7
Family composition and weight measurements (Kg)		
Average number of individuals per family		4
Average number of adults		2
Average number of children		2
Average weight of childbearing age women ($n = 53$)		49.89
Average weight of adult men (≥ 12 years) ($n = 58$)		56.45
Average weight of children (from 5│−12 years old) ($n = 24$)		24.45
Average weight of children (2│−5 years) ($n = 42$)		14.07
Fish consumption estimative (grams)		
	Weekly Intake	Daily Intake
Adult men (45%)	1517.2	216.75
Childbearing age women (35%)	1180.1	168.58
Children 5│−12 years old (15%)	505.7	72.25
Children aged 2│−5 years (5%)	168.6	24.08

The questions about fish consumption revealed that 96% of the families consume fish regularly (≥ 3 times a week) and the most consumed species varied according to the season. During the rainy season, the most consumed species, in order of frequency related, are *surubim* (*Pseudoplatystoma* spp.), *barbado* (*Pinirampus pirinampu*), *aracu* (family Anostomidae), *tucunaré* (*Cichla* spp.), and *caratinga* (*Geophagus* spp.). The species most consumed in the dry season are *caratinga*, *curimatá* (*Prochilodus nigricans*), *surubim*, *pacu* (family Serrasalmidae), and *barbado*.

The average daily fish consumption estimates for the studied groups were the following: adult men consume 216.75 g (corresponding to 45% of the fish available for consumption), childbearing age women consume 168.58 g (35%), children over 5 years consume 72.25 g (15%), and children under 5 years consume 24.08 g (5%) (Table 2).

3.3. Health Risk Assessment

The analysis of the estimates reveals that the daily intake of methylmercury exceeds the reference limits recommended by the U.S. EPA [40] and FAO/WHO [41] in all scenarios built and in all studied population strata (Table 3). It means that in all hypothetical situations created in this study, the risk ratio estimates have values greater than 1.0. In summary, the Munduruku indigenous people living in the Middle-Tapajos River are at high risk of illness by the ingestion of mercury-contaminated fish. We can say that the less alarming risk ratio estimates (between 1.0 to 2.0) were observed in the population stratum represented by children aged 2 to 5 years, and by adults in general. Considering the safe dose proposed by FAO/WHO, risk ratio estimates under 2.0 were observed in children under 5 years old and adults in all hypothetical situations, except for the critical scenario. The risk ratio estimate for the critical scenario was 5.0 and 5.75 in children and adults, respectively (Table 3).

Table 3. Estimated of methylmercury intake dose and risk ratio in different scenarios, *Sawré Muybu* Indigenous Land, Pará, Amazon, Brazil, 2019.

Scenarios Constructed	Hg-intake Dose µg/kg bw/day	Risk Ratio		
		U.S. EPA	FAO/WHO (Women and Children)	FAO/WHO (Adults in General)
Scenario 1—Rainy Season				
Women of childbearing age	0.78	7.84	3.41	N.A.
Adult Men	0.89	8.91	N.A.	1.98
Children 5|–12 years old	0.69	6.86	2.98	N.A.
Children 2|–5 years	0.40	3.97	1.73	N.A.
Scenario 2—Dry Season				
Women of childbearing age	0.59	5.95	2.59	N.A.
Adult Men	0.68	6.76	N.A.	1.50
Children 5|–12 years old	0.52	5.20	2.26	N.A.
Children 2|–5 years	0.30	3.01	1.31	N.A.
Scenario 3—Current				
Women of childbearing age	0.73	7.29	3.17	N.A.
Adult Men	0.83	8.28	N.A.	1.84
Children 5|–12 years old	0.64	6.37	2.77	N.A.
Children 2|–5 years	0.37	3.69	1.60	N.A.
Scenario 4—Critical				
Women of childbearing age	2.28	22.76	9.90	N.A.
Adult Men	2.59	25.86	N.A.	5.75
Children 5|–12 years old	1.99	19.90	8.65	N.A.
Children 2|–5 years	1.15	11.53	5.01	N.A.

U.S. EPA = United States Environmental Protection Agency; FAO = Food and Agriculture Organization; WHO = World Health Organization.

In our opinion, the current scenario is the closest to the reality of fish consumption by the Munduruku indigenous villages, and it indicates that all population segments ingest mercury in quantities above what is considered acceptable or safe. According to the U.S. EPA, women of childbearing age, who represent the most vulnerable demographic group to the effects of methylmercury, ingest 7 times more mercury than the reference dose proposed by this agency. According to FAO/WHO, the ingestion is 3 times higher than the safe intake. The critical scenario represents the levels of exposure observed in approximately 5% of the Munduruku population. In this case, women of childbearing age ingest 10 times more mercury than the limit proposed by the FAO/WHO, and 23 times more mercury than the safe limit proposed by the U.S. EPA. The analysis of the mercury levels in hair of the Munduruku population revealed that, in fact, there are individuals which presented mercury levels above 20 µg/g (more details in Basta et al. [34]).

4. Discussion

Fish are not only an essential source of protein, but many species are also rich in polyunsaturated fatty acids that reduce cholesterol levels in the blood, reduce the risk of myocardial infarction, and promote cognitive development [42,43]. Some authors point out that the annual average consumption of fish is 23 kg per capita in the Brazilian Amazon [44]. Frequently, the fish intake of riverside communities exceeds 300 g per day, resulting in annual average consumption that could surpass 100 kg per capita [10,45,46].

Despite the undeniable nutritional potential of fish, contaminants such as methylmercury has provoked significant debate about the balance between risks and benefits associated with fish consumption. Hu et al. [47] in a meta-analysis suggest that hair mercury concentration of 2–3 µg/g might be considered as a threshold for risk of developing hypertension. Fillion et al. [30] investigated riverine communities in the Amazon and showed an odds ratio equal to 2.91 (CI 95% 1.26–7.28) for elevated systolic blood pressure among individuals with hair Hg levels above 10 µg/g. In addition to these studies, Salonen et al. [29], in a longitudinal study with Finnish men, concluded that hair mercury levels above 2.0 µg/g represent a risk 69% higher for an acute myocardial infarction. Besides that, the neurotoxic effects of methylmercury have been known for a long time, since the Minamata tragedy in the 1950s and 1960s. The cohort studies conducted in the Faroe Islands and New Zealand indicate that even in low doses, the consumption of mercury-contaminated fish during pregnancy can cause important cognitive alterations in children [48,49]. The mercury neurotoxic potential effects in children and adults of the Amazon have been reported in recent publications [50–54]. The most common effects in children are cognitive problems, neurodevelopmental impairment, and psychomotor disorders. In adults, decreased visual field, neurobehavioral, and motor coordination disorders are most frequently reported [27].

Given the current federal government's effort to create strategies to facilitate the invasion of protected areas in the Amazon by *garimpeiros* and mining industries, it is essential to clarify that the contamination of fish by mercury and all related health damages are caused (or intensified) by exploitation of gold. Many studies have already shown mercury contamination in the fauna of the Tapajós River Basin at least two decades ago [55–65]. Dórea et al. [59] detected mean mercury levels in piscivorous fish of 0.578 µg/g and 0.052 µg/g Hg in non-piscivorous in the upper Tapajós basin, whilst Brabo et al. [56] investigated fish contamination in the Sai Cinza region, also inhabited by indigenous Munduruku. They observed that the piscivorous species had mean mercury levels of 0.293 µg/g, while the non-piscivorous species had average mercury levels equal to 0.112 µg/g. These studies corroborate the present results that the mean mercury levels detected in piscivorous species are about 4 times greater than non-piscivorous species, highlighting the methylmercury biomagnification. Indeed, piscivorous fish were the only trophic level where we found a positive relationship between fish size and total Hg concentration, indicating bioaccumulation. Therefore, the larger the size of piscivorous fish, the higher the mercury concentration in their tissues and thus the higher the health risk for people who eat the larger ones.

In Brazil, the National Health Surveillance Agency (ANVISA) establishes the maximum concentrations of mercury in fish tissues that are judged appropriate for commercialization. Resolution No. 42 establishes that the maximum limit for inorganic mercury in fish is 0.5 µg/g for non-predatory species and 1.0 µg/g for predatory species [66]. Reflection on the applicability of these concentration limits promotes questions. The first question is, why propose limits for inorganic-mercury species, when almost all mercury present in the fish muscle is methylmercury, an organic mercury form? The second question is, how effective is the use of mercury concentration limits in fish in protecting the health of the population that consumes this fish?

We believe that the National Health Surveillance Agency (ANVISA) resolution does not promote any regulatory or normative effects, since the limits proposed by this agency are basically a wrong adaptation of the limits recommended by FAO/WHO [67] (0.5 µg MeHg/g for non-piscivorous fish and 1.0 µg MeHg/g for piscivorous fish). Furthermore, it is vital to clarify that these limits established by the FAO/WHO were adopted in 1991 and do not consider health effects produced by the ingestion of methylmercury in the fish [67]. The calculations for defining these maximum limits were performed based on data of the average mercury levels in fish samples of different trophic levels. Unfortunately, these values are frequently cited as safe levels for consumption.

The people's diet is an extremely important cultural characteristic, as well as language and spiritualistic rituals. In indigenous communities, the inclusion of fish and other aquatic organisms as a diet items and the consumption frequency vary considerably among the groups living in the Amazon. The consumption of these items depends not only on the availability in the environment but also on the individual's preferences as well as cultural patterns. For example, the Yanomami people who live in the Auaris region in the extreme northwest of Roraima state, as well as the Yanomami living in Venezuela, rarely eat fish [68,69]. On the other hand, fish consumption among Munduruku indigenous people can be considered high (at least three meals per day), varying slightly between different groups [56,58,59]. Studies that focus on the characterization of indigenous people's diet face numerous difficulties, ranging from cultural and linguistic barriers to the choice of an effective method for quantifying the consumption of certain foods. Memory-based methods (recall method) about what was consumed by the family in the past 24 h or in the past few days generally produce over or underestimated data that rarely translate into reality and cause errors in estimates. Taking into consideration all the aspects exposed previously, it is extremely hard to measure during a study's fieldwork the quantity in grams of fish consumed by each person in a day and the number of daily meals that include fish (and other aquatic organisms such as fish, crabs, mollusks, shrimp, turtles, etc.). From this point of view, the present study proposed a methodology for estimating potential fish consumption based on the catching of fish by indigenous themselves and then recorded by field researchers. The time devoted to fishing and the catching strategies were defined based on the reports of Munduruku fishermen.

With this challenge to estimate the food intake in culturally differentiated communities in mind, the goal of this study was to simulate an ordinary fishing day for the head of a Munduruku household. Thus, the mean amount of fish caught on a typical fishing day represents the amount of fish that a Munduruku family consumes over a week. Since there is no electricity in the homes visited, neither a refrigerator nor any other way of preserving food, the "moquém" technique (which is a type of smoking) is used to conserve fish.

To assess the accuracy of the empirical methodology accomplished in this investigation for estimating fish consumption, the daily mercury intake doses calculated for the current scenario were compared to the mercury levels detected in hair samples of the Munduruku indigenous people in the studied communities (data available in Basta et al. [34]). The current scenario was built to represent the mercury exposure scenario that most closely matches the local reality. The estimated mercury daily intake in this scenario for adult men and women was 0.828 and 0.729 µg/bw kg, respectively. The mean mercury level in male hair was 8.83 µg/g (SD: 4.56) and in women of childbearing age, the mean hair mercury level was 7.71 µg/g (SD: 3.88). If we consider that the intake of 0.1 µg/bw kg/day corresponds to hair mercury levels of 1.0 µg/g [39], the calculation of the amount of mercury intake daily is well-matched with the mercurial concentration detected in hair samples. Children from 5 to 12 years old also had a mercury daily intake dose matching with the levels of mercury in hair. The intake dose was estimated at 0.64 µg/bw kg/day and the average level of mercury in hair was 7.62 µg/g (SD: 5.44). Only the population stratum constituted by children aged 2 to 5 years did not indicate compatibility between intake and concentration in hair. In this case, the daily intake was estimated at 0.37 µg/bw kg/day and the average concentration in hair was 6.68 µg/g (SD: 3.44). Most likely, the difference found may be due to the influence of other routes of exposure, besides to fish consumption, such as breastfeeding and remnants of intrauterine transfer. However, there is a possibility that fish consumption was underestimated by our team for this age group.

The risk ratio estimated in this study indicates that there is no safe consumption of fish by the Munduruku population in any of the scenarios created for counterfactual analysis. Comparing the mercury intake doses in the different scenarios, we observed that mercury ingestion during the rainy season is higher than in the dry season. This result reflects the mercury levels detected in the most consumed fish species in this season of the year, according to reports by the study participants. In the rainy season, according to the interview reports, 60% of fish most consumed by the Munduruku families are piscivorous and therefore have higher levels of mercury.

According to the safety parameters proposed by FAO/WHO [41] and U.S. EPA [40], the entire study population is at risk of becoming ill due to the consumption of methylmercury contaminated fish. It is important to remember that the safe intake doses proposed by these international agencies were calculated from data produced in longitudinal studies. The dose of FAO/WHO [41] (PTWI: 1.6 µg MeHg/Kg bw/week) was derived from data produced in Seychelles, Faroe Islands, and New Zealand cohort studies. The dose recommended by U.S. EPA [40] was based only on the findings of the Faroe Islands cohort. However, the longitudinal studies mentioned above considered populations that differ strongly from the Amazonian populations and, probably, present mercury exposure thresholds for toxic health outcomes quite different from the indigenous communities.

The native people of the Brazilian Amazon are neglected by the State, which often becomes evident from the difficulty in accessing health services, the lack of sewage sanitation, and the high prevalence of many infectious diseases and child stunting. Besides this, the Amazonian ecosystem sees several risk factors for human exposure to mercury alongside each other which combine to create a uniquely dangerous situation. These factors include the presence of natural mercury in the soil as well as the development of activities that significantly change the mercury biogeochemical cycle in the region (e.g., artisanal gold mining, industrial gold mining, construction of dams and hydroelectric plants and agribusiness, which promotes forest burning and deforestation). This becomes evident that the development of a longitudinal study involving different population groups in the Amazon, such as indigenous, riverine, and urban populations, is especially important. Only after a long-term study will it be possible to estimate safe doses of mercury intake for the Amazonian population.

5. Conclusions

The current gold mining activity in the Middle-Tapajós Region is causing environmental devastation, social conflict, and increasing mercury levels in the environment. This activity causes mercury accumulation in fish, especially in piscivorous. Consequently, the population living in this region consumes contaminated fish and compromises their health. The present study revealed that the fish collected in the rivers that cross the *Sawré Muybu* Indigenous Land have mercury concentrations with the potential to harm the health of the Munduruku population, particularly women of childbearing age and children. In all of the scenarios created for counterfactual analysis, the estimated risk ratios are greater than 1.0, indicating that the intake of mercury by the groups studied is higher than the limits proposed by health agencies. However, we highlight that fish is an important element of Munduruku culture and is an essential animal protein for riverside and indigenous populations across the Amazon. The mercury contamination observed in fish and the indigenous Munduruku is a direct consequence of gold mining and the Brazilian authorities' longstanding refusal to condemn this activity, threatening the health and rights of the native peoples. Therefore, we refute the current policies of the Brazilian federal government regarding the permission of mining in Indigenous Land. In conclusion, we recommend the immediate closure of illegal gold mining in the Brazilian Amazon, the principal cause of mercury contamination in the region.

Author Contributions: Proposal design, study design, and methodology, A.C.S.V., G.H. and P.C.B.; Fieldwork data collection, A.C.S.V., J.G.B., A.N.S.A. and P.C.B.; Laboratory analysis, J.G.B., A.N.S.A., H.N.M.M., G.H., I.M.J. and M.O.L.; Writing—original draft preparation, A.C.S.V., G.H. and P.C.B.; Writing—review and editing, A.C.S.V., G.H., P.C.B. and S.S.H.; Supervision, obtaining resources, and project management, P.C.B. and S.S.H. All authors have read and agreed to the published version of the manuscript.

Funding: This research received no external funding.

Institutional Review Board Statement: The study was conducted in accordance with the guidelines of the Declaration of Helsinki and was approved by the Research Ethics Committee of the National School of Public Health at Oswaldo Cruz Foundation (REC/ENSP) and the Brazilian National Research Ethics Commission of the National Health Council (CONEP/CNS), CAAE: 65671517.1.0000.5240, with Opinion No. 2.262.686 favorable to its performance. In compliance with Convention No. 169 of the International Labor Organization (ILO), the study began with a pre-study consultation, carried out in August 2019, during a visit to the villages, in which two authors (S.S.H. and P.C.B.) and local indigenous leaders participated. At the time, the study objectives were presented and discussed (https://www.youtube.com/watch?v=oFEYEGxNmns&t=704s accessed on 3 March 2021). After answering questions and obtaining approval for the proposal by the communities, we received support from the coordination of the Special Indigenous Sanitary District of the Tapajós River through the multidisciplinary indigenous health team to carry out the study. In addition, the interviews and data collection started only after the participants had their questions answered and given formal consent in the Informed Consent Form (ICF) by the children's guardians.

Informed Consent Statement: Informed consent was obtained from all subjects involved in the study. Written informed consent has been obtained from the patients to publish this paper.

Data Availability Statement: Data sharing not applicable.

Acknowledgments: Through chiefs Juarez Saw, Jairo Saw, and Valdemar Poxo, and the leader Alessandra Korap, we thank the Munduruku people for the trust placed in our team and the support in carrying out the research. On behalf of Cleidiane Carvalho Ribeiro dos Santos we thank the team from the Rio Tapajós Indigenous Special Sanitary District, who spared no efforts to support us in all stages of the fieldwork. In particular, we thank nurses Alan Marcelo Simon and Lygia Catarina de Oliveira. We thank João Paulo Goes Pereira for mercury analysis in the fish samples. We also thank Marcelo Oliveira-Costa from the WWF-Brasil for financial and technical support.

Conflicts of Interest: The authors declare no conflict of interest. The funders had no role in the design of the study; in the collection, analyses, or interpretation of data; in the writing of the manuscript, or in the decision to publish the results.

References

1. FAO. *The State of World Fisheries and Aquaculture*; FAO: Rome, Italy, 2020; ISBN 978-92-5-132692-3.
2. Kawarazuka, N.; Béné, C. Linking small-scale fisheries and aquaculture to household nutritional security: A review of the literature. *Food Secur.* **2010**, *2*, 343–357. [CrossRef]
3. Hicks, C.C.; Cohen, P.J.; Graham, N.A.J.; Nash, K.L.; Allison, E.H.; D'Lima, C.; Mills, D.J.; Roscher, M.; Thilsted, S.H.; Thorne-Lyman, A.L.; et al. Harnessing global fisheries to tackle micronutrient deficiencies. *Nature* **2019**, *566*, 378–382. [CrossRef]
4. Funge-Smith, S.; Bennett, A.A. Fresh look at inland fisheries and their role in food security and livelihoods. *Fish Fish.* **2019**, *20*, 1176–1195. [CrossRef]
5. Fluet-Chouinard, E.; Funge-Smith, S.; McIntyre, P.B. Global hidden harvest of freshwater fish revealed by household surveys. *Proc. Natl. Acad. Sci. USA* **2018**, *115*, 7623–7628. [CrossRef] [PubMed]

6. Béné, C.; Steel, E.; Kambala, L.B.; Gordon, A. Fish as the "bank in the water": Evidence from chronic-poor communities in Congo. *Food Policy* **2009**, *34*, 108–118. [CrossRef]
7. McIntyre, P.B.; Liermann, C.A.R.; Revenga, C. Linking freshwater fishery management to global good security and biodiversity conservation. *Proc. Natl. Acad. Sci. USA* **2016**, *113*, 12880–12885. [CrossRef] [PubMed]
8. Welcomme, R.L. *River Fisheries*; FAO: Rome, Italy, 1985; ISBN 978-92-5-102299-3.
9. Jézéquel, C.; Tedesco, P.A.; Bigorne, R.; Maldonado-Ocampo, J.A.; Ortega, H.; Hidalgo, M.; Martens, K.; Torrente-Vilara, G.; Zuanon, J.; Acosta, A.; et al. A Database of freshwater fish species of the Amazon basin. *Sci. Data* **2020**, *7*, 96. [CrossRef] [PubMed]
10. Isaac, V.J.; Almeida, M.C. *El Consumo de Pescado en la Amazonía Brasileña*; FAO: Rome, Italy, 2011; ISBN 978-92-5-307029-9.
11. Isaac, V.J.; Almeida, M.C.; Giarrizzo, T.; Deus, C.P.; Vale, R.; Klein, G.; Begossi, A. Food consumption as an indicator of the conservation of natural resources in riverine communities of the Brazilian Amazon. *An. Acad. Bras. Ciências* **2015**, *87*, 2229–2242. [CrossRef] [PubMed]
12. Begossi, A.; Salivonchyk, S.; Hallwass, G.; Hanazaki, N.; Lopes, P.; Silvano, R.A.M.; Dumaresq, D.; Pittock, J. Fish consumption on the Amazon: A review of biodiversity, hydropower and food security issues. *Braz. J. Biol.* **2019**, *79*, 345–357. [CrossRef] [PubMed]
13. Prestes-Carneiro, G.; Béarez, P.; Bailon, S.; Py-Daniel, A.R.; Neves, E.G. Subsistence fishery at Hatahara (750-1230 CE), a pre-Columbian central Amazonian village. *J. Archaeol. Sci. Rep.* **2015**, *8*, 454–462. [CrossRef]
14. Prestes-Carneiro, G.; Béarez, P.; Shock, M.P.; Prümers, H.; Betancourt, C.J. Pre-Hispanic fishing practices in interfluvial Amazonia: Zooarchaeological evidence from managed landscapes on the Llanos de Mojos savanna. *PLoS ONE* **2019**, *14*, e0214638. [CrossRef]
15. Fearnside, P.M. Social impacts of Brazil's Tucuruí Dam. *Environ. Manag.* **1999**, *24*, 483–495. [CrossRef]
16. Nevado, J.B.; Martín-Doimeadios, R.R.; Bernardo, F.G.; Moreno, M.J.; Herculano, A.M.; Do Nascimento, J.L.M.; Crespo-López, M.E. Mercury in the Tapajós River basin, Brazilian Amazon: A review. *Environ. Int.* **2010**, *36*, 593–608. [CrossRef]
17. Hallwass, G.; Lopes, P.F.; Juras, A.A.; Silvano, R.A.M. Fishers' knowledge identifies environmental changes and fish abundance trends in impounded tropical rivers. *Ecol. Appl.* **2013**, *23*, 392–407. [CrossRef] [PubMed]
18. Arrifano, G.P.; Martín-Doimeadios, R.C.R.; Jiménez-Moreno, M.; Ramírez-Mateos, V.; Da Silva, N.F.; Souza-Monteiro, J.R.; Augusto-Oliveira, M.; Paraense, R.S.O.; Macchid, B.M.; Nascimento, J.L.M.; et al. Large-scale projects in the amazon and human exposure to mercury: The case-study of the Tucuruí Dam. *Ecotoxicol. Environ. Saf.* **2018**, *147*, 299–305. [CrossRef] [PubMed]
19. RAISG. 2018. Available online: https://www.amazoniasocioambiental.org/pt-br/radar/mapa-inedito-indica-epidemia-de-garimpo-ilegal-na-panamazonia/ (accessed on 3 March 2021).
20. Silva-Junior, C.H.L.; Pessôa, A.C.M.; Carvalho, N.S.; Reis, J.B.C.; Anderson, L.O.; Aragão, L.E.O.C. The Brazilian Amazon deforestation rate in 2020 is the greatest of the decade. *Nat. Ecol. Evol.* **2021**, *5*, 144–145. [CrossRef] [PubMed]
21. Baird, I.G.; Silvano, R.A.M.; Parlee, B.; Poesch, M.; Maclean, B.; Napoleon, A.; Lepine, M.; Hallwass, G. The downstream impacts of hydropower dams and indigenous and local knowledge: Examples from the Peace–Athabasca, Mekong, and Amazon. *Environ. Manag.* **2021**, *67*, 682–696. [CrossRef] [PubMed]
22. Ferrante, L.; Andrade, M.B.T.; Leite, L.; Silva-Junior, C.A.; Lima, M.; Coelho-Junior, M.G.; Da Silva Neto, E.C.; Campolina, D.; Carolino, K.; Diele-Viegas, L.M.; et al. Brazils Highway BR-319: The road to the collapse of the Amazon and the violation of indigenous rights. *J. Geogr. Soc. Berl.* **2021**, *152*, 65–70. [CrossRef]
23. Malm, O. Gold mining as a source of mercury exposure in the Brazilian Amazon. *Environ. Res.* **1998**, *77*, 73–78. [CrossRef] [PubMed]
24. Kalamandeen, M.; Gloor, E.; Johnson, I.; Agard, S.; Katow, M.; Vanbrooke, A.; Ashley, D.; Batterman, S.A.; Ziv, G.; Holder-Collins, K.; et al. Limited biomass recovery from gold mining in Amazonian forests. *J. Appl. Ecol.* **2020**, *57*, 1730–1740. [CrossRef]
25. Ferrante, L.; Fearnside, P.M. Brazil's new president and "ruralists" threaten Amazonia's environment, traditional peoples and the global climate. *Environ. Conserv.* **2019**, *46*, 261–263. [CrossRef]
26. Siqueira-Gay, J.; Soares-Filho, B.; Sanchez, L.E.; Oviedo, A.; Sonter, L.J. Proposed legislation to mine Brazil's indigenous lands will threaten Amazon forests and their valuable ecosystem services. *One Earth* **2020**, *3*, 356–362. [CrossRef]
27. Crespo-Lopez, M.E.; Augusto-Oliveira, M.; Lopes-Araújo, A.; Santos-Sacramento, L.; Yuki Takeda, P.; Macchi, B.M.; Do Nascimento, J.L.M.; Maia, C.S.F.; Lima, R.R.; Arrifano, G.P. Mercury: What can we learn from the Amazon? *Environ. Int.* **2021**, *146*, 106223. [CrossRef]
28. Lacerda, E.M.D.C.B.; Souza, G.D.S.; Cortes, M.I.T.; Rodrigues, A.R.; Pinheiro, M.C.N.; Silveira, L.C.D.L.; Ventura, D.F. Comparison of visual functions of two Amazonian populations: Possible consequences of different mercury exposure. *Front. Neurosci.* **2020**, *13*, 1428. [CrossRef] [PubMed]
29. Salonen, J.T.; Seppänen, K.; Nyyssönen, K.; Korpela, H.; Kauhanen, J.; Kantola, M.; Tuomilehto, J.; Esterbauer, H.; Tatzber, F.; Salonen, R. Intake of mercury from fish, lipid peroxidation, and the risk of myocardial infarction and coronary, cardiovascular, and any death in eastern Finnish men. *Circulation* **1995**, *91*, 645–655. [CrossRef] [PubMed]
30. Fillion, M.; Mergler, D.; Passos, C.J.S.; Larribe, F.; Lemire, M.; Guimarães, J.R.D. A preliminary study of mercury exposure and blood pressure in the Brazilian Amazon. *Environ. Health* **2006**, *5*, 1–9. [CrossRef]
31. Vasconcellos, A.C.S.; Barrocas, P.R.G.; Ruiz, C.M.V.; Mourão, D.D.S.; Hacon, S.D.S. Burden of Mild Mental Retardation attributed to prenatal methylmercury exposure in Amazon: Local and regional estimates. *Cienc. Saude Coletiva* **2018**, *23*, 3535–3545. [CrossRef] [PubMed]
32. Poulin, J.; Gibb, H.; Prüss-Üstün, A.; World Health Organization. *Mercury: Assessing the Environmental Burden of Disease at National and Local Levels*; World Health Organization: Geneva, Switzerland, 2008.

33. Bose-O'Reilly, S.; McCarty, K.M.; Steckling, N.; Lettmeier, B. Mercury exposure and children's health. *Curr. Probl. Pediatric Adolesc. Health Care* **2010**, *40*, 186–215. [CrossRef]
34. Basta, P.C.; Viana, P.V.S.; Vasconcellos, A.; Périssé, A.; Hofer, C.; Paiva, N.S.; Kempton, J.W.; Ciampi de Andrade, D.; Oliveira, R.A.A.; Achatz, R.W.; et al. Mercury exposure in Munduruku indigenous communities from Brazilian Amazon: Methodological background and an overview of the principal results. *Int. J. Environ. Res. Public Health* **2021**, *18*. in press.
35. Santos, G.M.; De Mérona, B.; Juras, A.A.; Jégu, M. *Peixes do Baixo Rio Tocantins: 20 Anos Depois da Usina Hidrelétrica Tucuruí*; Eletronorte: Brasília, Brasil, 2004; p. 216.
36. Santos, G.M.; Ferreira, E.J.G.; Zuanon, J.A.S. *Peixes Comerciais de Manaus*; Ibama/PróVárzea: Manaus, Brazil, 2006.
37. Akagi, H.; Suzuki, T.; Arimura, K.; Ando, T.; Sakamoto, M.; Satoh, H.; Matsuyama, A. *Mercury Analysis Manual*, 105th ed.; Ministry of the Environmental: Tokyo, Japan, 2004. Available online: http://nimd.env.go.jp/kenkyu/docs/march_mercury_analysis_manual(e).pdf (accessed on 21 November 2019).
38. da Silva, S.F.; de Oliveira Lima, M. Mercury in fish marketed in the Amazon triple frontier and health risk assessment. *Chemosphere* **2000**, *248*, 125989. [CrossRef]
39. World Health Organization. *Guidance for Identifying Populations at Risk from Mercury Exposure*; Mercury Publications: Geneva, Switzerland, 2008.
40. U.S.-EPA. *Reference Dose for Methylmercury*; U.S. Environmental Protection Agency: Washington, DC, USA, 2000.
41. FAO/WHO. Evaluation of certain food additives and contaminants: Sixty-first report of the Joint FAO/WHO Expert Committee on Food Additives. In Proceedings of the Joint FAO/WHO Expert Committee on Food Additives (JECFA), Rome, Italy, 10–19 June 2003.
42. Domingo, J.L. Omega-3 fatty acids and the benefits of fish consumption: Is all that glitters gold? *Environ. Int.* **2007**, *33*, 993–998. [CrossRef]
43. Sidhu, K.S. Health benefits and potential risks related to consumption of fish or fish oil. *Regul. Toxicol. Pharmacol.* **2003**, *38*, 336–344. [CrossRef] [PubMed]
44. Arruda, M.C.F. *Avaliação Dos Indicadores da Política de Pesca do Programa Zona Franca Verde: Perspectivas Econômicas e Ambientais*; Universidade Federal do Amazonas: Manaus, Brasil, 2017.
45. Cerdeira, R.G.P.; Ruffino, M.I.; Isaac, V.J. Consumo de pescado e outros alimentos pela população ribeirinha do lago grande de Monte Alegre, PA-Brasil. *Acta Amaz.* **1997**, *27*, 213–227. [CrossRef]
46. Batista, V.D.; Isaac, V.J.; Viana, J.P. *Exploração e Manejo Dos Recursos Pesqueiros da Amazônia. A Pesca e os Recursos Pesqueiros na Amazônia Brasileira*; Ibama/ProVárzea: Manaus, Brasil, 2004; pp. 63–151.
47. Hu, X.F.; Singh, K.; Chan, H.M. Mercury exposure, blood pressure, and hypertension: A systematic review and dose–response meta-analysis. *Environ. Health Perspect.* **2018**, *126*, 076002. [CrossRef] [PubMed]
48. Weihe, P.; Grandjean, P.; Jørgensen, P.J. Application of hair-mercury analysis to determine the impact of a seafood advisory. *Environ. Res.* **2005**, *97*, 201–208. [CrossRef] [PubMed]
49. Crump, K.S.; Kjellström, T.; Shipp, A.M.; Silvers, A.; Stewart, A. Influence of prenatal mercury exposure upon scholastic and psychological test performance: Benchmark analysis of a New Zealand cohort. *Risk Anal.* **1998**, *18*, 701–713. [CrossRef]
50. Santos Serrão de Castro, N.; de Oliveira Lima, M. Hair as a biomarker of long-term mercury exposure in Brazilian Amazon: A systematic review. *Int. J. Environ. Res. Public Health* **2018**, *15*, 500. [CrossRef] [PubMed]
51. Reuben, A.; Frischtak, H.; Berky, A.; Ortiz, E.J.; Morales, A.M.; Hsu-Kim, H.; Pendergast, L.L.; Pan, W.K. Elevated hair mercury levels are associated with neurodevelopmental deficits in children living near artisanal and small-scale gold mining in Peru. *Geo. Health* **2020**, *4*, e2019GH000222.
52. Costa Junior, J.M.F.; Lima, A.A.D.S.; Rodrigues Junior, D.; Khoury, E.D.T.; Souza, G.D.S.; Silveira, L.C.D.L.; Pinheiro, M.D.C.N. Emotional and motor symptoms in riverside dwellers exposed to mercury in the Amazon. *Rev. Bras. De Epidemiol.* **2017**, *20*, 212–224. [CrossRef]
53. Marques, R.C.; Bernardi, J.V.; Abreu, L.; Dórea, J.G. Neurodevelopment outcomes in children exposed to organic mercury from multiple sources in a tin-ore mine environment in Brazil. *Arch. Environ. Contam. Toxicol.* **2015**, *68*, 432–441. [CrossRef] [PubMed]
54. Marques, R.C.; Bernardi, J.V.; Cunha, M.P.; Dórea, J.G. Impact of organic mercury exposure and home delivery on neurodevelopment of Amazonian children. *Int. J. Hygen Environ. Health* **2016**, *219*, 498–502. [CrossRef] [PubMed]
55. Malm, O.; Castro, M.B.; Bastos, W.R.; Branches, F.J.; Guimarães, J.R.; Zuffo, C.E.; Pfeiffer, W.C. An assessment of Hg pollution in different goldmining areas, Amazon Brazil. *Sci. Total Environ.* **1995**, *175*, 127–140. [CrossRef]
56. Brabo, E.D.S.; Santos, E.D.O.; Jesus, I.M.D.; Mascarenhas, A.F.; Faial, K.F. Mercury levels in fish consumed by the Sai Cinza indigenous community, Munduruku Reservation, Jacareacanga County, State of Para, Brazil. *Cad. Saúde Pública* **1999**, *15*, 325–332. [CrossRef]
57. Roulet, M.; Lucotte, M.; Canuel, R.; Farella, N.; Courcelles, M.; Guimaraes, J.R.; Amorim, M. Increase in mercury contamination recorded in lacustrine sediments following deforestation in the central Amazon. *Chem. Geol.* **2000**, *165*, 243–266. [CrossRef]
58. de Oliveira Santos, E.C.; de Jesus, I.M.; da Silva Brabo, E.; Loureiro, E.C.B.; da Silva Mascarenhas, A.F.; Weirich, J.; Cleary, D. Mercury exposures in riverside Amazon communities in Para, Brazil. *Environ. Res.* **2000**, *84*, 100–107. [CrossRef]
59. Dórea, J.G.; Barbosa, A.C.; Ferrari, Í.; De Souza, J.R. Fish consumption (Hair Mercury) and nutritional status of Amazonian Amer-Indian Children. *Am. J. Hum. Biol. Off. J. Hum. Biol. Assoc.* **2005**, *17*, 507–514. [CrossRef]

60. Telmer, K.; Costa, M.; Angélica, R.S.; Araujo, E.S.; Maurice, Y. The source and fate of sediment and mercury in the Tapajós River, Pará, Brazilian Amazon: Ground-and space-based evidence. *J. Environ. Manag.* **2006**, *81*, 101–113. [CrossRef]
61. Hacon, S.; Barrocas, P.R.; Vasconcellos, A.C.S.D.; Barcellos, C.; Wasserman, J.C.; Campos, R.C.; Azevedo-Carloni, F.B. An overview of mercury contamination research in the Amazon basin with an emphasis on Brazil. *Cad. Saúde Pública* **2008**, *24*, 1479–1492. [CrossRef] [PubMed]
62. Passos, C.J.S.; Da Silva, D.S.; Lemire, M.; Fillion, M.; Guimaraes, J.R.D.; Lucotte, M.; Mergler, D. Daily mercury intake in fish-eating populations in the Brazilian Amazon. *J. Expo. Sci. Environ. Epidemiol.* **2008**, *18*, 76–87. [CrossRef]
63. Faial, K.; Deus, R.; Deus, S.; Neves, R.; Jesus, I.; Santos, E.; Brasil, D. Mercury levels assessment in hair of riverside inhabitants of the Tapajós River, Pará State, Amazon, Brazil: Fish consumption as a possible route of exposure. *J. Trace Elem. Med. Biol.* **2015**, *30*, 66–76. [CrossRef]
64. Freitas, J.S.; Lacerda, E.; Maria, C.; Rodrigues, D., Jr.; Corvelo, T.C.O.; Silveira, L.C.L.; Souza, G.S. Mercury exposure of children living in Amazonian villages: Influence of geographical location where they lived during prenatal and postnatal development. *An. Acad. Bras. Ciências* **2019**, *91*. [CrossRef] [PubMed]
65. Lino, A.S.; Kasper, D.; Guida, Y.S.; Thomaz, J.R.; Malm, O. Total and methyl mercury distribution in water, sediment, plankton, and fish along the Tapajós River basin in the Brazilian Amazon. *Chemosphere* **2019**, *235*, 690–700. [CrossRef] [PubMed]
66. Brasil. Resolução RDC n°42. *Dispõe sobre o Regulamento Técnico MERCOSUL Sobre Limites Máximos de Contaminantes Inorgânicos em Alimentos*; Diário Oficial da União da República Federativa do Brasil: Brasília, Brasil, 2013.
67. FAO/WHO. Joint FAO/WHO Expert Committee on Food Additives (JECFA), Report of the Tenth Section, Rotterdam, The Netherlands 4 to 8 April 2016. Available online: http://www.fao.org/fao-who-codexalimentarius/sh-proxy/en/?lnk=1&url=https%253A%252F%252Fworkspace.fao.org%252Fsites%252Fcodex%252FMeetings%252FCX-735-10%252FReport%252FREP16_CFe.pdf (accessed on 22 June 2020).
68. Holmes, R. Non-dietary modifiers of nutritional status in tropical forest populations of Venezuela. *Interciencia* **1984**, *9*, 386–390.
69. Dufour, D.L. Diet and nutritional status of Ameridians: A review of the literature. *Cad. Saúde Pública* **1991**, *7*, 481–502. [CrossRef] [PubMed]

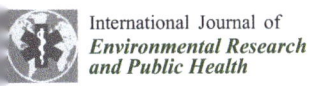

International Journal of
Environmental Research and Public Health

Article

Analyzing Spatial Patterns of Health Vulnerability to Drought in the Brazilian Semiarid Region

Júlia Alves Menezes [1,*], Ana Paula Madureira [2], Rhavena Barbosa dos Santos [1], Isabela de Brito Duval [1], Pedro Regoto [3], Carina Margonari [4], Martha Macêdo de Lima Barata [5] and Ulisses Confalonieri [1]

1. Transdisciplinary Study Group on Health and Environment René Rachou Institute–Oswaldo Cruz Foundation, Avenida Augusto de Lima, 1715, Barro Preto, 30190-009 Belo Horizonte, MG, Brazil; rhavena.santos@gmail.com (R.B.d.S.); isabelafbrito@gmail.com (I.d.B.D.); uconfalonieri@gmail.com (U.C.)
2. Department of Biosystems Engineering, The Federal University of São João del-Rei, Praça Dom Helvécio, 74, Fábricas, 36301-160 São João del-Rei, MG, Brazil; apmadureira@ufsj.edu.br
3. Postgraduate Program of Meteorology, National Institute for Space Research, Rodovia Presidente Dutra Km 39, 12630-000 Cachoeira Paulista, SP, Brazil; pedro.regoto@yahoo.com.br
4. Leishmaniasis Study Group René Rachou Institute–Oswaldo Cruz Foundation, Avenida Augusto de Lima, 1715, Barro Preto, 30190-009 Belo Horizonte, MG, Brazil; carina.souza@fiocruz.br
5. Postgraduate Program of Public Health and Environment, National School of Public Health–Oswaldo Cruz Foundation, Rua Leopoldo Bulhões, 1480, Manguinhos, 21041-210 Rio de Janeiro, RJ, Brazil; baratamml@gmail.com
* Correspondence: menezes.jalves@gmail.com

Citation: Menezes, J.A.; Madureira, A.P.; Santos, R.B.d.; Duval, I.d.B.; Regoto, P.; Margonari, C.; Barata, M.M.d.L.; Confalonieri, U. Analyzing Spatial Patterns of Health Vulnerability to Drought in the Brazilian Semiarid Region. *Int. J. Environ. Res. Public Health* **2021**, *18*, 6262. https://doi.org/10.3390/ijerph18126262

Academic Editors: Rejane C. Marques, José Garrofe Dórea and Rafael Junqueira Buralli

Received: 5 May 2021
Accepted: 25 May 2021
Published: 9 June 2021

Publisher's Note: MDPI stays neutral with regard to jurisdictional claims in published maps and institutional affiliations.

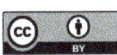

Copyright: © 2021 by the authors. Licensee MDPI, Basel, Switzerland. This article is an open access article distributed under the terms and conditions of the Creative Commons Attribution (CC BY) license (https://creativecommons.org/licenses/by/4.0/).

Abstract: Health determinants might play an important role in shaping the impacts related to long-term disasters such as droughts. Understanding their distribution in populated dry regions may help to map vulnerabilities and set coping strategies for current and future threats to human health. The aim of the study was to identify the most vulnerable municipalities of the Brazilian semiarid region when it comes to the relationship between drought, health, and their determinants using a multidimensional index. From a place-based framework, epidemiological, socio-economic, rural, and health infrastructure data were obtained for 1135 municipalities in the Brazilian semiarid region. An exploratory factor analysis was used to reduce 32 variables to four independent factors and compute a Health Vulnerability Index. The health vulnerability was modulated by social determinants, rural characteristics, and access to water in this semiarid region. There was a clear distinction between municipalities with the highest human welfare and economic development and those municipalities with the worst living conditions and health status. Spatial patterns showed a cluster of the most vulnerable municipalities in the western, eastern, and northeastern portions of the semiarid region. The spatial visualization of the associated vulnerabilities supports decision making on health promotion policies that should focus on reducing social inequality. In addition, policymakers are presented with a simple tool to identify populations or areas with the worst socioeconomic and health conditions, which can facilitate the targeting of actions and resources on a more equitable basis. Further, the results contribute to the understanding of social determinants that may be related to medium- and long-term health outcomes in the region.

Keywords: vulnerability; drought; health; social determinants; rural population; Brazil

1. Introduction

The importance of socio-economic status and other underlying living conditions of the population has been considered relevant to public health policies and the reduction of health inequalities worldwide, especially after the Commission on Social Determinants of Health established by the World Health Organization in 2005 [1–4]. This approach recognizes the interaction between social, economic, cultural, ethnic, psychological, environmental, and behavioral factors that influence the occurrence of health problems and their risk factors in the population, creating health inequities among different strata. Recently, these determinants have been analyzed from the perspective of disaster risk reduction, since they influence and overlap the different elements that make up the risk, such as vulnerability, exposure, and adaptation, affecting the outcomes related to disasters and health of the population [5–8].

As are health outcomes and their determinants, the vulnerability to natural disasters is shaped by underlying risk factors such as poverty, urbanization, gender, and, more recently, climate change. Understanding that different types of hazards produce distinctive health burdens is then central to adequately design multi-sector measures to reduce disaster risks, although this might be a difficult task of implementing in extensive events such as droughts [6]. Although droughts are not the most common type of disaster, it was responsible for the highest number of deaths worldwide between 1900 and 2019 (about 30%) and has in a changing climate an additional risk factor [9]. In fact, critical changes in precipitation and temperature are expected for places already marked by this event, even if the target of warming up to 1.5 °C to 2 °C is reached [10].

Understanding how possible interactions between drought and health take place at the regional level is then essential to map risks and vulnerabilities, assisting in the agreement on adaptation and preparedness measures that contribute to reducing future risks from disaster and climate change to human health [11–13]. However, monitoring the outcomes of mid-to-long-term events such as drought makes evidence on the direct and indirect impacts scarce [6,8,13–18]. Most of them are indirect and long-lasting with multiple causal pathways, which hinders the establishment of a clear health-drought association due to, in part, the silent evolution of the event and its diffuse spatial distribution [14,16,19–21].

While scarce, epidemiological evidence shows the impacts of drought on human health ranging from an increase in infectious diseases to mental health deterioration [8,13,14,16–18,21–25]. A worldwide review from Stanke et al. (2013) [16] observed effects related to nutrition (e.g., mortality and malnutrition), water-borne diseases (e.g., cholera, algae bloom), and vector-borne diseases (e.g., malaria, dengue). Local studies have shown possible effects related to nutritional deficiencies, mental health, water and air quality, compromised quality and access to health services, and slower gains in population health, perpetrating long-lasting consequences of drought to human well-being [8,14]. Water and food security, social capital, and social determinants have also been related to health vulnerability to droughts in different regions, including semiarid places [14,15,21,26–28]. However, especially in Brazil, these studies are often limited to the biophysical and epidemiological impacts of disasters, failing to produce a bigger picture on the theme [8,13–15,17,29–31].

In this sense, the use of indices focused on understanding health risks in all its dimensions may be valid for a better understanding of the distribution of local health outcomes and can add valuable information to identify health vulnerabilities useful for disaster risk reduction [32]. Indices related to social vulnerability, human health, climate change, and infectious diseases are a common practice in disaster risk and public health approaches, adding to the comprehension of important underlying health risks, highlighting inequalities in the epidemiological profiles of populational groups, and prioritizing public health resources for slow onset disasters in specific areas [14,27,32–42].

The present study can add a multidimensional perspective to this context, highlighting complex interactions basing the drought–health relationship in Brazil, as it brings together the perspectives of environmental disasters, social determinants, and possible health effects in an index useful for vulnerability analyses. The findings might provide evidence of the underlying health–drought connections in the Brazilian Semiarid municipalities, a region considered the most inhabited semiarid area on the planet (more than 22 million people). Based on a multivariate analysis, this study proposes (i) to identify how some important determinants of health related to drought are grouped and distributed; (ii) to identify vulnerable populations by creating a relative vulnerability index that produce a spatial view of the health–drought patterns in the region.

2. Materials and Methods

2.1. Study Area

The Brazilian Semiarid region is situated mainly in the Northeastern part of the country, being delimited based on the following dominant semiarid climatic conditions: (i) average annual rainfall below 800 mm; (ii) aridity index of up to 0.5 (water balance between precipitations and potential evapotranspiration); and (iii) drought risk greater than 60%. It has 22,598,318 inhabitants (about 12% of the Brazilian contingent), underperforming the other regions in key indicators such as illiteracy, infant mortality, and poverty [14]. In addition to this social context is the scarcity of natural resources and the poor agricultural and livestock production, negatively affecting the living conditions of communities, which have in subsistence farming one of their main economic activities [13,30,31]. The rainfall has a strong space–time variability (concentrated in 3–4 months) and low total annual volumes (average accumulated precipitation less than 600mm year-1, which are more reduced in the interior parts of the region) [43–45]. Droughts are a chronic phenomenon registered since at least the 16th century, the most recent lasted from 2010 to 2016 [46]. Large-scale phenomena like El Niño and La Niña are often associated with exceptionally dry or wet episodes in the region [46]. The present study was based on the 2005 delimitation, which includes 1135 municipalities in nine states of the federation—most of which are located in the Northeast region of the country, while a few occupy the northern part of the state of Minas Gerais (Figure 1).

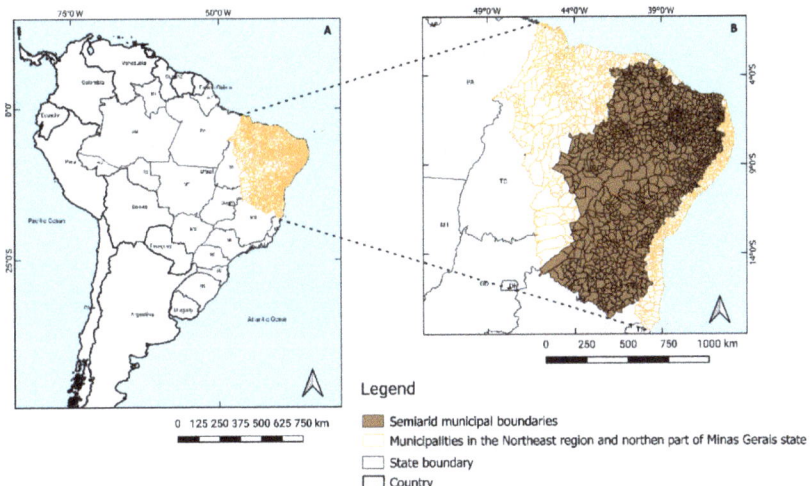

Figure 1. Limits of the study region—Brazilian Northeast region and part of Minas Gerais state (**A**), and the Semiarid municipalities (**B**). The 1135 municipalities studied are located mainly in the Northeast region of the country, but also occupy part of the northern portion of the state of Minas Gerais, in the Southeast region (85 municipalities). Adapted from: [31].

2.2. Conceptual Framework

In public health, vulnerability represents a multidimensional construct comprising several biophysical, sociocultural, political, institutional, and economic factors that converge at the community and individual levels to influence health outcomes. It also represents a dynamic process that acts to modulate the capacity of populations or systems to cope with adverse impacts of extreme events, being influenced by underlying factors known as determinants of health [1,13,31,47,48]. In the literature of disasters, these health determinants are considered key in understanding population level outcomes following disasters, and are known as determinants of vulnerability [48,49]. These key conditions help in understanding existing vulnerability prior to disasters, which can also be exacerbated after a disaster, fulfilling priority one in the Sendai Framework of addressing disaster risk from location-based information [7,48,49].

Considering these key concepts, an explanatory model was developed for the Brazilian Semiarid region. Figure 2 represents the possible and complex interactions that are established between sociodemographic, environmental, and health aspects in the context of droughts. It is noticed that the health effects occur slowly and mostly indirectly so that the vulnerability of the population is shaped by factors such as location in the geographical space, the subsistence economy, and the lack of government investment in mitigation and assistance measures that may impact health [27,50]. In general, changes in rainfall and temperature affect the quantity and the quality of the water available for consumption, producing a cascading scenario of food and social insecurity, damage to health infrastructure or human resources, and other health issues that can modulate the epidemiological profile of the population. The direct and indirect impacts arising from drought influence other determinants of health (e.g., socio-economic vulnerability), as well as being influenced by them, resulting in changes in the population's health status.

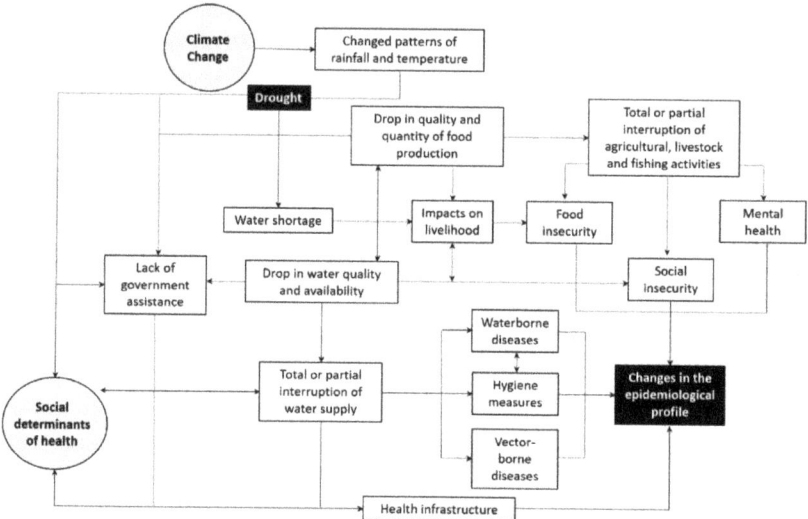

Figure 2. Conceptual framework on the links between drought, health, and the environmental and social determinants. Adapted from: [8,16,27].

2.3. Vulnerability Data

The 32 indicators were compiled, and their sources are shown in Table 1. A municipal scale was chosen, comprising 1135 study units in the Brazilian Semiarid region. The initial categorization of variables was based on the structure proposed by Ebi & Bowen (2016) [28] to explore the main health vulnerabilities in the context of extreme weather events, namely, socio-environmental, socio-economic, and health status/health systems. The criteria for inclusion of variables were: (i) to demonstrate a literature basis of the relationship between health, its determinants, and vulnerability to drought, and (ii) be available on systematic and freely accessible platforms (i.e., public, governmental, or private).

Table 1. Description of the variables and indices.

Dimension	Indicator	Variable	Source
Socio-economic	Income below the poverty line	% of households with per capita nominal monthly income (BRL) of up to 1/2 minimum wage in 2010	Demographic census–IBGE
	Per capita income	Value in BRL of average household income per capita in 2010	
	Ratio between rural and urban population	Resident population whose household situation was rural in 2010	Demographic census–IBGE
		Resident population whose household situation was urban in 2010	
	Population with complete primary education or more	% population aged 15 years or older with a completed 2nd elementary school or more in 2010	
	Illiterate population	% population aged 15 years and older with no education in 2010	
	Survival probability	Likelihood of a newborn child living up to 40 years if the level and pattern of mortality by age of the 2010 Census remain constant throughout life	Atlas of Human Development in Brazil
	Illiterate female heads of household	% of households in which the woman was responsible and illiterate in 2010	Demographic census–IBGE
	Dependency ratio	% of people living in households with a dependency ratio > 75% in 2010	Atlas of Human Development in Brazil
	Unemployment rate	Unemployment rate of people aged 16 years and older in 2010	Demographic census–IBGE
	Population employed in agriculture	% of the employed population in the agricultural sector aged 18 years or older in 2010	Atlas of Human Development in Brazil
	Municipal population engaged in family farming	% of establishments presenting a declaration of suitability to PRONAF (National Program for Strengthening Family Agriculture) in 2017	Agricultural Census–IBGE
	Rural establishments where the producer is an association member	% of establishments in which the producer is associated with a cooperative or class entity in 2017	Agricultural Census–IBGE
	Rural establishments with irrigated agriculture	% of establishments with irrigated agriculture in 2017	Agricultural Census–IBGE
	Rural establishments with access to water	% of establishments with rivers/streams protected by riparian forest in 2017	Agricultural Census–IBGE
	Rural population with access to water technology	Number of rural households served by water access technologies (i.e., consumer cisterns, storage tanks) in 2019	National Semiarid Institute–INSA
Socio-environmental	Demographic density	Resident population in 2017	IBGE
		Municipal area in km^2	National Semiarid Institute–INSA
	Drought index	SPI-12 frequency and duration. Methodology adapted from [48]. Standardized Precipitation Index (SPI) is the most commonly used indicator worldwide for detecting and characterizing meteorological droughts, based on a comparison of observed total precipitation amounts for an accumulation period of interest (e.g., 1, 3, 12, 48 months)	CHIRPS
		Number of drought events recorded between 2003 and 2015	National Water Agency—ANA
	Change in agricultural participation in gross domestic product (GDP)	Gross change in income obtained through work in the rural area between 1999 and 2012	National Semiarid Institute—INSA
	Population with access to sanitation	% of households with general sewerage or septic tank in 2010	Demographic census—IBGE
	Population with access to piped water	% of households with public water supply in 2010	

Table 1. Cont.

Dimension	Indicator	Variable	Source
Health conditions and systems	Dengue index	Incidence rate, temporal trend, and proportion of cases between 2001 and 2015. Adapted from [26,31]	DATASUS
	Hepatitis A index		
	Asthma admissions rate	Hospital admission rate, temporal trend, and proportion of cases between 2001 and 2015. Adapted from [26,31]	
	Malnutrition admissions rate		
	Skin infections admissions		
	Mental disorders admissions		
	Diarrhea admissions		
	Admissions sensitive to primary care	% of hospitalizations for conditions sensitive to primary care in 2015 (a set of health problems for which the effective action of primary care would decrease the risk of hospitalizations)	
	Infant mortality up to 5 years	Probability of dying between birth and the exact age of 5, per 1000 children born alive in 2010	Atlas of Human Development in Brazil
	Number of beds/inhabitants	Total outpatient, emergency, intensive care, and hospitalization beds per 1000 inhabitants in 2015	DATASUS
	Health professionals per inhabitant	Number of registered health professionals in the public and private sectors per 1000 inhabitants in 2015	
	% population covered by health insurance	Number of health plan beneficiaries that contain hospital and/or outpatient segmentation, and may also contain dental assistance in 2015	National Supplementary Health Agency
		Estimated population in 2015	IBGE

2.4. Multivariate Analysis

An exploratory factor analysis was performed in order to obtain groups of indicators more correlated with each other. This type of multivariate procedure is used to obtain latent variables (factors) that would not be observed directly in the data set, allowing the creation of scales or indexes through its output scores [51,52].

The entire database was prepared to replace missing or no variation values as required by statistical procedure. In the case of missing values, the mean value of the variable was used, which did not change its distribution. All information was normalized by the minimum–maximum method to present the same scale—the minimum value is transformed into a 0, the maximum value is transformed into a 1. Model adequacy measures comprised the subject–item ratio, sample size, Bartlett sphericity, and Kaiser–Mayer–Olkin tests [53–57]. The extraction method used was the Iterated Principal Factor (IPF), indicated when the multivariate normality of the variables is not met [55]. Orthogonal (varimax) and oblique (oblimin) methods were chosen for rotation. For the factors retention, the following rules were followed: Kaiser criterion, scree plot, and parallel analysis as quantitative methods, in addition to the gradual elimination of factors (stepwise) and the interpretability of the results [51,52,58]. The data analysis for this paper was generated using SAS® Studio Software, Version 3.8 (SAS Institute Inc., Cary, NC, USA) [59].

2.5. Indices and Maps

The standardized scoring coefficients created by the SAS® during the factor analysis were used as weights to generate a Health Vulnerability Index (HVI) in drought situations. The normalized variables were multiplied with the assigned weights to construct separate indices for each common factor, using the regression method with the following formula:

$$I_j = \sum_{i=1}^{k} b_i \left[\frac{a_{ji} - x_i}{s_i} \right] \quad (1)$$

where, I is the index value of the factor, b is the standardized scoring coefficient (weights), a is the indicator value, x is the mean indicator value, s is the standard deviation, i is the indicator, and j is the specific municipality. Thus, an underlying index of vulnerability, per municipality, was created considering only the indicators that comprised each factor. All indices were normalized using the minimum–maximum method.

A simple additive model of the four factors was used to generate the HVI, with no weights assigned, allowing each factor to contribute equally to the overall vulnerability score [38]. It being an exploratory analysis, the approach of equal weights was chosen because there was no prior assumption about the importance of each factor for the overall sum. A cardinality adjustment was performed to demonstrate the influence of each factor on the final vulnerability [38,52,60,61]. For this purpose, the relationship of the indicators with the vulnerability and the value of their factorial loads was analyzed, being adopted mainly, but not exclusively, the limits of 0.7 or 0.5.

The QGis software, version 3.10 "A Coruña", was used to spatialize the indices in choropleth maps and allow a visualization of their regional distribution. The maps varied between 0 and 1, indicating a comparative scale from the lowest to the highest vulnerability, respectively, for the municipalities of the Semiarid.

3. Results

The model's adequacy measures were satisfactory. The subject–item ratio was 32:1, and Bartlett's sphericity test ($p \leq 0.001$) and Kaiser–Mayer–Olkin test (KMO = 0.82) presented values suitable for analysis. The Cronbach's alpha value was 0.7 (most of the variables demonstrated robust internal consistency with Cronbach's alpha ≥ 0.6 for each). The four-factor solution showed consistent results between the initial sample ($n = 1135$) and the random samples ($n1 = 567$ and $n2 = 568$), demonstrating the stability and reliability of the initial solution.

Four common factors were retained, a result converged in all quantitative methods (Kaiser factor, parallel analysis, and scree plot). Together, these factors explained 84.4% of the variance observed for the 32 indicators included. An oblimin rotation verified low correlations between the factors [62]. Hence, the varimax rotation model (i.e., assumes independent factors) proved to be more appropriate since one of the aims of this work was to generate indices for each Semiarid municipality. The results for factor analysis are shown in Table 2.

Health and its social determinants represented the first common factor with the highest proportion of explained variance (51.8%). Some living and socio-economic conditions of the municipalities of the Semiarid region that, in the public health context, are known to influence the occurrence of health problems and its risk factors were highlighted. These conditions are mainly related, but not limited, to income, education, and quality of life, features with loads greater than 0.5. While the highest per capita income and higher education were positively related to the factor, other important indicators were negatively related: occupation in agriculture, low income, and low education. Therefore, the cardinality of the factor has been reversed to reflect the greater vulnerabilities in places with poor socio-economic and health conditions.

Rural Economy and access to water represented those municipalities with higher prevalence of rural activities, explaining 13.2% of data variance. The municipalities with the highest proportion of rural households with water related technologies were those in which the availability of the water supply system is lower, increasing overall vulnerability. Although the existence of water technologies represents less susceptibility to drought, a data analysis on this factor reveals this indicator positively correlating to the rural population and the drought index, but negatively relating to irrigated farming and piped water, pointing out the most critical locations from the point of view of water scarcity. Thus, this factor was considered to increase vulnerability.

Table 2. Factor names, indicators, percentage of explained variance, factor loads, and cardinality.

Factor Name	Indicator	Factor Loading	Explained Variance (%)	Cardinality
Health and its social determinants	Average household per capita income	0.803	51.8	+
	% population with complete primary education or more	0.705		
	% population covered by health plans	0.488		
	Survival probability	0.469		
	Demographic density	0.448		
	% of households with access to sanitation	0.427		
	Health professionals per 1000 inhabitants	0.421		
	Dengue index	0.393		
	Skin infections admissions	0.337		
	Hepatitis index	0.245		
	Mental disorders admissions	0.203		
	Infant mortality	−0.438		
	Dependency ratio	−0.459		
	% of the population employed in agriculture	−0.666		
	% households with monthly income per capita up to $\frac{1}{2}$ salary	−0.685		
	% population illiterate	−0.693		
Rural economy and access to water	% rural households with water related technologies	0.639	13.2	+
	Rural urban ratio	0.456		
	Drought index	0.397		
	Unemployment rate	−0.315		
	% rural establishments with irrigation	−0.319		
	% change in agricultural participation in GDP	−0.354		
	% households with access to piped water	−0.707		
Health problems and infrastructure	Asthma admissions	0.783	10.1	+
	Undernutrition admissions	0.569		
	Diarrhea admissions	0.520		
	Admissions sensitive to primary care	0.520		
	Beds per 1000 inhabitants	0.387		
Rural structure and social capital	% family farming establishments	0.615	9.2	+
	% rural establishments associated with a cooperative or class entity	0.418		
	% establishments with water resources	0.312		
	% of households with female heads of household illiterate	−0.540		

Factor 3 represented health problems and infrastructure with 10.4% of the explained variance. It indicates those municipalities where the burden of hospitalizations for health conditions that may be related to droughts is greater, as well as demonstrates the effectiveness of the care provided to the population (i.e., beds and primary health care). Hospitalizations for conditions related to drought phenomena in the scientific literature—asthma, malnutrition, and diarrhea (the first with the highest load)—and admissions sensitive to primary care, were grouped together, all with positive loadings. Another less relevant information was the number of beds per 1000 inhabitants. All the characteristics observed in this factor increase vulnerability in drought contexts, except the number of beds, hence the cardinality was positive.

Finally, the fourth factor was related to the characteristics of rural establishments, named as rural structure and social capital (explained variance of 9.2%). The main attributes were the prevalence of family farming with a positive load and households headed by illiterate women with a negative load. The interpretation of this factor indicates that the places where there is a greater participation of family farming are those where there is some social organization, properties with a watercourse and fewer women as breadwinners. Although it seems contradictory to hold a positive cardinality for this factor, family farming is very important in rural semiarid regions, as it represents a low productivity activity focused on subsistence and is very susceptible to droughts, which is why this factor was considered to increase vulnerability.

The spatial distribution of the factors, as well as the HVI are shown in Figure 3. There is a large regional difference in the distribution of vulnerability between the four factors. Health and its social determinants were found to be underdeveloped throughout the Semiarid region, with municipal clusters presenting values greater than 0.8 in the extreme west towards the north, and at the eastern border towards the south. The municipalities with lower values in the index were dispersed. For rural economy and access to water (Factor 2) there is a general reduction of vulnerability, where most of locations ranged from

0.2 to 0.6. Clusters of municipalities with low values prevailed in the southern and northern regions, while municipalities with less developed rural economies concentrated in the western and northeastern parts. A similar situation was observed for health problems and infrastructure, in which vulnerability was punctual, especially in the center–south portion. Most municipalities were placed in categories of lesser vulnerability, with groups less vulnerable to health issues in the southern and northern parts of the Semiarid region. Factor 4, in which the conditions of rural establishments were highlighted, showed a tendency to increased vulnerability from the eastern border, which assembled vulnerabilities below 0.3, and a dispersion of the highest scores towards the northern, central–western, and southern areas. It is worth mentioning that in this factor, the eastern belt, of lesser vulnerability, represents those municipalities in which there is a greater concentration of illiterate female breadwinners, with little rural social articulation and poorly developed family farming, that is, they are more urbanized or present commercial agriculture, at the expense of subsistence farming.

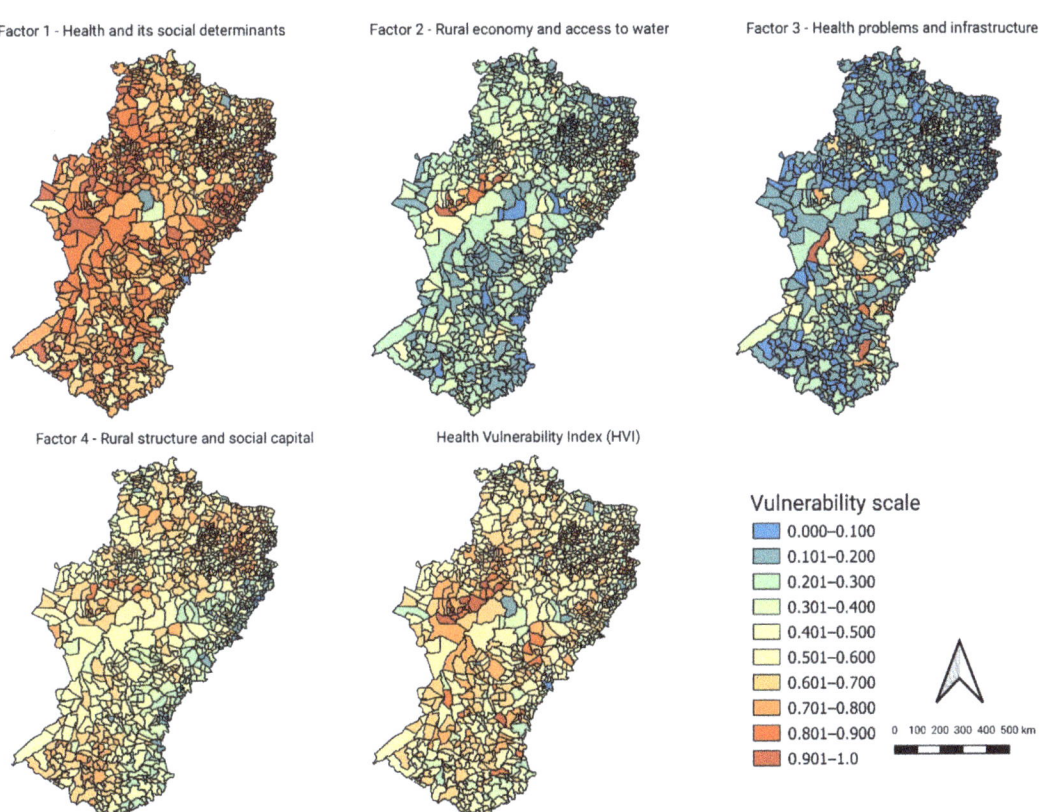

Figure 3. Spatial distribution of the Health Vulnerability Index (HVI) and its factors for municipalities of the Brazilian Semiarid region ranging between 0 and 1 (0 represents lesser vulnerability and 1 greater vulnerability).

The HVI represents the results of the additive model and reflects some of the patterns found in the factors individually. There was a tendency for high scores to be concentrated in the central–western and other clusters in the northeastern and southern portions. However, it is perceived a modulation of the different aspects of vulnerability in the HVI through the "compensation" between the factors, which seems to have leveled the extremes. Thus, although for health and its social determinants (Factor 1), the highest vulnerability scores prevailed across the Semiarid region, with special attention to the extremes of the border (eastern–western), the other factors modulated the final vulnerability by presenting lower vulnerability scores for many of these critical regions. All the index scores are available at a data repository [63].

4. Discussion

4.1. Rural and Social Characteristics Influencing Health Vulnerabilities

The literature on vulnerability, health and droughts in Brazil has been growing in recent years, but the discussion on health determinants of disasters and drought vulnerabilities is still scarce [8,13–15,29,31,64]. In this sense, the present study proposed an index of health vulnerability in drought situations (HVI) based on social, economic, epidemiological, and environmental indicators that, assembled in factors, elucidated some health determinants, based mainly on publicly available information for all the Semiarid municipalities.

In general, the configuration of the factors of this study showed rural characteristics in a remarkable aggregation with worst living conditions. In Factor 1, the population employed in agriculture was opposed to higher levels of education and average income per capita, while aligning to income below the poverty line and illiteracy. Factor 2 showed conditions such as drought, rural population, and water technologies in a opposite direction of access to irrigated agriculture and access to piped water. This might explain why the municipalities with the highest values in this index presented a higher proportion of cisterns and other forms of water storage. In Factor 4, family farming showed greater weight in the definition of the factor, a condition considered extremely susceptible to environmental hazards such as drought, while antagonistic correlating to women heads of households, a predominant situation in urban areas of the Brazilian Northeast [31]. All these findings point to the possibility of rural subsistence conditions acting as a predictor of increased health vulnerability and poor quality of life in the region. Furthermore, it allows differentiating the municipalities between those with predominant urban characteristics, where rural economies are better developed (commercial agriculture), and those essentially rural, with subsistence farming as major activity.

Similar findings were reported by several authors in the region [31,65–67]. Hummell, Cutter, & Emrich (2016) [39], when replicating the Social Vulnerability Index (SoVI®) in Brazil, observed that the population employed in agricultural activities and livelihood was linked to greater social vulnerability and less developed areas. In the same sense, the National Institute of the Semiarid (INSA), while monitoring the desertification process in the region from a model considering institutional, economic, and social drivers, pointed out as prone to desertification, the same areas indicated as the most vulnerable in Factors 1 and 4, therefore less liable to commercial agriculture [68]. These locations were the ones where social determinants of health presented impoverished and the family farming prevailed.

Although the Northeast, where most of the Semiarid is located, has made improvement in its socio-economic conditions, health sector activities, and supply services since the 2000s, investments and the expansion of economic activity maintained the historical trend of concentration in state capitals and in traditional regional hubs [69]. This has produced inequalities in access to agricultural technology and resources, concentrating these assets in environmentally and economically prosperous areas, while those with predominance of subsistence agriculture face greater difficulties imposed by drought. Thereby, these locations end up demanding more social and political articulation to ensure better living conditions and commercial competition, which might explain why the social organization indicator is positively correlated to family farming in Factor 4. Additionally, the indicator of irrigated agriculture, by showing to be inversely correlated to the rural population and the incidence of drought in Factor 2, shows that this type of technology is not available or is not viable for the places most vulnerable to drought in the Semiarid. Indeed, family farming is more common in smaller tracts of land in the region and is based primarily on rainfed systems, an activity very vulnerable to water scarcity and characterized by low levels of productivity, which makes small farmers highly vulnerable to drought impacts [70].

However, irrigation proved to be effective in managing risks in the context of drought in Northeast, where families in possession of this asset were less likely to experience food insecurity than families without irrigation [71].

These findings align with other studies showing that, both globally and in Brazil, the rural population is often more exposed to drought hazards than urban populations [26,72]. Rural households are at greater risk of chronic food insecurity than families in urban areas, for example [73,74]. Overall, rural societies earn lower incomes and may be more dependent on natural resources and the local economy, being particularly susceptible to climate hazards [26,38,39,71]. In drought situations, the cycle of reducing subsistence, decreasing income, and increasing prices of agricultural products, in a scenario of low rural technologies as observed in the Semiarid, is seen as a driver of food insecurity in this populational group [30].

The deprivation of access to drinking water is another problem added to this resource scarcity scenario, where the countryside is usually the most affected area. This condition was demonstrated in Factor 2, in which access to piped water has been shown to be inversely related to the rural population and to the greater incidence of droughts. Several government and civil society programs have sought to minimize the effects of drought by making water tank truck operations and water storage programs a commonplace. Programs such as "cisterns", "one million cisterns", and "one land two waters" have been implemented to provide access to water for human consumption and food production, engaging simple and low-cost social technologies [29,75]. However, such efforts have not been enough to tackle the reality experienced by agricultural families, since the poor water quality provided by tank trucks and cisterns, is combined with other problems such as lack of sanitation, with significant health repercussions.

Worldwide, health indicators tend to vary according to the social gradient, being less favorable in groups of lower socio-economic levels, whether measured by income, education, occupation, or social class [3,48,76–79]. These indicators are often related in an "ecological level", in which spatial clusters show areas with a high income level offering good coverage of sanitation services, health facilities and education with high populational density [80–82]. This relationship was observed in Factor 1 of the present study. A polarization was observed between locations with more concentration of wealth, population, and human well-being (e.g., higher income, education, health coverage, and sanitation), and places with limited resources, where residents with lower quality of life and health are found (e.g., lower income, illiteracy, higher agriculture labor force and infant mortality).

This distinction highlights persistent intra-regional discrepancies in the Semiarid, albeit this region is considered quite homogeneous in its socio-economic and health levels [3,13]. This can be explained by the region's development profile, influenced by the migration of labor force to large regional hubs. In these places, the population density was not accompanied by the expansion of public services infrastructure, fostering urban agglomerations with poor living standards than the national average, while the countryside remained lacking investments [83]. However, underneath this apparent homogeneity, local dissimilarities still emerge as identified by other authors for economic, land use, and health indicators [13,14,84–87]. Factor 1 ends up locally reflecting this bigger picture where poor human well-being and social/health inequalities are observed for the whole Semiarid region, strongly distancing it from the patterns observed for other Brazilian regions, while highlighting its local differences.

Regarding health issues, the municipalities with the highest level of health care development were those with the best socio-economic performance (observed in the Factor 1 arrangement). Health professionals per capita and coverage of private health plans showed a positive correlation with indicators such as average income, higher education, access to sanitation, and lower infant mortality rate. On the other hand, some of these characteristics have been positively correlated to morbidity indicators such as dengue, hepatitis, mental disorders, and skin infections, even though featuring small loads. This fact seems to demonstrate that even the most prosperous Semiarid areas, in which the social determinants of health have shown better scores, still lack investment in health care and health promotion actions. Yet, recent socioenvironmental changes such as urbanization, population growth, poverty, and climate change pose an additional risk to the proper management of impacts related to extreme events as droughts, since they could modify the emergence and transmission of infectious diseases and other health problems [88,89].

Although Factor 3 has been shown to be quite homogeneous regarding the distribution of health problems and infrastructure across the municipalities, poor values were observed in the center–southern portion. In these places, the health outcomes that may be related to drought represented a great burden to the health system, with higher admission rates. However, the availability of beds with positive loads suggests that these municipalities are also able to offer more complex health services. On the other hand, high loads were obtained for hospitalizations sensitive to primary care, showing that many health problems are transferred to more complex levels when they should be addressed at the entrance level of the system. It highlights the current deficiencies in primary care and the likely overloading of secondary care, contributing to a lower resolution of local health services. These municipalities may also have a reduced capacity to respond and cope with extreme weather events due to the great burden on the health system, since other common health outcomes not directly related to droughts, such as hypertension and diabetes, are managed mainly at primary care levels.

The Unified Health System (SUS) represents the only assistance structure for a large part of the Semiarid population, mainly for rural, which still face recurring difficulties in accessing health care services [3,15,90–92]. The infrastructure and health care networks, at its different levels of complexity, shape to a certain extent the assistance available to the public along to the allocation of resources in Brazil. Primary care is present in almost all municipalities, while secondary and tertiary levels are available in regional or large urban centers. Such an arrangement fosters local inequalities in the allocation of financial and human resources, as well as in the availability of medical and hospital services, equipment, and instruments. This generates a shortage of physicians and other specialties in small rural areas and in primary care levels, while concentrating specialists in the private sector of large urban hubs [69,91,92]. As small municipalities are predominant in the Semiarid, health services and access to them are restricted to more prosperous regional hubs with better conditions for attracting and retaining health professionals, which also provide better infrastructure, better collective working conditions, higher income level, and higher quality of life [29,90,93]. It is possible that such aspects contributed to the spatial homogeneity of Factor 3.

4.2. Social Determinants at the Borders, Rural Aspects in the Inland Regions

Spatial analysis proves to be an important instrument in assessing the impact of social processes and structures in determining disaster vulnerabilities, highlighting the municipalities in which health determinants—environmental, economic, and social—must be better analyzed. Starting from an overview of the HVI, the highest values were shown to be continuously grouped on the eastern and western borders, where the municipalities with the least social and economic development are located. At the same time, most municipalities remained in intermediate categories of vulnerability in HVI—between 0.3 and 0.7—demonstrating a homogeneity of health conditions and its determinants as observed by other authors [13,39]. This arrangement causes the municipalities of the Semiarid region as a whole to present a widespread fragility of the health system, somewhat demonstrable by the worst health conditions observed amid the resident population, which are not shared by other non-semiarid municipalities in Brazil [14]. This pattern is also apparent in other indices or studies adapted to the Brazilian reality such as the Municipal Human Development Index, the SoVI® and others [13,14,39,94,95]. Usually, intermediate levels of development and vulnerability prevail in the Semiarid, with a general worse performance when compared to the rest of the country.

The factors that presented the most dispersed vulnerabilities in the semiarid territory were the health and social determinants and the rural structure, with the first presenting a greater homogeneity in the spatial distribution of the highest vulnerabilities. This lack of clear differences was expected due to the unfavorable socioeconomic conditions of the Semiarid as a whole, which comprised central characteristics of the social determinants of health grouped precisely in Factor 1. The opposite could be observed for Factors 2 and 3, in which the spatial pattern of lesser vulnerabilities prevailed in the territory.

A general pattern of poor values grouped on the frontiers for health and its social determinants index (Factor 1), while the other factors modulated the final vulnerability (HVI) by presenting lower vulnerability scores was observed. An overlap between the areas of greatest vulnerability in each factor was evident, except for Factor 3. Consistently, a group of municipalities in the western portion of the Semiarid was amongst the largest categories of vulnerability of health and its determinants, rural economy, and rural structure, stressing the need for investments in adapting to droughts regarding the socio-economic and water access levels. These localities comprised small towns, with a high dependence on external revenues (i.e., those coming from other sources such as the state and union), with low income from work, high rates of infant mortality and with medium to high levels of previous droughts records [13,96].

In Factor 2, where the most vulnerable categories represented the places where there is a greater rural population, with a reduction in agricultural participation in GDP, less irrigation and less access to piped water, there is an intersection with the greatest vulnerabilities of the health and its social determinants. Similarly, the spatialization of Factor 4 reveals the highest values associated with the municipalities with the greatest percentage of family farming, although with some type of social organization (western part), locations where Factor 1 also presented high scores. Thus, western, eastern, and northeastern parts of the region represent places where the health of populations, in its various aspects, may be more affected in the context of drought, lacking social investments, with poor quality of life, low income, and precarious access to water that increase their vulnerability to drought.

Similar conclusions were reported by Vieira et al. (2020) [31] regarding vulnerability of the drylands. The authors showed that physical characteristics of dry regions do not necessarily imply high social vulnerability, but rather a historical political environment that defines the social construction of risk associated with droughts in Brazil. The fact that the drought indicator was not among the largest loads in Factor 2 points in the same direction—although the whole Semiarid experiences the impacts of droughts at diverse intensities, are the aspects of infrastructure, services, employment, income, and social conditions more important in shaping the HVI. These conditions are probably a consequence of both poor management and reduced political will in facing the recurrent droughts of the region, rather than a consequence of the climate hazard itself. However, the current scenario can be greatly exacerbated by the ongoing climate change, given that changes in annual-mean air temperature are projected higher for the Brazilian Northeast than globally, demonstrating that local impacts can be much stronger [97]. Sectors already weakened, such as food and water security, as well as small-scale agriculture, can be strongly impacted by warming above 4 °C due to increased temperatures and reduced precipitation, increasing the vulnerability of smallholder livelihoods in municipalities supported by subsistence agriculture [97].

Interestingly, the HVI spatial pattern was remarkably similar to the risk index constructed by Sena et al. (2017) [13] for the Semiarid considering drought situations. The similarities also encompass the distribution of their vulnerability and access to piped water indices, which presented extensive overlap with the health and social determinants index of the present study. This corroborates the factors pointed out here as fundamental to shape health vulnerabilities to droughts in the Brazilian Semiarid and to help in reducing existing hazards, while creating resilience to future ones. Key factors that must be tackled at the populational level to lessen drought impacts before and after its occurrence were highlighted.

However, some limitations of the study should be addressed. They refer mainly to (i) the weighting scheme used to calculate the HVI and (ii) the use of secondary data and its systematization. It is acknowledged that different methods lead to significantly different results, directly affecting the value of the index and shifting considerable the ranking of the municipalities under study [98–100]. This is important when dealing with vulnerability indices and its implication to decision making, as different spatial vulnerability pattern related to the chosen methodology may be used by different actors (e.g., authorities, planners, and emergency services) [98]. However, even though there is a lot of discussion about the robustness of the different weighting schemes available, the HVI methodology can be a good starting point in supporting the Semiarid municipalities to ascertain the similarities and differences in their relative levels of health vulnerability. Regarding the data limitation, SUS official data refer mainly to the public sphere, which, although comprising most of the information, does not express the totality of the health indicators in the region. Another aspect is the contemporaneity of socio-economic data, which, despite being systematically updated, may have long-term intervals between your publications (e.g., census editions). It is possible that the use of more recent indicators provides a better representation of health vulnerability in the context of drought. However, this update is feasible from the release of new data, adding to the HVI and its factors an ability to demonstrate the evolution of health vulnerabilities overtime.

5. Conclusions

This study developed a health vulnerability index for the Brazilian Semiarid region from a factor analysis that showed the connections between different aspects influencing the health vulnerabilities in the context of drought. Investment in improving education, employment and income, healthcare facilities, family rural production, and access to water proves essential to ensure the quality of life and health of the population. Moreover, the conformation of the factors made it possible to distinguish the municipalities between those with subsistence characteristics and those with developed commercial agriculture, with marked differences in human well-being. The simple approach of the method helps understand the dynamics of the relationship between health and its determinants, as well as contribute to the spatial visualization of the associated vulnerabilities. The results might support decision making on drought risk reduction as the identified determinants are modifiable underlying conditions, which are linked to medium to long-term health outcomes arising from disasters.

It is believed that the built indices can serve as a guiding tool for decision making at regional levels, helping to reduce risk and increase local resilience of the public health sector. Monitoring the changes that are anticipated in the indices proposed here, from its systematic update, can secure the adequate management of health outcomes more related to drought in the Brazilian Semiarid. Future directions point to need of continued efforts in examining the health–drought nexus in the region, bringing together stakeholders and policy-makers' perspectives to build a local fit approach to tackle health vulnerabilities in the context of the ongoing climate change. Further, an extension of the study is possible as the region presents now a more recently political delimitation, which comprises 1262 municipalities distributed throughout 10 Brazilian states. This might help in a more rational and direct application of the HVI in guiding regional policy practices in the region.

Appropriate policies to ensure the improvement of health determinants and drought vulnerabilities are needed, mainly those related to rural areas and human well-being. Furthermore, the capillarity of the health sector shows itself crucial in various governmental instances, as it enriches the debate about the most visible or long-term impacts associated with droughts. It also assists other sectors whose actions directly affect the quality of life of the population, such as agriculture, water management, and social protection, enabling people to increase control over, and to improve, their health.

Author Contributions: Conceptualization, J.A.M., M.M.d.L.B. and U.C.; Data curation, J.A.M.; Formal analysis, J.A.M. and A.P.M.; Funding acquisition, U.C.; Investigation, J.A.M., R.B.d.S., I.d.B.D. and P.R.; Methodology, J.A.M. and A.P.M.; Supervision, M.M.d.L.B. and U.C.; Validation, R.B.d.S. and I.d.B.D.; Visualization, C.M.; Writing—original draft, J.A.M., R.B.d.S., I.d.B.D. and P.R; Writing—review and editing, A.P.M., C.M., M.M.d.L.B. and U.C. All authors have read and agreed to the published version of the manuscript.

Funding: This research was funded by the National Institute of Science and Technology for Climate Change Phase 2 under CNPq, grant number 465501/2014-1; Fundação de Amparo à Pesquisa do Estado de São Paulo (FAPESP), grant number 2014/50848-9; and the National Coordination for High Level Education and Training (CAPES), grant number 88887.136402/2017-00. The APC was funded by the National Institute of Science and Technology for Climate Change Phase 2.

Institutional Review Board Statement: Not applicable.

Informed Consent Statement: Not applicable.

Data Availability Statement: The data presented in this study are openly available in Mendeley repository at [http://dx.doi.org/10.17632/vfvrr97zb4.1].

Acknowledgments: The authors are grateful to René Rachou Institute—Oswaldo Cruz Foundation for the technical support, and the National Institute of Science and Technology for Climate Change Phase 2 for the administrative and financing support.

Conflicts of Interest: The authors declare no conflict of interest.

References

1. World Health Organization. *Closing the Gap in a Generation: Health Equity through Action on the Social Determinants of Health. Final Report of the Commission on Social Determinants of Health*; World Health Organization: Geneva, Switzerland, 2008.
2. Lucyk, K.; McLaren, L. Taking stock of the social determinants of health: A scoping review. *PLoS ONE* **2017**, *12*, e0177306. [CrossRef] [PubMed]
3. Rasella, D.; Machado, D.B.; Castellanos, M.E.P.; Paim, J.; Szwarcwald, C.L.; Lima, D.; Magno, L.; Pedrana, L.; Medina, M.G.; Penna, G.O.; et al. Assessing the relevance of indicators in tracking social determinants and progress toward equitable population health in Brazil. *Glob. Health Action* **2016**, *9*, 29042. [CrossRef] [PubMed]
4. Pedrana, L.; Pamponet, M.; Walker, R.; Costa, F.; Rasella, D. Scoping review: National monitoring frameworks for social determinants of health and health equity. *Glob. Health Action* **2016**. [CrossRef] [PubMed]
5. Gray, L. Social determinants of health, disaster vulnerability, severe and morbid obesity in adults: Triple jeopardy? *Int. J. Environ. Res. Public Health* **2017**, *14*, 1452. [CrossRef]
6. Nomura, S.; Parsons, A.J.Q.; Hirabayashi, M.; Kinoshita, R.; Liao, Y.; Hodgson, S. Social determinants of mid-to long-term disaster impacts on health: A systematic review. *Int. J. Disaster Risk Reduct.* **2016**, *16*, 53–67. [CrossRef]
7. Lindsay, J.R. The determinants of disaster vulnerability: Achieving sustainable mitigation through population health. *Nat. Hazards* **2003**, *28*, 291–304. [CrossRef]
8. Alpino, T.A.; de Sena, A.R.M.; de Freitas, C.M. Disasters related to droughts and public health—A review of the scientific literature. *Cienc. Saude Coletiva* **2016**, *21*, 809–820. [CrossRef]
9. Centre for Research on the Epidemiology of Disasters—CRED EM-DAT—The International Disaster Database. Available online: https://public.emdat.be/ (accessed on 10 January 2020).
10. Masson-Delmotte, V.; Zhai, P.; Pörtner, H.-O.; Roberts, D.; Skea, J.; Shukla, P.R.; Pirani, A.; Moufouma-Okia, W.; Péan, C.; Pidcock, R.; et al. (Eds.) IPCC Summary for policy makers. In *Global Warming of 1.5 °C. An IPCC Special Report on the Impacts of Global Warming of 1.5 °C above Pre-Industrial Levels and Related Global Greenhouse Gas Emission Pathways, in the Context of Strengthening the Global Response to the Threat of Climate Change*; World Meteorological Organization: Geneva, Switzerland, 2018; p. 32, ISBN 1496354044.
11. Obermaier, M.; Rosa, L.P. Mudança climática e adaptação no Brasil: Uma análise crítica. *Estud. Av.* **2013**, *27*, 155–176. [CrossRef]
12. Wilhite, D.A.; Sivakumar, M.V.K.; Pulwarty, R. Managing drought risk in a changing climate: The role of national drought policy. *Weather Clim. Extrem.* **2014**, *3*, 4–13. [CrossRef]
13. Sena, A.; Ebi, K.L.; Freitas, C.; Corvalan, C.; Barcellos, C. Indicators to measure risk of disaster associated with drought: Implications for the health sector. *PLoS ONE* **2017**, *12*. [CrossRef]
14. Sena, A.; Barcellos, C.; Freitas, C.; Corvalan, C. Managing the health impacts of drought in Brazil. *Int. J. Environ. Res. Public Health* **2014**, *11*, 10737–10751. [CrossRef]
15. Sena, A.; Freitas, C.; Feitosa Souza, P.; Alpino, T.; Pedroso, M.; Corvalan, C.; Barcellos, C.; Carneiro, F. Drought in the Semiarid Region of Brazil: Exposure, Vulnerabilities and Health Impacts from the Perspectives of Local Actors. *PLoS Curr.* **2018**. [CrossRef]
16. Stanke, C.; Kerac, M.; Prudhomme, C.; Medlock, J.; Murray, V. Health effects of drought: A systematic review of the evidence. *PLoS Curr.* **2013**, *5*, 1–40. [CrossRef]

17. Coêlho, A.E.L.; Adair, J.G.; Mocellin, J.S.P. Psychological responses to drought in northeastern Brazil. *Interam. J. Psychol.* **2004**, *38*, 95–103.
18. McCann, D.G.C.; Moore, A.; Walker, M.-E. The water/health nexus in disaster medicine: I. Drought versus flood. *Curr. Opin. Environ. Sustain.* **2011**, *3*, 480–485. [CrossRef]
19. Vins, H.; Bell, J.; Saha, S.; Hess, J.J. The mental health outcomes of drought: A systematic review and causal process diagram. *Int. J. Environ. Res. Public Health* **2015**, *12*, 13251–13275. [CrossRef]
20. Organização Pan-Americana da Saúde (OPAS). Atuação do Setor Saúde Frente a Situações de Seca. In *Série Desenvolvimento Sustentável e Saúde*; Ministério da Saúde: Brasília, Brazil, 2015.
21. Yusa, A.; Berry, P.; Cheng, J.J.; Ogden, N.; Bonsal, B.; Stewart, R.; Waldick, R. Climate Change, Drought and Human Health in Canada. *Int. J. Environ. Res. Public Health* **2015**, *12*, 8359–8412. [CrossRef]
22. OBrien, L.V.; Berry, H.L.; Coleman, C.; Hanigan, I.C. Drought as a mental health exposure. *Environ. Res.* **2014**, *131*, 181–187. [CrossRef]
23. Lima, E.d.A.; Firmino, J.L.d.N.; Gomes Filho, M.F. A relação da previsão da precipitação pluviométrica e casos de dengue nos estados de Alagoas e Paraíba nordeste do Brasil. *Rev. Bras. Meteorol.* **2008**, *23*, 264–269. [CrossRef]
24. Londe, L.d.R.; Coutinho, M.P.; Gregório, D.; Torres, L.; Santos, L.B.L.; Soriano, É. Desastres relacionados à água no Brasil: Perspectivas e recomendações. *Ambient. Soc.* **2014**, *17*, 133–152. [CrossRef]
25. Marcynuk, P.B.; Flint, J.A.; Sargeant, J.M.; Jones-Bitton, A.; Brito, A.M.; Luna, C.F.; Szilassy, E.; Thomas, M.K.; Lapa, T.M.; Perez, E. Comparison of the burden of diarrhoeal illness among individuals with and without household cisterns in northeast Brazil. *BMC Infect. Dis.* **2013**, *13*, 65. [CrossRef]
26. Lohmann, S.; Lechtenfeld, T. The Effect of Drought on Health Outcomes and Health Expenditures in Rural Vietnam. *World Dev. Vol.* **2015**, *72*, 432–448. [CrossRef]
27. Confalonieri, U.E.C.; Lima, A.C.L.; Brito, I.; Quintão, A.F. Social, environmental and health vulnerability to climate change in the Brazilian Northeastern Region. *Clim. Change.* **2014**, *127*, 123–137. [CrossRef]
28. Ebi, K.L.; Bowen, K. Extreme events as sources of health vulnerability: Drought as an example. *Weather Clim. Extrem.* **2016**, *11*, 95–102. [CrossRef]
29. Damasceno, N.P.; Khan, A.S.; Lima, P.V.P.S. Desempenho da saúde pública no semiárido brasileiro. *Rev. Ibero-Am. Ciências Ambient.* **2018**, *9*, 171–187. [CrossRef]
30. Alvala, R.; Cunha, A.P.; Brito, S.S.B.; Seluchi, M.E.; Marengo, J.A.; Moraes, O.L.L.; Carvalho, M.A. Drought monitoring in the Brazilian Semiarid region. *An. Acad. Bras. Cienc.* **2019**, *91*, e20170209. [CrossRef] [PubMed]
31. Vieira, R.M.d.S.P.; Sestini, M.F.; Tomasella, J.; Marchezini, V.; Pereira, G.R.; Barbosa, A.A.; Santos, F.C.; Rodriguez, D.A.; do Nascimento, F.R.; Santana, M.O.; et al. Characterizing spatio-temporal patterns of social vulnerability to droughts, degradation and desertification in the Brazilian northeast. *Environ. Sustain. Indic.* **2020**, *5*, 100016. [CrossRef]
32. Chan, E.Y.Y.; Huang, Z.; Lam, H.C.Y.; Wong, C.K.P.; Zou, Q. Health vulnerability index for disaster risk reduction: Application in belt and road initiative (BRI) region. *Int. J. Environ. Res. Public Health* **2019**, *16*, 380. [CrossRef]
33. Menezes, J.A.; Confalonieri, U.; Madureira, A.P.; Duval, I.d.B.; do Santos, R.B.; Margonari, C. Mapping human vulnerability to climate change in the Brazilian Amazon: The construction of a municipal vulnerability index. *PLoS ONE* **2018**, *13*, e0190808. [CrossRef]
34. Vommaro, F.; Menezes, J.A.; Barata, M.M.d.L. Contributions of municipal vulnerability map of the population of the state of Maranhão (Brazil) to the sustainable development goals. *Sci. Total Environ.* **2020**, *706*, 134629. [CrossRef]
35. Asmall, T. The Adverse Health Effects Associated with Drought in Africa: Working towards Developing a Vulnerability Index. Master's Thesis, Queen's University, Kingston, ON, Canada, 2020. Available online: http://hdl.handle.net/11427/32447 (accessed on 21 April 2021).
36. Secretaria Municipal de Saúde de Belo Horizonte. Índice de Vulnerabilidade da Saúde. Available online: https://prefeitura.pbh.gov.br/sites/default/files/estrutura-de-governo/saude/2018/publicacaoes-da-vigilancia-em-saude/indice_vulnerabilidade2012.pdf (accessed on 21 April 2021).
37. Debortoli, N.S.; Camarinha, P.I.M.; Marengo, J.A.; Rodrigues, R.R. An index of Brazil's vulnerability to expected increases in natural flash flooding and landslide disasters in the context of climate change. *Nat. Hazards* **2017**. [CrossRef]
38. Cutter, S.L.; Boruff, B.J.; Shirley, W.L. Social Vulnerability to Environmental Hazards. *Soc. Sci. Q.* **2003**, *84*, 242–261. [CrossRef]
39. Hummell, M.B.d.L.; Cutter, S.L.; Emrich, C.T. Social Vulnerability to Natural Hazards in Brazil. *Int. J. Disaster Risk Sci.* **2016**, *7*, 111–122. [CrossRef]
40. Khan, F.A.; Salman, A. A simple human vulnerability index to climate change hazards for Pakistan. *Int. J. Disaster Risk Sci.* **2012**, *3*, 163–176. [CrossRef]
41. Pastrana, M.E.O.; Brito, R.L.; Nicolino, R.R.; de Oliveira, C.S.F.; Haddad, J.P.A. Spatial and statistical methodologies to determine the distribution of dengue in Brazilian municipalities and relate incidence with the health vulnerability index. *Spat. Spatiotemporal. Epidemiol.* **2014**, *11*, 143–151. [CrossRef]
42. Sullivan, C.; Meigh, J. Targeting attention on local vulnerabilities using an integrated index approach: The example of the climate vulnerability index. *Water Sci. Technol.* **2005**, *51*, 69–78. [CrossRef]

43. Silva, V.D.R.P. On climate variability in Northeast of Brazil. *J. Arid Environ.* **2004**, *58*, 575–596. [CrossRef]
44. Marengo, J.A.; Alves, L.M.; Bessera, E.A.; Lacerda, F.F. Variabilidade e mudanças climáticas no semiárido brasileiro. In *Recursos Hídricos em Regiões Áridas e Semiáridas*; Instituto Nacional do Semiárido—INSA: Campina Grande, Brazil, 2011; pp. 385–422, ISBN 9788564265011.
45. De Oliveira, M.B.L.; Santos, A.J.B.; Manzi, A.O.; Alvalá, R.C.d.S.; Correia, M.d.F.; de Moura, M.S.B. Trocas de energia e fluxo de carbono entre a vegetação de Caatinga e a atmosfera no Nordeste Brasileiro. *Rev. Bras. Meteorol.* **2006**, *21*, 378–386.
46. Marengo, J.A.; Alves, L.M.; Alvala, R.; Cunha, A.P.; Brito, S.; Moraes, O.L.L. Climatic characteristics of the 2010–2016 drought in the semiarid Northeast Brazil region. *An. Acad. Bras. Cienc.* **2018**, *90*, 1973–1985. [CrossRef]
47. World Health Organization. *Operational Framework for Building Climate Resilient Health Systems*; World Health Organization: Geneva, Switzerland, 2015; ISBN 978 92 4 156507 3.
48. Phibbs, S.; Kenney, C.; Severinsen, C.; Mitchell, J.; Hughes, R. Synergising public health concepts with the sendai framework for disaster risk reduction: A conceptual glossary. *Int. J. Environ. Res. Public Health* **2016**, *13*, 1241. [CrossRef]
49. United Nations International Strategy for Disaster Reduction (UNISDR). *Sendai Framework for Disaster Risk Reduction 2015–2030*; UNISDR: Geneva, Switzerland, 2015.
50. Confalonieri, U.E.C. Variabilidade climática, vulnerabilidade social e saúde no Brasil. *Terra Livre* **2003**, *1*, 193–204.
51. Sakaluk, J.K.; Short, S.D. A Methodological Review of Exploratory Factor Analysis in Sexuality Research: Used Practices, Best Practices, and Data Analysis Resources. *J. Sex Res.* **2017**, *54*, 1–9. [CrossRef]
52. Holand, I.S.; Lujala, P.; Rod, J.K. Social vulnerability assessment for Norway: A quantitative approach. *Nor. Geogr. Tidsskr.* **2011**, *65*, 1–17. [CrossRef]
53. Hair, J.F.; Black, W.C.; Babin, B.J.; Anderson, R.E. *Multivariate Data Analysis*, 7th ed.; Pearson: Harlow, UK, 2014; ISBN 978-1-292-02190-4.
54. Cattell, R.B. *The Scientific Use of Factor Analysis in Behavioral and Life*; Plenum: New York, NY, USA, 1978.
55. Fabrigar, L.R.; Wegener, D.T.; MacCallum, R.C.; Strahan, E.J. Evaluating the use of exploratory factor analysis in psychological research. *Psychol. Methods* **1999**, *4*, 272–299. [CrossRef]
56. Gorsuch, R.L. *Exploratory Factor Analysis*, 2nd ed.; Lawrence Erlbaum Associates: Hillsdale, MI, USA, 1988; ISBN 978-0898592023.
57. MacCallum, R.C.; Widaman, K.F.; Zhang, S.; Hong, S. Sample size in factor analysis. *Psychol. Methods* **1999**, *4*, 84. [CrossRef]
58. Fabrigar, L.R.; Wegener, D.T. *Understanding Statistics: Exploratory Factor Analysis*; Oxford University Press: New York, NY, USA, 2012.
59. SAS Institute Inc. *SAS® Studio 3.8: User's Guide*; SAS Institute Inc.: Cary, NC, USA, 2018.
60. De Sherbinin, A.; Bardy, G. Social vulnerability to floods in two coastal megacities: New York City and Mumbai. *Vienna Yearb. Popul. Res.* **2015**, *13*, 131–166. [CrossRef]
61. Thornton, P.K.; Jones, P.G.; Owiyo, T.; Kruska, R.L.; Herrero, M.; Orindi, V.; Bhadwal, S.; Kristjanson, P.; Notenbaert, A.; Bekele, N. Climate change and poverty in Africa: Mapping hotspots of vulnerability. *Afr. J. Agric. Resour. Econ.* **2008**, *2*, 24–44.
62. Tabachnick, B.G.; Fidell, L.S. *A Practical Approach to Using Multivariate Analyses*; Pearson: Boston, MA, USA, 2012.
63. Menezes, J.A.; Madureira, A.P.; Santos, R.B.D.; Duval, I.D.B.; Regoto, P.; Margonari, C.; Confalonieri, U. *Data for: Analyzing Spatial Patterns of Health Vulnerability to Drought in the Brazilian Semiarid Region*; Mendeley Data, V1; Elsevier: Amsterdam, The Netherlands, 2020. [CrossRef]
64. Freitas, C.; Silva, D.; Sena, A.; Silva, E.; Sales, L.; Carvalho, M.; Mazoto, M.; Barcellos, C.; Costa, A.; Oliveira, M.; et al. Desastres naturais e saúde: Uma análise da situação do Brasil. *Cien. Saude Colet.* **2014**, *19*, 3645–3656. [CrossRef]
65. Bortolotto, C.C.; De Mola, C.L.; Tovo-Rodrigues, L. Qualidade de vida em adultos de zona rural no Sul do Brasil: Estudo de base populacional. *Rev. Saude Publica* **2018**, *52*, 4s. [CrossRef]
66. Instituto Brasileiro de Geografia e Estatística—IBGE. *Pesquisa Nacional de Saúde 2013: Percepção do Estado de Saúde, Estilos de Vida e Doenças Crônicas*; Fiocruz, IBGE, Ministério da Saúde: Rio de Janeiro, Brazil, 2014.
67. Moreira, J.P.d.L.; de Oliveira, B.L.C.A.; Muzi, C.D.; Cunha, C.L.F.; Brito, A.d.S.; Luiz, R.R. A saúde dos trabalhadores da atividade rural no Brasil. *Cad. Saude Publica* **2015**, *31*, 1698–1708. [CrossRef]
68. Instituto Nacional Do Semiárido—INSA. Portal da Desertificação: Dados e Indicadores do Semiárido Brasileiro. Available online: https://portaldadesertificacao.insa.gov.br/ (accessed on 21 April 2021).
69. De Albuquerque, M.V.; d'Ávila Viana, A.L.; De Lima, L.D.; Ferreira, M.P.; Fusaro, E.R.; Iozzi, F.L. Regional health inequalities: Changes observed in Brazil from 2000–2016. *Cienc. Saude Coletiva* **2017**, *22*, 1055–1064. [CrossRef]
70. Cunha, A.M.P.d.A.; Brito, S.S.d.B.; Rossato, L.; Célia dos Santos Alvalá, R.; Carvalho, M.A.; Zeri, M.; Cunningham, C.; Paula dos Reis Maciel, A.; Soares Andrade, E.; Marcia da Silva Pinto Vieira, R.; et al. Avaliação de indicador para o monitoramento dos impactos da seca em áreas de pastagens no Semiárido do Brasil. *Rev. Bras. Cartogr.* **2017**, *69*, 89–106.
71. Lemos, M.C.; Lo, Y.J.; Nelson, D.R.; Eakin, H.; Bedran-Martins, A.M. Linking development to climate adaptation: Leveraging generic and specific capacities to reduce vulnerability to drought in NE Brazil. *Glob. Environ. Chang.* **2016**, *39*, 170–179. [CrossRef]
72. Christenson, E.; Elliott, M.; Banerjee, O.; Hamrick, L.; Bartram, J. Climate-related hazards: A method for global assessment of urban and rural population exposure to cyclones, droughts, and floods. *Int. J. Environ. Res. Public Health* **2014**, *11*, 2169–2192. [CrossRef]
73. Tibesigwa, B.; Visser, M. Assessing gender inequality in food security among small-holder farm households in urban and rural South Africa. *World Dev.* **2016**, *88*, 33–49. [CrossRef]

74. Tibesigwa, B.; Visser, M.; Collinson, M.; Twine, W. Investigating the sensitivity of household food security to agriculture-related shocks and the implication of social and natural capital. *Sustain. Sci.* **2016**, *11*, 193–214. [CrossRef]
75. Articulação Semiárido Brasileiro—ASA. *Propostas da Sociedade Civil Para Garantia de Acesso à Água às Populações Rurais do Semiárido*; Semiárido—Caderno de Debates; Articulação Semiárido Brasileiro—ASA: Recife, Brazil, 2019. Available online: https://www.yumpu.com/pt/document/read/62697726/frente-parlamentar-propostas-da-sociedade-civil-para-a-garantia-do-acesso-a-agua-as-populacoes-rurais-do-semiarido (accessed on 21 April 2020).
76. Adler, N.E.; Boyce, W.T.; Chesney, M.A.; Folkman, S.; Syme, S.L. Socioeconomic Inequalities in Health: No Easy Solution. *JAMA* **1993**, *269*, 3140–3145. [CrossRef]
77. Kunst, A.E.; Geurts, J.J.M.; Van Den Berg, J. International variation in socioeconomic inequalities in self reported health. *J. Epidemiol. Community Health* **1995**, *49*, 117–123. [CrossRef]
78. Szwarcwald, C.L.; de Souza-Júnior, P.R.B.; Esteves, M.A.P.; Damacena, G.N.; Viacava, F. Socio-demographic determinants of self-rated health in Brazil. *Cad. Saúde Pública/Ministério da Saúde Fundação Oswaldo Cruz Esc. Nac. Saúde Pública* **2005**, *21*, 54–64. [CrossRef]
79. Almeida, G.; Sarti, F.M.; Ferreira, F.F.; Diaz, M.D.M.; Campino, A.C.C. Analysis of the evolution and determinants of income-related inequalities in the Brazilian health system, 1998–2008. *Rev. Panam. Salud Publica* **2013**, *33*, 90–97. [CrossRef]
80. Carstairs, V. Deprivation indices: Their interpretation and use in relation to health. *J. Epidemiol. Community Health* **1995**, *49*, S3–S8. [CrossRef]
81. Barcellos, C.d.D.; Sabroza, P.C.; Peiter, P.; Rojas, L.I. Organização Espacial, Saúde e Qualidade de Vida: Análise Espacial e Uso de Indicadores na Avaliação de Situações de Saúde. *Inf. Epidemiológico SUS* **2002**, *11*, 129–138. [CrossRef]
82. Yang, K.; LeJeune, J.; Alsdorf, D.; Lu, B.; Shum, C.K.; Liang, S. Global distribution of outbreaks of water-associated infectious diseases. *PLoS Negl. Trop. Dis.* **2012**, *6*, e1483. [CrossRef]
83. Da Silva, J.M.C.; Leal, I.R.; Tabarelli, M. *Caatinga—The Largest Tropical Dry Forest Region in South America*, 1st ed.; da Silva, J.M.C., Leal, I.R., Tabarelli, M., Eds.; Springer International Publishing: Cham, Switzerland, 2017; ISBN 9783319683386.
84. Da Silva, T.C.G.; Silva, C.C.M.; Paes, N.A. Mortalidade dos Adultos por Doenças Cardiovasculares e Fatores Associados no Semiárido Brasileiro. *Rev. Espaço Para Saúde* **2015**, *16*, 74–86. [CrossRef]
85. Szwarcwald, C.L.; de Souza Júnior, P.R.B.; Marques, A.P.; de Almeida, W.d.S.; Montilla, D.E.R. Inequalities in healthy life expectancy by Brazilian geographic regions: Findings from the National Health Survey, 2013. *Int. J. Equity Health* **2016**, *15*, 141. [CrossRef]
86. Rufino, I.A.A.; Da Silva, S.T. Análise das relações entre dinâmica populacional, clima e vetores de mudança no Semiárido Basileiro: Uma abordagem metodológica. *Bol. Ciencias Geod.* **2017**, *23*, 166–181. [CrossRef]
87. Duarte, M.M.S. Cobertura das Ações de Vigilância da Qualidade da Água para Consumo Humano e Indicadores de Vulnerabilidade nos Municípios do Semiárido Nordestino, Universidade de Brasília. 2018. Available online: https://1library.org/document/zln3e3lq-cobertura-vigilancia-qualidade-indicadores-vulnerabilidade-municipios-semiarido-nordestino.html (accessed on 21 April 2021).
88. Weiss, R.A.; McMichael, A.J. Social and environmental risk factors in the emergence of infectious diseases. *Nat. Med.* **2004**, *10*, S70–S76. [CrossRef]
89. Hacon, S.d.S.; Costa, D.; Siqueira, A.S.P.; Pinheiro, S.d.L.; Gonçalves, K.S.; Oliveira, A.; Barcellos, C. Vulnerabilidade, riscos e impactos das mudanças climáticas sobre a saúde no Brasil. In *Modelagem Climática e Vulnerabilidades Setoriais à Mudança do Clima no Brasil*; Ministério da Ciência, Tecnologia e Inovação: Brasília, Brazil, 2016; pp. 387–456.
90. De Oliveira, A.P.C.; Gabriel, M.; Dal Poz, M.R.; Dussault, G. Desafios para assegurar a disponibilidade e acessibilidade à assistência médica no Sistema Único de Saúde. *Cienc. Saude Coletiva* **2017**, *22*, 1165–1180. [CrossRef] [PubMed]
91. Garnelo, L.; Lima, J.G.; Rocha, E.S.C.; Herkrath, F.J. Acesso e cobertura da Atenção Primária à Saúde para populações rurais e urbanas na região norte do Brasil. *Saúde Debate* **2018**, *42*, 81–99. [CrossRef]
92. Massuda, A.; Hone, T.; Leles, F.A.G.; De Castro, M.C.; Atun, R. The Brazilian health system at crossroads: Progress, crisis and resilience. *BMJ Glob. Health* **2018**, *3*, 1–8. [CrossRef] [PubMed]
93. Hone, T.; Rasella, D.; Barreto, M.; Atun, R.; Majeed, A.; Millett, C. Large reductions in amenable mortality associated with brazil's primary care expansion and strong health governance. *Health Aff.* **2017**, *36*, 149–158. [CrossRef]
94. Instituto de Pesquisa Econômica Aplicada—IPEA. *Atlas da Vulnerabilidade Social nos Municípios Brasileiros*; Costa, M.A., Marguti, B.O., Eds.; IPEA: Brasília, Brazil, 2015; ISBN 978-85-7811-255-4.
95. Programa das Nações Unidas para o Desenvolvimento—PNUD; Instituto de Pesquisa Econômica Aplicada—IPEA; Fundação João Pinheiro—FJP. *Índice de Desenvolvimento Humano Municipal Brasileiro*; PNUD: Brasília, Brazil, 2013.
96. Instituto Brasileiro de Geografia e Estatístca—IBGE. Cidades@. [No Date]. Available online: https://cidades.ibge.gov.br/ (accessed on 20 April 2020).
97. Marengo, J.A.; Cunha, A.P.; Soares, W.R.; Torres, R.R.; Alves, L.M.; de Barros Brito, S.S.; Cuartas, L.A.; Leal, K.; Neto, G.R.; Alvalá, R.C.S.; et al. Increase Risk of Drought in the Semiarid Lands of Northeast Brazil Due to Regional Warming above 4 °C. In *Climate Change Risks in Brazil*; Nobre, C., Marengo, J., Soares, W., Eds.; Springer: Cham, Switzerland, 2019; pp. 181–200.

98. Papathoma-Köhle, M.; Cristofari, G.; Wenk, M.; Fuchs, S. The importance of indicator weights for vulnerability indices and implications for decision making in disaster management. *Int. J. Disaster Risk Reduct.* **2019**, *36*, 101103. [CrossRef]
99. Willis, I.; Fitton, J. A review of multivariate social vulnerability methodologies: A case study of the River Parrett catchment, UK. *Hazards Earth Syst. Sci* **2016**, *16*, 1387–1399. [CrossRef]
100. Becker, W.; Saisana, M.; Paruolo, P.; Vandecasteele, I. Weights and importance in composite indicators: Closing the gap. *Ecol. Indic.* **2017**, *80*, 12–22. [CrossRef]

MDPI
St. Alban-Anlage 66
4052 Basel
Switzerland
Tel. +41 61 683 77 34
Fax +41 61 302 89 18
www.mdpi.com

International Journal of Environmental Research and Public Health Editorial Office
E-mail: ijerph@mdpi.com
www.mdpi.com/journal/ijerph

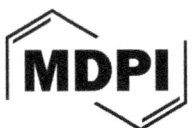

www.ingramcontent.com/pod-product-compliance
Lightning Source LLC
LaVergne TN
LVHW070237100526
838202LV00015B/2138